Dedicated to Evelyn Lebby and in memorium to Janet Schmitz
Two loving, caring and devoted mothers.

CONTENTS

PREFACE

Neuroimaging technology is advancing rapidly and, with the change from film to digital, has become much more accessible to medical and allied health care professionals. Only a few decades ago, brain imaging was only capable of providing low-resolution images of substantial pathology such as hydrocephalus or large strokes; it was was not helpful in evaluating more subtle neurological conditions. Currently, brain imaging can provide evidence of subtle neuropathology, disruption of cellular water diffusion, changes in blood flow, perfusion and oxygenation, integrity and direction of axonal pathways, metabolic functioning, and even the changes in electrical potentials at the millisecond resolution, within a three-dimensional matrix of brain tissue. With increased access to brain imaging techniques and with the greater technological sophistication of available scans come increased responsibility for evidence-based use and improved understanding of what brain imaging can and cannot provide to clinical decision-making. Not too long ago, a clinician was only required to differentiate between density differences on a CT or between only two types of MRI, a T1- or a T2-weighted image. Today, clinicians are expected to interpret imaging data derived from a variety of CT techniques and multiple MRI sequences.

This guide was written with the clinician in mind. It is written at a level appropriate to a reader with a working knowledge of brain functioning but with limited experience or formal education in the clinical use of brain imaging. The text is intended for non-radiologist professionals who currently use, or would like to integrate, brain imaging within their clinical practice. Professionals such as neurologists, neuropsychologists, and general practitioners, including hospitalists, family physicians, and pediatricians, as well as medical and graduate-level students, residents, and interns will find this guide to be a valuable resource. Evidence-based information within this guide will assist clinicians in more appropriately and competently determining which type of brain scan to order given a specific symptom constellation, set of diagnostic questions, or patient presentation. In addition, this text was written to provide a solid foundation of brain imaging information necessary to enable the non-radiologist to more competently interpret and use brain imaging in the clinic. Throughout this guide, the author has attempted to balance the necessary technical information on brain imaging with real-life, pragmatic knowledge useful to a clinician working with patients who have brain-based disorders.

This guide provides information regarding the clinical use of neuroimaging technologies, including the types of scans currently available, the risks and benefits associated with the different techniques, the limitations involved in interpreting imaging data, and the clinical application of imaging data as they relate to a variety of brain pathologies and conditions. The discussion of basic anatomical neuroimaging techniques includes all common sequences of CT and MRI. For example, CT sequences include, but are not restricted to, two- and three-dimensional presentation and reconstruction, contrast and non-contrast imaging, and CT angiography (CTA) and ventriculography, for visualizing blood vessels and ventricles. Different parameters are also used for highlighting specific tissue, such as bone windowing. MRI sequences discussed here include, but are not restricted to, T1, T2, FLAIR, PDI, DWI, GRE, GRE-EPI, SWI, cube, propeller, MRA, MRV, TOF, and FIESTA. Contrast and non-contrast procedures are also discussed using a variety of different MRI sequences. Advanced functional neuroimaging techniques covered in this text include, but are not restricted to, MRS, fMRI, SPECT, PET, and MEG-MSI. Additional imaging techniques such as brain ultrasound and angiography are also discussed within this text.

The goal of this guide is to assist the reader in developing clinical skills related to the use of brain imaging in the clinic; thus the guide covers a range of topics related to brain imaging. The book begins with a discussion on the general use of brain imaging, including the positive and negative consequences of showing or discussing brain pathology with the patient and family, and the limitations of the technology. Readers will then learn basic techniques that are helpful in the interpretation of a variety of different types of brain images used to assess common pathological conditions.

Basic neuroanatomy is covered from the perspective of brain imaging, to assist the reader in identifying key anatomical structures, pathways, and systems. Clinical examples involving traumatic and nontraumatic pathologies to the brain are also provided, to facilitate understanding of how brain pathology appears on a variety of imaging techniques and sequences. Some of the conditions discussed include traumatic brain injury, strokes, demyelinating disorders, infections, hypoxic conditions, brain tumors, developmental conditions, and projectile injuries, such as gunshot wounds. Many of the clinical examples include descriptions of the type and severity of the brain pathology, functional deficits or limitations exhibited by the patients, and outcomes following treatment.

Finally, the guide ends with a brain atlas comprising both MRI and CT images, to serve as a reference when viewing brain scans in the clinic.

ACKNOWLEDGMENTS

I would like to thank my colleagues for their willingness and effort dedicated to the review of this guide. General review of this work was conducted by Randy Mack, M.P.T.; Hitha Amin, M.D.; Errol Leifer, Ph.D.; and Jennifer Crocker, M.D. Technical review was conducted by Fred Laningham, M.D., and Raymond Valenzuela Jr., R.T. In addition, I extend thanks to E. Mark Haacke, Ph.D.; Kenneth Laxer, M.D.; Lucian Maidan, M.D.; Margaret Verrees, M.D.; and Joseph Sullivan, M.D., for their contribution of images to this guide, their expert counsel and encouragement during the production of this work. I extend appreciation to Marc Schneider, production editor, Oxford University Press.

I acknowledge the permission that was kindly granted to publish three-dimensional images from the 3D brain atlas originally created by AXS Biomedical Animation Studio, Incorporated, as part of the *3D Brain*, an interactive atlas of the human brain created for Cold Spring Harbor's Dolan DNA Learning Center. The *3D Brain* is available as a free iPhone/iPad app and online at Genes to Cognition (G2C) Online. Images © 2005–2009, Cold Spring Harbor Laboratory. All rights reserved.

In addition, I acknowledge the permission that was kindly granted by Somso, Inc., to use pictures of their brain model BS 25 within the neuroanatomy chapter (Chapter 3).

I would like to extend thanks to Dr. Errol F. Leifer, my dear friend, professional colleague and clinical partner, for his support and generosity. I also wish to acknowledge my family, friends and colleagues for their patience, encouragement and much needed humor, in particular Dan Sniffin, John Barclay, Brian Ponte, Blair Cunnings and Ambros Morales. My deepest appreciation is extended to my patients and families for their courage, compassion and generosity.

Most importantly, I thank and acknowledge my wife and partner in life, Kathy, for all of her patience and understanding during the writing of this guide. It is clear that without the support and encouragement from Kathy, along with our pups Dolce and Gabbana, this work would never have been completed.

Paul C. Lebby

INTRODUCTION

Learning about brain imaging can be a daunting task. With rapid advances in technology and the constant addition of new techniques, developing a solid foundation of knowledge about brain imaging can seem overwhelming to even the most experienced clinician. Not only must the clinician understand the basic differences between the various types of brain scans, but must also develop an ability to interpret images, differentiate features on an image that are clinically meaningful from those that are irrelevant or artifact, and also become adept at communicating information obtained through imaging in a manner understandable by the patient, family or other health care providers. This guide has been designed to maximize your learning by gradually building on a basic clinical and anatomical foundation, progressing to more technical knowledge regarding imaging techniques, and ultimately integrating material via the presentation of a variety of traumatic and non-traumatic clinical cases.

Many of the examples in this guide are derived from technologies common to most medical centers, and readily available to most clinicians. Some examples are taken from older technologies using photographic film as was used prior to the advent of digital media. Other images were obtained from more current digital systems providing both two-dimensional and three-dimensional graphical representations of the brain. The older images were included in this guide as many medical centers around the world still use such technology, and even if your center has updated equipment, you may be asked to review older films from many of your aging patients. Most examples in this guide are drawn from current, state-of-the art, cutting-edge technologies in order to provide you examples of what is currently available, even if not at your particular center. As much as possible, clinical examples are provided using common sequences available to most clinicians, in addition to some more advanced imaging protocols to give you a full appreciation of techniques available to you. It is important to understand that brain imaging technology is advancing rapidly, with new techniques becoming available every few years. As such, it is recommended that you become aware of the techniques available to you in your particular area or clinical setting, and not just rely on the older sequences such as basic T1 or T2 MRI. As newer sequences become available, be sure to integrate information about the scans, including the clinical strengths and weaknesses of the new sequences with the knowledge and skills you develop from this guide.

It is recommended that you progress through this guide in order of the presented chapters, or at a minimum, you read the first four chapters prior to spending time reviewing the clinical chapters five and six. The foundation information provided within the first four chapters will assist you in fully appreciating the clinical cases, and optimize your interpretation and integration of pathological processes and the presentation of such on brain scans. If you already view brain images as part of your clinical role, it is strongly recommended that you read chapters one, two and four first, then progress to the anatomical chapter three and the pathological examples in chapters five and six. Chapters one, two and four provide critical information regarding the interpretation of brain scans by a non-radiologist for clinical purposes, including limitations of the technology, features that may be misleading or artifacts, in addition to the impact that the images can have on a patient or family.

Chapter one provides information helpful in determining when and how to use brain images in the clinic. The decision to use brain images as a source of additional clinical information can seem straightforward and simple, although should not be taken lightly. Many important issues should be considered prior to using brain images for clinical purposes. Without a basic understanding, their use can result in erroneous conclusions, or the dissemination of information that is misleading or inaccurate. Failing to take into account the limitations of the technology, or the accuracy of imaging data can result in poor clinical formulation or the development of a non-optimal treatment regimen. In addition, at times it can be highly beneficial and advantageous to show brain scans to patients, families or care providers, while other times presentation of images may not be recommended, or can even be harmful or disruptive to patient care. Consideration of both the medical and psychological impact of brain scans depicting trauma is critical when determining whether to show images, which images from a series should be shown, and also when determining if the images may be misleading or result in emotional trauma or confusion. Chapter one covers many of these issues and considerations, and guides the reader in determining how and when images are best utilized within a clinical setting.

Chapter two provides the reader a basic tutorial on how to interpret information presented on a brain scan. Even with an increasing number of different imaging sequences available to a clinician, following a few basic guidelines can assist in the interpretation of most common images. Chapter two introduces the primary image planes and the effects of variations in acquisition and presentation plane on image appearance. Assessment of head placement in the scanner is important in accurate interpretation of brain scans and can significantly change the appearance of common anatomical structures. In addition, the appearance of both normal and pathological tissues or processes can differ across a variety of scanning techniques, resulting in confusion and difficulty assessing for injury. Chapter two presents a basic guideline to follow when viewing brain scans, especially helpful early in the learning process. Because some brain structures change with early development, and pathology often changes appearance over time, an understanding of the temporal influences on brain imaging is critical when viewing scans. The interpretation of neuroimaging is complex and can lead to a number of diagnostic pitfalls. Chapter two covers some of the more common pitfalls that you may encounter when using brain images to facilitate your clinical decision making.

Chapter three covers neuroanatomy from the perspective of brain imaging. Unlike neuroanatomy presented in a standard format, in radiology one must often view brain structures using two-dimensional slices oriented orthogonally. Some workstations allow for three-dimensional viewing, although these are not commonly available to the general clinician. In chapter three, the reader is introduced to the primary brain structures and regions presented as a series of two-dimensional slices, each color-coded with reference lines and crosshairs to assist you in identifying anatomical structure on all three primary image planes. Images with a green border have an axial orientation and were derived from a slice represented by a green line on the images from the alternate planes (coronal and sagittal). Similarly, red borders and reference lines represent coronal slices and blue borders and reference lines represent slices obtained on the sagittal plane.

Primary anatomical landmarks are introduced, and include the ventricles and white matter tracts. As anatomical regions are presented, they are discussed in relation to the landmarks formed from the ventricles and white matter pathways. As primary structures are discussed, spatial and functional information is provided to assist the clinician in integrating anatomy and functional pathology. Examples of pathologies involving many of the structures are included to facilitate understanding of the effects of damage to the key structures or systems. Areas covered in Chapter three include, but are not restricted to the cortical regions of the right and left hemispheres, subcortical nuclei of the basal ganglia and limbic system, diencephalic structures of the thalamus and hypothalamus, in addition to midbrain and hindbrain structures of the mesencephalon, pons, cerebellum and brain stem. Other structures that are more diffusely distributed such as white matter pathways, ventricles and the vascular system are also included within chapter three. Two-dimensional brain images, two and three-dimensional brain graphics, images taken from a brain model, pictures of dissected brain slices and graphical illustrations are included to assist you in fully developing your ability to identify neuroanatomical structures or regions on brain scans.

Chapter four may be considered one of the more complex chapters in this guide and covers the technology used by the various scanning systems. Although an understanding of how an image is produced may not be critical to your clinical role, understanding the technology becomes important when interpreting complex cases, or when deciding which of the many imaging techniques and sequences will provide the most salient information relating to a particular clinical question. For example, choosing between CT and MRI can appear simple, although requires consideration of many strengths and weaknesses of each system. Static or anatomical scans may be adequate for some disorders, although for a better understanding of pathology, diffusion-based or functional imaging techniques may be recommended. CT is often the scan of choice for conditions involving the cranium, or for emergency situations, with MRI being more often used for outpatient or follow-up imaging of soft tissues such as brain parenchyma. MRS, SPECT or PET may be the technique of choice for questions regarding the metabolic integrity of particular tissues, while DTI may be necessary to fully evaluate white matter pathways around a tumor or following trauma. Decisions regarding the use of CT should balance the advantages offered by the technology such as very rapid image acquisition and safety for those with ferromagnetic implants, with the negative effects of exposing the patient to a dose of ionizing radiation, especially in small adults and children. Higher resolution images may be available using MRI, although the extremely strong magnetic field leads to concerns about safety for the patient and staff, especially in emergency situations. Both CT and MRI can produce images of bone, soft tissue and blood vessels, and the positive versus negative aspects of each system should be considered prior to use. A variety of CT and MRI sequences are discussed with examples of their use for a variety of pathological conditions. Technologies other than CT and MRI are also introduced, such as ultrasound and angiography, in addition to functional techniques using PET, MEG and SPECT. As a general rule, with complex cases, the use of a combination of techniques provides the most accurate and the clearest picture of a patient's condition or pathology.

Chapters five and six provide examples of common conditions encountered in a clinical setting. Chapter 5 covers injuries resulting primarily from physical trauma to the brain such as contusions, diffuse axonal injuries, hemorrhages, post-traumatic edema and encephalomalacia.

Chapter 6 covers conditions mostly unrelated to physical trauma, such as infections, neoplasms, hypoxemia and neurodevelopmental syndromes. It is important to consider the considerable overlap between conditions presented in chapter 5 and chapter 6, and understand that many conditions from one chapter may include pathologies from the other and vice versa. The conditions presented in chapter five and six are by no means mutually exclusive, and the organization was chosen only to assist you in your learning.

Chapter 7 provides a brain atlas containing MRI and CT images arranged in the three primary orthogonal orientations of axial, coronal and sagittal. For each slice, color-coded images with reference lines are used, and follow the same format as that used in the previous chapters, particularly chapter three. As you read this guide, it may be helpful to refer to chapter 7 as a reference when viewing clinical examples provided throughout this work. Chapter 7 can also be used as a basic brain atlas when viewing scans in the clinic, and will be especially helpful for those without a strong neuroanatomy background.

Because this is a guide to brain imaging, most clinical examples were chosen because of their ease of interpretation. Many cases that you may encounter in the clinic will be less obvious, subtle or even ambiguous compared to those in this guide. However, the primary features will be similar to those presented here, with the severity and extent of injury differing from case to case. When in doubt, consult a radiologist or clinician more familiar with the type of pathology being assessed. The clinical examples presented in Chapters 5 and 6 were selected based on a variety of criteria. The primary focus was to use exemplar cases that were neither too subtle nor too obvious. Cases that are very subtle are difficult to visualize using only a few static images, and may be missed by many readers. Cases that are obvious do not require close inspection or analysis on the part of the viewer and can result in a passive approach to learning. To facilitate skill acquisition, many of the examples chosen represent pathologies that are readily evident, but not always obvious without close inspection. Where appropriate, arrows are used to assist you in identifying specific image features relevant to the case, or useful in your clinical interpretation and learning. Where arrows are not used, it should not be difficult for you to visualize the regions of interest based on the anatomical descriptions, the specific slice choices and the use of reference lines and crosshairs.

Brain Imaging

1 THE CLINICAL APPLICATION OF BRAIN IMAGING

Neuroimaging technology is advancing rapidly and, with the change from film to digital imaging, has become much more accessible to a variety of professionals. Only a few decades ago, brain scans were capable of providing evidence of substantial pathology but were not helpful for more subtle neurological conditions. Brain imaging sequences currently provide evidence of subtle neuropathology, disruption of cellular water diffusion, compromised blood flow, perfusion or oxygenation, integrity and direction of axonal pathways, metabolic functioning, and electrical activity at the millisecond resolution within the three-dimensional matrix. Modern advanced neuroimaging has changed how brain scans are used in the clinic. With advances in technology and increased access to sophisticated brain imaging, clinicians carry a greater responsibility to understand what brain imaging can and cannot offer to clinical decision-making. Over the next few decades, evidence-based use of brain imaging and a basic understanding of the technology will likely become the norm, not the exception.

ACCESS TO BRAIN IMAGING

For many years, access to brain scans was limited by the logistics of transporting large sheets of film from one location to another. Film was stored in a radiology department, where a file technician could retrieve the film from a storage file-room. Film could be checked out by the clinician, or it could be duplicated using photographic systems so that copies could be kept or mailed as needed. This process was often slow and inefficient, especially if key staff were not available. Given the inconvenience to the busy clinician, radiology reports accessible in the patient file were usually reviewed in lieu of personal review of the films. Although radiology reports have been available in medical records for decades, the amount and type of information provided within the reports often related more to the pathological processes and the anatomical structures involved than to the clinical significance of such findings. To a trained eye, actual review of radiology films can provide critical information not available within a radiology summary.

Access to brain scans is improving rapidly, and recent changes in how brain scans are recorded has allowed for a variety of presentation modalities. With the transition from film or analog recordings to digital data storage, brain scans can be stored and accessed via computers running a variety of image-reading programs. Computers connected to hospital networks via wired or even wireless systems can access brain scans within seconds of them being completed. Scans can be loaded onto CD or DVD disks for mailing or be stored with a patient's medical records. Currently, several systems are available that enable access to neuroimaging via the use of smart phones or tablet devices, all via secure, encrypted wireless networks.

Not only has access improved dramatically with the transition to digital recording, but the way in which scans are viewed has also changed. With film, one had to display large sheets of images on light boxes and view brain slices as individual images. To form a three-dimensional representation, one had to mentally reconstruct the images in order from the bottom of the brain to the top (axial), from the front of the brain to the back (coronal), and from one side to the other (sagittal). Many clinicians had great difficulty with such visualization and found it almost impossible to mentally construct an internal three-dimensional representation using single two-dimensional slices. Even those with a strong background in neuroanatomy and years of experience could find it a daunting task figuring out the specific location of a lesion on sheets of film.

Digital imaging of the brain has made the task of visualizing structures and pathology much simpler, enabling more clinicians to use neuroimaging in their daily clinical practice. Using a computer pointing device, such as a mouse, one can now fluidly move through the thin slices of brain in a manner that allows the clinician to effortlessly create a percept of three-dimensional brain structures. This is not unlike the perception of motion created in cartoons by sequencing many images in rapid succession, or in movies by rapidly sequencing consecutive image frames. This "structure from motion" or "kinetic depth effect" is most evident when rotating a semitranslucent brain to visualize blood vessels or even when viewing the cranium. As a static image, the blood vessels lack perceived structure in three-dimensional space and appear as a collection of white lines on a two-dimensional plane. If a vessel runs parallel to the image plane, it can appear very clear. However, if the vessel runs perpendicular to the image plane, only part of the vessel will be visible, and the size of the vessel will be difficult to appreciate. Using a computer to rotate the matrix of vessels around the horizontal or vertical axis, one can obtain a wonderful view of all vessels.

Conversely, the appearance of a normal scan should not be interpreted to mean that there is no injury to the brain. A brain scan read as "normal" only indicates that any possible damage is not of the extent or type made visible using current technology.

ADVANTAGES OF USING BRAIN IMAGING IN THE CLINIC

Digital brain imaging can provide information regarding the extent and severity of an injury, the areas of the brain most affected, changes over time, prognosis, and most importantly, critical data to facilitate patient care. Not only has digital image processing allowed non-radiologists to more easily interpret brain scans, it has also allowed patients and care providers to "see" the pathology in their head.

Sometimes, visualization of damage can provide a level of understanding regarding the type, severity, or extent of pathology that would be otherwise unobtainable. It is important to consider that the developments in digital image processing have both advantages and disadvantages for the clinician, and care is required when considering the use of such technology. For example, digital imaging can provide clues regarding the extent of an injury, but it also can be misleading and give the appearance of more damage or pathology than is actually present. The following sections provide a summary regarding what digital imaging can provide the clinician, in addition to some cautionary issues relating to the limitations of imaging data.

Clues Regarding Extent of Injury

Large injuries are easy to appreciate and are often visible on a variety of brain scans. Even microscopic injuries that are too small to be detected by current imaging systems, may often be evident on a scan due to the microbleeds and swelling that accompany them. Knowing the approximate size of an injury can be helpful in formulating a clinical picture of the patient and when considering prognoses and expected long-term therapeutic needs.

Caution is warranted when estimating the size or significance of an injury using brain scans. Edema can extend from a small area of damage, giving the impression that the injury involves more brain than in actuality. Blood can obscure a small injury that is clinically relevant, preventing accurate assessment of damage. Large extra-axial bleeds, such as epidural hematomas that form between the skull and dura, can appear devastating on a brain scan but may not result in any permanent injury to brain tissue.

Clues Regarding Type of Injury

Clinical history may not be the most reliable way to assess the type of injury to the brain. This is especially important when the presentation of the patient does not match the documented clinical history. This was the case with a child who was taken to the emergency department following a relatively minor head injury with a short period of confusion but no loss of consciousness. The child rapidly deteriorated before discharge from the emergency department, precipitating rapid intubation to protect his airway and imaging to assess for an etiology. Brain imaging revealed that the symptoms were not directly related to the head injury but were related to a secondary process. The mild physical trauma to the brain resulted in severe bilateral vasospasm of the patient's middle cerebral arteries, resulting in extensive damage to both hemispheres. Without the imaging, the vascular compromise would not have been discovered, the use of medications to minimize the effects of the vasospasm would not have been used, and there would have been no clear explanation for the poor outcome following a relatively mild brain injury. Epidural hematomas often do not result in obvious neurological symptoms for several minutes to hours following an injury and can easily be missed in an emergency department. Without imaging, it is difficult to determine whether a patient has an evolving epidural bleed or just a concussion. This becomes a critical issue for many patients, as epidural hemorrhages can become rapidly fatal if not treated prior to brain herniation.

Sometimes the initial injury to the brain is so obvious that clinicians may discount the effects of secondary processes in formulating opinions regarding a patient's condition or prognoses. Review of brain imaging may be focused on the effects of the primary injury, with less attention allocated to the effects of other factors that influence a patient's care and ultimate outcome. Secondary factors can involve the effects of infection, hypoxia, herniation of brain tissue, compromised vascular functioning, or even damage from toxic substances released by brain tissue following injury. Prior to brain scanning, many of these processes were suspected but not confirmed in a patient presenting with symptoms inconsistent with the initial trauma. With brain scanning becoming more readily available to clinicians, secondary processes can be assessed and monitored throughout recovery, with treatments modified as necessary. Active involvement of the clinician in viewing a patient's scans may mean the difference between a patient sustaining unnecessary injury to the brain from secondary processes and the patient receiving treatment in a timely manner to prevent such injury.

Clues to Location of Injury or Pathology

Information from a radiology report may identify general areas of the brain or common anatomical structures that were damaged, although often fail to provide specific details relevant to the clinician. For example, an injury may be described as involving the "frontal lobe," or "left occipital lobe," but the specific location of the injury may not be provided. Just within a frontal lobe the injury could conceivably involve the orbital or medial frontal structures, Broca's area, the motor cortex for the face, torso, arms, legs or feet, or it could involve the premotor cortex, frontal eye fields, or regions of the heteromodal lateral cortices. Occipital lobe damage may be at the pole influencing primary foveal vision or be more anterior, influencing lateral visual regions or inferior/superior influencing vision above/below fixation. Damage to the occipital lobes may even be within the secondary or tertiary regions, resulting in syndromes of visual processing but not vision per se (i.e., Balint's syndrome or visual agnosia). Each of these areas has a different function and can result in a variety of therapeutic needs and expected prognoses.

PEARL Be cautious about assuming that injuries evident on a brain scan are the most clinically meaningful or relevant ones. Sometimes less obvious injuries that are difficult to appreciate on a scan can be most important for clinical purposes. Value your clinical assessment and findings, even if they do not match the obvious areas of damage on a brain scan.

PERIL Focusing only on the pathology evident on brain scans may result in your missing clinically relevant findings relating to other areas of the brain. Contrecoup injuries can fall into this category, with many functional deficits being unrelated to the primary area of impact. The injury at the point of impact (coup) may be obvious on the scan because of the contusion, presence of blood, and swelling. However, the injury caused by the brain bouncing off the opposite side of the skull (contrecoup) may be less evident on the scan but more clinically meaningful.

It is not uncommon in closed-head injuries for the patient to exhibit symptoms that do not correspond to anatomical areas of visible injury on brain imaging. Bleeding into the brain due to the tearing of small blood vessels is relatively easy to visualize on a brain scan. However, the anatomical region with the blood may not be the most damaged tissue and you should not automatically assume that the primary area of bleeding is the most useful in predicting outcome or a treatment plan. Damage to other areas of the brain, even without evidence of bleeding on brain imaging, may be more disabling to the patient.

Some neuropathological processes may not be evident on brain imaging, even though the condition causes severe seizure disorders and treatment requires removal of the affected cerebral hemisphere. It is important to consider that a brain scan read as "normal" does not imply that there is no pathology to the brain, only that the pathology is not of the type, extent, or severity apparent using current neuroimaging technologies. When explaining why a brain scan may appear normal but the patient has clear neurological deficits, it is often helpful to use a tree analogy. Microscopic damage to the brain is akin to the loss of a few leaves from an oak tree in the middle of a field. A brain scan is like someone looking at the tree from across the large open field. With the loss of only a few leaves, the tree may appear "normal" and full of leaves. This is because the viewer is unable to appreciate the gaps in the leaves from such a long distance. Even as leaves fall, the gross structure of the tree may appear unchanged for quite some time. Over time, and with increasing loss of leaves, the appearance of the tree may change and the bare branches and skeletal structure will become easier to appreciate. The same is true with microscopic damage to the brain. When "looking from a distance," with a brain scan microscopic losses are not apparent, and the brain can appear normal. Over time, and with gradual atrophy of brain cells, the appearance of the brain may change, just as is true with the oak tree.

Normal Brain Scans Do Not Imply Normal Brain
Brain scans may appear normal or suggest only small areas of damage despite possible extensive microscopic pathology. Similarly, brain imaging of a patient with extensive axonal injury may appear normal even when the patient is experiencing profound deficits in functioning.

With current technology, brain scans are capable of imaging larger anatomical regions but not microscopic structures. Brain scans image "trees" and "forests," not "leaves."

Clues Regarding Prognosis and Expected Functional Outcome

One of the most difficult questions posed to a clinician treating a person with a brain injury relates to the patient's functional prognoses. "Will he be normal?" "Will she be able to drive?" "How long until she recovers?" are all questions heard many times by specialists working with patients with brain injuries. Although these types of questions are difficult to answer with high accuracy, information provided by brain scans can assist in formulating prognostic opinions. Brain scan evidence of profound, widespread infarction and encephalomalacia suggests a poor long-term prognosis. In contrast, an epidural bleed may give the appearance of severe injury with a large hematoma and distortion or compression of the brain, but prognosis may be very good as long as the mass effect and pressure are adequately controlled. Small focal injuries within the multimodal cortices of the frontal and parietal lobes can be relatively benign with respect to functional outcome, but widespread diffuse axonal injuries can result in significant loss of functional abilities. When brain scans suggest damage to the deeper structures of the brain stem and reticular pathways, prognosis is usually less positive and can be quite variable. A patient with minimal damage to the lateral cortex but significant damage to the deeper subcortical structures may remain in a prolonged vegetative or minimally conscious state for many months or years without notable recovery. Ava's case example, highlights how radiological information can be helpful when discussing a reasonable prognosis and expectations for recovery.

CLINICAL EXAMPLE
Ava: Traumatic Brain Injury

Ava was injured when a roof collapsed and a piece of concrete crushed her skull. The injury resulted in severe damage to much of her left hemisphere, with mild to moderate diffuse injury to her right hemisphere. Ava's primary symptoms included global aphasia with mutism, dense right hemiparesis, and emotional lability. She could interact with her environment in a superficial manner but not purposefully to achieve functional goals. She was fully dependent for all of her needs and was unable to communicate using verbal means. Ava was discharged from the hospital after many months of intensive care and medical rehabilitation. John, Ava's husband, spent the next few years searching for a "cure" for her inability to communicate verbally. John found some treatments on the Internet that were reported to "help autistic children talk." The treatments involved dietary supplements, vitamins, special diets, and other alternative health programs. After several years without notable improvement in verbal and adaptive functioning, it was clear that Ava would likely be dependent for the rest of her life.

Review of brain scans taken a few days prior to replacement of the bone flap that was removed to allow for swelling suggested that extensive atrophy had taken place, with almost no left-hemisphere tissue remaining (Figure 1-1). Note, the left hemisphere is shown on right side of the CT image in Figure 1-1. John wanted to know if the treatments he had found for autistic children would be helpful in the recovery of her cognitive and language abilities. After reviewing the CT scans with John, and following a discussion regarding how the brain is unable to "replace the tissue that was lost from her brain," he realized the catastrophic nature of her condition and gained a more realistic opinion regarding her long-term prognosis. Without the "pictures of holes in her brain," John would have had a more difficult time understanding the extent of Ava's injury and might have spent more time and money on "cures" that did not make sense given her medical situation.

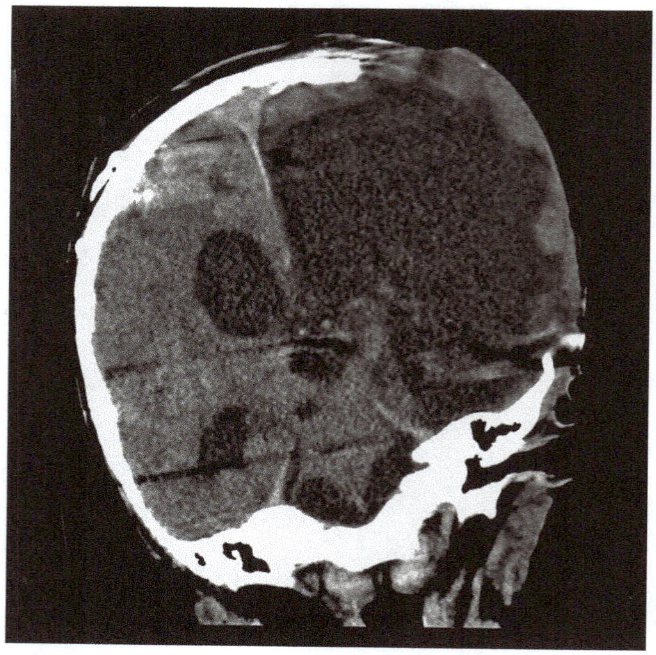

Figure 1-1 Case example Ava: CT showing severe trauma and extensive atrophy of brain tissue.

After showing brain scans to patients and family members, it is not unusual for them to remain confused. There is a common misconception that we do not use all of our brain, and with damage, noninjured areas will take over the functioning of the injured areas. It is not unusual for a patient or family member to believe that we "only use 20% of our brain" and ask if the other 80% will do the functioning for the damaged tissue. Responding to this line of questioning without becoming too complex is often the key to assisting patients and family members in understanding the effects of the injury. It is helpful to show areas of the brain that likely sustained diffuse microscopic injury and those areas that sustained severe damage. When considering the effects of traumatic injuries to the brain, you may wish to relate the surface of the brain to an agricultural area with many different types of orchards. Diffuse damage can be described as thinning an apple orchard by taking out every 10th tree. When an orchard is thinned, the initial result is a gap in the canopy that was once filled by the removed tree. Over time, the surrounding fruit trees receive more water and sunlight, their branches grow to fill the gap, and the hole in the canopy closes. Such growth takes approximately 2 years to complete. In the brain, when cells die the surviving cells increase their dendritic branching, making new connections with the cells around them. Just like fruit trees, the new dendritic growth takes about 2 years or more to complete and is the primary way through which the brain heals and compensates for microscopic loss of brain cells. When there is severe damage, the injury can be described as "clear-cutting" a section of orchard or even an entire orchard. In this case, surrounding areas are not designed to compensate for the loss of tissue, just as almond orchards around a clear-cut apple orchard will not suddenly begin producing apples. Just as you wouldn't expect the almond trees to produce apples, you would not expect thalamic cells to take over functioning of the hippocampus. Although remaining cells in a particular region may branch and compensate for lost cells, it is less likely that cells from other regions will take over the functions. Some adaptation of cells is possible, especially in young children, and within the distributed areas of cortex such as the frontal and parietal lobes (tertiary cortical regions), with less adaptation being evident after 1 to 2 years of age and within the primary cortical regions and subcortical nuclei.

At times, brain scan findings do not provide enough information to assist in predicting a patient's prognosis. Many factors influence patient outcome following an injury to the central nervous system. Medical complications such as post-traumatic seizures or infections can change a patient's outcome from good to bad very quickly. Cognitive and behavioral factors involving impulsivity, poor judgment, depression, slowed thought processes, and confusion can substantially increase risk of additional injury following discharge from a hospital setting. A patient's support network can also significantly influence outcome, irrespective of the severity of injury suggested by the brain scan.

In the next case example, Angelino's brain scans and rapid recovery during his rehabilitation suggested that he would do well after discharge from the hospital. His outcome was not predicted by his brain scans but by secondary medical complications.

CLINICAL EXAMPLE
Angelino: Gunshot Wound

Angelino was shot in the head while traveling in the back of an automobile; he was not the intended victim and was just in the wrong place at the wrong time. The bullet, measured on CT to be 9 mm in caliber, traveled some distance and through the side of the car before entering his brain just above his left eye. Because the projectile had slowed significantly before entering Angelino's brain, it did not produce the extensive injury often seen from a gunshot wound. The slow-moving bullet pushed through his soft brain tissue, leaving a clean wound channel from his left frontal lobe to his right parietal lobe. Directly below and above the path of the projectile, brain tissue appeared normal on imaging. In addition, tissue around the channel appeared mostly uninjured. Angelino quickly recovered from his injury and after only a few weeks of rehabilitation returned home with his family. Angelino returned to full-time schooling in a regular education classroom only a few weeks after his injury. During a follow-up examination, he presented with normal cognitive abilities, behavior, and emotional functioning. His mother had no concerns regarding his functioning and indicated that she believed he had returned to his baseline functional levels in all activities. Angelino appeared to be extremely lucky in that the path of the bullet traveled through distributed cortex and spared critical white-matter pathways and deeper subcortical nuclei. His residual deficits involved some minor motor limitations on his left side.

Shortly following discharge from the hospital, Angelino began to exhibit symptoms consistent with a common cold or the flu. His symptoms escalated over a day or two and he eventually required hospitalization. A CT scan suggested that there was an infection within the wound channel. The infection was so severe that within a couple of days the infection had destroyed much of his frontal cortex. There was a large abscess, extensive swelling, and increased pressure causing midline shift from his left frontal lobe across to the right side of his brain. Within a few days, Angelino progressed to brain death and ultimately passed away 2 days before Christmas. Angelino's mother, although distraught from losing her son, indicated that she always remembered being told that he may do very well unless there was a medical complication involving seizures, infection or additional injury. Angelino's case highlights how factors other than those identified on initial brain imaging can be important to a patient's outcome.

> Even when brain imaging suggests a positive prognosis, it is important to discuss medical complications that may change a patient's outcome.

Clues Regarding Time Course for Recovery

Estimating the time course for recovery during the post-acute period can be relatively simple. The rate of recovery from a brain injury following resolution of the acute processes is mostly constant across patients with similar type, severity, and extent of injury. After several months, future recovery is primarily related to the speed at which cells can form new dendrites and connections or produce new myelin. The rate of brain recovery begins relatively rapidly a few weeks following an injury, with the rate of improvement slowing after approximately 6 months and leveling off but continuing for several years after approximately 9 to 12 months. Estimating the time course for recovery during the first few weeks can be much more challenging, especially while the patient receives critical-care intervention. Information available from brain imaging can assist the clinician in estimating future progress and in treatment planning. If the brain scans suggest that only minimal functional gains can be expected during inpatient rehabilitation, discharge home may be seen as an option earlier in the course of recovery. If, however, the brain scans suggest limited disruption to primary cortical regions, with dysfunction being related to inflammation of white-matter tracts, diffuse edema, or brain stem swelling, a patient may be kept in the hospital longer with the hope that reduced inflammation or swelling will result in substantive changes in functioning and increased benefit of rehabilitative care.

In general, diffuse injuries to the brain result in a more gradual recovery course than that with focal injuries. Brain scan evidence of diffuse axonal injury can suggest that the patient will transition through an initial stage of low arousal or awareness to protracted recovery that is rapid at first but slows after several months. In contrast, focal injuries may result in a more rapid recovery of functioning but with residual loss to a narrow range of abilities related to the area of damage. Focal injuries to the brain stem or reticular activating system can result in loss of consciousness, prolonged vegetative state, or a minimally conscious state for weeks, months, or even years. With less severe damage, the patient may "wake up" cognitively in a period of only a day or two, followed by rapid recovery of functioning. Such injuries have been referred to as, "light-switch injuries," because recovery happens quickly as if a light switch were turned on.

In the next case example, Ninette's brain scans suggested damage to her brain stem without substantive injury to the rest of her brain, with her recovery course being consistent with a light-switch injury.

CLINICAL EXAMPLE

Ninette: Traumatic Brain Injury

Ninette was hit by a piece of wood that fell from the side of a truck. She sustained a posterior basilar skull fracture and a small contusion to her brain stem. The remainder of her brain appeared uninjured on CT and MRI sequences. Ninette remained in the intensive care unit for almost 2 weeks—intubated, ventilator-dependent, and nonresponsive to stimulation. Once she was medically stable on room air, she was transferred to the rehabilitation unit. Within a week, Ninette began to show signs of increased arousal, with consistent responses to stimulation and those around her. In a period of approximately 2 days, Ninette progressed from a minimally conscious state to one in which she was interacting, solving mental problems, and fully participating in her therapy regimen. Recovery was rapid, and she was discharged home 2 weeks later with ongoing outpatient therapy for some residual motor limitations. Because of her brain scans, Ninette's family received appropriate counsel regarding her condition, her possible outcome from worst case to best case scenarios, as well as her expected or most likely prognosis and time course for recovery.

Concrete Information for Families

Families receive a lot of confusing information during the early stages of brain recovery. In the intensive care unit, discussion often relates to whether the patient will survive or not. Patients are often not aware of their condition and may be unconscious due to the injury or sedative intervention. In the intensive care unit, family members are often in crisis mode, functioning at an emotional level more than a cognitive level. During this period, family members may not be receptive to details regarding functional prognosis or future deficits, as the focus is on keeping the patient alive and medically stable. Because of the difficulty of predicting outcome during the critical-care stage, any details are qualified as being speculative or an educated guess. Once the patient has been transferred to an acute care or rehabilitation unit, discussion changes from one of survival to one of functional recovery and adaptation to long-term deficits. It is on the acute care units that patients and family members become more receptive to detailed discussions about the implications of the injury to future functioning. The use of brain scans during the acute-care stages of recovery can become an important component of patient and family education. Brain scans can provide concrete visual information regarding how the brain was affected by an injury. When brain scans appear mostly normal, such visual information can provide comfort and reassurance to family members. Brain scans that demonstrate severe injury to large areas of tissue can assist others in their understanding of the severity and extent of the injury. Patients and family members often struggle to deal with ambiguous or limited information regarding a brain injury. The use of brain imaging by a knowledgeable clinician can go a long way toward providing objective and clinically meaningful information.

The use of brain imaging is helpful not only in an acute-care hospital setting but also when seeing patients in an outpatient clinic. This is especially true when a patient or family members have limited understanding of the causes of long-term changes in behavior or abilities following discharge from the hospital. Although information about long-term prognosis and residual deficits may have been communicated during hospitalization, several months later there may be little retention of the details. It is not uncommon for patients or family members to be genuinely surprised about changes in functioning many months following discharge, even if the issues were discussed in detail during the hospitalization. Having the brain scans available during follow-up visits enables the clinician to readdress the information and to do so during a time of less anxiety and emotional stress for the patient of family. Discussion of the brain injury and review of brain imaging may be even more helpful at follow-up than before discharge. During follow-up clinic visits, any residual functional, behavioral, or cognitive concerns can be directly related to the findings on brain scans, thus providing a concrete explanation to the patient and family.

Sometimes review of previous brain imaging can help explain later difficulties, even when there has been no acute injury for years, as demonstrated in the following example. An intellectually intelligent 21-year-old presented in the clinic with immaturity, poor judgment, impulsivity, attentional difficulties, and mildly disrupted executive functioning, seeking an explanation for failure to progress in college. Review of his past medical history revealed a brain injury as an infant. Further review of his brain scans suggested severe trauma to his orbital and medial frontal lobes, with no obvious injury to the rest of his brain. His performance on neuropsychological assessment and his described difficulties were highly consistent with that expected given his previous injury. Presentation of the images with an explanation of why he was having difficulty led to a clear discussion about what he could do to compensate for his limitations. His difficulties were instantly transformed from being "psychological" or "behavioral" in origin and a reflection of his "personality" to being organically mediated and amenable to compensatory strategies. Also helpful for this patients was the discussion of the axiom "A brain injury may explain inappropriate behavior but it should never be used to excuse the behavior." Consequences, both positive for appropriate behavior and negative for inappropriate behavior, are critical when working with a patient who has a brain injury. In regard to this patient, once a concrete explanation had been provided by the use of the brain scans, it was important to ensure that the patient did not use the injury as an excuse for failure or inappropriate behaviors. Emphasis was placed on techniques that could be used by the patient to overcome the difficulties relating to his previous injury. Alice's case, discussed below, involved a similar use of previous brain scans in an outpatient clinic, even though she had never sustained a traumatic brain injury.

CLINICAL EXAMPLE
Alice: Frontal Dysplasia

Alice, a delightful 9-year-old girl, was referred for neuropsychological evaluation because of "behavioral problems at school." In brief, several times a day Alice would be sent to the principle of the school for disruptive behaviors such as anger outbursts, violent episodes, throwing objects, verbal profanity, and a general inability to control her mood and actions. The school had recently transferred her to a home-hospital program in lieu of expulsion given her many suspensions without improvement in behavior. Alice's mother noted that she had always been like this, even as an infant. Review of Alice's medical records revealed that she had received a CT and MRI scan within the first 2 weeks of life and again at 5 years of age. The imaging report indicated a "frontal extra-axial fluid collection without mass effect or acute hemorrhage." When asked about the imaging results, her mother reported being told that there was a small amount of fluid outside of the brain and that it did not require any medical treatment. She was under the impression that the amount of fluid was about a quarter of an inch and that this had nothing to do with her child's problems.

Neuropsychological examination suggested severely impaired cognitive functioning within all domains, with Alice having an age equivalency of approximately 4 years, less than half her chronological age. Her mother agreed with this impression, reporting that Alice functioned at a level below that of her 5-year-old sibling. In addition, Alice had a severe form of attention deficit/hyperactivity disorder (ADHD) with an almost complete inability to focus her attention for more than a few seconds without becoming distracted. Impulsivity was pervasive during her evaluation and noted to be a concern for her safety. When discussing her difficulties, Alice reported "hating getting angry," and it was clear that she disliked losing her temper. She added that she "wished it would not happen." When asked why she becomes so upset, she explained, "I don't know, it just happens and I feel bad afterwards."

When asked about what she knew about Alice's brain development, her mother reported that she had not been told anything about brain development, only that there was a small collection of fluid outside of the brain, at the front. She did not understand how the collection of fluid could have anything to do with her child's problems and, after seeing many specialists, was becoming frustrated. Through use of a brain model, the functioning of the frontal lobes was explained to Alice's mother, in particular the regions responsible for behavioral and emotional control and attentional functioning.

Upon review of her brain imaging, it was clear that the majority of Alice's frontal lobes had not developed and that much of the tissue was distorted with areas of dysplasia. Figures 1-2A–C provide a series of axial CT images at different levels clearly showing the extra-axial fluid collection in the frontal area. Although the lack of normal frontal lobe mass is evident on the CT scans, the MRI series in Figures 1-2D–F showing axial, coronal and sagittal views respectively, allow for clearer identification of the disrupted frontal lobe strucures.

There was a frontal fluid collection, although this was due to a dysplastic and schizencephalic frontal lobe. The fluid collection was extra-axial and did not exert a mass effect on the brain. In addition, there was no evidence of acute hemorrhage, just as the

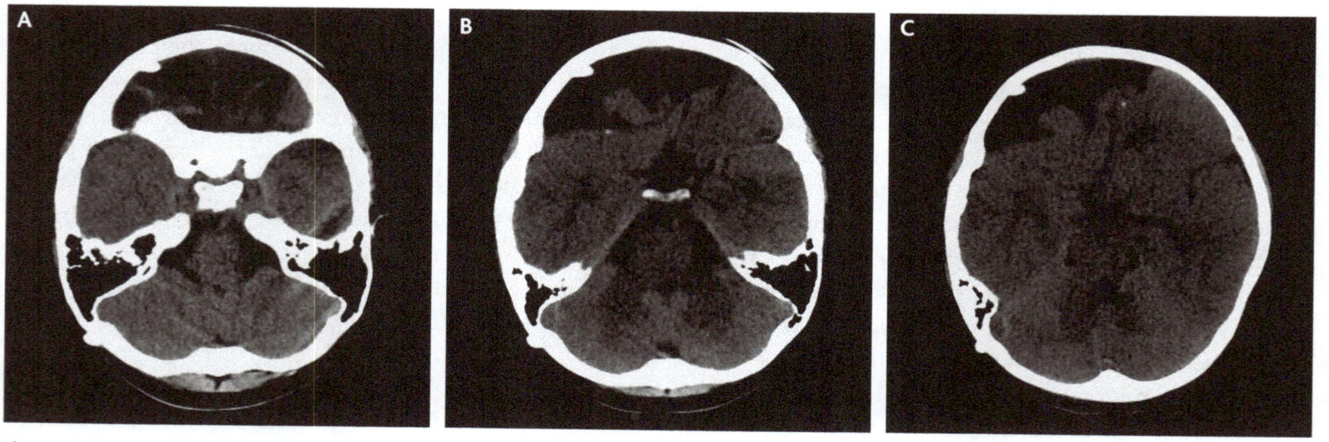

Figures 1-2A, B, and C Case example Alice: CT series.

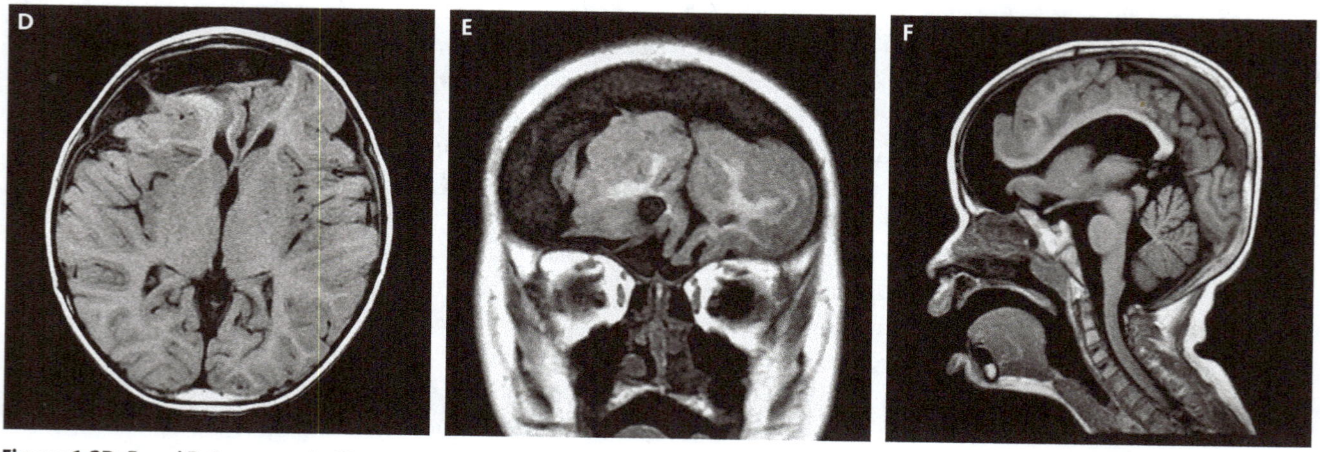

Figures 1-2D, E, and F Case example Alice: MRI series.

radiology report had mentioned. However, the report failed to describe the lack of frontal development obvious upon review of the images. The images were likely interpreted on the basis of the referral question of "ruling out acute pathological processes" that may require medical intervention. If the referral question had requested an explanation for her behavioral and cognitive difficulties, it would likely have included relevant details regarding the morphology of the brain from a neurodevelopmental perspective. The referral question regarding acute pathology resulted in the radiologist and the clinician approaching the child's care from two different levels of acuity: one focused on critical care issues relating to intracranial pressure and hemorrhaging, the other on an explanation for disrupted development and functioning.

When the brain scans were shown to Alice's mother, with an explanation of the effects of the disrupted frontal lobe neurodevelopment, she immediately appeared relieved that finally someone had provided her an explanation for her child's difficulties. She reported knowing for years that "Alice was a good child who is unable to control her behaviors," but she had never received a reasonable explanation for Alice's difficulties. With this new knowledge, it was easier for Alice's mother to plan an appropriate approach to helping her, with a combination of psychotherapeutic and pharmacological interventions, and with a better understanding of the difficulties her child was experiencing. Knowing about Alice's disrupted development also precipitated a new plan at school, as she was now documented as having a neurological condition and was not just viewed as a "bad child" or one with "behavioral issues."

Showing brain scans to a patient or family can make the injury more real, concrete, and understandable. This may result in a more realistic understanding and, ultimately, acceptance of the condition. However, showing scans may also result in a loss of hope and feelings of helplessness or dismay, especially if the scans show severe injury to the brain. Consider the possible consequences of showing brain scans to a patient or family, before doing so. Take into consideration the following to help you decide on whether or not to show the scans:

- Will showing the scans result in improved understanding and reduced emotional trauma? Concrete visual information about an injury may assist in understanding. If denial or poor understanding is disrupting patient care, the images may assist in communicating the extent of injury and provide a more realistic expectation for family participation in the patient's care.
- Will showing the images assist the family in understanding the patient's long-term care needs or expected outcomes.
- Who is your audience? You may wish to show family members the scans but not younger children or cognitively impaired adult patients who are unable to process the information or who may become traumatized.
- What does your audience already know or believe about the injury?
- Have the scans been shown to the patient or family by another clinician?
- Do the scans look "good" or "bad," and do they fit with your clinical impressions and prognosis?
- Will showing the scans be misleading or confusing?
- Are there artifacts on the scan that can be misinterpreted by the viewer?
- Will showing the scans result in excessive emotional difficulties for the viewer?
- Will showing the scans result in feelings of hopelessness, which can lead to reduced goals and poor compliance with therapeutic interventions?

LIMITATIONS: WHAT NEUROIMAGING OFTEN DOES NOT PROVIDE THE CLINICIAN

With increased access to brain imaging, along with improved technology, one can begin to view neuroimaging as a clinical panacea, a solution for any brain-related condition or question. However, the utility of brain scans is actually quite limited, and their use should be based on a specific need or question. As discussed above, brain scans can provide a wealth of information highly valuable to a clinician. However, sometimes brain scans are less useful to the clinician and may even be misleading or cause unnecessary emotional distress for the patient or family. It is important to consider the limitations of brain imaging and what they are unable to provide the clinician or patient. For example, with few exceptions, brain imaging cannot provide a measure of functioning, information regarding electrochemical processes or pathologies, or a precise etiology for the patient's symptoms.

Brain imaging does not measure a patient's functioning

With few exceptions, brain scans do not provide a measure of brain functioning, and no brain scan has the ability to measure a patient's actual functional abilities. The best measure of a person's functioning comes from a clinical evaluation. General mental status examinations are the standard in most institutions, although they provide only limited information regarding higher cognitive functioning or the ability to perform complex self-help skills. Examinations by neurology or physiatry/physical medicine and rehabilitation specialists can provide additional information on cognitive, motor, or sensory functioning. Neuropsychological evaluations can provide a detailed picture of complex cognitive, motor, perceptual, emotional, and behavioral functioning. More focused evaluations by speech-language, physical, and occupational therapists can provide even more detailed information about a patient's functioning.

Although information provided by brain imaging can guide specialist evaluations, a clear connection between radiology findings and a patient's functioning is not always evident. It is not unusual for a patient to present with notable functional limitations without radiological evidence of pathology, and, conversely, some patients with clear pathology on imaging may perform at normal or near-normal levels. In addition, there are times when subtle injuries to the brain cause marked deficits, whereas the same injury may not affect the functioning of a different person. For example, a mild frontal stroke in a highly productive professional who must rely on exceptional executive functioning involving organization, conceptual flexibility, complex and divided attention, and sophisticated problem solving may prevent the person from returning to his or her premorbid position. However, a similar stroke in someone who does not rely on highly developed executive abilities may not result in substantive compromise to normal functioning, and return to premorbid levels may be rapid.

In the next case example, Robert had a mild stroke in his right frontal lobe but exhibited no substantive limitations upon return to his regular work and family obligations.

CLINICAL EXAMPLE
Robert: Stroke

Robert was hospitalized for a spontaneous right frontal hemorrhage. Review of brain scans 2 days after his stroke suggested that he would experience significant functional deficits following discharge from the hospital. However, upon examination during a 3-month follow-up clinic visit, Robert reported functioning at premorbid levels and had no complaints. On examination, performance was commensurate with his educational and work background, without marked limitation or deficit involving his basic cognitive abilities. Mild deficits were noted for speed of processing and rapid switching of mental concepts, although such abilities were not critical for Robert's daily functioning. Robert had returned to work on a ranch and was caring for his family without difficulty. This is a case where Robert's brain scans suggested that he would experience deficits in functioning, due to the extent of hemorrhage. However, his mild loss of executive functioning was inconsequential to Robert and of no concern given the demands of his job and family commitments. If Robert had been someone who relied on higher cognitive abilities and rapid speed of mental processing, such as a pilot, his injury would have been much more disabling and would likely have prevented return to work.

Robert's example highlights the need to consider the relevance of radiology findings to a person's background, goals and expectations for return to premorbid functioning. Often, minor findings on brain scans may be meaningless at the functional level, although evident at the anatomical level. With the use of ever increasing magnet strength, new MRI sequences are able to detect microbleeds once only visible using microscopes. The relevance of such findings on a brain scan should be considered by the clinician as they relate to the patient's clinical needs. The question of whether such findings are clinically or functionally relevant to the specific patient may determine the extent to which such findings influence treatment decisions or patient consultation. Should a patient who is functioning within normal limits and at premorbid baseline levels be shown microbleeds in the brain? Or should the patient be counseled that he or she had a brain injury, has made a good recovery, and can expect additional healing over the next few years? By showing the scans, the clinician runs the risk of the bleeds being overinterpreted by the patient and ultimately affecting future outcomes. By not showing the scans, the clinician runs the risk of the patient underestimating the brain injury and putting himself or herself at risk of another injury post-discharge. There may be no right or wrong answer regarding nonclinically relevant findings on brain imaging; what is important is that consideration be given to the specific goals of showing the images and to the possible effects on the patient when doing so.

In young children, pathology that is clearly evident on brain imaging may not be clinically relevant because of the age of the child. Damage to some areas of the developing brain may not disrupt functioning until the child is much older. If damage occurs in areas of the brain that have not fully developed or are not currently required for functioning, a child may not exhibit deficits normally associated with those structures. For example, a frontal-lobe injury in an infant may not result in impaired cognitive functioning; the frontal lobes have not yet fully matured, and the child would not be expected to think abstractly, have intact executive abilities, or reason conceptually. However, as the child matures and expectations for frontal-lobe functioning increase, deficits relating to the early injury may become more evident. This was the case with Katie, a toddler who underwent surgical resection of a tumor via a right frontal-lobe approach.

CLINICAL EXAMPLE

Katie: Neoplasm Resection via the Right Frontal Lobe

Katie underwent surgery as a toddler to remove a midline brain tumor from above the third ventricle (Figures 1-3A–C). A right frontal-lobe approach was used, most easily visualized on the left side of Figure 1-3D. The surgery resulted in a relatively large cavity through her right lateral frontal lobe from the surface to the third ventricle and through the anterior portion of the corpus callosum. Interestingly, 6 months following her surgery, neuropsychological examination suggested high-average performance in all areas assessed. Her behavior and affective presentation was unremarkable, and her parents had no concerns regarding her abilities. Even with the post-resection frontal cavity and injury to her corpus callosum, Katie acted and functioned at an advanced level for her age.

Review and discussion of Katie's brain scans took into account her developmental age and the areas of the brain involved. Even with the large cavity in her frontal lobe including the corpus callosum (Figures 1-3D–F), her parents were counseled that Katie's functioning would likely remain age-appropriate for a few more years, although she might experience difficulties as she matured. They were further counseled that a "good recovery" over the next few years did not mean that she would not have any problems relating to her frontal-lobe and corpus callosum damage later in life. The brain scans were used to help the parents understand the effects of the surgery on current functioning as a toddler as well as on future development. They were instructed to closely monitor Katie's preschool and grade-school performance and to schedule a follow-up evaluation if they became concerned. These discussions prepared the parents for the future, and the review of the brain scans helped them understand why their child was at risk of future difficulties, even though she appeared to have made a full recovery from her surgery.

Long-term monitoring of Katie revealed that she began to have difficulties when she started first grade. This is a time when expectations for sustained attention, integrated reasoning, executive abilities, and behavioral control increase commensurate with her age and a time when she had to begin relying on frontal-lobe functioning to be successful in school.

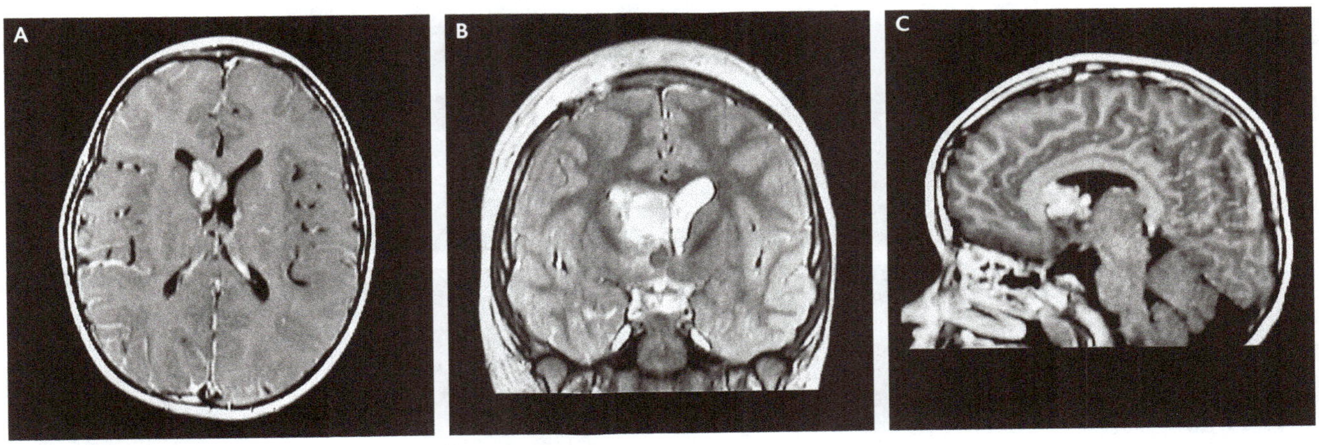

Figures 1-3A, B, and C Case example Katie: Preoperative MRI series.

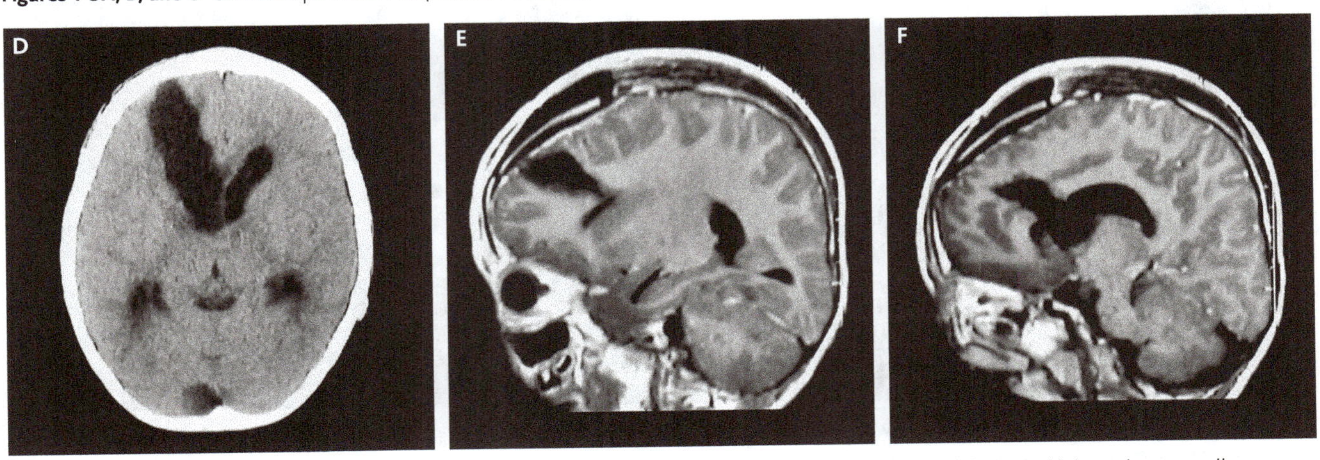

Figures 1-3D, E, and F Case example Katie: Postoperative CT and MRI showing resection channel through the right frontal lobe and corpus callosum.

Abnormal Brain Scans with Normal Functioning

It is not unusual for a brain scan to appear abnormal whereas the patient is asymptomatic and has normal functioning. Benign arachnoid cysts, neuroglial cysts and some very slow-growing cystic neoplasms can develop over many years without disruption of functioning, especially if they form during the fetal or neonatal period. Figure 1-4A shows a large area of cyst within the left temporal and parietal lobes that appears to have been present for many years. Very slow-forming cysts and space-occupying lesions can allow the brain the opportunity to adapt and form around the lesion over many years, resulting in the person being asymmtomatic and presenting

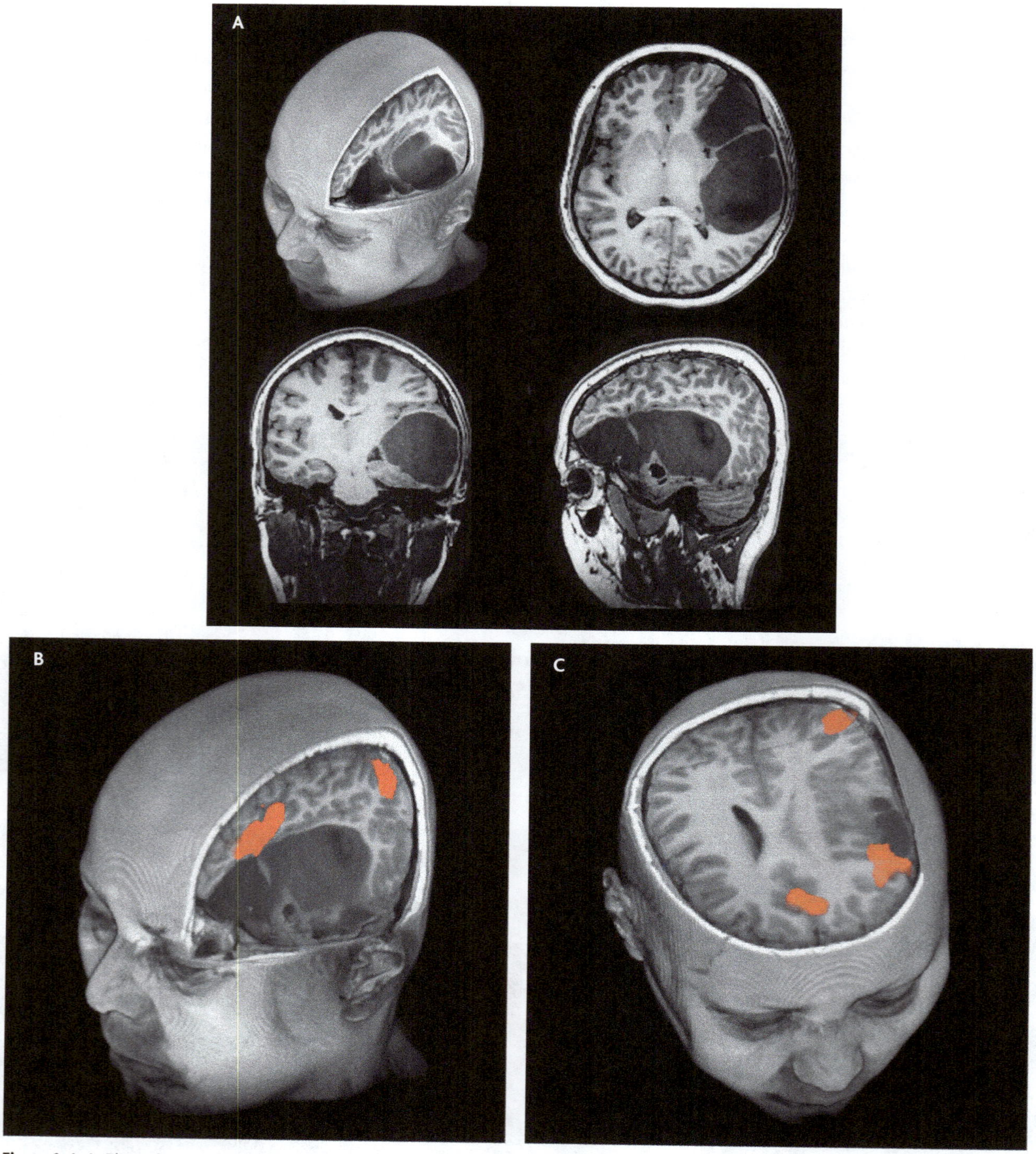

Figure 1-4 A: Three-dimensional cutout view with two-dimensional axial, coronal and sagittal images showing the benign left hemisphere cyst. **B and C:** Three-dimensional cutout views showing the results of fMRI brain mapping suggesting displacement of healthy cortical tissue.

(Continued)

(Continued)

with normal functioning. This was the case with the patient who's brain is depicted in Figure 1-4A. Following the serendipituous finding of the left hemisphere cyst during a routine study related to a mild closed head injury, brain mapping via functional MRI (fMRI) was performed to localize primary cortical areas responsible for motor, sensory and language functioning (Figures 1-4B–C). Results from the mapping (red) confirmed that the respective cortices had been displaced by the cyst, but were still fully functional. It is important to consider that imaging findings may not correlate with a patient's functioning, especially with long-standing conditions such as slowly developing cysts or lesions.

Brain imaging may not provide information about electrochemical processes

With a few exceptions, brain scans are unable to provide useful information regarding changes in the electrical or chemical processes of the brain. Sometimes, changes to the brain's electrical status and chemistry can be inferred from physical correlates such as swelling or loss of tissue density, although direct measures are mostly unavailable. Because normal neural functioning is highly dependent on electrochemical processes at the cellular level, substantive disruption of a person's functioning may be apparent even without evidence of pathology on a brain scan. Over time, however, electrochemical processes that cause damage to the brain can be detected as the gross anatomical structures begin to atrophy.

CLINICAL EXAMPLE

Sarah: Rasmussen's Encephalitis

Sarah's initial brain scans were read as normal, although she experienced profound disruption to her functioning as a result of partial status epilepticus. Even with her normal-appearing brain scans, Sarah experienced severe disruption to her memory, receptive and expressive language skills, reasoning, and general adaptive functioning. Sarah was experiencing almost constant partial seizures over her left hemisphere, with increasing frequency and duration eventually becoming epilepsia partialis continua. Electroencephalography (EEG) and follow-up brain imaging suggested that Sarah had Rasmussen's encephalitis, a condition that ultimately required surgical removal of her left hemisphere. Over time, subtle changes to her brain became apparent on brain imaging, with gradual atrophy of her left hemisphere. Sarah underwent a left-sided hemispherectomy, which stopped her seizures and any progression of her encephalitis. For several weeks following her surgery, Sarah was globally aphasic and failed to exhibit any signs of symbolic thought. She appeared to respond to pictures, so they were incorporated into her treatment regimen as much as possible. Happy faces were used to indicate "yes," and sad faces were used to indicate "no." Eventually Sarah improved and was able to use a few single words to communicate. However, even years after her surgery Sarah continued to rely on behavioral and physical means to communicate because of her inability to express herself verbally. Verbal comprehension was similarly disrupted, as were other cognitive abilities related to left-hemisphere functioning.

Pre- and Post-Surgery Brain Scans

The MRI images for Sarah suggest slight atrophy of her left hemisphere, shown on the right side of the scans. The atrophy is so subtle that it is only evident on close inspection. Note the size of the right and left hemispheres, or the distance from the lateral surface to the medial intrahemispheric fissure. Computer software enables clinicians to place reference lines on images, with recording of the length. This allows for accurate measurement of anatomical structures, or, in this case, the right and left hemispheres. An example of a T1 image with (Figure 1-5A) and without (Figure 1-5B) reference lines is included below, with a post-surgery CT (Figure 1-5C) to show the extent of surgical intervention necessary for this child. The dark area on the CT is the cavity from the left-hemisphere resection. T1 ultrafast spoiled gradient echo (FSPGR) MRI sequences were used, as they provide clear gray–white differentiation and good contrast for anatomical structures.

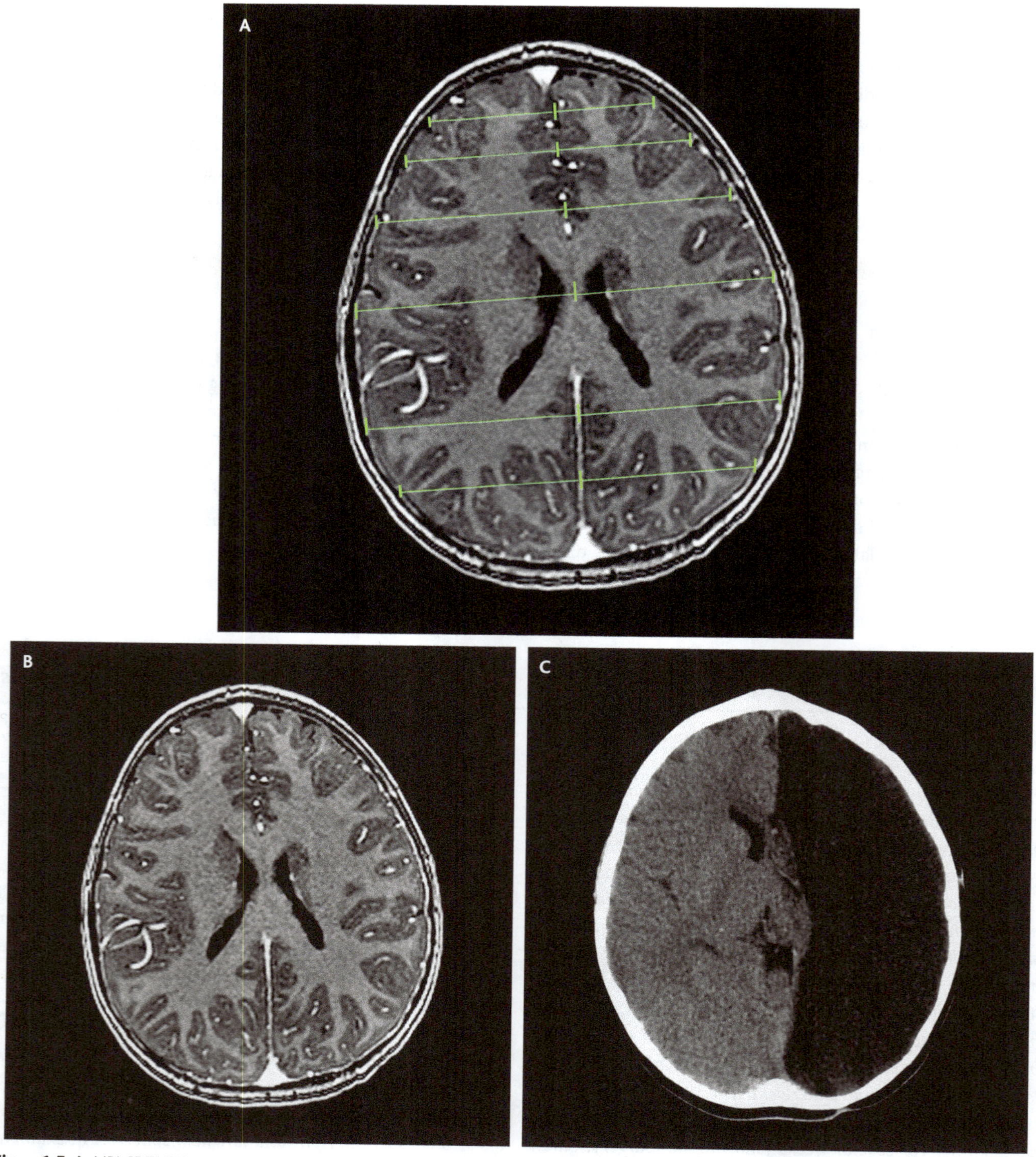

Figure 1-5 **A:** MRI CE T1 FSPGR With Reference Lines. **B:** MRI CE T1 FSPGR Without Reference Lines **C:** Postoperative CT.

Brain imaging does not provide direct visualization of microscopic injury

Even with advances in technology and notable gains in image quality, brain scans are still unable to resolve anatomy at the microscopic or cellular level. Microscopic damage can be inferred from features on a scan, although not directly viewed. Given the lack of microscopic resolution, it is not uncommon for a patient to present with significant functional limitations but without radiological evidence for this. Having "normal" brain scans with deficient functioning can be confusing for many patients and family members and can be perceived as contradictory. In addition, without radiological evidence of injury, some symptoms may be attributed to psychological, emotional, or behavioral etiologies when they actually stem from organic brain pathology. Explaining the limitations of brain imaging can go a long way toward resolving confusion and formulating more accurate differential diagnoses. With treatment regimens being dependent on accurate differential diagnoses, determination of the relevance of a "normal" brain scan can make the difference between appropriate and inappropriate clinical care.

Although microscopic cellular structure is still not visible on brain scans, current high magnet strength MRI systems do have the spatial and contrast resolution to allow visualization of small cortical areas in order to assess for abnormal cellular organization or dysplasia.

Brain scans often do not provide information regarding the etiology of damage

Brain scans generally show the results of an injury or pathological process but not the process itself. Even though some causes of central nervous system injury are obvious from the clinical history and markers on brain images, there are many occasions when brain scans are not helpful in determining a specific etiology. Infectious or toxic processes can result in significant brain damage and functional deficits without providing information regarding the cause of the pathology. Although scans are often ordered as part of a normal neurological workup, many patients presenting with neurological or psychiatric conditions are found to have normal brain imaging. Similarly, many children with developmental delays are shown to have normal brain scans, even though their functional deficits suggest marked neurological compromise.

Often, the pathological process can be inferred from specific markers on the brain scan. For example, hypoxic injury can be inferred from diffuse swelling in addition to focal damage to the basal ganglia or watershed area. Traumatic brain injuries are often quite obvious on brain imaging and are suggested by evidence of edema, tearing or damage to brain parenchyma and blood vessels, especially those between the skull and dura (epidural hematoma), between the dura and brain surface (subdural or subarachnoid hemorrhages), or within the brain tissue (intraparenchymal hemorrhages). Diffuse damage at the junction of the gray and white matter or within the corpus callosum may also suggest physical trauma to the brain. However, even when physical trauma is suggested by the scans, it may not be possible to determine precisely what caused the injury, especially without a clear clinical history. Large areas of hemorrhage can imply a stroke, although the feeding vessel or specific cause of the bleed may not be apparent on neuroimaging. There are times when neuroimaging suggests rupture of blood vessels, although following the stroke it is not possible to determine whether it was a normal vessel, vascular malformation, or aneurysm that ruptured. By the time the patient is scanned, the blood and edema may prevent any visualization of residual vessel tissue at the core of the stroke, making accurate assessment of etiology impossible.

One difficulty with determining etiology using brain imaging stems from the fact that neuroimaging only provides a picture of damage, with different pathologies looking remarkably similar on a brain scan. Determining if a lesion is neoplastic, parasitic, or infectious may not be possible using a single brain scan, although it becomes easier with a combination of sequences. If few sequences are available, clinical history and findings on examination become the best clue to the cause of a specific pathology on a brain scan. The two axial sequences shown in Figure 1-6 appear similar and suggest that the patients sustained similar injuries to their left frontal lobe regions, shown at the front and on the right side of the images. However, the etiologies for the two patients were vastly different, with one patient sustaining a traumatic brain injury from her head hitting the windshield of a car (Figure 1-6A), and the other patient sustaining injury to her brain due to bacterial encephalitis (Figure 1-6B).

Brain scans do not treat the patient

Brain scans are not therapeutic per se, although may guide therapy and treatment regimens. Because imaging has become an integral tool for many clinicians, patients and families frequently view neuroimaging as a therapeutic modality. During the acute stages of recovery, treatment may be highly dependent on findings from brain scans. For example, a patient with fluctuating intracranial pressure and who is at risk of herniating may require multiple brain scans for assessment of the efficacy of external ventricular drains, ventriculoperitoneal shunts, medications,

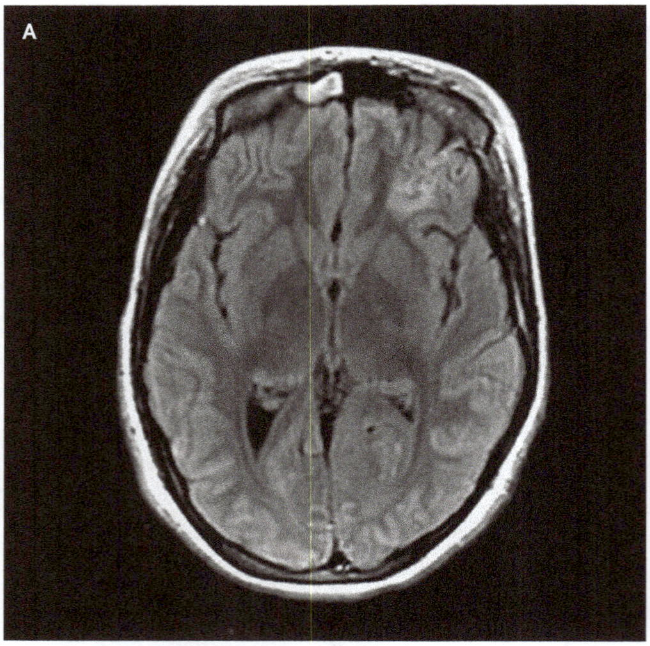

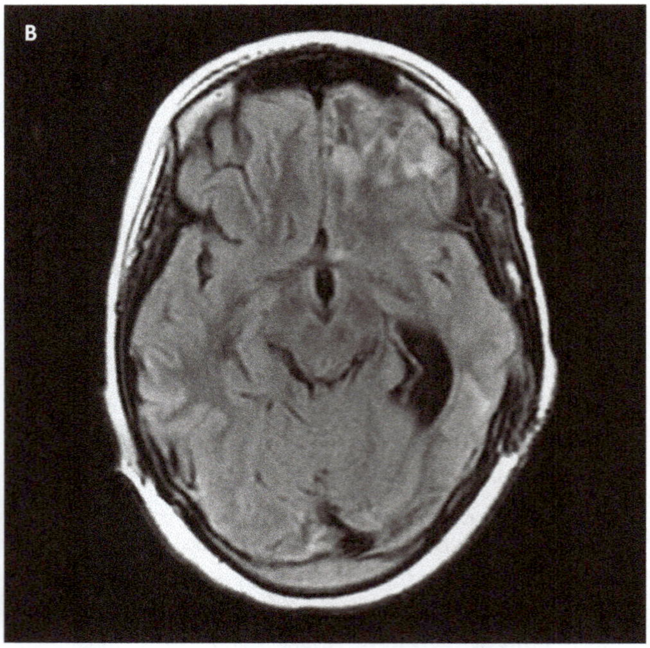

Figure 1-6 **A:** Traumatic Brain Injury **B:** Encephalitis.

or other surgical or medical interventions. Even though multiple brain scans are used during the early stages of treatment, it is important to remember that the brain scans themselves do not provide any therapeutic value to the patient; brain imaging can guide treatment but cannot provide it. Once a patient has been medically stabilized, neuroimaging may not be critical to patient care, and imaging studies are no longer ordered. Interestingly, although this is a sign of recovery, the lack of imaging can become a concern for family members. For example, in the next case example, the patient's husband had difficulty discriminating between diagnostic techniques such as neuroimaging and medical treatment or therapies for his wife.

CLINICAL EXAMPLE
Vicki: "Are you going to do another brain scan?"

Vicki was injured during a motor vehicle collision, sustaining severe trauma to her brain. Recovery followed the usual course, with several weeks of critical-care intervention in the intensive care unit, followed by several weeks of inpatient medical rehabilitation once she was stabilized. After a couple of weeks in rehabilitation, the initial rapid gains in functioning slowed and progress became more gradual. After discharge, she continued to improve for many months, but with the expected slowing of recovery at approximately 6 to 9 months post-injury.

Shortly following her injury, Vicki had undergone CT examination in the emergency department and MRI examination upon admission to the intensive care unit. Because of the difficulty controlling her increased intracranial pressure and the use of multiple techniques such as external ventricular drains, craniotomies, and medications, Vicki was sent for brain imaging every couple of days. Upon transfer to the medical rehabilitation unit, she received one more CT to ensure that the pressure had resolved and to plan for the replacement of the craniotomy bone flap. Vicki's husband was asked each time to provide consent for the imaging studies and had began to consider them a critical part of her care. When no more scans were required, Vicki's husband had difficulty understanding why the treatment team was not doing all that they could to treat her.

During the time when Vicki's recovery stabilized and slowed, no more scans were ordered. Unfortunately, Vicki's husband attributed her slowing progress to the reduced number of brain scans, which is not surprising given that the two were temporally linked. Every time treatment team members met with Vicki's husband they were asked, "When is she going to have another brain scan?" When told that she did not need one he became concerned that this would slow her recovery. Even after many explanations that neuroimaging was diagnostic and not therapeutic, the concern continued. Three months after discharge during Vicki's rehabilitation follow-up visit, the team was not surprised when the first question from the husband was "When are you going to do another brain scan?"

It is important to communicate the reason for brain scans with family members, who may see them as causal or treatment related in a patient's early recovery instead of a tool to monitor pathological processes such as bleeding, edema and intracranial pressure, ventricular size, or risk of herniation.

SHOWING DAMAGE ON BRAIN IMAGES MAY NOT BE RECOMMENDED

Be cautious when determining whether or not to show brain scans to patients or family members. Avoid developing the habit of always reviewing brain scans with patients or care providers as if this were a necessary component of your clinical role. Although the presentation of brain scans can provide significant clinical benefits, doing so can also cause undue emotional and psychological distress to the patient or family members. While visual evidence of injury may be helpful in breaking through denial or unrealistic expectations, there are times when denial and unrealistic expectations are beneficial to a patient's recovery. Shortly after a severe injury, denial and unrealistic goals can help family members cope with the trauma and focus on the positive. Over time, and with increasing interactions with the patient, most family members come to their own realization about the patient's deficits and likely long-term needs.

A parent of a young man who eventually passed away from his condition provides an excellent example of how denial can slowly change to realization and acceptance over several weeks to months. Tyler's mother was at his bedside during his initial critical-care hospitalization. Although he had a severe form of meningoencephalitis and he was in critical condition, her initial question was "When can he go back to playing football?" Showing the brain scans and describing his prognosis at this point would not have helped Tyler or his mother. Instead, the brain scans were not shown to her and she was told that it would be easier to determine when he could return to football once he was out of critical condition. This exchange allowed his mother to continue to hope and to reflect on the possibility of him returning to a sport that he loved and excelled at, in addition to providing her some comfort.

Removing hope is often counterproductive, especially during the early stages of brain recovery. Unfortunately, with severe neurological conditions, the showing of brain scans may be all that is required for family members to lose hope. For example, a patient paralyzed by severe trauma to the motor cortex or pathways may perform better in rehabilitation and improve faster with the unrealistic goals of returning to full able-bodied functioning. This is a situation in which showing a large hole where motor pathways used to be will likely result in hopelessness, emotional disruption, and reduced effort in therapy. When a patient discovers that limited recovery is expected on the basis of brain imaging data, he or she may just "give up" or become resolved to his or her "fate." Hope and goals facilitate effort; showing patients their brain imaging may remove their hope and goals and result in reduced effort. Just as is true with family members, over time, a realization of the permanence of deficits sets in, and this may be a more appropriate time to show the scans and answer questions about the injury. Interestingly, although patients and family members may have been told that deficits will likely be permanent, until they view pictures of the damage, the realization of the magnitude of damage is often limited. The old saying "A picture is worth a thousand words" rings true with brain injuries, thus the clinician must give careful consideration to the effects that the images may have on the patient and family.

Clinicians who view brain scans on a regular basis may underestimate the emotional impact of viewing a loved one's brain directly following severe injury. Professionals review brain scans from a scientific or intellectual perspective, not from an emotional or personal perspective. Brain scans become analogous to laboratory results or objective test findings. Patients and family members do not have the same background when viewing scans and are less likely to evaluate the images from a scientific or intellectual perspective. In addition, without knowledge of which image features are normal versus abnormal, it is difficult for patients or family members to make sense of what they see. Even normal features on a brain scan can quickly be interpreted incorrectly and result in beliefs that the patient is more "damaged" than in actuality. The most common mistake made by nontrained viewers of brain scans involves the "big black holes in the brain." Frequently, patients or family members will gasp as they first see the brain scans, not because they detected the damage or pathology but because they saw the ventricles and immediately thought that the "black holes" were damage. This imposes a duty on those presenting brain scans to fully explain what is to be shown, what is normal or inconsequential, and what represents injury *before* showing the images.

A useful approach is to use a brain model to first describe how the images represent slices of tissue in three different planes. Then, using the model or pictures, the clinician can describe the ventricles and explain how they will appear on the images (black for CT and T1, white for T2, etc.), so that the viewer is not shocked by the appearance of the "holes." Then the pathology is described and how such pathology appears on the various scans being used. This approach will prepare patients and family members for what they are about to see. For example, to prepare potential viewers of a scan for a patient with significant swelling, they may be instructed that the swelling will appear darker than other tissue, but not black; all this means is that the tissue is swollen, just like a thumb that is swollen after being hit accidently by a hammer. With T2 and T2 fluid attenuated inversion recovery (FLAIR) images, inflammation can appear as bright areas on a scan, something that can also be misinterpreted. Preparing viewers by explaining how inflammation will appear, as well as the possible effects of the inflammation on prognosis, will enable the viewers to benefit from seeing the scans and may prevent the initial shock of seeing the bright areas. Artifacts, especially those caused by metallic objects or movement, should be described to the potential viewers before showing the scans. It is natural for a clinician to ignore imaging artifacts, knowing that they are clinically meaningless, but naïve viewers may interpret them as indication of greater damage than is actually present.

PEARL Preparing a viewer by explaining what they are about to see on a series of brain images will go a long way toward minimizing confusion, improving understanding, and preventing misinterpretation.

PERIL Be cautious about showing brain scans when you don't have the time to prepare the viewer, respond to questions, or discuss the relevance of the findings to the patient's condition.

Often, too little information can be worse for a patient or family than no information at all. Showing brain scans without taking the time to explain clinically relevant or even irrelevant findings can result in the viewer interpreting the imaging results incorrectly. For instance, in the next case example, the patient's wife was shown brain scans without a discussion regarding what she was viewing and their relevance to her husband's clinical condition.

CLINICAL EXAMPLE

Cameron: Stroke with Coiling

Cameron suffered a stroke due to an aneurysm rupture and was treated with placement of a coil to embolize the damaged vessel and prevent further bleeding. Shortly after the procedure, the vascular surgeon presented the brain scans to Cameron's wife. Two weeks later, after Cameron was transferred to the acute care floor, his wife was asked if she had any questions about Cameron's condition and treatment plan. She indicated that she was extremely worried about the massive damage to Cameron's brain. She was informed that there was very little damage to Cameron's brain and that the surgery was very successful in preventing injury to critical brain structures. She was also informed that given the relatively small size of the hemorrhage and the rapid treatment that Cameron received, in addition to his excellent early recovery, he might not experience any significant functional limitations after a few months of recovery. Cameron's wife was surprised by this information and reported that she had seen a very large area of damage on his brain scans when they were shown to her by his surgeon. Review of the brain scans suggested only minimal damage to brain tissue, with otherwise normal-looking brain structures. Upon further discussion with his wife, and having her point out what she thought was damage on the scans, it became clear that Cameron's wife had not been provided enough information to allow her to fully understand what the surgeon was trying to tell her.

First, the neurosurgeon had informed her that the white areas were blood and that the dark area was where the brain was injured by the stroke. He had not spent time explaining that the skull would also appear white and that sections of the cranium would appear to be "inside the brain." In addition, he had not explained that cerebral spinal fluid in the ventricles would appear dark and that this is normal.

While viewing the CT scan shown in Figure 1-7, Cameron's wife interpreted the ventricles as tissue loss caused by the stroke, and the areas of bone as pools of blood. This gave the impression that her husband had experienced a massive injury to both sides of his brain and would be severely brain damaged. In addition, the surgeon had pointed to the part of the brain showing the coil, indicating that this was "from the surgery." Because of metallic

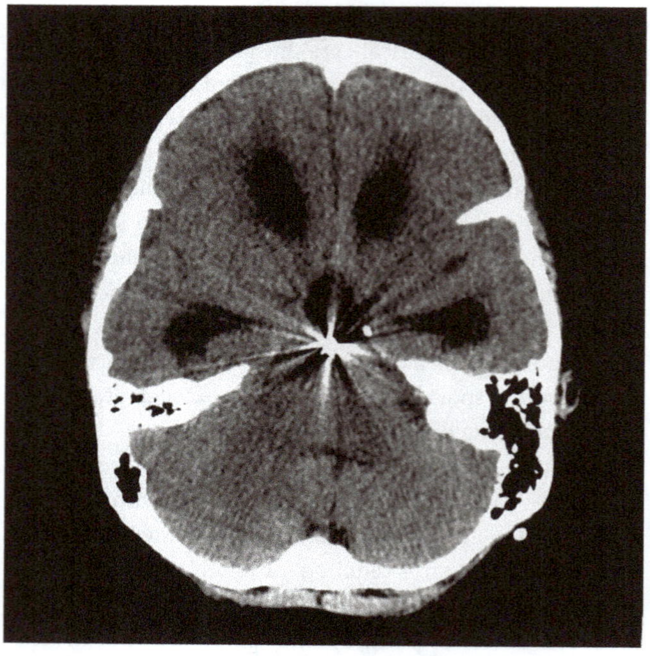

Figure 1-7 Case example Cameron: CT showing the ventricles, bone and metallic artifact from the coil that were misinterpreted by Cameron's wife.

artifact on the CT, the area around the surgery site appeared profoundly damaged to Cameron's wife, with the metallic part of the coil being interpreted as more blood in his brain.

Since meeting with the surgeon and reviewing the brain scans, Cameron's wife was extremely anxious and worried that her husband would never regain function, given the extent of injury. When doctors told her that he was expected to make a good recovery, she did not believe them because the images she had seen were more influential to her beliefs than what she was being told.

Not only can too little information be confusing, but too much can prevent efficient and accurate communication. There is a tendency to cover every aspect of a brain injury when meeting with patients or family members. However, they may be receptive to only one or two key points, especially given the complexity of brain injuries. With the stress of having to watch a loved one recover from an injury or illness, combined with the difficulties of navigating the world of medicine, many people do not have the mental or emotional resources to deal with massive amounts of technical information. The complexities of brain injury are difficult to understand for students studying the neurosciences in a quiet classroom. It should come as no a surprise when patients and family members struggle to understand a patient's condition during a time of great emotional crisis. Throw brain imaging into the mix, and the likelihood that the viewer will become overwhelmed and unresponsive to the information increases. This is especially true if the clinician does not take the time to ensure accurate understanding of the imaging findings.

Just as compassion and empathy are critical when giving bad news to patients or loved ones, the same care should be used when first showing brain scans. Once severe brain trauma has been viewed, the full impact of the trauma can become apparent, and hope may quickly fade. Such images may affect how the viewer interacts with the patient for years to come. Depression and hopelessness can follow the realization that brain damage is permanent, especially if the injury is seen and not just described. Thus, consider those who care for the patient, and their situation. For example, if a child was injured when unsupervised, would seeing the injury result in additional guilt for the parent? If an injury is severe, consider the possibility that the patient's loved ones may become depressed or overwhelmed by the information. They may try to escape their emotional pain by becoming less involved in the patient's care or less responsive to hospital staff. Different people process information about a personal or loved one's injury in different ways. Get to know your audience before subjecting them to the possible trauma of having to "see the injury."

Medical Literacy

Take into consideration the medical literacy of your audience when presenting brain scans to patients or family members. Medical literacy relates to the capacity of the receiver to understand medical information presented to them. Medical literacy can be affected by educational, cultural, socioeconomic, spiritual, or others aspects of a person's background. Those who do not speak the native language of the clinician are at additional risk of misinterpreting neuroradiology-based information. When discussing a medical condition, all of these factors must be taken into account. Showing "pictures of the damage" should never be viewed as a way to compensate for limitations involving medical literacy or language-based communication. Neuroimaging data should be treated with the same care as any other medical information and, at times, even more seriously, given the indelible memories that pictures can produce.

WHAT TO DO WHEN THE PATIENT OR FAMILY MEMBERS ASK TO SEE THE BRAIN SCANS

Showing relatively intact brain scans tends to pose fewer clinical concerns than when asked to show brain scans with obvious evidence of pathology. For the cases in which the images clearly show profound brain injury, consideration of the negative impact of doing so should guide clinical decisions. At times, it is helpful to educate the patient or others about the relevance of the scans to the patient's care, current status, and prognosis. For example, shortly after an injury the scans may appear relatively normal, even though it is clear from other clinical data that the patient sustained severe neurological damage. This might be a good opportunity to explain that the brain scans do not provide a clear picture of the damage and that they could be misleading. If the patient or family still wants to see them, be sure to discuss the limitations of the radiological data, the relevance to the patient's care, and why the scans may not seem to fit with the clinical status of the patient.

There are occasions when it is helpful to show some image sequences but not others. Because various brain imaging techniques illustrate brain structures or pathology in different ways, the clinician may wish to select a series of images that best illustrates the patient's condition without providing misleading information or information that may result in confusion or distress. Choosing which scans to show and which scans to leave unseen is akin to making decisions regarding which specific lab values or medical information to disseminate during clinical consultation with the patient and loved ones. The decision of which images to show may come down to something as simple as determination of the images that will communicate the necessary information, but not so much information that the message gets lost, with the audience being more confused after the discussion than before it. If it is clear that the audience is prone to emotional distress during meetings, it may be less traumatizing to them if the CT scans are presented first, then the T1 images, and then the T2 or T2 FLAIR sequences, which are often best for showing pathology. Beginning with images that show the damage less clearly and gradually moving to those on which the damage is obvious may help the patient and family to slowly acclimate and come to terms with the injury in a more gradual manner. Such a progression can also provide the clinician with more opportunity to discuss the injury in a manner that gradually builds, at the same time monitoring the responses and readiness of the audience to more details. Sometimes, it may be necessary to show some sequences one day and follow up with other sequences a day or two later when the patient or family have had some time to process the previous details and have had time to formulate new questions and concerns.

It is very helpful and almost always necessary to briefly review the images before sitting down with a family to discuss the findings. A prior review will give the clinician time to reflect on which scans would be most helpful in communicating the desired message, which scans may not be helpful or may even be misleading, and how to explain the pathology depicted in the images. Prior review will also give the clinician an opportunity to determine an appropriate presentation order, given the audience and goals of the meeting.

Before scheduling the meeting, be sure that you fully understand what the scans show and do not hesitate to seek consultation from a radiologist or other specialist if there is any question as to the relevance of findings. Differentiating clinically relevant findings from artifact can be difficult without years of experience and can result in one providing incorrect information to families or other clinical professionals. Interpreting images "on the fly" during a discussion with family members is not the time to be considering whether a finding is clinically meaningful, is just an artifact of the technology, or is within normal limits for the patient's age.

It is better to put off showing the scans than show them before a personal review or if you do not have the time to explain different features on the images or counsel the viewers on the clinical implications of the findings.

When Neuroimaging Suggests Pathology Without Deficits in the Patient

Neuroimaging has advanced rapidly over the past few decades, with current MRI sequences being much more sensitive to damage than only a few years ago. With susceptibility-weighted imaging using high-strength magnets, microhemorrhages once only visible using a microscope can now be visualized on a brain scan. With some very mild traumatic brain injuries or even concussions, patients recover rapidly and may show no evidence of compromised brain functioning during everyday activities or even on sensitive neuropsychological evaluations. However, it is possible that microbleeds can be detected using very high-strength susceptibility-weighted MRI scans. This is the opposite problem than has been historically the case. In the past, imaging was unable to detect damage that resulted in functional deficits.

We are rapidly approaching a time when brain scans will be able to detect pathological markers in the brain of a patient without functional deficit. Each clinician will need to decide whether it is beneficial to a patient or family to show scans with subtle microscopic hemorrhages after a concussion or very mild brain injury, even when the patient recovers fully from the incident. Clinicians should consider whether showing the scans of microbleeds may result in lowered expectations, an assumption by the patient and family that there is significant brain damage, or the self-fulfilling prophecy in which performance declines as a function of the psychological response to the images, not because of any clinically or functionally relevant damage to the brain.

WHAT TO REQUEST WHEN WRITING ORDERS FOR BRAIN IMAGING

The radiologist has the expertise to determine which specific combination of sequences would best assist in discriminating normal tissue or processes from those that are pathological. Radiologists consider issues pertaining to the yield or usefulness of a particular sequence, the need for sedation or introduction of contrast agents, the patient's medical condition and ability to tolerate the procedures, and the time required to complete the sequences. Balancing the number of sequences with the need for specific information, the radiologist will determine which specific set of sequences is critical and which may be helpful but not necessary.

Time Required in the Scanner

If a patient is unable to remain in the scanner for long periods of time without sedation and sedation is contraindicated, a few high-yield sequences may be acquired in lieu of a full battery of tests. Remember, each sequence can take anywhere from a couple of minutes to between 5 and 10 minutes to acquire on most MRI systems. Some high-resolution sequences can take 15 minutes or more to acquire, such as 1024 × 1024 pixel MRA sequences using a 3T system. There is a balance between the time needed to obtain imaging data and the tolerance of the patient or accessibility of the scanner. In theory, each patient could be scanned for hours to generate massive quantities of neuroimaging data, although usually less than 30 minutes is required to obtain more than enough information for most clinical conditions.

When time in the scanner is restricted by concerns of pain, discomfort, or other medical issues, the radiologist may determine which sequences are absolutely critical and which ones may be helpful but would not provide important critical information. A brief scanning session is also indicated for medically fragile patients requiring almost constant intervention from staff, something that is difficult to coordinate with image acquisition in an MRI. CT has the benefit of extremely rapid acquisition times, with some being less than a second, but most require a few minutes. However, for acute-care and complex diagnostic cases, CT may not have adequate spatial or contrast resolution, especially for soft tissues such as brain parenchyma. In addition, CT necessitates exposure to ionizing radiation, and a determination should be made regarding the expected yield for the scan versus the exposure risk for the patient.

In busy centers, the radiologist may not become aware of the sequences acquired until he or she reviews the images. Image reading can take place some time after the patient has left the scanner and returned to the inpatient unit or, for outpatients, has left the building. The standard protocol is for radiology staff to receive a physician order for imaging. If the order is specific, the technicians may just run the sequences as requested by the physician. If the order is more general, they will likely consult with the physician or radiologist to determine which sequences should be performed. Errors occur when orders do not contain a referral question or concern, there is too little information in the referral, or the goals for the study are not adequately communicated to the radiology team. Often, it is better to request a CT or MRI for a specific clinical goal, such as "evaluate for increased intracranial pressure" or "evaluate for pathology that may be causing chronic headaches." In these cases, the radiologist will be consulted regarding the best combination of sequences to use to achieve the goal.

At times, miscommunication can result in a lack of information critical for patient care. For instance, following a brain injury, a patient was sent for an imaging study. The resident was counseled that gradient echo (GRE) or gradient echo-echo planar imaging (GRE-EPI) and susceptibility-weighted imaging (SWI) sequences would be helpful in detecting petechial hemorrhages and microbleeds resulting from diffuse injury to the brain. Instead of ordering "MRI brain injury series to include GRE or GRE-EPI and SWI," the resident requested "GRE, GRE-EPI, and SWI due to brain injury." After the patient returned from the scanner, the images were reviewed by the radiologist, who asked the technicians why there were no standard sequences such as T1, T2, T2 FLAIR, and diffusion-weighted imaging (DWI) for this patient. The technicians indicated that the order only requested those three sequences, and

Writing Orders for Imaging Studies

Orders for brain imaging should include the reason for the study and the general protocol requested, in addition to any specific specialized sequences that may be available to the clinician. Some examples are as follows:

"MRI to assess for possible basal ganglia problem; patient has new onset movement disorder."

"MRI due to patient mental status deteriorating; use of contrast to be determined by radiologist."

"MRI brain injury series to assess for pathology following a closed-head injury. If available, please include GRE or GRE-EPI and SWI sequences to assess for hemorrhages."

"MRI brain tumor series with and without contrast to assess a large mass within the left parietal lobe evident on CT. If possible, please include MRS to compare the mass to normal tissue, diffusion imaging and DTI to visualize the integrity of the pathways around the mass."

"CT to assess ventricular size and rule out increased ventricular or intracranial pressure."

"CT to document the location of the external ventricular drain. There is concern that the tip is no longer in the right lateral ventricle."

they were correct. If they had not been so busy, they might have questioned the unusual request. However, that day they had patients scheduled back-to-back in the scanners and did not realize the mistake.

Radiologist Reports

Radiologists are trained to interpret images in order to formulate opinions regarding a patient's condition. Studies have demonstrated that interpreting or "reading" brain scans improves with experience; the more one evaluates brain scans, the better he or she becomes at interpretation. This means that the most accurate assessment of brain images comes from experienced radiologists and, in particular, neuroradiologists who specialize in brain imaging. Radiologists also possess expertise in determining which types of scans or scan sequences to use in order to most accurately answer the referral question. The role of discriminating normal tissue or processes from that which may be pathological falls on the shoulders of the radiologist. Radiologists dictate reports that are then made available to clinical staff. However, sometimes the information provided by the radiologist may not meet all of the needs of the clinical team. This is especially true if the clinician is seeking information that would be helpful in determining long-term prognosis or patient needs for future care, but the imaging requested was to assess for a critical-care issue such as hemorrhaging, ventricular dilation, or intracranial pressure. Radiologists are expected to review an ever-increasing number of scans and sequence types for each patient. In the past, a radiologist might have been required to review a few sheets of CT film for each patient. Today, radiologists may view hundreds of images from many different sequences, all during a short period of time. As such, the radiologist may assess the imaging series and dictate a report based on a narrow focus specific to the referral question, not general clinical issues that may be important to the practitioner.

Although a radiologist's report is helpful in identifying salient pathological markers or in answering the specific referral question, the information provided in the radiology report may not be as relevant to a patient's clinical presentation, general level of functioning, or prognosis. Critical medical information will take priority over information that may be helpful to the clinician but that is not germane to emergent or acute care. For example, if the scans are requested emergently for a patient with a "fall from a horse," the radiologist may initially look for evidence of bleeds or swelling that are of imminent medical concern and may require immediate treatment. The radiology report may not include information relating to more subtle injuries that can influence the patient's functioning and long-term outcome.

CLINICAL EXAMPLE

Ian: Traumatic Brain Injury

Ian was thrown from a horse, hitting his head on the ground. He was not wearing a helmet and sustained a traumatic brain injury. He was unconscious for approximately 15 minutes following the fall, with clear deficits involving cognition and his general mental-status upon waking. First responders transported him to a local hospital where a CT scan was ordered while receiving care in the emergency department. The CT report read as follows:

```
Right lateral skull fracture, linear and
  nondisplaced. Fracture extends from
  the temporal squamosa to the vertex.
3 mm right to left midline shift.
No extra axial hematoma or fluid
  collection.
No definite cerebral edema visualized.
Left supra-orbital and high frontal
  subarachnoid blood.
Large right lateral scalp hematoma.
```

This CT report provided critical information regarding Ian's acute-care needs but was not as helpful for explaining his symptoms once he transitioned from the intensive care unit to the general acute-care floor. This was not an omission or failure on the part of the radiologist but instead related to the goal of the evaluation: to assess for trauma requiring immediate medical attention. Explanation of future symptoms is outside the scope of such an evaluation or radiology report. In most situations, especially those that are trauma related, CT assessments are conducted to evaluate for critical medical complications. Primary attention is placed on indicators such as edema, bleeding, infarctions, increased intracranial pressure, and herniation. In Ian's case, the radiologist identified the primary medical concerns relating to the skull fracture, midline shift, and subarachnoid blood. Information was not provided for other areas of the brain that also showed evidence of injury. Because the information provided within the CT report failed to explain Ian's persistent mental-status changes, confusion, verbal dysfluencies, affective dysregulation, and fluctuations in arousal, his scans were personally reviewed using a more functional or clinical approach. In addition to the findings in the radiology report, there were also signs of bifrontal, orbital-medial contusions, diffuse axonal injury, and reduced tissue density surrounding the bony structures close to the temporal and orbital frontal lobes. An MRI brain injury series was ordered to provide additional information on Ian's injury. T2 and T2 FLAIR sequences showed extensive injury to Ian's orbital and medial frontal lobes and temporal poles.

Without personal review of the CT scans, the MRI series would not likely have been ordered. An accurate explanation for Ian's symptoms might not have been possible, and Ian would likely have been discharged home once medically stable. Cognitive, emotional, and behavioral difficulties were excessive given the report of injury from the original CT evaluation and were being attributed to personality and psychological disturbance. However, the bifrontal and bitemporal brain injury clearly evident on his MRI scans provided a reasonable explanation for his symptoms. Ian was transferred to the medical rehabilitation unit where he received therapeutic intervention and his family received much-needed education regarding his injury, the expected recovery course, and the effects of such damage on future functioning.

Information contained within a brain scan but not evident within the radiology report may make a significant difference to treatment planning or decisions of family members regarding a patient's care options. For example, decisions pertaining to the options of aggressive therapeutic treatment versus comfort or palliative care may be based almost entirely on the findings from MRI imaging but that were not described within a report (see Clinical Example Jan).

CLINICAL EXAMPLE
Jan: Stroke

Jan, a 79 year old patient underwent abdominal vascular surgery to treat a large arterial embolism but in the process suffered a left middle cerebral artery stroke. The radiology report indicated evidence of the stroke but provided no additional details regarding implications of the findings. Several days following her stroke, family members were asked about options for feeding, as the stroke had left Jan without the abilities to communicate verbally or eat or drink by mouth. Because of the stroke she had lost speech, oral-motor functioning, and even her gag reflex. Given the normal progress following a stroke, the family members were informed that Jan might appear much better in a few weeks and would be a candidate for inpatient rehabilitative care prior to discharge home. The family was given a few days to decide on feeding options for Jan, the primary consideration being one of surgically placing a tube into her stomach to supply nutrition.

Review of Jan's brain scans revealed significant damage to Broca's area, the motor cortex, and the basal ganglia bilaterally, left more than right, as well as evidence of the beginning stages of dementia. Additional information obtained from family members indicated that before her stroke, Jan had experienced difficulties with mobility and ambulation and suffered from severe and medically refractory back pain.

Some of the issues discussed with the family regarding options for Jan included, but were not restricted to, the following:

1. *Jan had previously stated that she did not want to live if she was unable to have a "normal" life.*
2. *Brain imaging revealed that she would most likely never regain the ability to talk fluently.*
3. *Brain imaging revealed that she would most likely never regain the ability to walk, especially given her pre-stroke difficulties with ambulation.*
4. *Brain imaging revealed that her deteriorating mental status pre-stroke was likely due to a neurodegenerative condition resulting in frontotemporal dementia, which would continue to disrupt cognitive and emotional functioning, with increasing difficulties over time.*
5. *With the new abdominal incision requiring 52 staples, Jan would experience abdominal pain in addition to her chronic back pain, due to being restricted to bed.*

The information from the scans was critical in assisting the family to make the decision to let Jan pass, instead of aggressively treating her condition. Information on the location and severity of the stroke, in addition to the effects of the stroke, was crucial in allowing the family members to come to a clear decision about treatment options. The information provided by the scans but not evident in the radiology report helped the family members decide to transition Jan from curative care to palliative or comfort care. Important in their decision was the understanding that Jan would likely never talk again or walk again and that she would likely continue to deteriorate mentally due to dementia.

Collaboration between the radiologist and the clinical practitioner is critical in providing the most comprehensive picture of a patient's condition. Accurate pathological and anatomical information from the radiologist can be used by the clinician to formulate an appropriate treatment plan and to determine reasonable goals. If the radiology report fails to explain clinical findings, as was the case with Ian, the clinician needs to personally review the images or discuss the discrepancy with a radiologist. As medical professionals, radiologists would rather spend time clarifying discrepancies between imaging findings and clinical presentation than having patient care compromised. Often a second look at a scan by a clinician or radiologist can result in findings that were not initially described in the report or noticed by the radiologist. When specific symptoms are present, it is even easier to re-evaluate brain scans, especially when critical anatomic structures are involved.

(Continued)

(*Continued*)

For instance, an MRI for an epilepsy patient was read as "normal" upon the initial review by the neuroradiologist. After the patient's seizures were localized to the right perisylvian region via EEG and magnetoencephalography (MEG), the radiologist was asked to take another look at the scans. A small area of cortical dysplasia was localized to the insula, deep in the right perisylvian region. Once the additional information was available to the radiologist, the area was much easier to identify; without the EEG and MEG information, and on initial review, the area appeared unremarkable.

ANATOMY VERSUS FUNCTIONING

Sometimes there is not a direct relationship between an injury to a specific part of the brain and expected functional deficits. The brain is composed of both focal and distributed functional units, with the organization being similar but not identical across individuals. Because of the small variability in brain anatomy, injury to the same part of the brain in two patients can result in different symptoms. Similarly, identical symptoms may be caused by injury to different brain locations. In regard to neuroimaging, two patients with the same clinical presentation may have different brain imaging results, and two patients with similar brain scan findings may have different clinical presentations. With such variability between individuals, it is not surprising that most clinicians have difficulty reconciling the functional implications of neuroradiology findings.

When considering the relationship between anatomical findings on neuroimaging and a patient's functioning, it can be helpful to view brain scans as simply photographs of an engine. When evaluating the functioning of an automobile, a photograph of the engine can provide some information but certainly does not provide critical information about the running of the vehicle. If you were buying a used car and wanted to know how well the engine ran, you could lift the hood and look at the engine. What can you learn by looking at the engine? You might note whether the engine looked new, appeared in good condition, or appeared old and damaged. You might notice some parts of the engine that are broken, worn-out, or even missing. However, you still would not know how well the engine ran or which of the car's features worked or did not work. This is not unlike reviewing a brain scan to determine the functioning of a brain. The brain scan can help identify areas that appear abnormal in comparison to those that appear more normal. However, the images provide little information regarding the actual functioning of the areas. With an automobile engine, a small amount of damage to the electrical system, not visible when lifting the hood, may prevent the engine from starting. Similarly, a small area of damage in the brain stem, not apparent on a brain scan, can prevent the patient from waking and from interacting with the environment. Using the same analogy, distributed yet mild damage involving the air intake or fuel system of an automobile may result in the car running poorly in the same way that diffuse damage to the brain can result in disrupted cognitive efficiency. In each of these cases, the diffuse damage may or may not be evident when lifting the hood of a car, or when reviewing a series of brain scans. To truly measure the functioning of a car engine one needs to go for a test drive, in the same way that a true measure of a person's brain functioning requires a clinical examination.

It is important to understand that any discrepancy between radiological findings and a patient's functioning may be due to "what is being measured." Put another way, brain scans and clinical assessments are based on different levels of analysis, with brain scans being anatomically based and assessments being functionally based. Do not dismiss your findings on examination just because they appear to conflict with radiological studies. Instead, look for a pattern of evidence across measures that may explain the patient's condition and account for any discrepancy between clinical and radiologic data. For example, if your patient presents with aphasia but has radiological findings suggesting no injury to the left hemisphere, but contusions to the right hemisphere, you may consider any of the following explanations: (1) your patient may be one of the few persons who has right-hemisphere dominance for language; (2) the right-hemisphere contusion may be the site of direct impact, but your patient also sustained a contrecoup injury to the left-hemisphere language regions that was not visible on the scans; (3) the aphasia is caused by swelling of the right hemisphere, putting pressure on the left-hemisphere language cortex; (4) your patient may not have aphasia but another condition such as elective mutism or a psychological or emotional response to the trauma or being in a hospital. Other explanations are feasible, and frequently multiple factors interact, some identifiable on the brain scans, others that are not.

Avoid relying too heavily on brain imaging, while minimizing the value of your clinical findings. Neuroimaging should be used to augment your clinical examination, not replace it. There is a tendency to view modern neuroimaging as a replacement for a solid clinical evaluation and diagnostic skill. With few exceptions, brain scans provide little information about a patient's functioning and can even distract the clinician from critical clinical details or from seeing what is really going on with the patient. Avoid using brain scan findings to explain all symptoms in a patient. Sometimes, the symptoms are unrelated to anything on the brain scans, even when the scans provide a reasonable explanation, which was the case with Jim (see clinical example).

CLINICAL EXAMPLE
Jim: Traumatic Brain Injury

Jim was highly agitated when he was transferred to the hospital. His imaging suggested bifrontal damage to his brain. The attending physician was concerned for his safety, thus restraints were used to prevent him from pulling at his nasogastric tube or intravenous lines. Sedation was used to calm Jim, as he became highly agitated every time he woke from the sedation. The agitation was explained by his frontal injury, clearly evident on neuroimaging. Upon personal review of the scans, assessment of the patient, and consultation with his treatment team, however, it became apparent that his agitation might not be due to his frontal injury but to his current environment and situation. The treatment team was counseled to assess for pain or discomfort caused by binding clothing, a full bladder or impacted bowel, or a headache resulting from some intracranial hemorrhaging. In addition, it appeared that some of the agitation was iatrogenic and being caused by the restraints. Staff initiated a bladder and bowel program and checked for any other causes of pain or discomfort. In addition, an evaluation was timed to coincide with Jim waking from the sedatives, and the restraints were removed. The patient was placed in a pool bed consisting of a mattress on the floor surrounded by padding to protect him. A one-on-one patient care technician was assigned to watch Jim to ensure that he did not pull out any of his lines. Even with the brain injury, Jim calmed and his agitation stopped. It became apparent that his agitation was caused by a combination of discomfort and restraint, combined with mental confusion, and was not simply due to his brain injury as evident on the brain scans. This is a case in which the brain imaging findings distracted the medical team from investigating the real cause of the symptoms; they relied too heavily on the brain scans and not enough on clinical assessment.

The goal of this chapter was to provide information that would be helpful in deciding when and how to use brain images in your work. A foundation of issues and concerns to be considered when using imaging in the clinic was presented. You may encounter issues that were not discussed in Chapter 1, especially those concerning complex medical or psychosocial cases. If you become concerned about how to use imaging data or which data to give to the family, seek counsel from a radiologist or colleague who may be familiar with your situation. As with many aspects of medicine, often there are no clear rules to follow regarding when and how to use medical information in your practice. Over time, experience can provide a guideline to follow, although exceptions will always be found. As a general rule, you will best be served by always considering the many positive and negative consequences of using brain scans in the clinic and in presenting them to patients and family members.

Once the decision is made to use brain imaging for treatment planning; communication with team members, patients, or families; and in determining prognosis and future care needs, you must be confident that your review of neuroimaging provides additional and accurate information critical to the clinical role. To ensure that your personal review of neuroimaging provides useful and accurate information and is not misleading or a source of confusion, it is important that you have basic competence in reading brain scans. Chapter 2 provides a basic tutorial for the interpretation and reading of brain scans. Guidelines in differentiating pathology from normal tissue or artifact are discussed, in addition to the effects of time on the appearance of pathology. Information is also provided to help you interpret three-dimensional space from two-dimensional image slices, including a guideline for determining the position of the patient's head in the scanner. If the head is not orthogonal to the gantry, the images of brain tissue can be confusing and even misleading, especially given that most pictures of the brain in anatomy books are presented using orthogonal planes showing the normal symmetry of structures. Because various brain-scanning techniques display tissue using different grayscale or color protocols, information is also provided to assist you in interpreting images produced by a variety of scanning technologies (CT versus MRI) or sequences (T1 versus T2). Chapter 2 also provides a basic guide to interpreting brain images but does not cover the technical aspects of the different technologies. A guide to the various imaging techniques, with their strengths and weaknesses, is provided in Chapter 4.

2

VIEWING AND INTERPRETING BRAIN SCANS

As is true with other clinical skills, reading and interpreting brain scans becomes easier with experience. When pathology is subtle, brain scans can look normal or have only a few indicators suggesting injury. When damage is severe, evidence on brain scans can be obvious to even the most inexperienced viewer. Difficulty interpreting brain scans often results when imaging findings are somewhere between these extremes; this is when experience and training become critical.

With experience, one can develop a conceptual schema for identifying normal brain tissue and a variety of pathological processes on different types of brain sequences. A solid understanding of how pathology appears on different sequences is critical to being able to utilize neuroimaging in the clinical role. For the non-radiologist, it is helpful to rely on some basic rules and concepts for reviewing brain scans. When the images are difficult to read or interpret it is strongly recommended that the clinician review them with a radiologist in order to fully comprehend and appreciate the information provided. This chapter will present basic information concerning the reading and interpreting of brain scans. Information will be presented in a general format and should be applicable to a variety of brain scans and sequences, unless indicated.

Structures in the central nervous system are presented on two-dimensional slices oriented either horizontally (*axial*), depicted in green; across the brain (*coronal*), shown in red; or vertically (*sagittal*), identified in blue (Figure 2-1).

To assist the reader, some of the examples have borders that are color coded using green for axial, red for coronal, and blue for sagittal. Color-coded lines on the images represent the location of a specific cut or slice on images with the same-colored border.

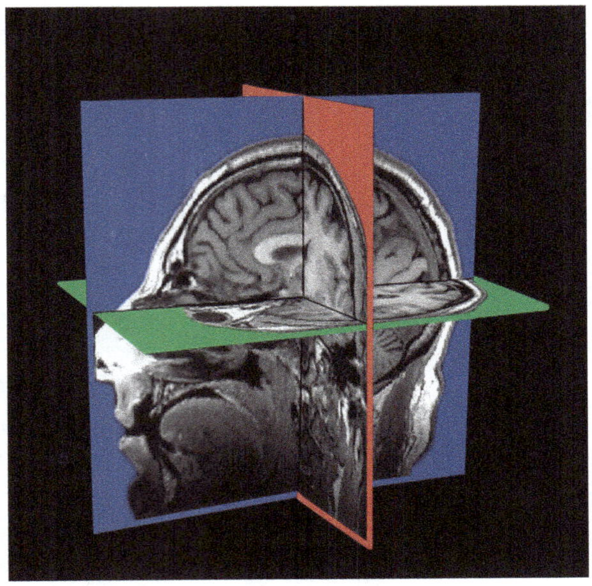

Figure 2-1 Primary slice orientations used in brain imaging

ORIENTATION AND IMAGE PLANE

With a few exceptions, brain scans involve the representation of three-dimensional space using a two-dimensional image plane. Some computer programs can present the imaging data as a three-dimensional representation, although this is primarily restricted to special radiology-based workstations. Currently, the ability to manipulate imaging data in three dimensions is not readily available to the general practitioner or basic workstations. Because most clinicians continue to rely on two-dimensional images presented on sheets of film or, more recently, computer or tablet screens, it is important to develop a solid understanding of how the brain is presented using a variety of orientations and image planes.

Axial or Horizontal Orientation

Axial images allow one to visualize the brain as a series of horizontal slices; the horizontal slices can be stacked on top of each other to compose the entire brain (Figures 2-2A–D).

Most axial slices on CT scans are created at an angle so that the image of the frontal lobes is more superior, or higher in the brain than the posterior structures. Put another way, the axial slice cuts through the brain at an angle that is not perpendicular to the vertical axis of the spine.

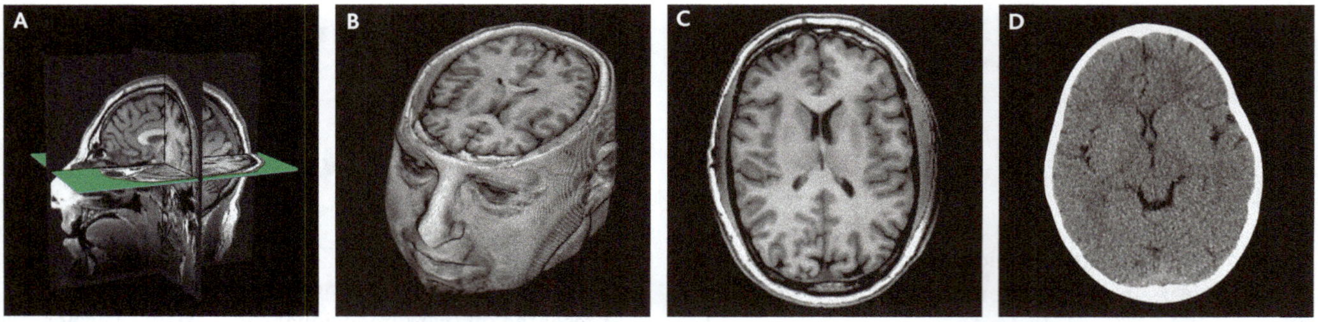

Figure 2-2 **A:** Color-coded slice. **B:** Three-dimensional MRI view. **C:** MRI. **D:** CT.

Figure 2-3 shows two axial images taken from the same patient on two different occasions. Both images were aligned so that the anterior frontal lobes are directly above the eye orbits. Since the acquisition angles were different, the only transected tissue common to both images is the orbital-frontal cortex. Moving away from the frontal lobes and toward the back of the brain, the dissimilarities between the images become more pronounced. This is expected given the differing acquisition angles resulting in diverging slices of tissue (green lines). Different slice angles become especially problematic when comparing scans taken on two different occasions to assess for changes over time.

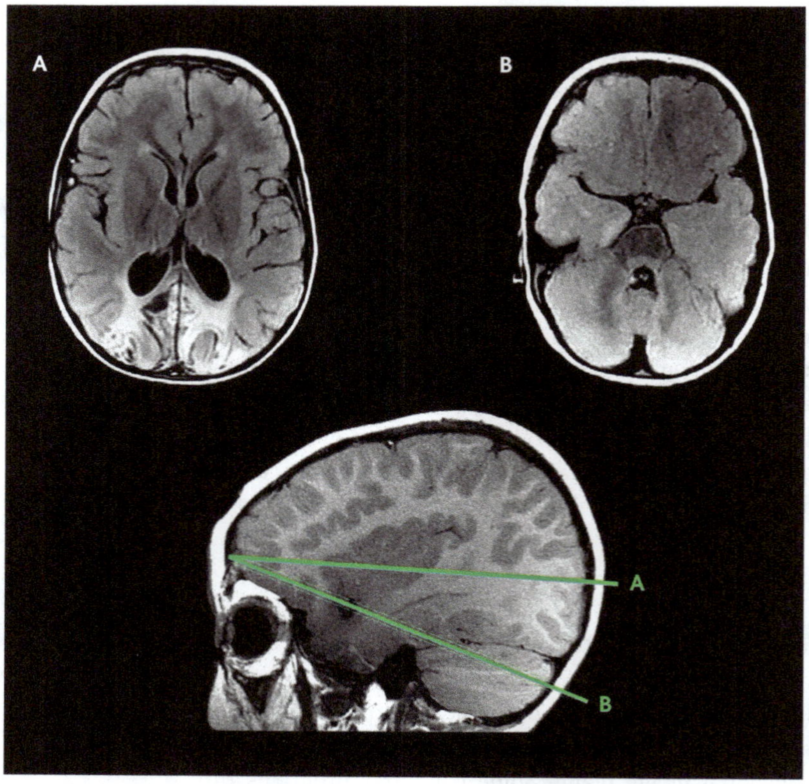

Figure 2-3 Axial images from the same patient, taken at two separate occasions, with different acquisition angles.

When first learning how to interpret brain images, it is important to remember that the use of different slice angles can result in added complexity. Scans acquired on two or more occasions may use a different slice angle and thus will look different.

As a guide, the axial series presented in Figures 2-4 through 2–7 were reformatted at increasing angles between perpendicular to the spinal axis and approximately 45 degrees from perpendicular, or between an axial and coronal plane. The images were reformatted and displayed using 10-mm slices beginning at the same level to allow for comparison. The effect of image plane is subtle between consecutive rows but profound between the horizontal and 45-degree series.

Axial Reformatting with Varying Slice Angles

Note: With increasing angle from perpendicular to parallel relative to the spinal axis, the images would be considered coronal, not axial.

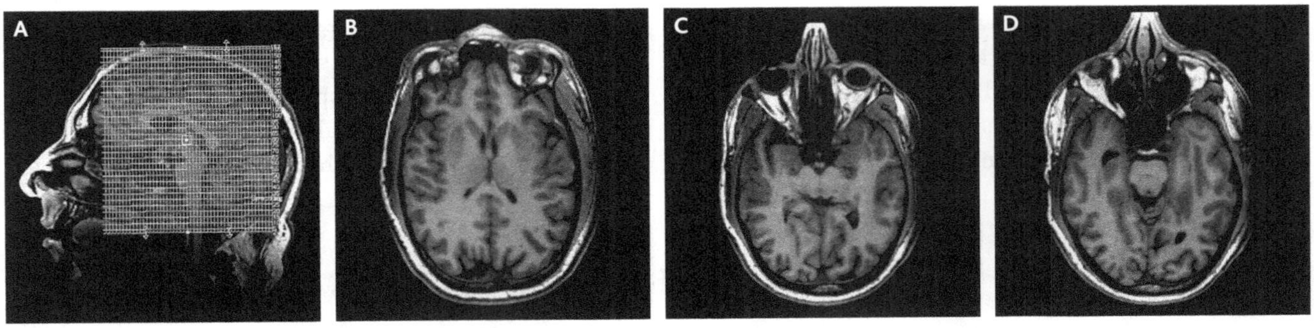

Figure 2-4 Horizontal or 90 degrees from the vertical spinal axis

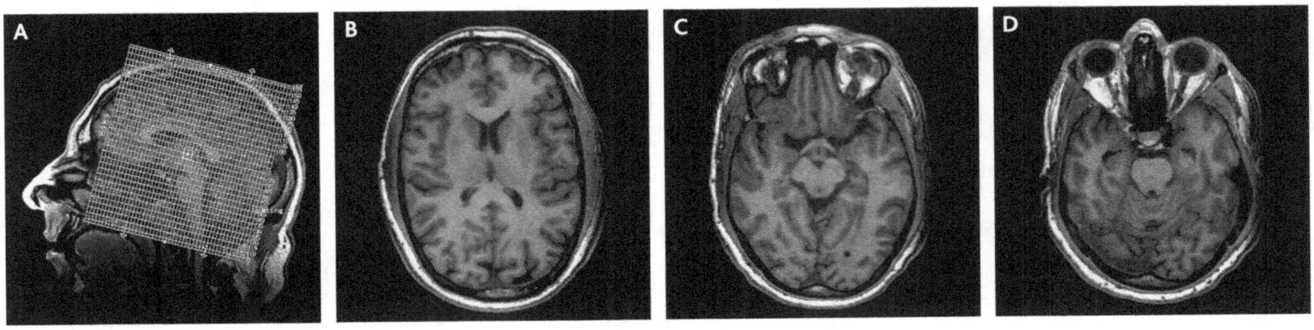

Figure 2-5 15 degree from horizontal or 105 degrees from the vertical spinal axis

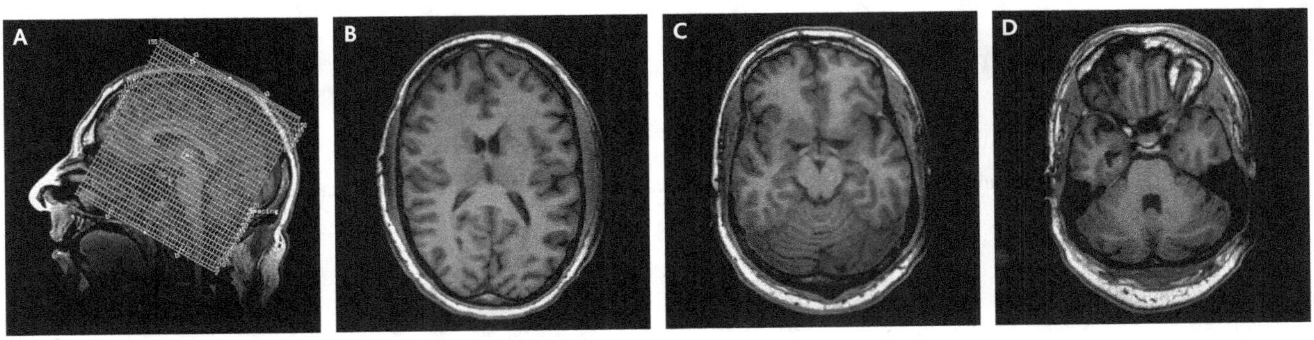

Figure 2-6 30 degrees from horizontal or 120 degrees from the vertical spinal axis

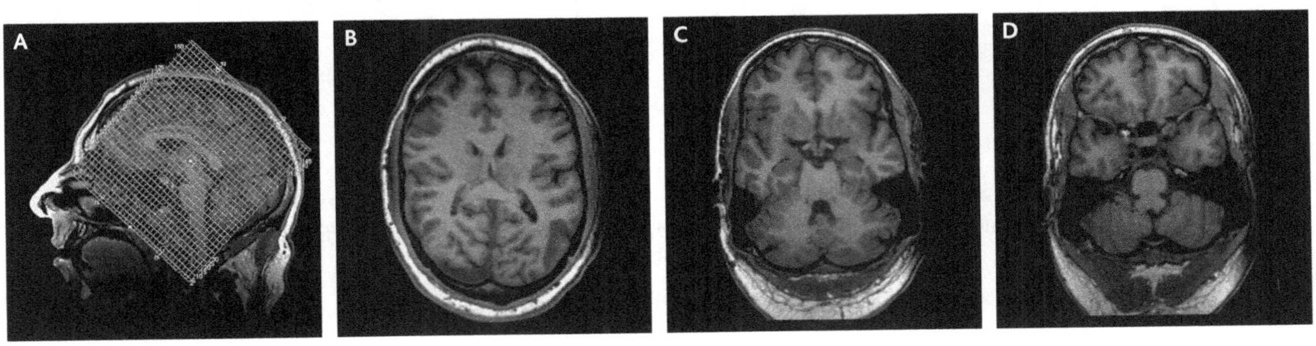

Figure 2-7 45 degrees from horizontal or 135 degrees from the vertical spinal axis

Coronal Orientation

Coronal images allow one to visualize the brain as a series of vertical slices from one side of the brain to the other, not unlike the slices of a loaf of bread. Stacking the images in front or behind each other will provide a full view of the brain (Figure 2-8a–d).

Coronal images are also acquired with varying slice angles. Sometimes the slice is vertical or parallel to the spinal axis (Figures 2-9a–d). Other times, slices are acquired between vertical and approximately 45 degrees between vertical and horizontal (Figures 2-10a–d). Note the different appearance of the images depending on the acquisition angle.

Sagittal Orientation

Sagittal images allow one to visualize the brain as a series of vertical slices oriented with the longitudinal plane of the brain. Mid-sagittal cuts separate the right and left hemispheres and show the structures located between the two hemispheres (Figures 2-11a–d). Paramedian or parasagittal slices are made using the same orientation but within either the right or left

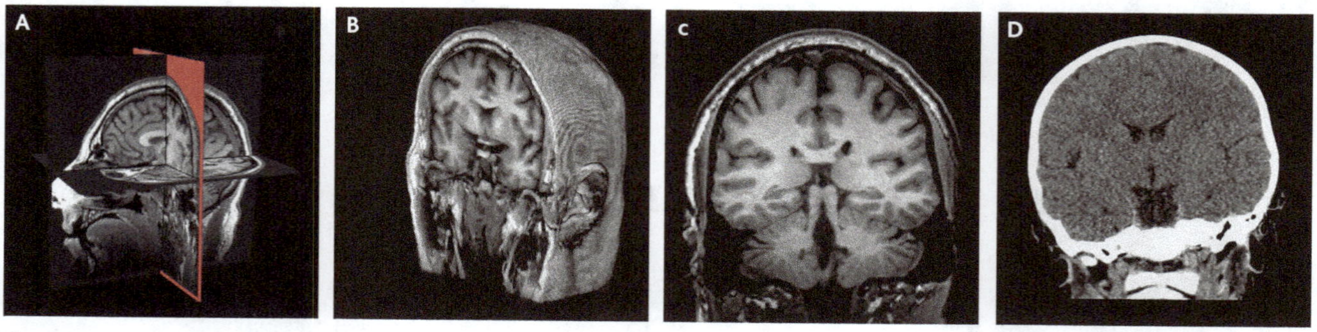

Figure 2-8 **A:** Color-coded slice. **B:** Three-dimensional MRI. **C:** Coronal MRI. **D:** Coronal CT.

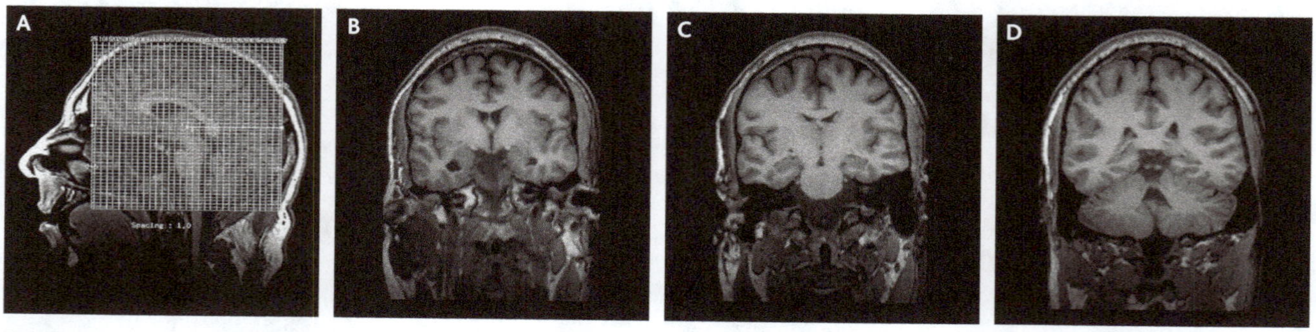

Figures 2-9A–D Coronal images acquired using an orientation equal to the vertical axis of the spinal cord, with slices organized from anterior (A) to posterior (D).

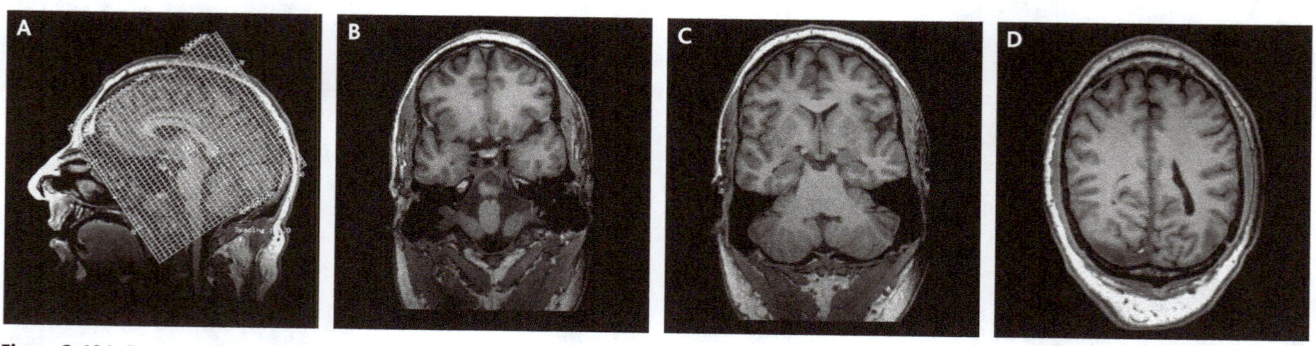

Figure 2-10A–D Coronal images acquired 35 degrees from the vertical axis of the spinal cord, with slices organized from anterior (A) to posterior (D).

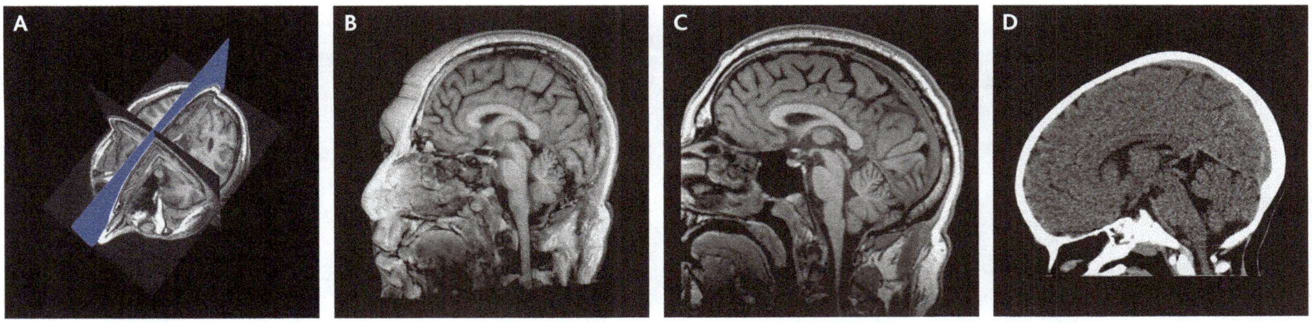

Figures 2-11A–D Mid-sagittal view. **A:** Color-coded slice. **B:** Three-dimensional MRI view. **C:** MRI. **D:** CT.

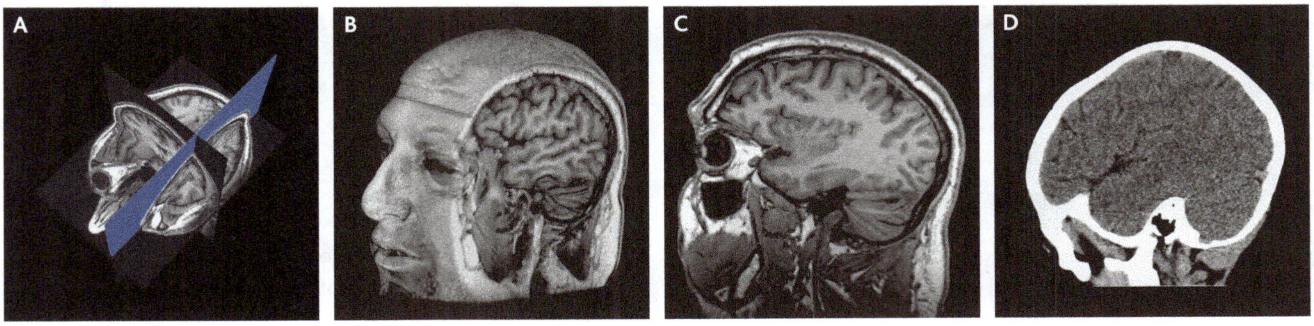

Figures 2-12A–D Para-median/sagittal view. **A:** Color-coded slice. **B:** Three-dimensional MRI view. **C:** MRI. **D:** CT.

hemisphere, not transecting the longitudinal fissure (Figures 2-12a–d).

WHEN RIGHT IS LEFT AND LEFT IS RIGHT

When first reviewing radiology films depicting images of the brain and spinal cord, it appears that the images are displayed "reversed" or as a "mirror image." On axial or coronal planes, the right side of the image depicts the left side of the brain, and the left side of the image shows the right side of the brain. The images are not reversed or mirrored; they are presented from the perspective of a clinician or viewer interacting with the patient. Interpreting radiology films of the brain and spinal cord from the perspective of a clinician interacting with a patient will help you minimize any confusion regarding right and left.

Some publications reverse radiology images in order to minimize reader confusion; they present the left hemisphere on the left side of the image and the right hemisphere on the right side. Because a primary goal of this guide is to assist you in interpreting radiology films and enable you to compare images from this text with those you may see in the clinic, all images in this text are presented in a standard radiology format.

When interacting with a supine patient from the foot of the bed, the left hemisphere is on the right side relative to the clinician's perspective, and the right hemisphere is located on the left side relative to the clinician's perspective. *Axial* images are displayed from the perspective of a patient lying on his or her back, with the clinician at the foot of the bed. If the clinician could see through tissue to view the brain, it would be as if the brain were being viewed from the bottom (Figure 2-13). Axial brain slices are acquired from this perspective, from bottom to top. The bottom-up perspective, or that of a clinician at the foot of the bed, means that the patient's right hemisphere will be displayed on the left side of the image, and the left hemisphere will be displayed on the right side of the image. This may be confusing at first, but if you always remember that axial images are taken from the perspective of you interacting with a patient lying supine in a bed, you should have less difficulty remembering this rule.

(Continued)

(*Continued*)

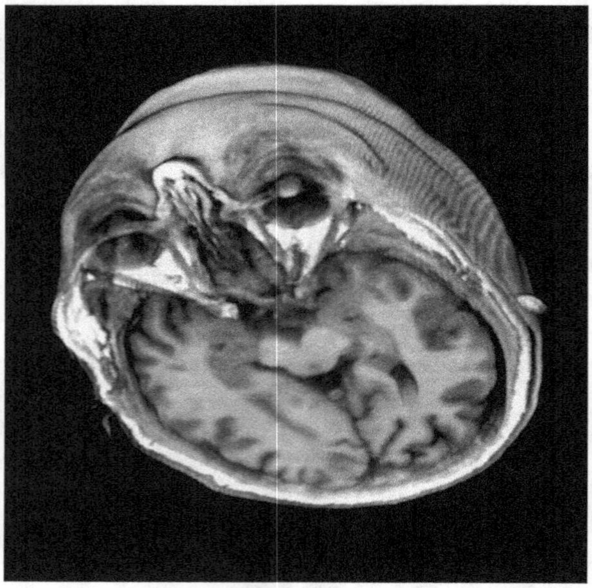

Figure 2-13 Three-dimensional axial image showing the standard bottom-up perspective.

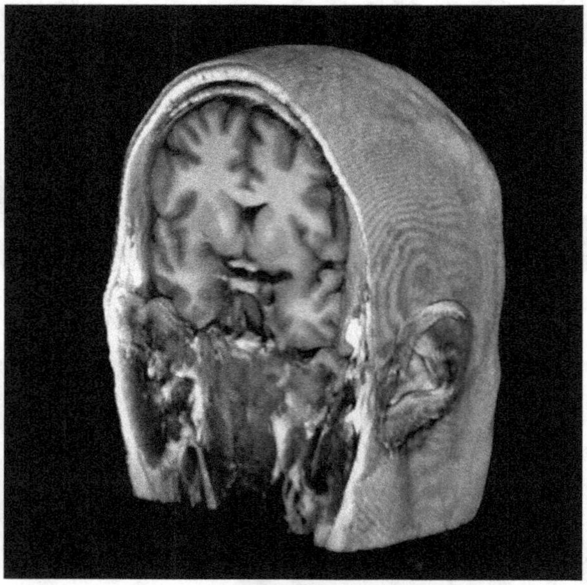

Figure 2-14 Three-dimensional coronal image showing the standard perspective as if facing the patient.

Coronal images are also displayed from the perspective of the clinician interacting with a patient. For coronal images, the clinician and the patient are facing each other with the patient's left hemisphere on the right side and the right hemisphere on the left side, as if the clinician were looking through the patient's face to the brain (Figure 2-14).

It is more difficult to determine right from left when viewing sagittal images. There is no standard protocol for the recording of sagittal slices by the scanner. Some scans "slice" the brain from left to right, and others from right to left. Because many images lack reference indicators relating to the specific hemisphere being viewed, *sagittal* sequences should be interpreted on the basis of additional information provided by the axial or coronal planes. The use of viewers that present all three planes simultaneously can assist you in determining the hemisphere being viewed on a particular sagittal cut.

BASIC CLINICAL INTERPRETATION

In any analysis of clinical findings, conclusions are often derived from a combination of "hard" or pathognomonic evidence and "soft" subjective or qualitative impressions. The interpretation of neuroimaging data follows a similar framework. At times there are clear pathognomonic signs evident on the brain scans. Other times, no clear pathological markers are evident, and the findings may be subtle or even ambiguous. With the heterogeneity and complexity of neurological conditions, especially those caused by trauma or infection, it is not uncommon for the imaging to have evidence of both hard and soft signs of pathology.

Just as is true for a clinical examination, when reviewing brain scans, interpretation of obvious pathology is much easier than that which leaves little to no visual evidence on imaging. It is important to consider that some features that appear to be obvious signs of abnormality may actually be unrelated to pathology and instead are an artifact or an anomaly that has little to no clinical relevance. It is critical for any clinician wishing to review brain images to understand how both normal and pathological tissue appears on a variety of sequences. It is also important for the clinician to be aware of the many artifacts that can appear on brain scans, as well as the many limitations of the technology used to provide images of the brain. Interpreting radiology images is dependent on pattern recognition, the ability to differentiate that which is normal from that which is pathological and from an artifact, all combined with the judgment and experience to evaluate the clinical importance of a particular finding.

Appearance of Brain Tissue on Different Types of Brain Scans

One of the more challenging aspects of reading brain scans derives from the fact that different imaging techniques or sequences display tissue in very different ways. For example, when viewing normal brain scans, the following appearance should be expected (Figure 2-15a–d):

Note: Pathological signs involving blood, edema, infection, and tissue damage can also have a different appearance on a variety of scan types or sequence.

Interpreting Findings on a Variety of Scans

The simplest way to interpret findings on a variety of different brain scans is to compare tissue being reviewed to that

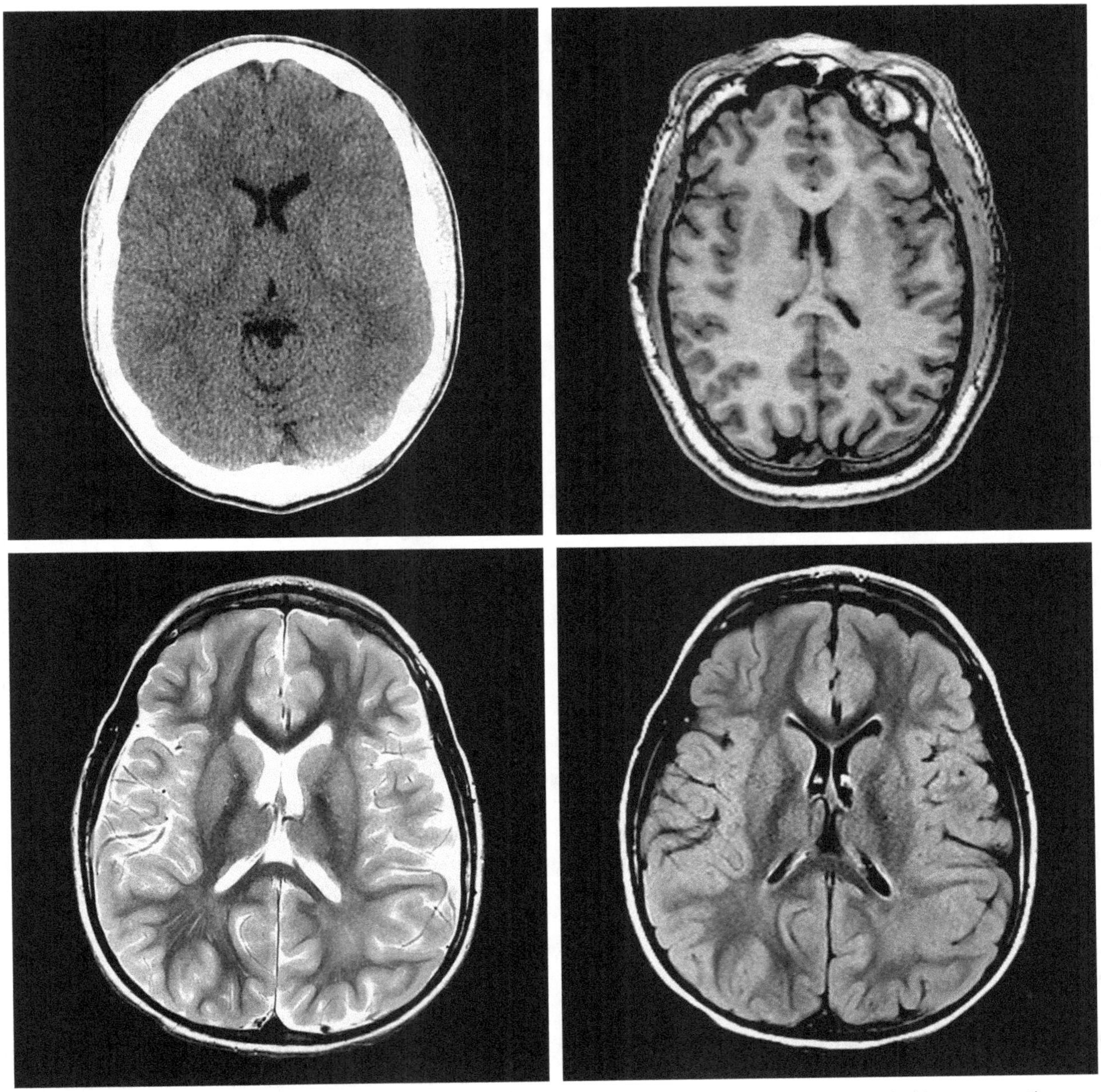

Figure 2-15 **A:** CT. Cerebral spinal fluid (CSF) is black; gray matter, or the neuron cell bodies, is displayed as light gray; and white matter, or the axon pathways, is displayed as dark gray. **B:** TI-weighted MRI. CSF is black; gray matter, or the neuron cell bodies, is displayed as dark gray; and white matter, or the axon pathways, is displayed as light gray. **C:** T2-weighted MRI. CSF is white; gray matter, or the neuron cell bodies, is displayed as light gray; and white matter, or the axon pathways, is displayed as dark gray. **D:** T2 FLAIR-weighted image. CSF is black; gray matter, or the neuron cell bodies, is displayed as light gray; and white matter, or the axon pathways, is displayed as dark gray.

of known appearance. A good place to begin would be to look at the primary fluid-filled cavities and note their appearance; the eyes and lateral ventricles are good options. Looking at the eyes and ventricles will give you an idea of how cerebrospinal fluid (CSF) should appear on a particular image sequence. Then review the primary areas of white matter and known areas of gray matter such as the cortical mantle to determine how such tissue will appear on the scan.

Contrast on a CT scan is based on tissue absorption of ionizing radiation. A brighter appearance reflects more absorption and a darker appearance, less. This is a carry-over from film days when x-ray images reflected the degree to which a sheet of film was exposed. On first review of a CT, note the appearance of the ventricles. The grayscale level of the ventricles gives a measure of low absorption or low density. Conversely, review of the bony structures of the calvarium will provide information regarding how high absorption, or high tissue density, should appear. Soft tissues such as brain parenchyma will have varying degrees of absorption, with white-matter tracts appearing darker on the CT than cortical regions and nuclei. Contrast between gray and white matter is poor because these soft tissues absorb similar amounts of ionizing radiation and have similar density levels. Pathology of the brain resulting in either increased or decreased density will appear either brighter or darker than normal tissue, respectively. For example, a dense tumor may appear brighter, and edema with increased water content will appear darker.

MRI scans are a little more complicated to read than CT imaging. CT grayscale values are based on density or absorption; MRI grayscale values are dependent on a variety of tissue properties and imaging parameters. However, some of the same principles that can be applied to the interpretation of CT images can also be used for MRI. In general, if the fluid cavities of the eyes and ventricles are white (T2 image), abnormal collections of fluid in the brain should also be white or lighter than similar surrounding tissue. It would then reasonably follow that if the eyes and ventricles are black (T1 image), abnormal collections of fluid in the brain should be black or darker than similar surrounding tissue. However, it is more complicated than this, especially given the frequent use of fluid attenuated inversion recovery (FLAIR) imaging. T2 FLAIR sequences are T2 images, but with the CSF signal attenuated. In this case, the eyes and ventricles will be black, but fluid accumulation in the tissue (edema) will appear brighter, just as is true for a regular T2 sequence.

PEARL When evaluating for pathology, compare areas of concern to other regions with a known appearance. Look for small regions that are darker or lighter than similar areas of tissue expected to have a similar appearance. With practice and experience, it becomes easier to identify areas that appear abnormal, no matter what type of scan you view. Comparing areas of concern to analogous regions of an unaffected hemisphere can often be a simple way to assess for pathology.

PERIL Comparing an area of concern to a region of similar tissue may highlight the differences but may not assist in your determination of pathology. If the two areas differ in their appearance, you must determine which area is pathological and which area is normal. Because the difference between two regions is relative, an area that appears pathological may be normal and vice versa. For example, when comparing two areas of cortex, one region may appear atrophied compared to the other, suggesting pathology in that region. However, the area appearing to have atrophy may be normal, and the comparison region may be edematous. Any comparison must take into account the many reasons for two regions of similar tissue appearing different, including normal variation and artifacts.

Use several image types or sequences when assessing for pathology

With CT scans, only a few options are available to change the way tissue appears on an image. Contrast agents can be used to highlight certain types of tissue or pathological processes, otherwise tissue that absorbs similar amounts of ionizing radiation will appear the same on the image. MRI scans provide an advantage over CT in their ability to produce a large variety of image sequences that highlight tissues or processes in different ways. In general, using a combination of MRI sequences can improve the viewer's ability to identify a variety of structures, tissues or pathological conditions. For anatomy, T1-weighted images are often better than T2, with a variety of special protocols using spoiled gradient echo T1 sequences having excellent resolution between gray and white matter, such as the BRAVO or FSPGR protocols by General Electric, the TFE SENSE protocol by Philips, or the MPRAGE protocols by Hitachi or Siemens. T2 images are often better for assessing damage or pathological processes, with T2 FLAIR images having advantages in differentiating normal CSF from post-injury edema or inflammation. Gradient echo (GRE) or susceptibility-weighted imaging (SWI) sequences are helpful in assessing blood, and diffusion-weighted images (DWI) enable assessement of cell integrity by identifying areas of restricted water diffusion. Perfusion images assist in identifying areas of reduced blood flow, and the use of both perfusion and diffusion sequences can assist in differentiating areas of infarct or cell death (reduced perfusion and diffusion) from areas that have reduced blood perfusion but are not yet infarcted and possibly salvageable.

To fully appreciate pathology, review a variety of MRI sequences and become familiar with more than just the traditional T1 and T2 studies. Over time, you will learn which types of sequences are best for the particular tissue or pathological process of clinical interest. Be aware that some types of pathology are not evident on some sequences but can be obvious on others.

PEARL Use the correct image type, sequence, or both for your specific question.

- For anatomy, use a T1-weighted MRI. T1 FLAIR sequences or specialized T1 protocols designed to give good gray-white differentiation such as BRAVO, FSPGR, TFE_SENSE or MPRAGE T1 sequences do an excellent job of differentiating gray and white matter and neuroanatomical structures.
- For pathology, use a T2-weighted image, especially a FLAIR sequence (T2 FLAIR). Diffusion images may be helpful for infarction, and GRE or SWI sequences are helpful in assessing for blood products.

PERIL Using the wrong scan or sequence can make it difficult to appreciate minor structural changes or mild pathological conditions.

- Small structures are difficult to identify on a T2 sequence but may be easy to see on a T1 image. Subtle inflammation may not be visible on a T1 image but may show up clearly on a T2 or T2 FLAIR sequence. Mild hypoxic injury may not be evident on T1 or T2 sequences but may be readily evident on diffusion-weighted images.

Know what to look for, but also be conservative in your interpretation

Having a general understanding of how pathology appears on a scan will assist you in identifying areas of concern. For example, when reviewing brain scans from a patient who sustained a traumatic brain injury, being cognizant of the general appearance of contusions, hemorrhages, and edema will assist you in searching for such markers. Similarly, when reviewing brain scans of someone who sustained a hypoxic injury, be prepared to assess for signs of edema, increased intracranial pressure, reduced gray-white contrast differentiation, or encephalomalacia depending on the timing of the image acquisition. Be cautious in this approach and conservative in your interpretation of pathology. As with many aspects of clinical diagnostics, there is a risk inherent in having a predetermined concept of what symptoms or pathology should be evident given a specific clinical history. There is a tendency to interpret pathology even in normal tissue, or look for anything that confirms one's clinical impressions and expectations. This is a particular concern when interpreting brain scans. Brain scans have a high degree of variability relating to the appearance of tissues and pathological markers. Equivocal findings are common when reviewing brain scans and should be considered as such. It is better to consider equivocal findings as nonconfirmatory than to overinterpret them because they "could be" pathological. Searching for pathology that matches specific symptoms may result in finding features on the images that fit the symptoms but are actually unrelated or clinically meaningless.

Symmetry as a Guide to Interpreting Brain Scans

With few exceptions, most major areas of the brain are symmetrical, appearing similar in either hemisphere. Some exceptions include the frontal gyri close to Broca's area, the planum temporale close to Heschl's gyrus and even the gross structure of the Sylvian fissure. These structures can be slightly asymmetrical because of the lateralized dominance for language. However, even the asymmetrical structures can appear relatively similar across hemispheres upon review of two-dimensional brain scans, making the asymmetry less problematic. An obvious asymmetrical appearance on a brain scan is usually a sign of pathology, and assessing for such can be an efficient way to initially review images.

Be cautious when interpreting asymmetry between the two hemispheres as pathology. Often, the asymmetrical appearance is an artifact of the way the head was positioned in the scanner. Other times, the asymmetry may be due to nonpathological incidental findings considered benign, such as an arachnoid cyst without clinical relevance. Scanning artifacts can also produce asymmetry unrelated to pathology.

CLINICAL EXAMPLE
Blair: Traumatic Brain Injury

Blair sustained a left frontal injury when he fell while taking a shower. During his hospitalization, he reported sustaining three previous head injuries while riding his skateboard. Initial review of neuroimaging revealed a small epidural hemorrhage to the left frontal region (Figure 2-16, arrow). The axial series also

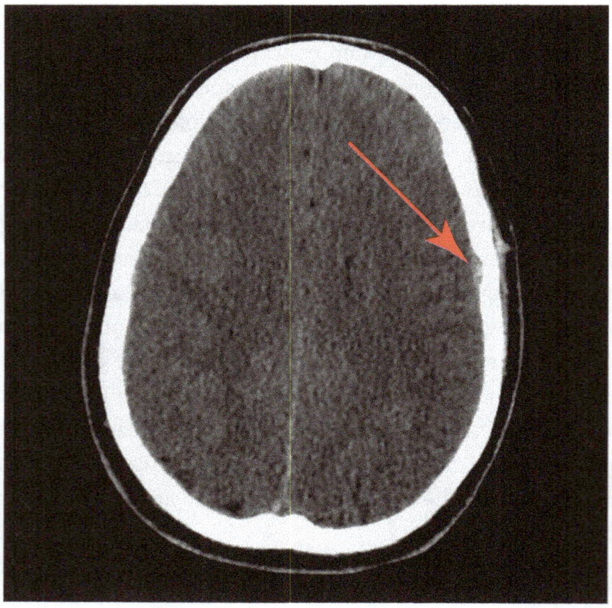

Figure 2-16 Clinical example Blair: small epidural hemorrhage to the left frontal region.

suggested an abnormal appearance to his left superior parietal region (Figure 2-17A–C, arrows), possibly relating to a developmental defect, or atrophy from previous injuries sustained while skateboarding.

More detailed review of the brain scans revealed that the falx appeared to be offset from the midline, with the offset being least evident at the level of the injury and becoming more pronounced as the cuts became more superior. If the offset falx was due to swelling, one would expect it to be greatest close to the level of the injury, becoming less evident as the slices become more superior or inferior. In addition, an offset falx, also called midline shift due to pressure, would result in compression and effacement of the lateral sulci-gyri patterning, something that is not evident on these images. The offset falx is not midline shift but an artifact of the head orientation during image acquisition. The head was not exactly perpendicular to the axis of the scanner and was leaning to one side. When the head is not perpendicular to the axis of the scanner or is leaning, the image slices through sulci and gyri at a different angle on one side of the brain than on the other. In Blair's case, this gave the appearance of asymmetry and atrophy to the superior parietal lobe on the left, but not on the right.

Observing the position of the falx will not always provide clues regarding the head position in the scanner, although at times it is helpful. Other clues concerning the head position in the scanner can be obtained from a review of a few basic anatomical structures known to be symmetrical between the right and left hemispheres.

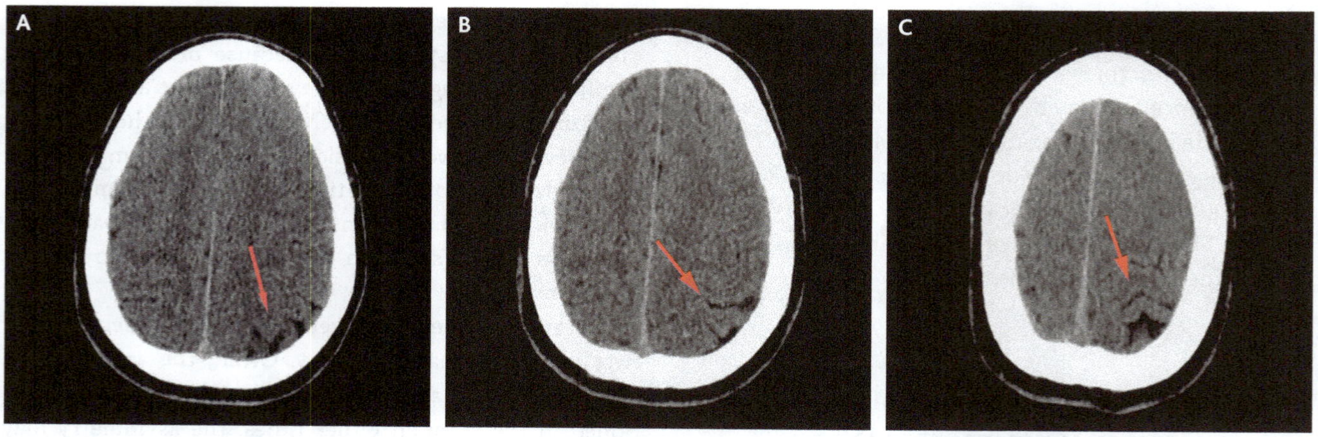

Figure 2-17 Clinical example Blair: superior axial series showing the area appearing abnormal in the left superior parietal lobe.

> Before evaluating symmetry to assess for pathology, it is critical that you assess whether the image was acquired with the head orthogonal to the scanner axis. If the head was resting at an angle, axial slices will not cut through the two hemispheres at the same height, and coronal slices will not show equivalent areas of the right and left hemispheres.

Evaluating Head Position in the Scanner

Look at the eyes

With few exceptions, the eyes are generally located at an equivalent height and horizontal offset within the cranium. The appearance of the eyes can provide valuable information about the orientation of the head in the scanner. If the head was tilted during data acquisition, the eyes will appear asymmetrical, with one appearing larger than the other. If the eyes appear symmetrical on the vertical and

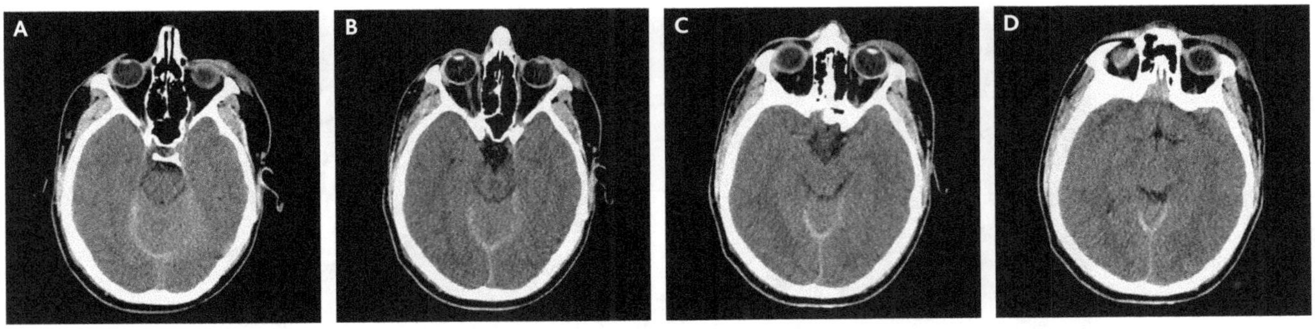

Figures 2-18A–D Axial series. Note asymmetry of the eyes on these axial images. Moving from Figure 2-18A to 2-18D, the slices were acquired from increasingly superior levels. Note that the right eye on the left side of the image is full in Figure 2-18A, with the left eye being only partially captured at the most inferior aspect of the globe. However, with the slices moving superiorly, the sequences passes through both eyes, and by Figure 2-18D the very top of the right eye and a greater amount of the left eye (right side of the image) are captured. Although the brain tissue on the images appears relatively symmetrical, it is important to realize that the slice is cutting through tissue that is higher (more superior) on the left side of the image and lower (more inferior) on the right side of the image.

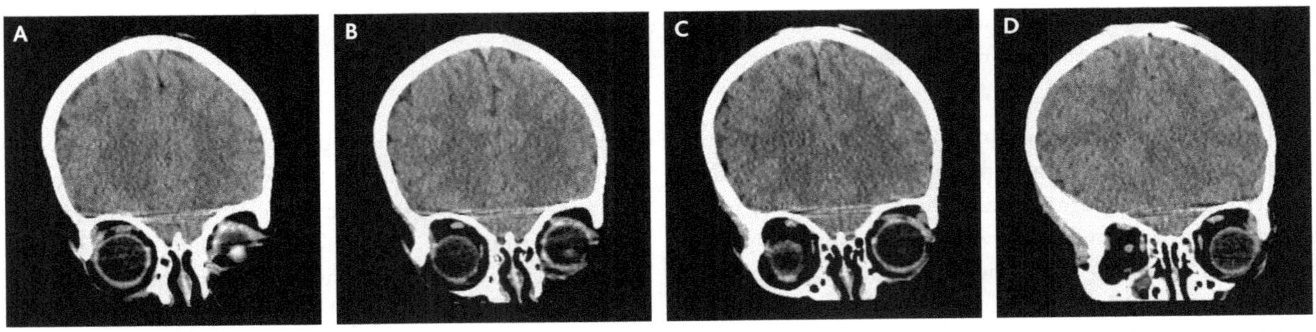

Figures 2-19 Coronal series. Note how the eyes do not appear symmetrical on the coronal images. The head was rotated slightly in the scanner, and the images have acquired data from different levels of the brain along the anterior–posterior axis.

horizontal planes, you can conclude that most major areas of the brain should also appear symmetrical between the right and left hemispheres. It is helpful to review multiple images when using the eyes as a measure of head position in the scanner. If the head was tilted in the scanner, a series of axial images will slice through the eyes at different levels along the inferior–superior axis (Figures 2-18A–D). If the head was rotated relative to the scanner, coronal images will slice through the eyes at different locations along the anterior–posterior axis (Figures 2-19A–D).

PEARL If the eyes are symmetrical, you know the head was level in the scanner.

Axial images are useful to assess tilting of the head relative the scanner axis.

Coronal images are useful to assess rotation of the head relative to the scanner axis.

Tissue directly above the eyes is frontal lobe.

Tissue directly behind the eyes is temporal lobe.

PERIL If the eyes are not symmetrical, the head was not level in the scanner and brain tissue will not be presented symmetrically. Any observed asymmetry may be misinterpreted as pathology. Prior to a determination of pathology-based asymmetry, the general angle of head tilt and rotation must be assessed and taken into account.

Look at the bones of the skull

The skull can also give clues regarding the orientation of the head in the scanner. When the head is not perpendicular to the scanner axis, horizontally oriented axial slices will cut through different parts of the skull on the right and left hemispheres, respectively (Figures 2-20A and B). This is also true for rotation of the head relative to the scanner axis.

Look at the bilateral structures that are commonly symmetrical

A brief review of the major bilateral structures of the brain can provide additional information about the orientation of the head in the scanner. The easiest structures to review for symmetry are the basal ganglia, thalami, or the

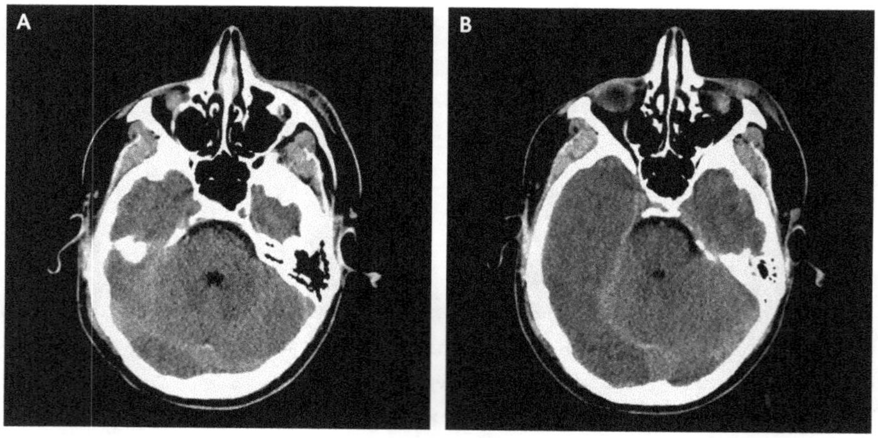

Figure 2-20 A: In this image there appears to be significant asymmetry around the temporal lobes and less asymmetry at the back of the brain. To the untrained eye, such asymmetry could suggest damage or problems with the development of the brain. However, the asymmetry is caused by the axial slice cutting through the right side of the picture, or left hemisphere, at a lower point than on the left side of the picture, or right hemisphere. The slice is cutting through the top of the temporal bone on the left side of the picture, and through the body of the temporal bone and auditory structures on the right side of the image. **B:** This image was acquired from a more superior position and shows the complete right temporal lobe on the left side and the superior margin of the temporal bone on the right side of the image.

white-matter pathways running through the deeper structures such as the internal capsule (Figures 2-21A and B). Larger areas of white matter and the ventricles may not be symmetrical, and caution is warranted when using these structures to assess head orientation during acquisition. The least symmetrical structures involve the sulci and gyri of the cortical surface.

Exercise caution when using symmetry as a guide

Structural differences may be apparent between the right and left hemispheres but have no clinical relevance. Figure 2-22 shows a notable asymmetry between the right and left hemispheres that was caused by a benign left anterior temporal lobe cyst, likely present since early brain development. Prior to this patient's closed-head injury, he was completely asymptomatic, graduating from college with honors. Note how readily the cyst can distract the viewer and make it more difficult to notice the small left parietal subdural hemorrhage (arrow). There is also a right temporal subdural hemorrhage consistent with a contrecoup injury. Other areas of the brain are relatively symmetrical, such as the white-matter tracts, midbrain, bones around the eyes, and the eyeballs. The eyes are relatively similar in size, which suggests that the asymmetrical appearance of the brain is not related to

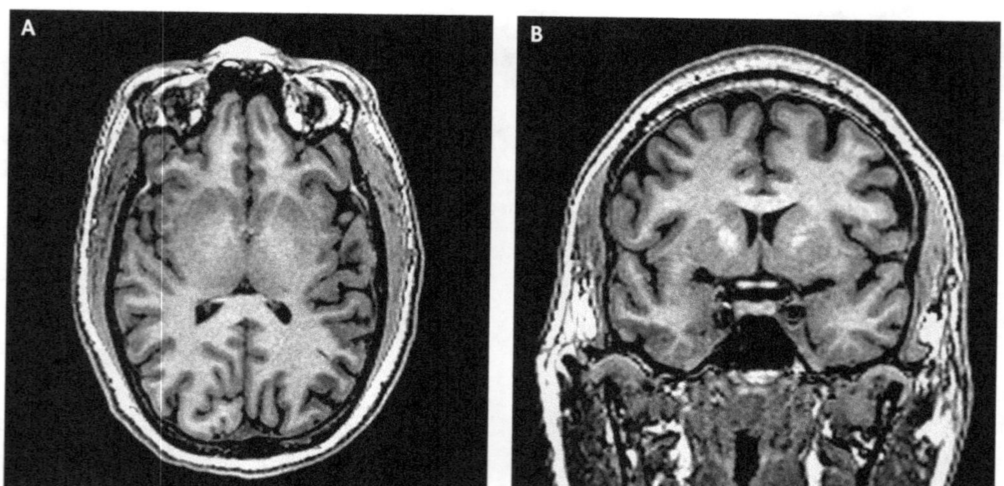

Figures 2-21A and B Note the symmetry of the deep gray-matter structures of the basal ganglia and thalamus. Also note how the sulci–gyri pattern is not symmetrical, a reason to avoid using the cortex to assess for head tilt or rotation in the scanner.

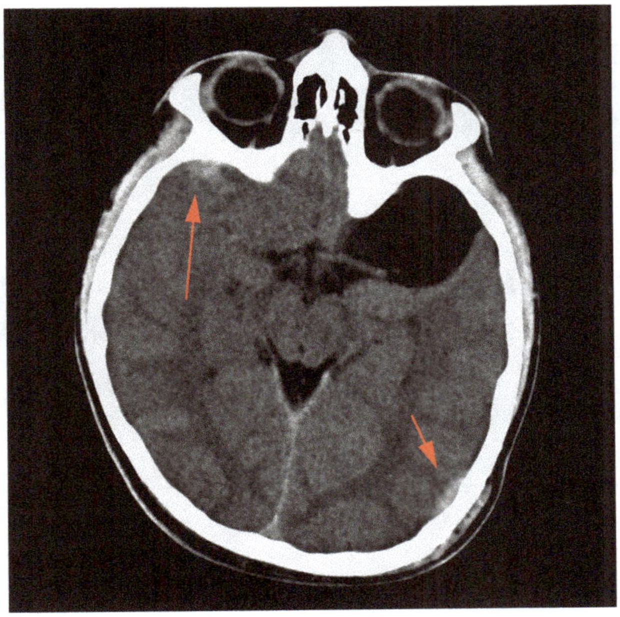

Figure 2-22 CT showing a benign left anterior temporal lobe cyst that distracts from the subdural hemorrhages (arrows).

how the head was angled in the scanner but is related to tissue in one hemisphere being different from tissue in the other.

If you have a good idea of what the patient's pathology should look like before viewing the scans, less time is needed to formulate appropriate conclusions. In the example shown in Figure 2-22, knowing that the patient experienced a closed-head injury with impact to the left parietal-occipital region should lead you to look for hemorrhage or contusion at the point of impact as well as in the area across from the impact, or contrecoup region. Knowing the patient's medical history should minimize the degree to which you become distracted by the benign cyst and thus miss the clinically relevant findings.

Multiple pathologies can produce asymmetry of the brain

When asymmetry is evident and not explained by head orientation, scanner artifacts, or benign conditions, you must then consider which of several pathologies may be causing the asymmetry. For example, when the general sulci–gyri pattern appears markedly different between the two hemispheres, consider the effects of edema or atrophy. If one side of the brain has the appearance of prominent sulci compared with that of the other, it is natural to assume that the hemisphere is atrophic. However, there are actually several feasible explanations for one hemisphere appearing more shriveled than the other. First, the side with the prominent sulci may be atrophied, especially if there was unilateral damage to that hemisphere several weeks prior to image acquisition. Another feasible explanation is that the side that appears more "wrinkled" may be within normal limits for the patient's age but appears atrophied when compared with a swollen opposite hemisphere. The relative difference between the hemispheres can give the impression that the prominence of the sulci is greater than it actually is. Checking the fluid-filled cavities in the brain such as the ventricles and cisterns may assist you in determining which side is abnormal and whether the side without prominent sulci is edematous. Another explanation is that steroids may have been used as part of the patient's treatment regimen. Steroids will have a greater effect on normal tissue than on swollen tissue, shrinking the normal side enough to give the appearance of asymmetry (see Clinical Case Natasha).

CLINICAL CASE
Natasha: Asymmetry Resulting from Steroid Use

The effects of systemic medications such as steroids would be expected to affect the brain globally, with changes being symmetrical across hemisphere. However, steroids affect nonedematous tissue more than edematous tissue. In this clinical case, Natasha suffered a stroke resulting in swelling of her left hemisphere. Steroids were used to control the swelling and prevent herniation or the need for surgical intervention. Initial review of brain scans suggested left-hemisphere edema with possible right-hemisphere atrophy (Figures 2-23A–C). On the scans the left hemisphere appears swollen, with compression and effacement of the cortical sulci and extra-axial fluid spaces. The right hemisphere has the appearance of atrophy, with prominent sulci-gyri patterning especially around the Sylvian fissure and insular cortex. However, this appearance is not related to atrophy but is a function of the steroids affecting the nondamaged right hemisphere more than the swollen left hemisphere.

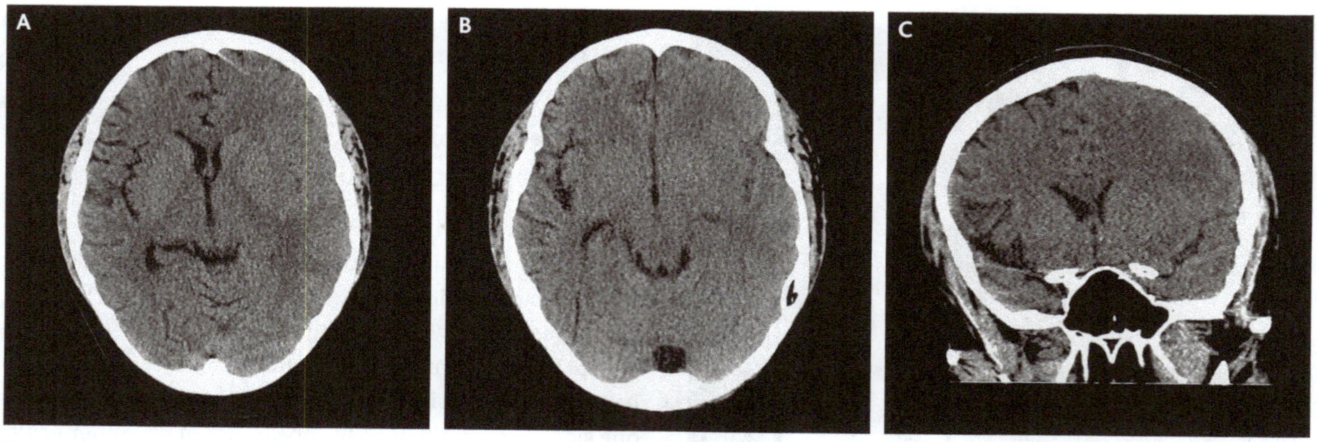

Figure 2-23A–C Clinical case Natasha: left hemisphere edema with the appearance of right hemisphere atrophy.

Artifacts can produce asymmetry on an image

It is not uncommon for imaging artifacts to produce asymmetry, which may then be interpreted as pathology. For example, the transection of tissue such as dura or blood vessels can give the appearance of asymmetry on an image and, thus, injury to the brain. Because of the acquisition angle used to produce slices of the brain, it is not unusual for an image to show tissue that has been transected at an angle. When dura is transected along the length instead of across, it can give the appearance of pathology (Figure 2-24A). When the transection is evident on one side of the image but not the other, it can result in misinterpretation of the findings. Transection of bone on one side and not the other can also produce asymmetry (Figure 2-24B), leading to incorrect interpretation of pathology.

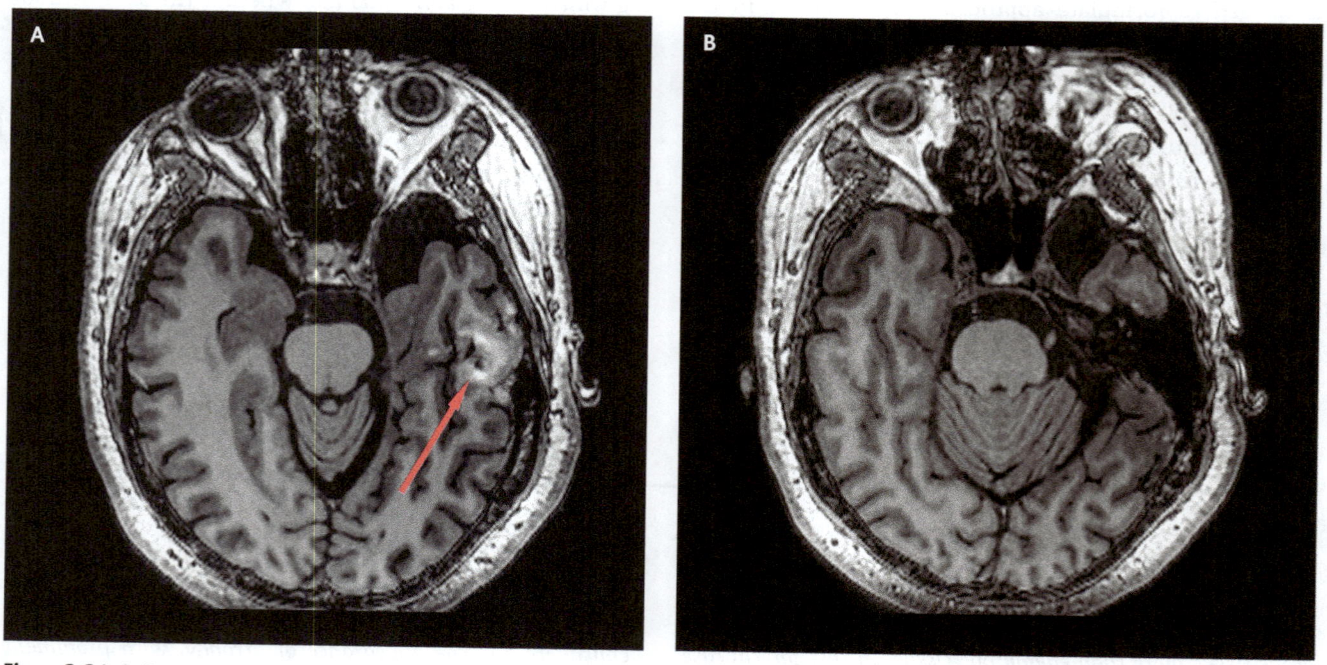

Figure 2-24 **A:** Transection of dura. The bright area could be interpreted as blood, but it is actually transection of the meningeal layers. **B:** Transection of bone due to asymmetry of the head in the scanner, the acquisition angle, and thickness of the image slices. The darker area within the left temporal region is actually caused by the transection of bone and is unrelated to pathology.

The transection of tissue along the longitudinal axis or sagittal plane can also result in interpretive errors when the slice is not aligned with the brain. If the head is not vertical during acquisition, a sagittal slice down the longitudinal fissure may be at a slight angle relative to the fissure. This results in some parts of the medial cortical surface being transected while others parts are not. The transection of some brain structures but not others can result in the appearance of pathology where none exists. In Figure 2-25A, the gyri within the medial occipital lobe (arrows) appear brighter than that of the medial parietal and frontal lobes, suggesting pathology. However, the brighter appearance is due to the sagittal slice transecting the cortical mantle of the occipital lobe but not the rest of the hemisphere, as evident on Figures 2-25B and 2-25C. The blue lines indicate the location of the acquisition slice used for Figure 2-25A. Note how the slice transects the medial occipital cortex but not the frontal cortex on Figure 2-25B and the inferior occipital cortex but not the superior parietal cortex on Figure 2-25C.

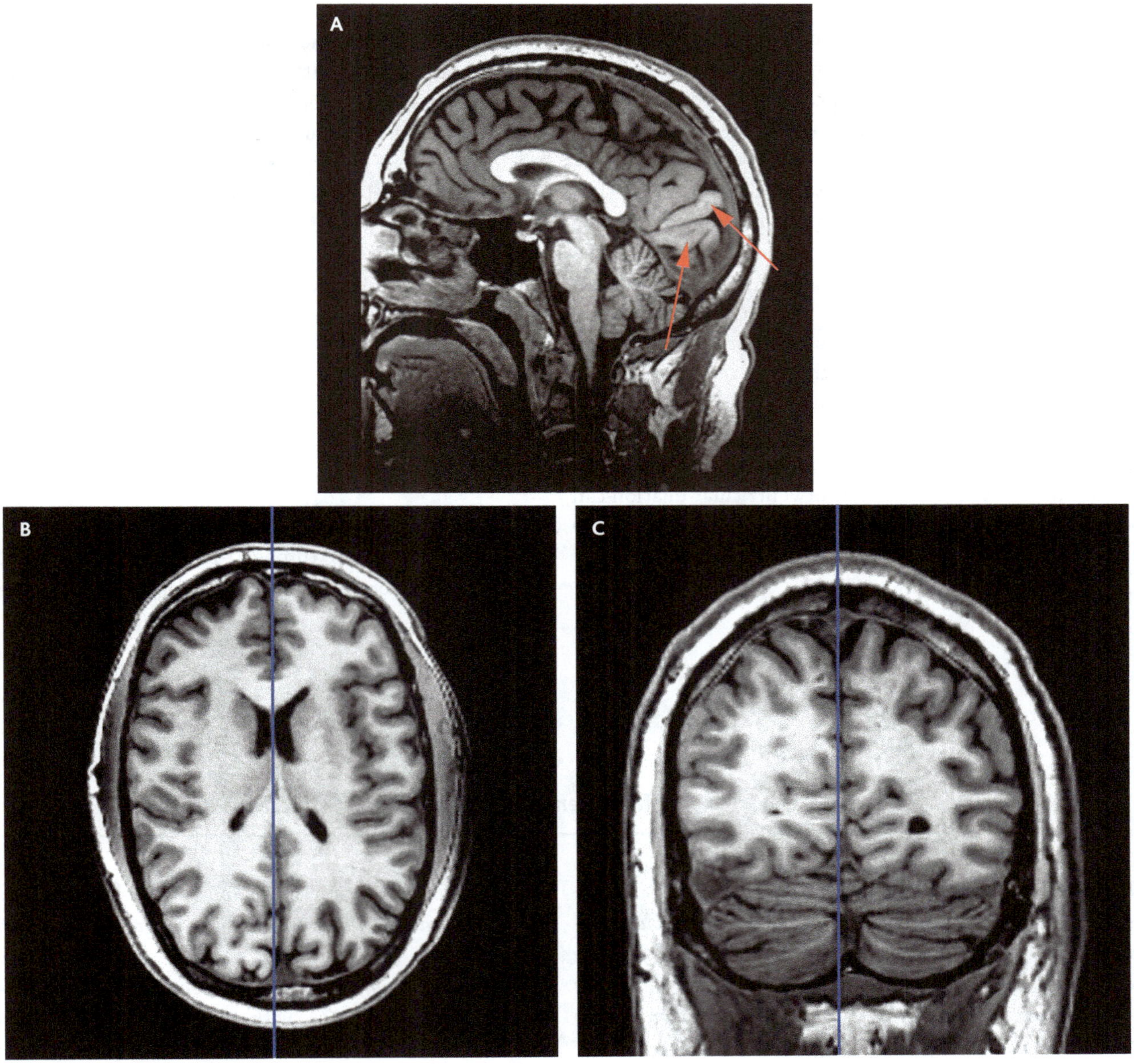

Figure 2-25A–C Inconsistent transection of tissue along the longitudinal axis due to the head being tilted in the scanner.

Ventricular Dilation and Compression

The appearance of the ventricles on brain imaging can provide the clinician with information on a variety of pathological processes or conditions. It is important to consider the size of the ventricles when viewing brain scans; ventricles that are too small or too big can signify pathology.

Large ventricles with effacement of fissures and sulci suggest high-pressure hydrocephalus. Increased intraventricular pressure can result from a variety of causes, the two most common being obstructive (noncommunicating) hydrocephalus or communicating hydrocephalus. Obstructive, or noncommunicating hydrocephalus is caused by a blockage in the flow of CSF through the ventricular system. Communicating hydrocephalus is caused by reduced absorption of CSF by the arachnoid granulations.

When pressure within the ventricles increases they dilate, compressing surrounding tissue. With increasing compression of tissue, the risk of permanent damage escalates. Damage first occurs to the periventricular white matter and then areas of subcortical and cortical gray matter. As brain tissue becomes compressed there is also a reduction in blood perfusion through the capillary beds, a condition that can result in hypoxic ischemic injury. Squeezing of brain tissue can also result in the downward herniation of the brain stem through the foramen magnum. Reversal of symptoms caused by the effects of ventricular dilation can be quite remarkable, as long as the pressure on brain tissue does not build to critical levels or is not left elevated for extended periods of time.

How much ventricular dilation can a person sustain without symptoms?

The amount of ventricular dilation that a person can tolerate is a difficult question to answer and is dependent on a variety of factors. If the increase in ventricular size is slow, building over years, the ventricles can become very large without notable neurological symptoms. This is called normal pressure hydrocephalus. However, if the increase in ventricular size takes place more rapidly, once compensatory mechanisms become exhausted, intracranial pressure will increase rapidly. With rapid increases in ventricular and intracranial pressure there is often a rapid deterioration of neurological functioning. With high intraventricular and intracranial pressure, small changes in ventricle size may lead to a profound deterioration of a patient's mental status and neurological condition. For example, with a change of less than 1 millimeter measured at the third ventricle and less than 2 millimeters at the lateral ventricles, Mark (see Clinical Example) deteriorated from having intact mental status and cognitive and functional abilities to being inconsistently obtunded, disoriented, and globally encephalopathic (see Figures 2-26 and 2-27).

Obstructive (Noncommunicating) Hydrocephalus

A frequent cause of high-pressure hydrocephalus is obstruction in the flow of CSF through the ventricular system. The most common locations for obstruction to CSF flow are at

CLINICAL EXAMPLE

Mark: Ventricular Dilation with Increased Intracranial Pressure

Neuropsychological testing of Mark at the time of initial image acquisition (Figures 2-26A and B) suggested intact basic cognition, intellect, orientation, arousal, and ability to perform activities of daily living. There was mild diminution of memory and executive functioning, although not of the magnitude to disrupt normal everyday functioning.

With just a slight increase in ventricular size and pressure (Figures 2-27A and B), Mark's functional abilities rapidly deteriorated. Mark was inconsistently obtunded with excessive lethargy, low levels of arousal, and an inability to participate in examination. He had no insight into his condition and lacked basic orientation, reasoning ability, judgment, and safety awareness.

Note the minimal increase in ventricular size between Figures 2-26A and 2-27A, with an increase of 0.9 mm at the third ventricle, and Figures 2-26B and 2-27B, with an increase of 1.5 mm at the lateral ventricles. Prior to making comparisons such as these, it is important to ensure that the images being compared have relatively consistent slice positions, angles, and head positions in the scanner.

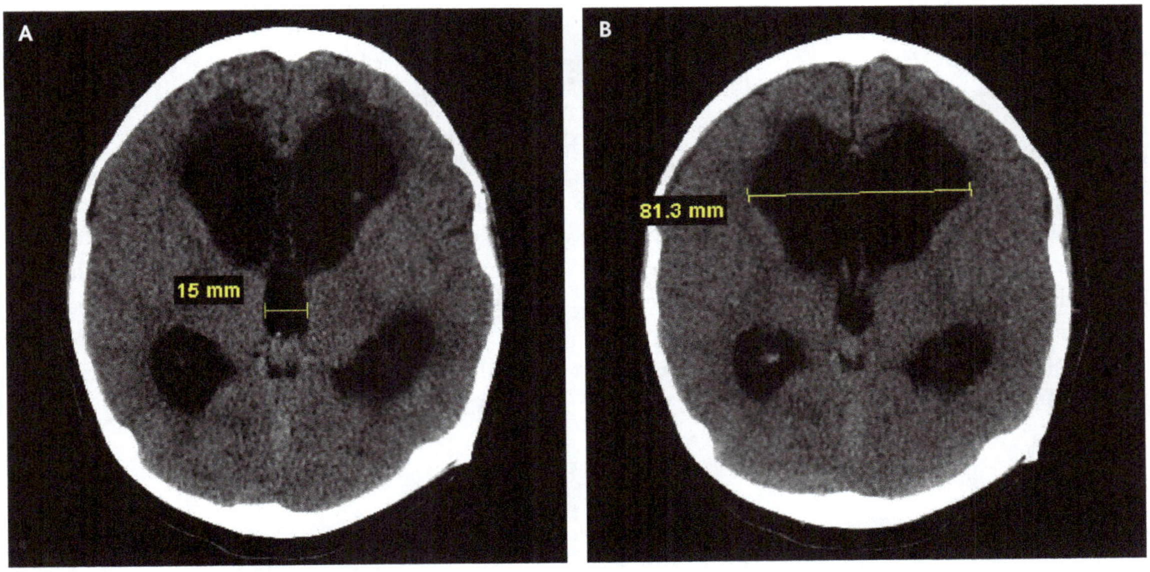

Figure 2-26A and B Clinical example Mark: initial image showing ventricular size with intact functioning.

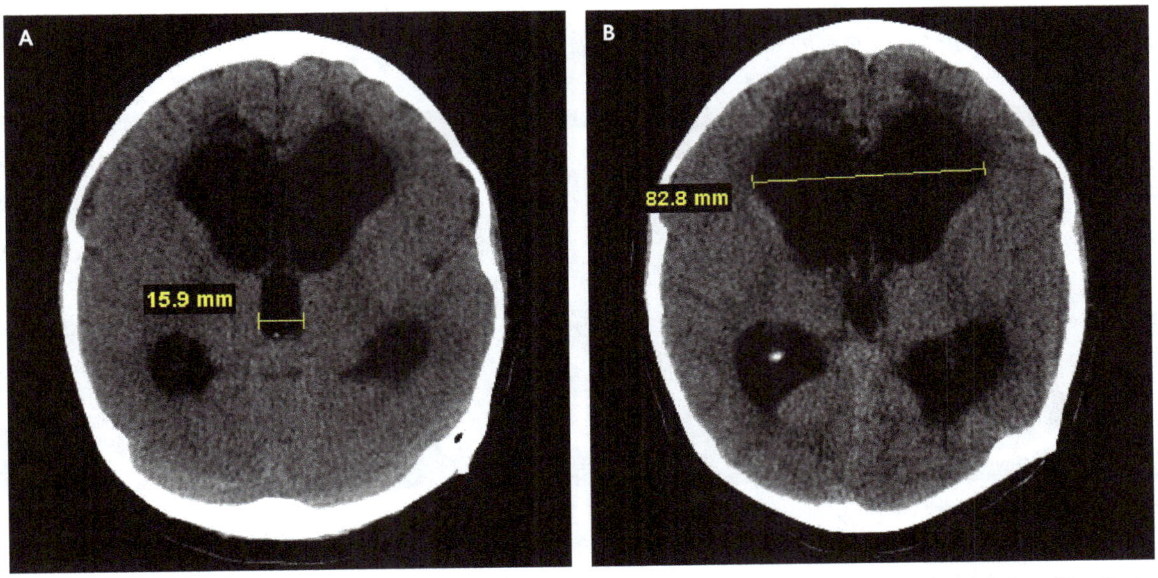

Figure 2-27A and B Clinical example Mark: image showing slight increase in ventricular size and pressure resulting in deterioration of functioning.

the base of the lateral ventricles at the foramena of Monro, at the third ventricle, at the cerebral aqueduct of Sylvius, at the fourth ventricle, or at the foramina of Luschka or Magendie.

Communicating Hydrocephalus

High-pressure hydrocephalus can also be caused by inadequate absorption of CSF by the arachnoid granulations, a condition referred to as communicating hydrocephalus. In this condition, there is no obvious obstruction in flow of CSF through the ventricular system, although the CSF is being produced faster than it is being reabsorbed. Communicating hydrocephalus can be caused by a variety of pathological processes, including but not restricted to meningitis; blood within the CSF or subarachnoid space which disrupts the functioning of the arachnoid granulations; or reasons that are unknown, as in idiopathic or congenital hydrocephalus. Clinical example Mark, described above, involved a patient with communicating hydrocephalus that was believed to be caused by post-surgery blood blocking some of his arachnoid granulations. The blockage of the arachnoid granulations resulted in reduced CSF absorption, hydrocephalus, and increased intracranial pressure.

Normal-Pressure Hydrocephalus (Hydrocephalus ex vacuo)

Hydrocephalus ex vacuo, also called normal-pressure hydrocephalus, results from ventricular dilation due to loss of brain tissue. The loss of brain parenchyma frequently results from traumatic, infectious, or hypoxic injuries to the brain. Neurodegenerative conditions such as dementia, multiple sclerosis, or other degenerative processes can cause ventricular dilation without an increase in intraventricular pressure. Surgical resection of brain tissue or neoplasms can also result in ventricular dilation, especially if the periventricular white matter is involved.

Normal-pressure hydrocephalus can also be caused by chronic but stable communicating hydrocephalus in which intracranial pressure remains slightly elevated but not to the point that the patient becomes symptomatic. Over time, the brain compensates for the slightly increased intracranial pressure and reaches a state of equilibrium without overt signs of increased pressure such as headaches, vomiting, nausea, or changes in mental status.

CLINICAL EXAMPLE

Madison: Obstructive Hydrocephalus due to a Posterior Fossa Tumor

Madison had a juvenile pilocytic astrocytoma located in her cerebellum that put pressure on the cerebral aqueduct of Sylvius, resulting in hydrocephalus (Figures 2-28A–C and 2-29A–C).

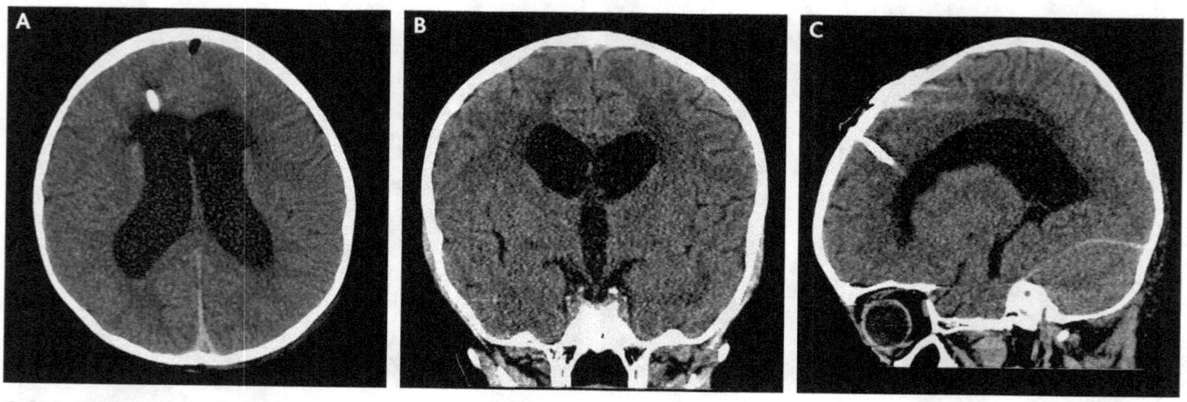

Figures 2-28A–C Clinical example Madison: CT series.

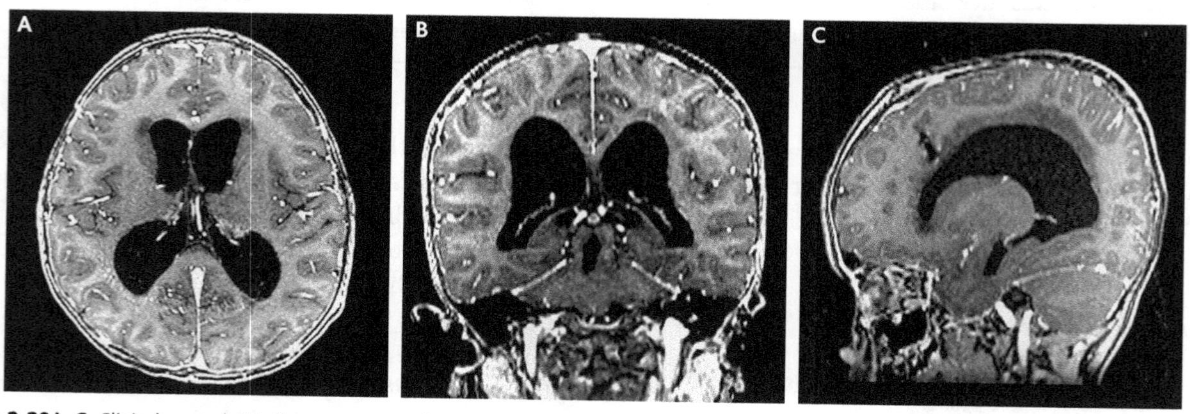

Figures 2-29A–C Clinical example Madison: contrast-enhanced TI series.

Trapped Fourth Ventricle

John was being treated for meningitis and arachnoiditis. He had marked inflammation around the cerebral aqueduct and below the fourth ventricle at the base of the brain. The inflammation and swelling resulted in a condition referred to as a "trapped fourth ventricle." Although some CSF could be pushed through the mostly closed cerebral aqueduct into the fourth ventricle, the CSF was not able to pass through the foramena of Luschka and Magendie into the subarachnoid spaces. John presented with signs of brain stem disruption due to pressure from the dilated fourth ventricle. He had nausea and vomiting several times an hour and was disoriented and at times obtunded, lacking the ability to interact with his environment. CT scans indicating the trapped fourth ventricle (Figures 2-30A and B) were critical in diagnosing the cause of his new symptoms and in scheduling appropriate surgical intervention. After drawing CSF from above and below the fourth ventricle, his condition improved and he was again able to interact with those around him. Without the CT scans, it would have been reasonable to believe that his deterioration of mental status and new onset of nausea and vomiting were the result of disease progression to his brain stem, not due to the pressure effect of the dilated fourth ventricle. CSF and ventricular disruption was not initially considered, as CSF pressure from the lateral ventricles was read as normal.

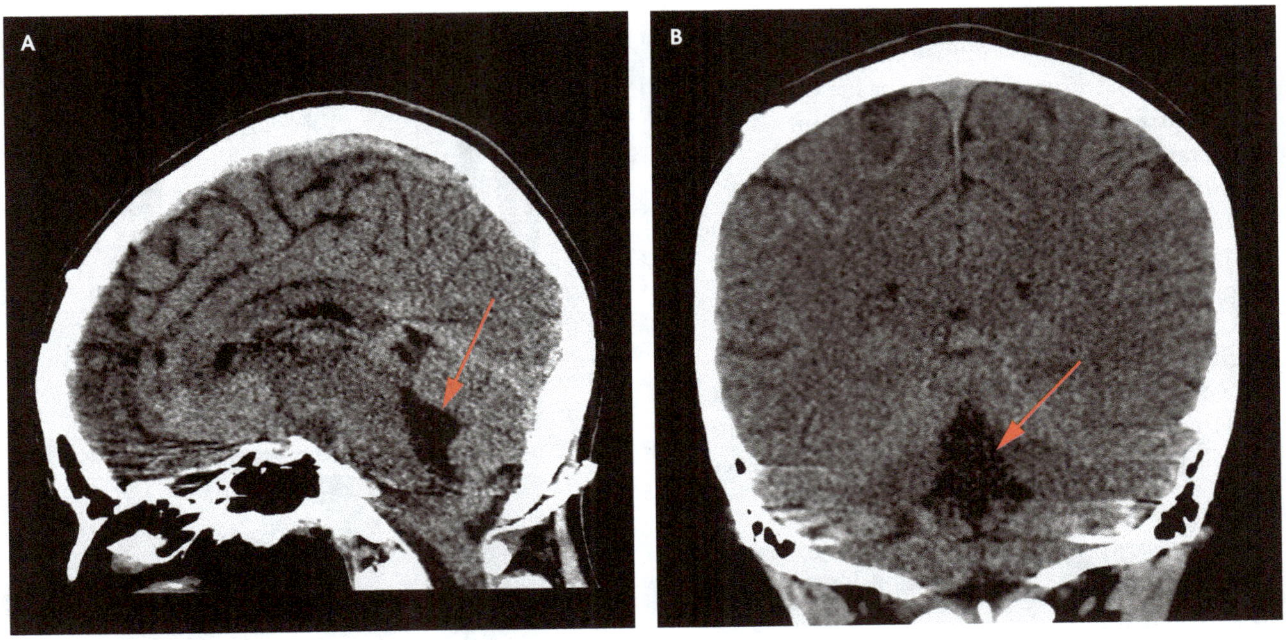

Figures 2-30A and B CT series showing the trapped fourth ventricle (arrows).

Transependymal Edema

When intraventricular pressure exceeds the limits of the ependymal lining of the ventricles, CSF is forced through the wall of the ventricles into the periventricular brain tissue, most often the white matter. Transependymal edema is most common around the frontal and posterior/occipital horns. Because some small amount of CSF leakage is normal within these regions, caution is warranted when differentiating between normal amounts of periventricular fluid and pathological transependymal edema. When first observing hypodensity or hypointensity on a CT or T1 image, or hyperintensity on T2 sequences around the frontal or occipital horns, it is important to consider that this may not be pathological. In addition, patients with normal-pressure hydrocephalus can have signs of CSF migration through the ventricular wall without clinical relevance.

On T2 sequences, transependymal edema appears as a rim of hyperintensity surrounding the lateral ventricles (Figure 2-31A). T2 FLAIR images are preferred when assessing transependymal edema, especially mild cases. The edema appears as a bright border of hyperintensity surrounding the ventricles (Figure 2-31B). On T1 sequences, mild transependymal edema can be difficult to appreciate. More severe transependymal edema appears as dark patches within the periventricular white matter surrounding the ventricles (Figure 2-31C).

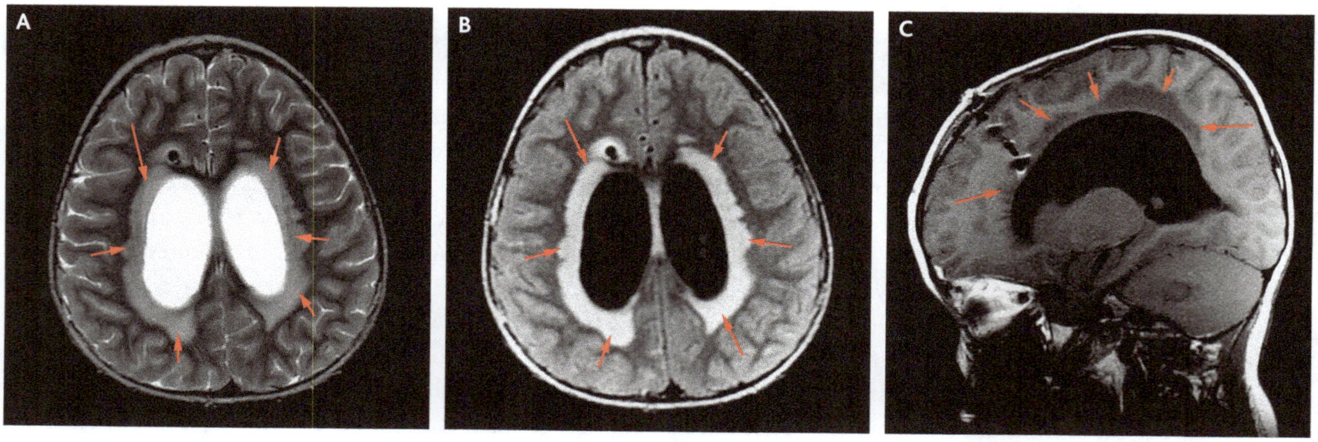

Figures 2-31A–C Transependymal Edema. **A:** T2 image. **B:** T2 FLAIR image. **C:** T1 image.

Small ventricles with effacement of cisterns, fissures, or sulci suggest diffuse edema (Figure 2-32). Diffuse edema can be life threatening if left untreated because of the increase in intracranial pressure and risk of downward herniation of the brain stem.

Large ventricles with prominent cisterns, sulci and fissures suggests diffuse atrophy to the brain (Figures 2-33A and B). When considering the effects of atrophy to brain tissue, it can be helpful to think of the brain as being like a doughnut left on a counter for several days. As the doughnut dries and the volume of dough decreases, the hole in the middle gets bigger while the outside circumference gets smaller. With diffuse atrophy to the brain, a similar phenomenon takes place: the ventricles or holes in the middle increase in size (ventricular dilation) and the outside diameter decreases.

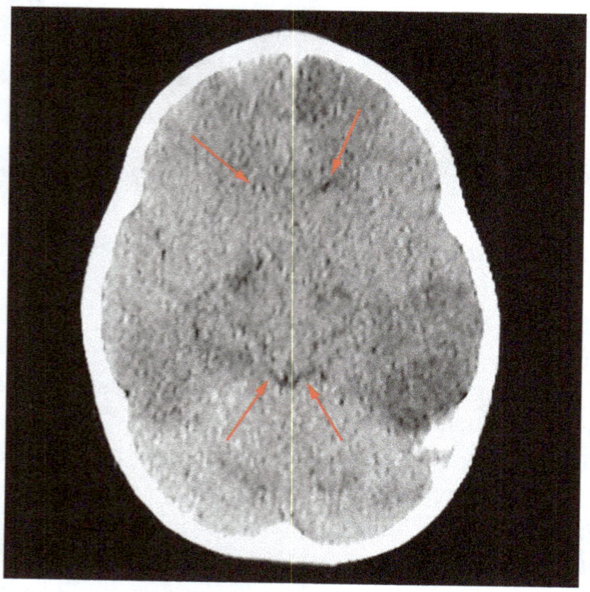

Figure 2-32 Small ventricles with effacement of cisterns, fissures, or sulci suggest diffuse edema.

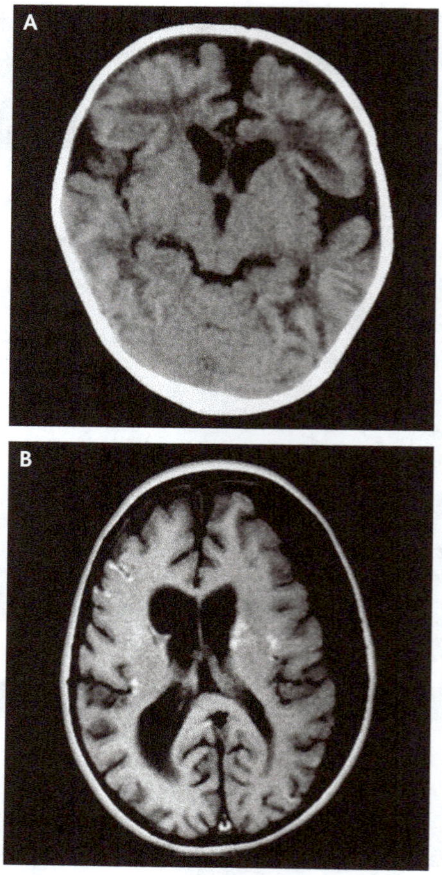

Figure 2-33 **A:** CT of diffuse atrophy secondary to a drowning incident resulting in prolonged hypoxic ischemic brain injury. **B:** MRI of diffuse atrophy, the left hemisphere showing more atrophy than the right hemisphere, due to a severe traumatic brain injury.

Ventricular Asymmetry

When mass effect is greater on one side of the brain than on the other, compression of the ventricles or cisterns will be asymmetrical. Asymmetrical compression of the ventricles or cisterns can be a useful way to localize areas of focal edema.

Figure 2-34 shows the appearance of asymmetrical compression of the lateral ventricles due to more swelling of the left hemisphere than of the right hemisphere.

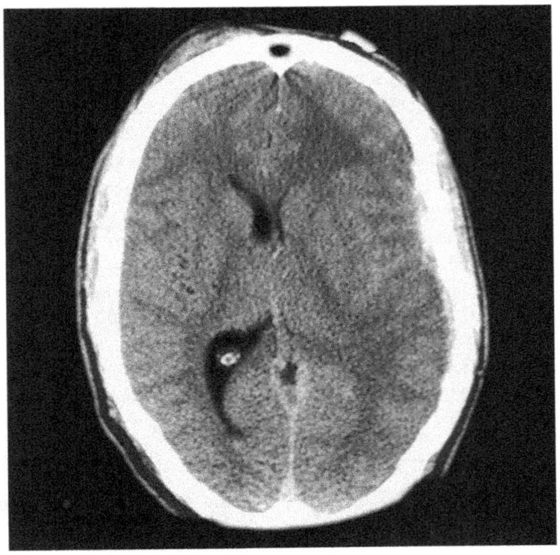

Figure 2-34 Asymmetric compression of the lateral ventricles.

> Diffuse dilation of the ventricles and cisterns in addition to increased prominence of the sulci suggests diffuse atrophy. However, the appearance may not be related to atrophy but instead the effects of medications. Steroids can cause an increase in the size of the ventricles and subarachnoid cisterns, an appearance that can be mistaken for atrophy. Caution is warranted when interpreting images from patients who have been on a long-term, high-dose steroid regimen.

Steroid Use

The use of steroids to treat pathologies of the brain is common, especially with space-occupying lesions or with swelling of tissue increasing the risk of herniation. The effects of steroids on brain tissue can lead to misinterpretation of scans and faulty assumptions of the extent and severity of damage. High-dose steroids can cause the brain to take on the appearance of atrophy, with prominence of the sulci–gyri patterning being diffusely evident. In patients who have sustained injury to the brain and are expected to have some degree of brain atrophy, the use of steroids may magnify the appearance of atrophy, leading to an overestimation of damage. Once steroids are discontinued, the brain may plump, changing the appearance on brain imaging to a level more representative of the sustained injury.

CLINICAL EXAMPLE
Sue: High-Dose Steroids

Sue was hospitalized for suspected encephalitis. Her functioning was mildly compromised and not of the magnitude to suggest severe damage to her brain. Subtle atrophy and mild prominence of extra-axial spaces was expected given the type of infection and Sue's age. However, the appearance on CT was concerning and suggested that Sue had sustained a significant

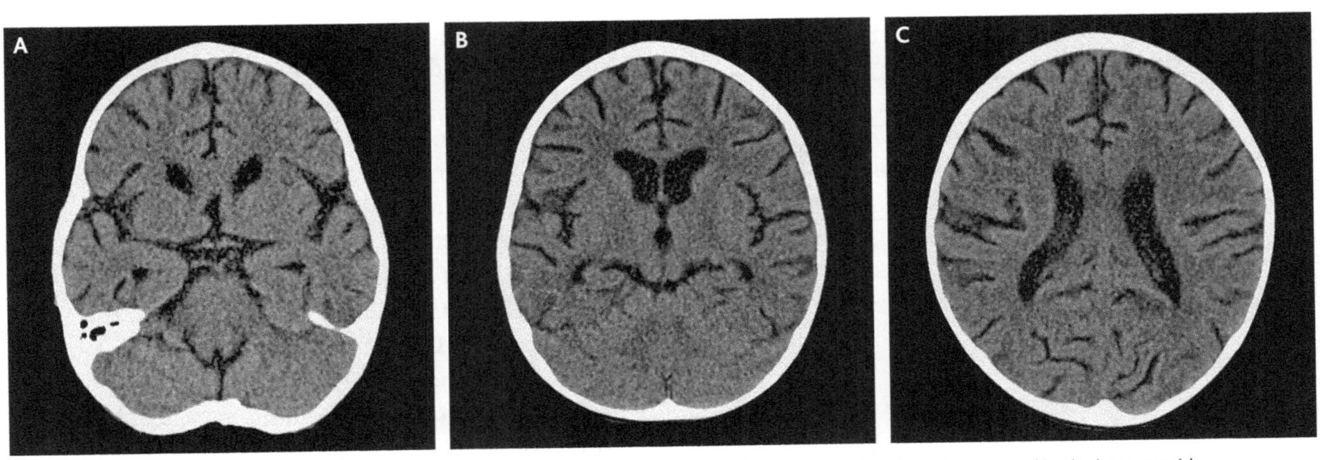

Figures 2-35A–C Clinical example Sue: CT series with the appearance of atrophy, likely exacerbated by long-term use of high-dose steroids.

injury to her brain, with notable diffuse atrophy. Clinically, the appearance on brain imaging was highly inconsistent with Sue's clinical presentation and recovery; she experienced only mild diminution of cognitive and functional abilities, with rapid recovery to premorbid levels. It was concluded that the appearance of "atrophy" was exacerbated by the effects of long-term, high-does steroids, and that the images did not truly represent the degree of damage to her brain (Figure 2-35A–C). This case highlights the importance of correlating brain imaging results with measures of functioning. When there appears to be a discrepancy between imaging results and a patient's functioning, further investigation may be necessary. It is important to consider all of the reasons for a particular appearance on brain imaging, not just those that are obvious or expected.

Thus in patients with known pathology and expected diffuse atrophy, it is important to remember that the use of high-dose steroids may exacerbate the atrophic appearance on imaging, giving the impression of greater damage to the brain than was actually sustained.

Guide to General Appearance of Different Tissues on Brain Images

When interpreting brain scans, it is important to understand how normal and abnormal tissue should appear. Even though different types of scans and sequences display tissue by means of a variety of grayscale values, a few general rules can be applied to make interpretation simpler (Tables 2-1 and 2-2).

TABLE 2-1 General Guideline to Appearance of Tissue on Common Brain Sequences

NORMAL TISSUE	CT	MRI T1	MRI T2
Gray matter	Light	Dark	Light
White matter	Dark	Light	Dark
CSF	Black	Black	White
Bone	White	Dark	Dark
Fat	Dark	White	Darker/varies
Air	Dark/black	Dark/black	Dark/black
Pathology			
Blood	See Table 2-3	See Table 2-3	See Table 2-3
Infarction	Dark	Dark	Light
Ischemia	Gray to dark	Gray	Gray
Edema	Dark	Dark	Light
Plaque	Gray	Dark	Light
Encephalomalacia	Dark	Dark	Bright
Gliosis	Light	Gray	Bright
Cyst	Dark	Dark	Bright

TABLE 2-2 General Guideline to Appearance of Tissue on T1 versus T2 MRI Sequences

	APPEARS DARK	APPEARS LIGHT
MRI T1	Inflammation Infection Hemorrhage (1–2 weeks) Edema (swelling) Infarction Encephalomalacia Tumor Calcification	Fat Hemorrhage (>3 <14 days) Protein-rich fluid Slow flowing blood Contrast agent (Gad) Laminar necrosis Cerebral infarction
MRI T2	Hemorrhage (<1 week or >2 weeks) Fibrous Tissue Protein-rich fluid Flow void	Inflammation Infection Infarction Encephalomalacia Hemorrhage (>7 <14 days) Edema (swelling) Gliosis

Temporal Effects on Appearance of Blood Products

As blood in the brain ages, the hemoglobin goes through a variety of stages (Table 2-3), each producing a different appearance on brain imaging (Table 2-4). For example, on CT scans, fresh bleeds may appear isodense or a shade similar to brain parenchyma. Over an hour or two, the appearance can change to become brighter than parenchyma. The blood can appear hyperdense and brighter for several days, gradually changing back to neutral with an isodense appearance after a week or more. After 2 or more weeks, the blood takes on a hypodense or darker appearance than that of brain parenchyma. Because most post-traumatic CT scans are conducted several hours after a bleed or within a day or two, most CT images portray blood brighter than surrounding parenchyma. Blood also changes appearance on MRI scans, although with the large number of sequences available, assessment of blood on MRI is much more complicated than that of blood on CT. Differentiating the subtle differences between new and old blood in the brain, especially on MRI, is outside of the scope of this text and is best left to an experienced radiologist.

Table 2-3 Stages of Blood Decomposition over Time (times are approximates)

Age of Bleed	Phase	Hemoglobin Form	Hemoglobin Location	Magnetic State
<14 hours	Hyperacute	Oxyhemoglobin	Intracellular	Diamagnetic
1–3 days	Acute	Deoxyhemoglobin	Intracellular	Paramagnetic
>3 days	Early subacute	Methemoglobin	Intracellular	Paramagnetic
>7 days	Late subacute	Methemoglobin	Extracellular	Paramagnetic
>14 days	Chronic	Ferritin/ hemosiderin	Extracellular	Paramagnetic

Table 2-4 General Guideline to Appearance of Blood on Common Brain Scans (times are approximates).

Age of Bleed	CT	MRI T1	MRI T2
Blood <14 hrs	Gray	Dark/gray	Light/white
Blood 1–3 days	Bright	Dark	Dark
Blood >3 days	Bright	Light	Gray
Blood >7 days	Bright to gray	Light	Light
Blood >14 days	Dark	Dark	Dark

Developmental Changes Evident on Neuroimaging

Developmental factors can result in a brain appearing abnormal, even when it is within normal limits for the patient's age. This is especially true for both the very young and the very old, in whom normal developmental and aging factors result in an appearance different from that of adolescents and adults.

Myelination

One of the primary differences between infant brains and those of older children and adults involves the degree to which the axons have myelinated. Myelination occurs at different rates and times throughout the brain, although it tends to follow a few general trends. Deeper brain structures achieve myelination earlier than more lateral brain structures, and posterior regions of the brain complete myelination before more frontal structures do.

Knowing what to expect on a brain scan based on an infant's age becomes a critical factor when assessing for pathology (Table 2-5). For example, abnormal T1 signal in the white matter is developmentally expected in a 2-month old child but not in a 10-month old child. Similarly, a CT scan of a 2-month-old may appear to suggest subcortical edema; the white matter appears darker than normally expected. However, the dark appearance is due to the lack of myelination at that age, not pathology.

Myelination Trends in Infants

Brain myelination follows the basic temporal course of "inside to outside" and "back to front."

Internal capsule	Posterior limb before anterior limb
Corpus callosum	Splenium before genu
Subcortical white matter	Occipital lobe before frontal lobe

T1 MRI: Birth to 1 Month

During the first month of postnatal life (gestational age of approximately 40 to 44 weeks), the posterior limb of the internal capsule should look brighter than other areas of white matter on a T1-weighted image (increased T1 signal from the fatty myelin). Similarly, the motor tracts from the cortex to the spine should also appear brighter, as should the midbrain, because of the early myelination of these pathways.

T1 MRI: 1 Month to 3 Months

From the first month to the third month of postnatal life (gestational age of approximately 44 to 52 weeks), the splenium of the corpus callosum and the occipital lobe pathways become myelinated. As such, T1 signals should be brighter in these areas as well as those that myelinated prior to this stage of development (such as the motor tracts).

T1 MRI: 3 Months to 6 Months

From three to 6 months of postnatal life (gestational age of approximately 52 to 64 weeks), the anterior limb of the internal capsule and the genu of the corpus callosum become myelinated, resulting in a brighter appearance on T1-weighted images. In addition, the anterior subcortical white matter myelinates, resulting in a somewhat normal-looking brain scan on T1 (white matter appears lighter than the gray matter across the entire brain). Generally, T1 images take on a normal appearance for myelin by two years of age.

T2 MRI

Prior to 6 months' postnatal life, T2 imaging has limited usefulness for white-matter studies. After 6 months of life,

TABLE 2-5 When Appearance of White Matter Generally Normalizes on T1 and T2 MRI Images (ages are approximates).

T1	T1	T1	T2	T2	T2	T2
Newborn	3 months	6 months	6 months	12 months	18 months	24 months
Posterior limb internal capsule	Posterior limb internal capsule	Posterior limb internal capsule	Posterior limb internal capsule	Posterior limb internal capsule	Posterior limb internal capsule	Posterior limb internal capsule
Motor cortex to corticospinal tract	Motor cortex to corticospinal tract	Motor cortex to corticospinal tract	Motor cortex to corticospinal tract	Motor cortex to corticospinal tract	Motor cortex to corticospinal tract	Motor cortex to corticospinal tract
Midbrain	Midbrain	Midbrain	Midbrain	Midbrain	Midbrain	Midbrain
	Splenium of corpus callosum	Splenium of corpus callosum	Splenium of corpus callosum	Splenium of corpus callosum	Splenium of corpus callosum	Splenium of corpus callosum
	Occipital lobes	Occipital lobes		Some genu of corpus callosum	Genu of corpus callosum	Genu of corpus callosum
		Anterior limb of internal capsule		Occipital lobes start	Occipital lobes	Occipital lobes
		Genu of corpus callosum		Some anterior limb of the internal capsule	Anterior limb of the internal capsule	Anterior limb of the internal capsule
		Subcortical white matter from occipital to frontal lobe		No frontal lobe subcortical white matter	Some frontal lobe subcortical white matter	Frontal lobe subcortical white matter
		Entire brain appears near normal on T1 imaging				Entire brain appears near normal on T2 imaging

T2 imaging becomes more useful as myelination continues. For the first 6 months of life, the pattern of myelin development on T2 imaging follows a pattern similar to that described above for T1 imaging, although, as myelin becomes brighter on T1 imaging it becomes darker on T2 sequences. Using T2 imaging techniques, the following basic rules apply.

T2 MRI: 6 Months to 12 Months

At 6 months, although the T1 image is close to normal, the T2 image may only appear normal in the posterior limb of the internal capsule and posterior corpus callosum (splenium).

T2 MRI: 12 Months to 18 Months

From 1 year of age, the anterior limb of the internal capsule and some occipital and frontal subcortical white matter tracts begin to appear normal.

Perinatal Hemorrhages

Newborn babies may appear to have pathology-related hemorrhages, but both subarachnoid and subdural blood is not uncommon in the newborn. As a general rule, subdural hematomas less than 4 mm in size, with resolution by 4 months of postnatal age, are normal in the newborn (Rooks et al., 2008). In their study of 46 neonates with hematomas, most of the hemotomas were less than 3 mm, and all were less than 4 mm. Most resolved by 1 month, and all resolved by 3 months. Infants from all types of delivery had subdural hematomas. Therefore, it was concluded that hematomas of 3 mm or less in a child under 3 months of age can be normal, but those over 4 mm in a child over 4 months of age should be considered pathological. For example, nonaccidental trauma should be considered when there is a subdural hemorrhage greater than 4 mm after 3 months of age or with other signs of trauma.

REFERENCE

Rooks, V. J., Eaton, J. P., Ruess, L., Petermann, G. W., Keck-Wherley J., & Pedersen, R. C. (2008). Prevalence and evolution of intracranial hemorrhage in asymptomatic term infants. *American Journal of Neuroradiology, 29*, 1082–1089.

T2 MRI: 18 Months to 24 Months

From 1 1/2 years to approximately 2 years of age, the anterior limb of the internal capsule, the anterior portion of the corpus callosum, and parts of the occipital lobe start to normalize on T2 imaging.

T2 MRI: 24 Months

At 2 years of age, T2 white-matter imaging begins to appear normal across the entire brain with the myelination of the subcortical frontal pathways. Even though myelination continues for years, especially in the frontal lobes, at approximately 24 months, it is usually complete enough to appear normal on T2-weighted images.

Temporal Effects on Appearance of Brain Scans

It is not possible to discuss the appearance of brain injury on neuroimaging without taking into account the dynamic nature of pathology. Both structural and chemical processes change over time following injury to the brain, with corresponding changes to the appearance of brain images.

Following damage, it is not uncommon for changes in brain structures and physiology to continue for many months. Acute changes often include bleeds and swelling due to both cytotoxic edema (cells accumulating fluid) and vasogenic edema (increased permeability of blood vessels). Inflammatory processes can take time to evolve and then gradually subside. Changes several weeks following an injury can result from resolution of swelling or inflammation and from slow breakdown of blood products, in addition to the slow process of tissue decomposition and atrophy.

Severely damaged brain tissue often goes through a gradual process from loss of metabolic activity to disruption of water diffusion, breakdown of the cellular integrity, and finally, atrophy and replacement by CSF. Each of these stages results in a different appearance on neuroimaging. For example, acutely following a severe traumatic brain injury, CT may be helpful in assessing for hemorrhage and swelling as well as skull fractures. As time progresses, T2 FLAIR images may be useful in assessing areas of primary damage; the tissue becomes hyperintense (T2 prolongation) and has a brighter appearance than that of noninjured tissue. Cytotoxic edema can develop rapidly over a period of just a few minutes to hours and is often evident on MRI diffusion-weighted imaging (DWI = bright; apparent diffusion coefficient [ADC] = dark). Later, often corresponding with the onset of infarction, vasogenic edema most evident in the white matter becomes apparent due to the increased permeability of capillary endothelia (vessel walls). Vasogenic edema has a different appearance on MRI diffusion-weighted images (DWI = bright; ADC = bright). Chronic ischemic tissue can also appear different on MRI diffusion-weighted imaging (DWI = dark; ADC = bright) because of unrestricted or isotropic diffusion resulting from tissue atrophy.

Other more sophisticated imaging may also assist in determining the specific stages of injury and pathological processes. Perfusion-weighted images (PWI) can give indirect evidence of cell death by highlighting areas of reduced blood perfusion resulting from lowered metabolic demand. Magnetic resonance spectroscopy (MRS), single photon emission computed tomography (SPECT), and positron emission tomography (PET) can also provide information relating to brain metabolic activity. Over longer periods of time, serial scans can give evidence of atrophy as the density of brain tissue declines (encephalomalacia) and there is a loss of cells (atrophy).

It is critical that certain rules are followed when using diffusion imaging to assess infarction or ischemia. For most situations, it is necessary to view both the diffusion-weighted sequences (DWI) and the apparent diffusion coefficient sequences (ADC). Because DWI sequences have a T2 weighting component, any bright areas on a T2 scan can also appear bright on the DWI image, irrespective of any disruption in diffusion. This phenomenon has been called "T2 shine-through." As a general rule, if there is T2 shine-through *and* restricted diffusion, the area will be brighter than that of T2 alone or DWI alone, sometimes called "light-bulb bright." Because disrupted diffusion appears dark on ADC images, a good way to differentiate T2 shine-through from reduced diffusion is to review the ADC map. A simple rule that fits most situations is the following.

(Continued)

(*Continued*)

With bright T2 and DWI, if the ADC map is dark or hypointense, it is likely disrupted diffusion; if the ADC map is neutral or isointense, it is likely shine-through; and if the ADC map is hyperintense or bright, it is likely vasogenic edema.

It is important to take into account the age of an injury when assessing pathology using diffusion sequences. As the extent of diffusion changes over time following brain injury, there are times when the T2, DWI, and ADC images suggest shine-through, although there was infarction of the tissue. This is because it can take several days after an infarction for the ADC sequence to change. As with many guidelines in medicine, it is helpful to have general rules, but it is critical to understand the limits, exceptions, and caveats to the rule.

Over time, and with experience, the determination of which types of imaging to review (CT or MRI) and which sequences will be most helpful (T1, T2, FLAIR, GRE, DWI, ADC, etc.) becomes much easier and even automatic.

PEARL Neuropathology is a dynamic process. Chemical changes such as edema and inflammation can continue for several weeks following an injury. Physical changes involving atrophy can continue for many months.

PERIL Avoid reviewing a brain scan taken close to the time of injury and assuming that all of the damage is visible. Over time, extensive injury can become apparent, even if the acute brain scans appear relatively unremarkable. Initially, the scan may only show diffuse swelling. A few days later the scan may look completely normal. Later the image may show the beginning of encephalomalacia as damaged brain tissue begins to break down. After several weeks to a few months the image may show extensive atrophy and the brain may look completely different from earlier scans. As brain tissue changes, the images change, leading to different clinical impressions and, ultimately, revision of prognoses and treatment options.

Use caution when assessing atrophy

Caution is warranted when interpreting an atrophic appearance on a brain scan. There are times when such an appearance is benign and does not suggest acute pathology. In addition, the condition may not affect the person's functioning, and the individual's abilities may fall well within normal limits for his or her age. With normal aging, the brain can appear more atrophied than expected, especially if the viewer is not familiar with the appearance of geriatric brain imaging. For example, Lucian received a brain scan after a fall. To a specialist familiar with younger brains the prominence of the sulci–gyri pattern on the images might suggest pathology. However, the scans were

CLINICAL EXAMPLE
Quinton: Nonaccidental Trauma

Quinton sustained severe damage to his brain due to nonaccidental trauma (NAT), previously referred to as shaken baby syndrome or Kempe's syndrome. Quinton was only 16 months old when he was injured; he never regained consciousness and eventually died from sepsis. Figures 2-36A–E are serial CT images of his severe diffuse traumatic injury, illustrating some of the more common changes seen over several weeks.

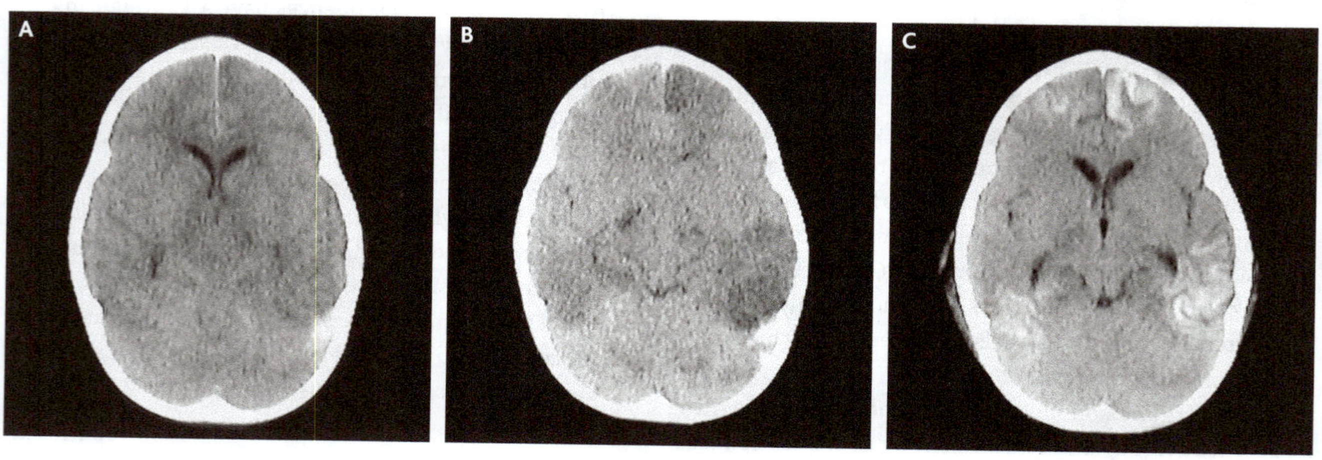

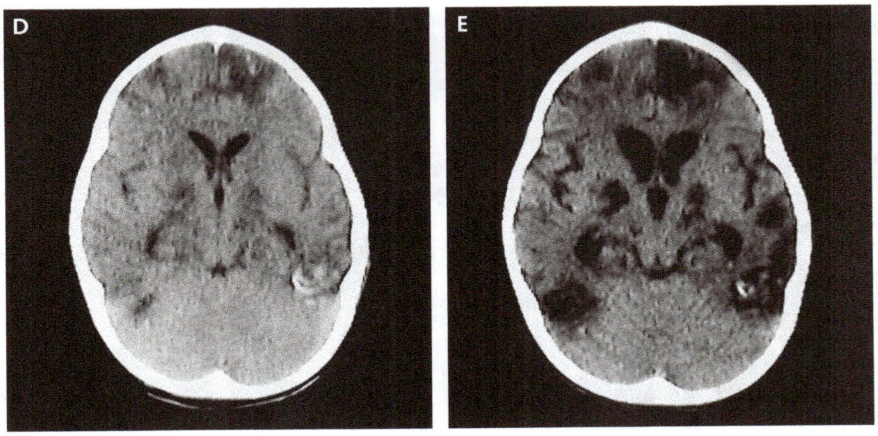

Figure 2-36 A: Clinical example Quinton: 24 hours post-injury. Cerebral edema is apparent with some loss of extra-axial fluid spaces and basal cisterns, raising the possibility of herniation. Extra-axial blood appears along the left side of the tentorium. There is low density to the cortex with scattered focal areas where the gray–white differentiation is attenuated, likely due to edema. **B:** Clinical example Quinton: 4 days post-injury. There is increased intracranial pressure, with additional loss of gray–white differentiation due to edema. Right frontal and temporal more than left frontal and temporal regions of low density are consistent with increased fluid content from the edema. **C:** Clinical example Quinton: 2 weeks post-injury. The intracranial pressure has resolved, as indicated by the better visualization of the ventricles and cisterns and of extra-axial spaces, most evident close to the Sylvian fissure and insula. Gray–white differentiation remains poor but has improved slightly commensurate with resolution of the edema. Bifrontal and biposterior temporal-occipital lobe damage is now becoming more apparent, with the bright appearance following the gyral pattern, suggestive of laminar necrosis and gliosis. **D:** Clinical example Quinton: 3 weeks post-injury. Slightly increased prominence of the Sylvian fissure is shown, with reduced density of brain parenchyma (darker). Encephalomalacia (brain tissue becoming softer) is now evident throughout the brain, especially frontal and posterior temporal-parietal. The deeper basal ganglia and thalamic structures have also become hypodense, suggesting significant injury. **E:** Clinical example Quinton: 4 weeks post-injury. There is ongoing diffuse atrophy with ventricular dilation due to loss of tissue and not increased intraventicular pressure. Increased sulci–gyri prominence is now evident, most notable within the Sylvian fissure and insular regions.

CLINICAL EXAMPLE
Meg: Traumatic Brain Injury with Atrophy

The extent and timing of atrophy can give clues to a patient's prognosis. Meg was crushed by falling lumber from a construction truck. Within a month after her injury, axial and coronal CT scans suggested almost complete loss of the right hemisphere, with atrophy and ongoing encephalomalacia of the left hemisphere (Figures 2-37A and B). Atrophy was expected to continue for some time after these scans were obtained. This catastrophic injury had severely damaged much of her brain, resulting in profound deficits for Meg. Because of the ongoing encephalomalacia, it could be concluded that additional atrophy would take place over the next month or two, even without ongoing pathological processes. Meg's mother was counseled that changes in the appearance of the brain scans were not due to ongoing pathology but to the effects of the previous trauma with ongoing absorption of damaged cells.

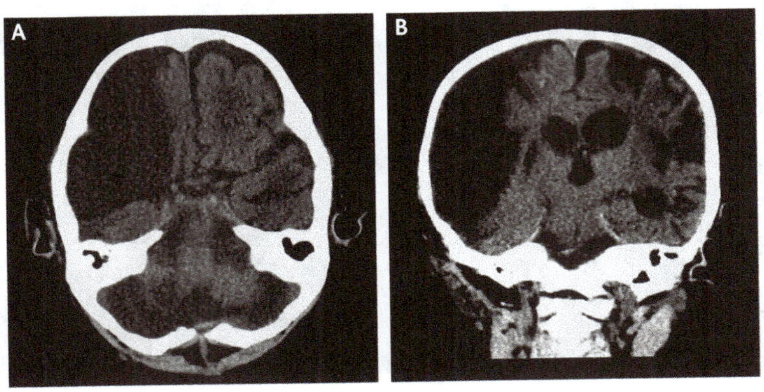

Figure 2-37A and B Clinical example Meg: axial and coronal CT images showing extensive atrophy.

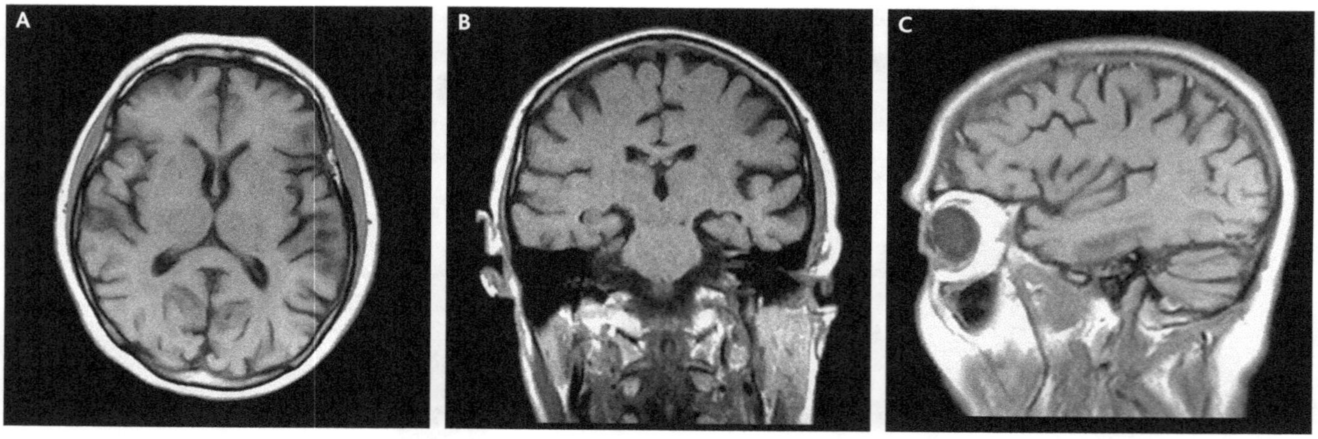

Figure 2-38A–C Brain scan appearing atrophied, although within normal limits for the 80 year old patient.

within normal limits for this geriatric patient in his 80s (Figures 2-38A–C). Lucian was functioning appropriate to his age and maintained an active life, without obvious deficits involving basic cognition, judgment, or self-help skills.

An atrophic appearance to the brain in an adult may be misleading and can suggest greater deficits than are actually evident. It is often not the extent of atrophy that is important but the age of the patient at the time of the injury or how much time has passed since the atrophic changes took place. If the cause of atrophy took place early in life, especially before 1 year of age, neural plasticity can compensate for tissue loss and functioning can become grossly normal (see Clinical Example Elliott).

CLINICAL EXAMPLE
Elliott: Previous Injury to the Brain

Elliott contracted encephalitis as a baby, resulting in significant diffuse damage to his brain. At 36 years of age, Elliott was referred for examination due to a refractory seizure disorder. Initial review of his brain scans revealed left medial temporal sclerosis but also an atrophic appearance to his brain (Figures 2-39A–C).

It was expected that his neuropsychological evaluation would demonstrate global cognitive and functional compromise commensurate with the appearance of his brain. However, his neuropsychological performance fell within normal limits for his age, with mild diminution of language skills but not of the extent to disrupt functioning.

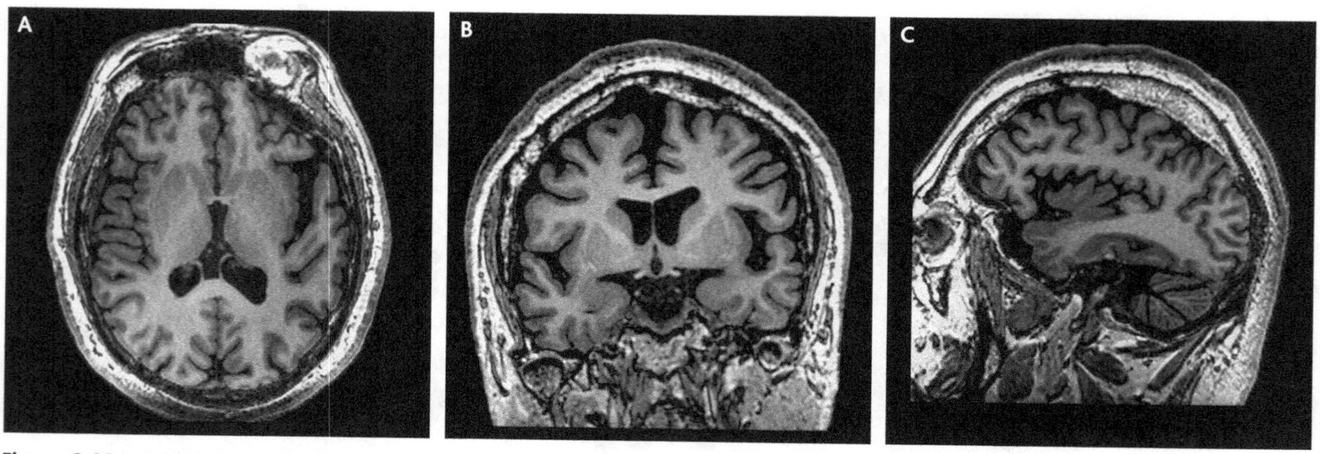

Figures 2-39A–C Clinical example Elliott: MRI T1 FSPGR series.

As part of his workup he was also to undergo a Wada evaluation necessitating continuous EEG recordings while each hemisphere of his brain was anesthetized one after the other to assess localization of language and memory functioning. Wada evaluation involves the introduction of a local anesthetic to the internal carotid distribution of the right or left hemisphere individually while the other hemisphere stays awake. This procedure enables the evaluation of language, memory, motor, and sensory-perceptual functioning of the nonanesthetized hemisphere. The EEG technologist was cautioned that his baseline EEG might show diffuse slowing, something frequently seen in those with global damage to the brain. However, his brain wave patterns were normal, with high-frequency, low-amplitude activity across all regions of this brain. It was further predicted that once either side of his brain was anesthetized during the Wada procedure, there would not be enough tissue on the other side to sustain full awareness and cognitive abilities; it was expected that he would either become obtunded or emotionally decompensate. Again, his performance during the Wada procedure was completely inconsistent with that expected; he remained awake, cooperative, interactive, and emotionally stable during examination and anesthesia of each hemisphere.

Apparently, Elliott's brain had recovered from his injury as a baby. The appearance of his brain many decades later was deceiving and resulted in incorrect clinical assumptions regarding expectations and functioning. The lesson to be learned from Elliott's case is that brain scans, with few exceptions, provide a picture of anatomical structures, not a measure of system functioning. Using the analogy from Chapter 1, Elliott's brain scan was the equivalent of a picture of an old, dirty car engine. The various evaluations were the equivalent of a series of test drives, which indicated that the car and engine functioned normally.

Temporal Effects due to Progression of an Illness

Traumatic or hypoxic injuries result in a relatively consistent pattern of changes to brain physiology over the first few weeks. Some brain conditions result in less consistent changes over time, with early imaging results being more difficult to interpret. For example, some forms of meningitis or encephalitis can result in changes to brain physiology many weeks after the onset of infection. In these cases, early review of brain imaging may be more useful in determining acute-care needs than long-term prognosis. Caution is warranted when reviewing brain scans involving infectious conditions, as imaging results obtained early in the process may be misleading. Some infectious processes such as coccidioidomycosis (cocci) meningitis or encephalitis can be difficult to treat, with complications such as hydrocephalus, inflammation, or infarction becoming evident many weeks after onset of the condition. Iatrogenic changes resulting from medication management can also cause injury to the brain many weeks after the start of medical care.

CLINICAL EXAMPLE
Tyler: Cocci Meningoencephalitis

Tyler was hospitalized with cocci meningitis. His initial brain imaging and early response to treatment were encouraging. Unfortunately, his infection progressed to involve brain structures in addition to the meningeal layers, resulting in meningoencephalitis. Once the infection had spread to his deep brain structures, there was a gradual deterioration of functioning over several weeks. Management of his infection and brain swelling included both medications and surgical intervention, although ultimately, neither were successful. Iatrogenic effects of the antifungal medications resulted in severe inflammation of the arachnoid layer, a condition called arachnoiditis.

Tyler's case highlights the importance of being cautious when predicting long-term prognosis from imaging acquired early in the course of an illness. In Tyler's case, the T2 FLAIR image acquired 2 weeks after hospitalization (Figure 2-40A) suggested a good prognosis. However, later studies were more representative of his condition and poor outcome (Figure 2-40B). Before using brain scans for long-term prognosis, consider the effects of illness progression and treatment.

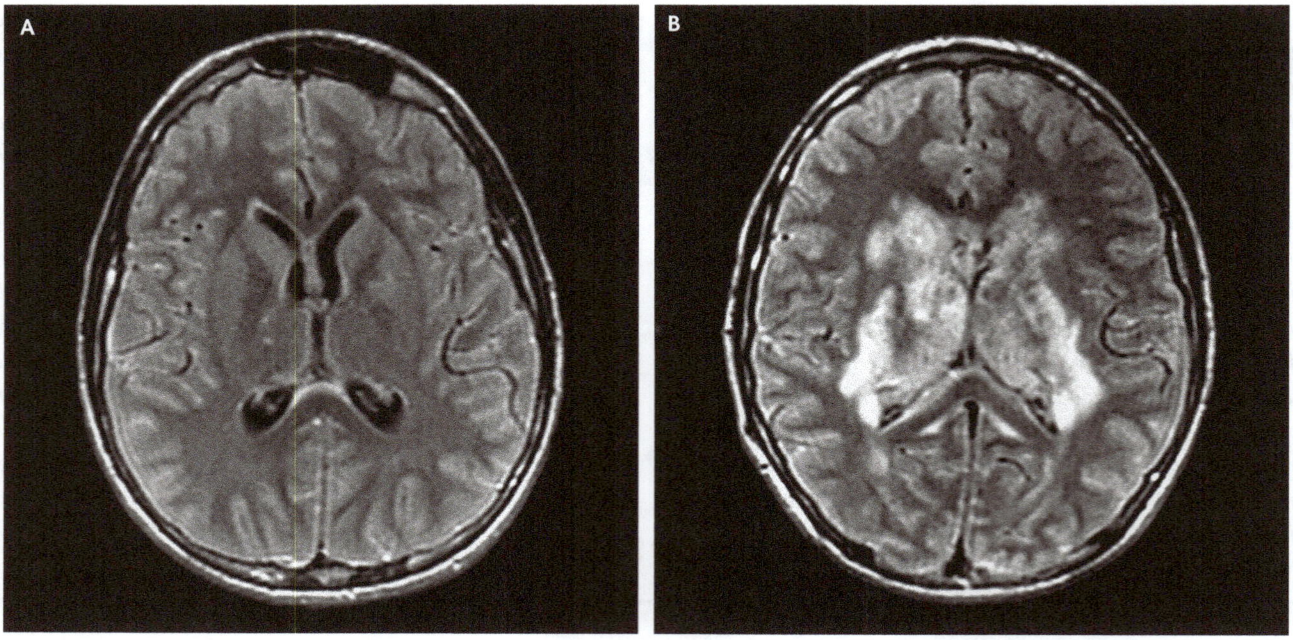

Figure 2-40 **A:** Clinical example Tyler: 2 weeks post–cocci infection. **B:** Clinical example Tyler: 6 weeks post–cocci infection.

Know what the imaging should look like before viewing it

When viewing brain scans with the goal of detecting pathology, it is helpful to formulate a concept of how the images should appear and what type of pathology might be expected. Forming a clear understanding of expected image appearance for a variety of pathologies using a number of different scans can take years of experience. It is not adequate to simply memorize tables providing such information; review of pathology on actual images is most beneficial. When first developing the ability to perform complex tasks, a degree of structure in the form of a workflow can be extremely helpful. As experience builds and one's abilities develop, rigid adherence to a highly structured workflow may not allow for the flexibility required to fully apply one's skills. When asked about their specific workflow when reviewing a series of scans, experienced radiologists generally indicate that they don't really think about a workflow; they just start with a specific scan and move on from there. For example, one radiologist reported, "I look at the T1 first because it is located on the screen to my left, and then I go from there. If I see something that looks like blood, I may jump to the GRE sequence, then to the FLAIR or DWI sequences. I really don't have a set workflow, I let the scans guide my approach."

One of the more difficult aspects of radiology interpretation relates to the difficulty of teaching others exactly what it is in a series of images that leads one to a specific conclusion. This is not unlike the elder clinician being able to recognize a subtle pattern of clinical findings as an unusual condition because of years of practicing "pattern recognition" but being unable to describe to medical students or residents what it was about the pattern that led to the diagnosis. Pattern recognition is critical in the interpretation of brain images and develops over years of experience and training. This is an area where a guide such as this will be unable to provide you with all of the information necessary to consistently recognize subtle patterns over a series of scans. The term *Aunt Minnie sign* has been used for many years to describe this phenomenon. The Aunt Minnie sign is based on a gestalt interpretation of findings, with a top-down approach of "seeing the whole" being more important than a bottom-up approach of analyzing the component details. "Aunt Minnie" conveys the experience of picking out a known aunt from a crowd of similar-appearing women. Finding Aunt Minnie in a crowd of other women who look like her and are dressed similarly is easy if you know her but is almost impossible if you don't know her, even when you have a basic description of her looks. Further, after seeing Aunt Minnie, it may be impossible to fully describe what it was about her features that made you recognize her out of all of the other women. The term has been attributed to two iconic radiologists from Children's Hospital Boston: Ed Neuhauser, M.D., who first coined the term, and Ben Felson, M.D., who popularized the term. Ironically, both deny ever having an aunt named Minnie (Hall & Griscom, 2008).

REFERENCE

Hall, F. M., & Griscom, N. T. (2008). Gestalt: Radiology's Aunt Minnie. *American Journal of Roentgenology, 191*(4), 1272.

Diagnostic Pitfalls of Neuroimaging

> "We see what we look for, and we recognize what we know."
>
> *Merrill C. Sosman, M.D. (1890–1959)*

Often there may be very little difference between a scan suggesting pathology and one read as normal. Findings on neuroimaging are frequently equivocal, with the radiologist having to make decisions qualified by statements such as "suggests, but is not conclusive" or "may be due to ..., although may also be a normal variant." As noted earlier, even imaging findings that appear definitive or pathognomonic may be of little clinical relevance. When viewing brain scans, it is important to understand the limitations of the technology, in addition to the limitations of the viewer. Following are some pitfalls that clinicians should avoid when assessing brain images from a clinical perspective.

Being Too Focused or Not Focused Enough

When viewing brain scans, there is a tendency to search for pathological signs that are expected and then stop searching once the "pathology" has been seen. This is not unlike the approach many take to clinical assessment. Given a clear history, a clinician may look for specific symptoms that match the patient's history or complaints and then fail to continue assessing for additional findings once the primary symptoms have been explained. However, the axiom "explanation does not imply etiology" becomes an important consideration when interpreting imaging findings. Put simply, just because the clinician discovers a cause for a symptom or condition does not mean that it is the only cause or even the primary one. From a clinical perspective, there may be multiple explanations for a particular symptom constellation, and discovering the correct one is critical to providing appropriate treatment and information to the patient and family. The same is true when reviewing brain scans. It is not uncommon for more than one feature on the scan to be viewed as an explanation for a particular condition, even though it may not be the primary factor or related to the condition. Thus during clinical examination, it is important to avoid the tendency to search for a finding that confirms one's clinical impressions and then stop the assessment. Likewise, when reviewing brain scans, it is important to avoid a confirmatory bias of looking for a finding that explains the symptoms and then moving on as if the assessment were completed.

When conducting diagnostic evaluations, clinicians are often taught two different approaches. One approach dictates that an evaluation take place without prior knowledge of the expected findings. This will minimize the chances of the clinician using a top-down bias to look for any findings that would confirm his or her expectations. The second approach posits that the clinician should focus the examination to a specific symptom constellation, or series of tests, based on prior knowledge about the patient's condition and expected findings. Both of these approaches have their advantages and disadvantages. The nonfocused or general approach has the advantage of allowing the clinician to evaluate all possible etiologies, instead of being narrowly focused on only a few findings. The disadvantage of this approach is that adequate attention may not be focused on the primary pathology, and if findings are subtle, they may be missed. The focused approach has the opposite problem. The advantage of the focused approach is the ability to do a very detailed evaluation regarding a specific condition or symptom constellation. The disadvantage is that other clinically relevant information may be missed because the examination is too narrow, the clinical equivalent of "tunnel vision." Ultimately, a combination of both a general and focused approach to interpreting brain scans will result in the most comprehensive assessment of neuroimaging. Unfortunately, with increasing time constraints imposed by a busy practice, there is a tendency for clinicians to rely too heavily on one or other of these approaches and not use both.

Pitfall: Being too focused and missing subtle but critical findings

Pitfall: Not being focused enough and failing to investigate subtle but relevant findings

Solution: Use both a general and focused approach to your assessment of brain scans.

If little is known about a patient's pathology, initially review the brain scans using a broad, general approach. Then, focus on specific areas of the brain in a systematic manner to ensure that you do not miss important information. For example, check for extra-axial and intraparenchymal bleeds, then check for edema or inflammation, then for disrupted diffusion, and so on until you have reviewed all areas of the brain and all common pathological processes.

If you have prior knowledge of the type, extent, and severity of a patient's brain injury, you may want to start by searching for the expected findings. However, then spend a few minutes reviewing other areas of the brain for additional types of pathology that may be missed. Sometimes, the smallest areas of damage cause the greatest functional deficits, especially if the damage involves subcortical nuclei or white-matter tracts.

Missing What Is Missing

Remember to look for what may be missing from the image to avoid "missing what's missing." We often spend so much time looking for pathological markers that we miss something that should be there but isn't. Common pathological features that may be missed without adequate attention include the following:

- Reduction in the gray–white differentiation, a sign of edema or encephalomalacia
- Effacement of the sulci–gyri cortical pattern, suggesting swelling
- A vessel that no longer appears on a CTA or MRA because of reduced blood flow
- Thinning or absence of the corpus callosum due to injury or abnormal brain development
- Absence of the septum pellucidum separating the two bodies of the lateral ventricles
- Structural damage obscured by edema or blood
- Loss of some cavities (ventricles, cisterns, aqueducts), suggesting mass effect on the brain
- No visible aneurysm on time-of-flight imaging, caused by loss of a flow signal within the aneurysm resulting from stagnant flow in the void
- Compromised cellular functioning at the microscopic or cellular level that is not visible on CT or most MRI sequences but may be evident on diffusion imaging

Missing Pathology in the Neutral Gray

Photography students are instructed to avoid having very bright or very dark features visible in the background of a picture. Bright or dark features attract visual attention and can distract the viewer from the subject of a photograph or a region of interest on a brain scan. In general, our eyes first look at the brightest part of a picture, then the darkest, and finally the neutral areas. The same is true for brain images; our eyes tend to first focus on the bright areas or the black areas and then the neutral gray. When pathology is subtle and located in the neutral gray or the parenchyma, it is easy to miss, especially if our attention is drawn to a bright or dark area away from the pathology.

CLINICAL EXAMPLE

Sarah: Stroke

Sarah had suffered a cerebral vascular accident affecting her right posterior cerebral artery, causing damage to her right medial occipital lobe. The stroke also resulted in diffuse brain swelling necessitating a frontal craniotomy to prevent herniation. Following resolution of the edema, her bone flap was

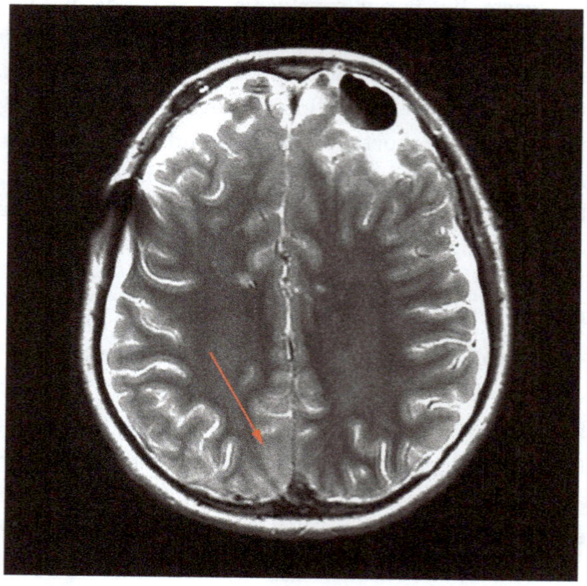

Figure 2-41 Clinical example Sarah: Note how easily the black area of pneumocephalus within the bright region of T2 hyperintensity draws your attention to the frontal lobes and away from the occipital lobes. The most clinically relevant injury to Sarah's brain involved the medial, and some lateral occipital cortex. Note the subtle T2 hyperintensity in the right medial occipital lobe (arrow).

replaced and she was transported to a rehabilitation facility. Upon initial review of her brain scans, the most salient feature was the bifrontal fluid and left frontal pneumocephalus caused by air under the bone flap (Figure 2-41). These findings were not a result of damage from the stroke but were secondary to the craniotomy.

Stop searching after finding an obvious abnormality

Almost without exception, traumatic, infectious, or hypoxic injuries to the brain involve more than one area or structure. Traumatic injuries resulting from physical forces with or without penetration can result in both focal and diffuse damage to brain tissue. Infectious or hypoxic conditions also result in a variety of severity levels across different regions of the brain and can be considered to involve both focal and diffuse components. Because of the heterogeneous nature of brain injury, one cannot assume that the first area of pathology is the only area of clinical concern. It is important to avoid becoming overfocused on the first signs of pathology and to continue reviewing the scans in order to rule out other regions that may be of clinical interest. Clinicians may be more likely to stop searching after finding the first obvious pathology when a patient's condition is neither severe nor mild. When there is severe damage to multiple areas of brain tissue, there is a tendency to search all areas of the brain to fully appreciate the extent of injury. When brain damage is mild and most of the brain structures appear within normal limits, a relatively quick review of the images may be adequate. However, for conditions that are between these extremes, there is a tendency to focus on the most salient region of pathology and conclude that it is the primary focus of interest. This can lead to the clinician prematurely stopping his or her search for pathology in other areas involving other tissues.

The tendency to stop searching after viewing the region of primary injury is greater when the main symptoms are consistent with that region. However, often there are other symptoms of clinical interest that are unrelated to the primary area of damage and that may not be readily accounted for on neuroimaging after a cursory review. When reviewing brain scans, it is important to remain undistracted by obvious pathology and to spend some time looking for more subtle signs of injury that may explain additional milder limitations in a patient's functioning. Conversely, if review of areas outside of the primary location of damage suggests additional pathology, it may be necessary to re-evaluate the patient for functional compromise related to those areas, which may have been missed during the initial assessment.

With subtle brain injury, rudimentary bedside neurological or mental-status examinations often fail to detect clinical findings relating to the injuries, and the patient's chart may simply indicate "neurologically intact." After discovering subtle findings on a brain scan that are separate from the primary region of injury, you may detect limitations in the patient in addition to the primary findings. If you stop your review of neuroimaging after finding the primary pathology, you will lose the opportunity to discover less salient areas of injury, which may be associated with subtle clinical symptoms in the patient. Sensitive assessment to evaluate such subtle limitations may make the difference between a comprehensive treatment plan for the patient and one that deals with only the primary deficits but not other problems restricting the functioning of the patient. Remember, the mild deficits may be more limiting to a patient than more obvious deficits, and failure to treat them may result in suboptimal recovery for your patient.

The following clinical cases involving Tatum and Kevin highlight the tendency to stop searching for pathology after finding the most obvious regions of damage as well as the value of extending one's review of scans to areas outside of the primary region of pathology. In each of these cases, the subtle clinical findings changed the patients' treatment plans, prognoses, need for accommodations, and interventions. The additional findings also enabled the provision of more comprehensive clinical information to the patients and their families, helping them make sense of their respective conditions.

CLINICAL EXAMPLE
Tatum: Viral Encephalitis

Tatum contracted viral encephalitis. Upon hospitalization and treatment, she appeared to show a relatively rapid recovery, and on bedside examination she had little difficulty interacting with staff and performing basic activities of daily living. The most obvious deficits from the infection related to her language functioning; however, she quickly recovered the ability to communicate verbally. Her parents described Tatum as being less talkative than before her illness. Following resolution of her viral infection and with medical stabilization, Tatum was discharged home with her parents.

Tatum was seen for a follow-up evaluation several weeks after discharge, and a new MRI series was acquired. At the time of her follow-up appointment, she was described as "becoming lost" in her own home and having difficulty with her vision. On assessment, she presented with intact visual processing ability, being able to describe and identify objects in a manner appropriate to her age without obvious difficulty. The only other complaint involved her affective state; she was described as emotionally labile, crying much of the time, and often becoming inconsolable.

Initial review of the brain scans revealed notable T2 FLAIR hyperintensities bilaterally within her visual association cortex. Damage was mostly localized to the medial cortex but also involved some lateral occipital cortex. Also remarkable on the images was the T2 hyperintensity of the bilateral occipital white matter, something that was not readily evident on imaging during her hospitalization. The "new" appearance of the white-matter T2 hyperintensity, most obvious on FLAIR sequences (Figure 2-42), suggested ongoing disruption of the white matter, possibly due to Wallerian degeneration or posterior reversible encephalopathy syndrome (PRES). The severity of the white-matter involvement with atrophy of the occipital poles indicated permanent injury more consistent with Wallerian degeneration than with PRES.

The damage to Tatum's visual association cortex explained the discrepancy between the difficulties described by her parents and the lack of findings on basic examination of visual acuity in the clinic. Bilateral damage to the medial occipital-lobe structures and secondary visual cortices can result in Balint's syndrome, a condition in which visual acuity and basic visual processing remain intact but higher-level visual processing required for spatial orientation, the perception of multiple visual features simultaneously, and the ability to integrate visual information with motor actions becomes disrupted. Although someone with Balint's syndrome can "see," they are unable to use the visual information functionally because of an inability to localize objects, relate what they see to personal space, or appreciate complex visual scenes. In effect, they become lost in their environment, unable to navigate visually or easily interact with the objects that they can "see."

Following review of the brain scans, the parents were asked to describe Tatum's visual difficulties in more detail. She was described as "becoming lost in her own home"; when she was only a few steps from her bedroom door, she was unable to find her bedroom from the living room. She was also noted to cry when asked to pick up objects from the floor and was unable to do so without assistance. Tatum was described as being perpetually scared and anxious, likely due to her feeling "lost" all of the time.

In Tatum's case, review of the brain scans enabled a more accurate description of her clinical condition and gave an explanation for her difficulties at home. The brain scans allowed for reconciliation of the discrepancy between her parent's report of visual difficulties and her "intact" basic visual acuity in the clinic.

After concluding that the damage on the brain scans was consistent with Tatum's symptoms, it would have been natural to cease reviewing the scans in detail and conclude that additional time spent with the scans would be unproductive. Not only were the areas of damage clearly evident on the scans, but they also fully explained the patient's symptoms. The expected yield from additional review of the images was low, as no other symptoms were evident on clinical examination or were described by Tatum's parents. However, additional review of the brain scans was conducted to ensure that nothing was missed. During the additional review of the scans, pathology was discovered in other areas of her brain. The T1 coronal sequences suggested right and left hippocampal atrophy consistent with bilateral medial temporal sclerosis (Figure 2-43).

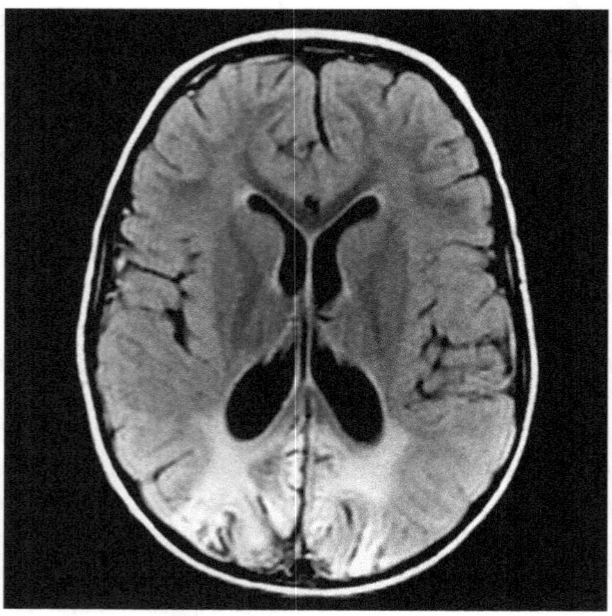

Figure 2-42 Clinical example Tatum: viral encephalitis T2 FLAIR sequence.

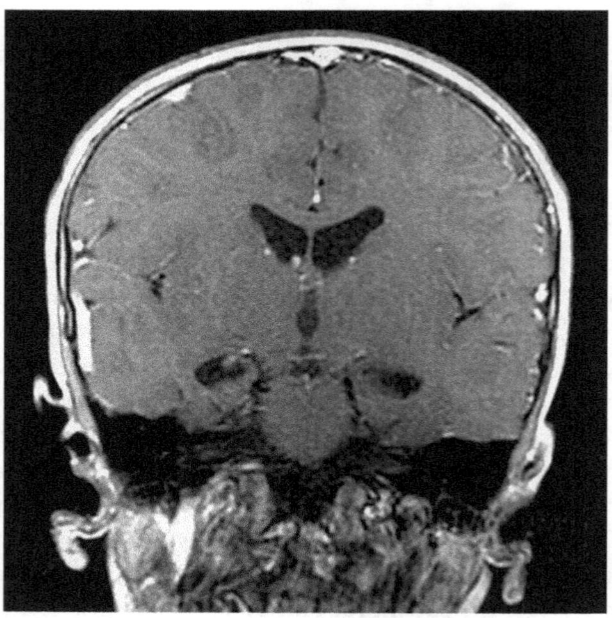

Figure 2-43 Clinical example Tatum: bilateral hippocampal damage T1 coronal sequence.

The finding of bilateral hippocampal atrophy was not initially identified, likely because the focus was primarily on the occipital lobe damage. In addition, there was no T2 hyperintensity in these structures, and they were difficult to appreciate using an axial image plane. Assessment of the T1 coronal and sagittal images was helpful in identifying the hippocampal damage. After observing the damage to her hippocampi, Tatum's parents were asked about Tatum's memory and learning ability. This line of questioning cued them to report that she had been unable to learn new information since her illness, something that had been a strength for her prior to the infection. Although she retained much of her previous learning, she did not appear able to consolidate new information, even with repetition and extra effort. Tatum was left with a severe anterograde amnestic condition requiring a higher level of supervision and educational instruction. Because of the retained old learning, Tatum's parents had concluded that her memory was fine, a frequent misunderstanding regarding the various forms of memory. Identifying the suspected hippocampal damage on imaging led to further investigation of Tatum's functioning and, ultimately, identification of unreported symptoms involving her memory. The additional information on Tatum's anterograde memory disorder changed her treatment plan in a significant way. Tatum required accommodations for her limited capacity to remember and learn, in addition to a structured program to assist her in compensating for her difficulties.

CLINICAL EXAMPLE
Kevin: Neoplasm

Kevin presented in the emergency room with complaints of persistent mild headache unresponsive to over-the-counter medications. The neurological and mental-status examinations were otherwise unremarkable, and he was described as being fully functional without limitation or deficit. Initially, the emergency room physicians wanted to discharge him with some prescription medications, even though Kevin insisted that his headaches were "not normal for him," a concern that precipitated a CT scan. The CT suggested a very large right-hemisphere neoplasm, with follow-up MRI suggesting extensive right-hemisphere peri-Sylvian involvement with mass effect, midline shift, and uncal herniation. Kevin was fast-tracked to neurosurgery service. Given the size of the tumor and the expected extent of resection, information regarding the lateralization of language was critical in considering a surgical approach. Wada evaluation was scheduled that afternoon and conducted the next morning.

Unfortunately, during the pre-injection angiogram for the right-hemisphere procedure, it was discovered that Kevin had a fetal posterior cerebral artery originating from the internal carotid (Figures 2-44A and B arrows). If the anesthetic were introduced to the internal carotid distribution, the backflow would result in anesthesia of the brain stem and respiratory arrest. As such, the right injection was not performed. A small minority of patients have some persistence of the fetal posterior cerebral artery, which originates at the internal carotid artery during the embryological stage of development. Normally, with ongoing development, the posterior cerebral artery will attach to the basilar artery, and the vessel between the internal carotid and the basilar shrinks to become the posterior communicating artery.

Left hemisphere injection and anesthesia suggested that Kevin's language was localized predominantly within the left hemisphere. The assessment also suggested memory functioning using only the right hippocampus was compromised, as expected given the infiltration of the tumor into the right hippocampal structures.

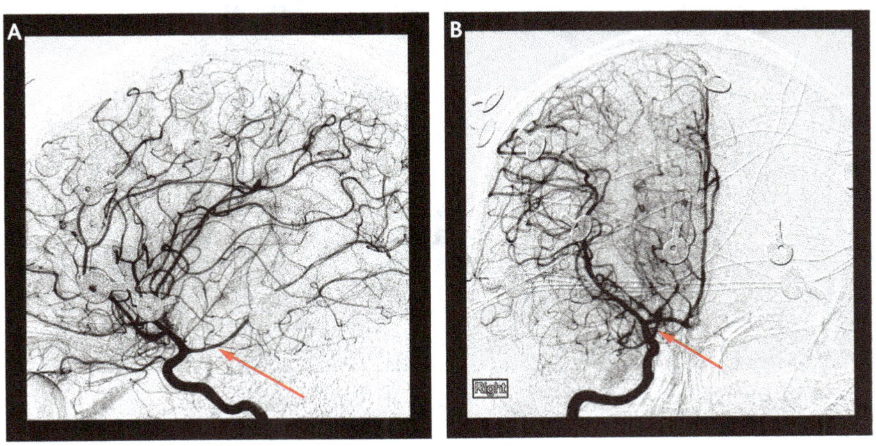

Figures 2-44A and B Clinical example Kevin: Angiography showing the fetal posterior cerebral artery originating from the right internal carotid distribution.

On the basis of the patient's reported normal memory functioning during his initial neurological examination and tumor involvement of the right hippocampal structures, it was assumed that the left hippocampus was fully functional. A healthy left hippocampus would suggest that resection of the tumor could be aggressive and include the right hippocampus without significant disruption of general memory. In addition, with the initial examination suggesting intact language, along with the Wada results suggesting left-hemisphere language representation, it was concluded that the surgery could take place without significant risk to language. This information also suggested that the resection could be relatively aggressive without severe harm to language functioning. It is important to consider that these conclusions were based on a review of the imaging data that was focused on the brain tumor, not structures that were some distance from the tumor boundary. As expected, given such obvious pathology, review of other areas of the brain was not as extensive as that of the neoplasm.

During additional, more detailed review of Kevin's brain scans, it became apparent that he likely had bilateral hippocampal damage, not just disruption of the right hippocampus due to tumor growth. When viewing brain scans, it is always important to consider the wisdom of the axiom, "you can have a cold and a broken leg at the same time, and they do not need to be related." Once the primary pathology has been observed, it is important to assess other structures that may be of clinical concern. In Kevin's case, additional review of his brain scans suggested possible medial temporal sclerosis of the left hippocampus (arrows), most evident on coronal T2 FLAIR sequences (Figures 2-45A–C).

The suspected left medial temporal sclerosis may have beeen unrelated to the tumor or possibly due to subclinical electrical disruption via the pathway that connects the two hippocampi, a concept referred to as "kindling." The suggestion of bilateral hippocampal damage upon further review of Kevin's MRI images resulted in a significant modification of his presurgical workup and, ultimately, his surgery.

The appearance of possible left hippocampal atrophy, with known dysfunction of the right hippocampus on Wada assessment, was inconsistent with the clinical findings of Kevin having fully intact cognitive functioning. Such inconsistency in clinical and radiological findings precipitated comprehensive neuropsychological evaluation of Kevin's cognitive abilities. Such evaluations are much more sensitive to subtle functional compromise than bedside mental-status or neurological examinations and can take several hours. Neuropsychological examination findings suggested deficiencies involving anterograde memory for both visual and verbal information, with performance falling below the first percentile for immediate, delayed, and recognition memory. Deficits were also evident for day-to-day activities, such as Kevin not remembering what he had eaten for lunch or what he had watched on television that afternoon, only a few hours before the assessment. The deficits were not related to attention, effort, affective disruption, or cultural or language barriers. This pattern of performance is highly suggestive of an organically based memory impairment related to disruption of both hippocampi and surrounding tissue.

The additional review of Kevin's MRI scans resulted in suspicion of possible bilateral hippocampal damage. This finding precipitated further examination of cognition and memory via neuropsychological assessment, which confirmed the suspicion of bilateral hippocampal compromise. The additional information ultimately resulted in a full re-evaluation of the surgical plan. It was decided that the surgery should be conducted in a manner to retain the right medial temporal-lobe structures. Given the poor memory performance using both hippocampi on neuropsychological examination as well as compromised performance on Wada examination using just the right hemisphere,

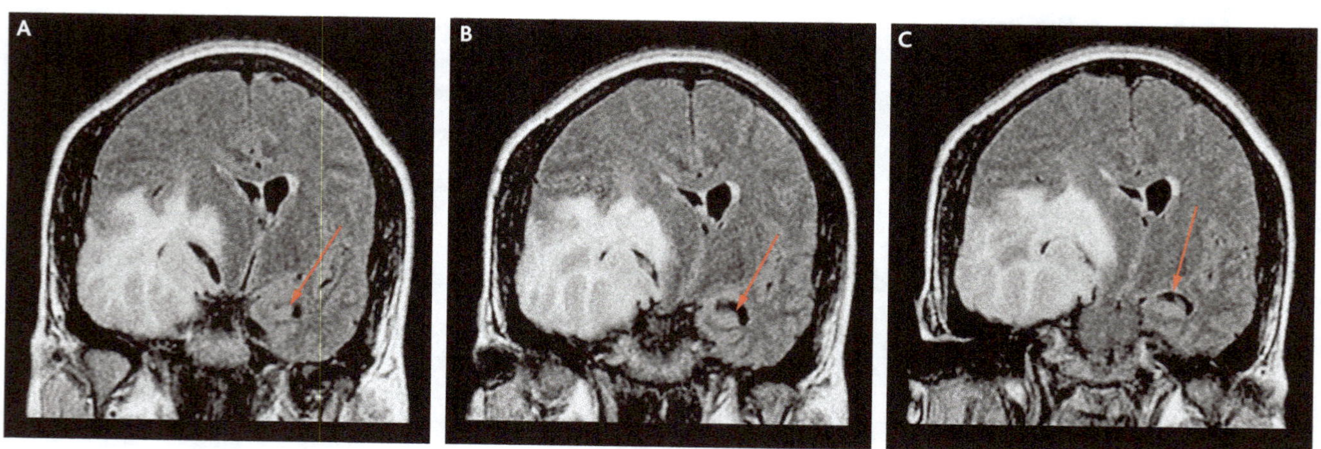

Figures 2-45A–C Clinical example Kevin: T2 FLAIR sequences moving from anterior (A) to posterior (C) showing medial temporal sclerosis involving the left hippocampus (arrows).

it was concluded that the left hippocampus was also likely compromised. Resection of the right hippocampal structures would most likely reduce memory ability even more and could result in greater anterograde amnesia, of the magnitude to prevent normal functioning. Retaining the right hippocampal structures allowed Kevin to retain premorbid memory functioning after his surgery, thus preventing a significant cognitive disability.

Tatum and Kevin's cases provide excellent examples of how one can become overly focused on the obvious pathology, resulting in a failure to give adequate attention to other areas of the brain. These case examples also demonstrate how the additional information provided by the secondary review of the scans can change one's clinical conclusions, treatment plan, prognoses, and decisions regarding appropriate interventions or accommodations. Those extra few minutes of image review following assessment of the primary or obvious damage can result in information critical to the clinician; information that can change a patient's life forever.

PEARL Most brain injuries involve pathology in a variety of tissues and anatomical structures.

Remember to look for pathological markers in a variety of brain areas and tissue types such as the meninges, white matter, gray matter, ventricles, and blood vessels, in addition to brain parenchyma.

PERIL Prematurely concluding that you have "seen the pathology," before searching for other clinically relevant markers, can result in your missing important additional findings. Don't stop evaluating the scan once you "find" the first evidence of pathology. Generally, the most obvious injury is the first seen by the viewer, although this injury may not be most clinically relevant. For example, a large epidural bleed may be immediately evident on the brain scan but have limited utility in clinical management once the bleed has been evacuated. Smaller petechial hemorrhages within the frontal lobes or subcortical white matter may severely disrupt the patient's functioning and, ultimately, his or her ability to be safely discharged home without rehabilitative services or supervision. As such, the smaller, easily missed markers of diffuse axonal injury may be more important to patient care than the larger bleed.

Consider all possible causes for a particular "pathological" appearance

Just as a car engine can look damaged but run well, it is not uncommon for brain scans to have the appearance of abnormality or damage, without functional deficit or clinical relevance. Many benign developmental conditions, such as cysts or vascular "abnormalities," can give the appearance of pathology but remain clinically benign. Most of the time, such anatomical anomalies remain undiscovered until the person receives a scan for other reasons, at which time the anomaly is discovered. It is important to take active steps to prevent becoming distracted by the anomaly and to instead focus on the clinically relevant features of the scan.

Many "pathological" signs may be present for nonpathological reasons. Interpreting nonpathological features as pathological will result in false-positive findings and clinical error. Examples of some conditions that mimic pathological processes include the following:

- Appearance of asymmetry or sulcal enlargement caused by the head being turned slightly in the scanner
- Mild T2 hyperintensity around the frontal horns of the lateral ventricles can suggest transependymal edema, although is often a normal occurrence in the nonclinical population.
- Incidental white-matter lesions in asymptomatic persons can be of little clinical relevance.
- Bright appearance on diffusion-weighted imaging but without disrupted diffusion, with the hyperintensity caused by T2 shine-through
- Contrast-enhancing ring suggesting a high-grade tumor, but actually due to a variety of processes such as an abscess, tuberculosis, demyelinating lesion, or chemo/radiation necrosis
- Appearance suggesting diffuse atrophy (ventricular dilation, prominence of the cisterns and sulci–gyri pattern) but which is the result of high-dose steroids, normal aging, or other nonpathological conditions
- Appearance of a lesion caused by imaging artifacts

PEARL A finding on a brain scan that offers a solid explanation for a particular clinical symptom may actually be unrelated to the symptom. Being able to put aside the finding and consider other alternative explanations may uncover the real reason for the symptoms. There is a tendency to interpret any abnormal appearance on a brain scan as being the explanation for a particular condition, even if the area involved is unrelated. This follows the incorrect assumption that "because there is brain damage, deficits or patient complaints must be related to that damage." However, an abnormal appearance on brain scans may be completely benign and unrelated to any complaints or concerns expressed by the patient. Do not become so focused on something that appears abnormal that you forget your basic skills as a clinician. It is important to understand that even excellent explanations may be incorrect or misleading, especially those related to static pictures of the brain: Explanation does not imply etiology.

PERIL Try to avoid using brain scans to search for a reason why a patient is experiencing symptoms. At times, even normal brain scans can appear abnormal for a variety of reasons or may show abnormalities that are benign or artifact. If you look for an explanation, you will be more likely to consider any abnormality on a brain scan as a cause for a symptom, even if there is no clinical relationship. Such assumptions can result in incorrect diagnostic conclusions, failure to provide appropriate treatments, and, ultimately, harm to the patient.

Pitfalls of Knowing the Neuropathology and Anatomy of the Injury

Although a strong background in neuroanatomy is exceedingly helpful when viewing brain scans, there are some pitfalls to be aware of that can result from too much reliance on anatomical knowledge. The most common clinical errors resulting from one's anatomical knowledge include the following:

- Assuming that all patients have the same anatomy. Intrasurgical brain mapping and, more recently, the use of functional imaging such as fMRI, MEG, PET, and SPECT have provided evidence that some degree of anatomical variability between persons is normal.
- Assuming that pathology will result in loss of functioning
- Assuming that pathology in a specific region will result in specific deficits normally attributed to that region
- Assuming that a patient with a "normal scan" will function normally and that one with an abnormal scan will have deficits
- Overpathologizing or looking for evidence of dysfunction in a patient in order to fit findings on a scan; interpreting normal variation in functioning as pathological just because if fits with your expectations from viewing the brain scans

Quality of Brain Imaging

Brain image quality is dependent on several characteristics of the scanning technology. Contrast and spatial resolution, noise and artifact suppression, and linearity all affect how an image appears. A change in any of the many scanning parameters will change the appearance of tissues on a brain scan. The goal of manipulating parameters is to provide an image that has the best contrast and spatial resolution for a particular tissue, substance or physiological process, while also maximizing the signal-to-noise ratio, or image quality. Adjustment of scanning parameters can have trade-offs, with improvements to some aspects of the image but degradation of others. For example, changing the parameters of a CT scan to highlight bone will result in excellent bone resolution but with a lower signal-to-noise ratio for soft tissues, degrading resolution or brain parenchyma. The trade-off is that an image of bone lacks soft-tissue resolution, and an image set for brain tissue lacks good bone resolution. Out of all the characteristics of brain imaging, the most disruptive to the viewer are those that involve image noise and artifacts.

At the simplest level, brain imaging involves the conversion of three-dimensional (3D) tissue to either a two-dimensional image formed from pixels or a three-dimensional matrix formed from voxels (3D pixels). Each pixel or voxel contains a value dependent on the type of sensor used to scan the patient. For example, values derived from a CT scan correlate with the absorption profile for the tissue (how much ionizing radiation is absorbed). The values from an MRI are based on a variety of tissue characteristics, such as the proton relaxation times corresponding to T1 or T2. The precision of a scan relates to the degree to which a particular pixel or voxel value actually represents or corresponds to the tissue characteristics being scanned. If the pixel value is affected by noise or artifact, the image ceases to be a true representation of the tissue being scanned.

The concept of signal detection suggests that there are four possible outcomes when one is attempting to detect a signal or pathology on a scan. The four signal-detection outcomes are indicted in Tables 2-6A and 2-6B.

TABLE 2-6A Signal Detection Theory Terminology

Hit	Correctly identifying a signal
Miss	Not detecting a signal that is present
False alarm	Incorrectly identifying a signal when one is not present
Correct rejection	Correctly failing to identify a signal when one is not present

TABLE 2-6B Signal Detection Theory Decision Options

	SIGNAL/ PATHOLOGY = PRESENT	SIGNAL/ PATHOLOGY = ABSENT
Viewer decision = present	Hit	False alarm
Viewer decision = absent	Miss	Correct rejection

When there is a strong signal, with little noise or artifact (high signal-to-noise ratio), the chances of a hit or correct rejection increase, and the chances of error involving a miss or false alarm decrease. When the signal is weak and there is a lot of noise or artifact (low signal-to-noise ratio), the chances of error increase (miss or false alarm), while the chances of correctly identifying the signal (hit) or correctly determining that there is no signal (correct rejection) decline.

Noise and artifacts reduce the clarity of an image, which may result in a failure to appreciate a small lesion (miss). Conversely, if the viewer mistakenly interprets noise or an artifact as evidence of pathology, he or she has also erred and produced a false alarm. Large lesions are more readily interpreted and result in more hits and correct rejections. However, even large features can be related to noise or artifact and require consideration from the viewer.

DICOM Viewers

There are a variety of software packages available to view DICOM images. DICOM stands for **D**igital **I**maging and **Co**mmunications in **M**edicine and is the standard format for storing, transmitting, and viewing medical images. Although each DICOM viewer works a little differently, they all have similar features.

When learning to interpret brain scans using sheets of film, no image adjustments were possible. The best view that could be achieved was to hold the sheets of film up to a variety of light sources in order to highlight a specific structure or pathology. Most of the time, film was viewed using a light-box, a device that produced relatively uniform light across the sheet of film. With the change to digital images, the ability to adjust the image appearance on a computer screen has become a critical component to viewing radiology images. One of the more useful features of a DICOM viewer is the ability to control contrast and brightness of an image. This tool allows one to adjust the contrast and brightness of images in order to highlight certain aspects of the scan, especially when wishing to assess darker or lighter areas over those that are neutral gray.

It is critical that you remain aware of how the DICOM viewer adjustments can affect your interpretation of the images and the relevance of findings. For example, a failure to take into account the contrast/brightness settings when interpreting gray–white differentiation may lead you to over- or underinterpret the findings. Because the gray–white differentiation on a brain scan is dependent on the contrast differences between tissues, any change of contrast/brightness by the viewer can either attenuate or exaggerate the apparent difference between the tissues. In addition, when considering the appearance of pathological tissues, be aware that changing the DICOM settings may also change the appearance of the tissue. For example, when assessing tissue density differences on a CT scan or inflammation on a T2 sequence, contrast or brightness adjustments can attenuate or exaggerate the pathological appearance. In general, the DICOM settings can make light areas look brighter, and dark areas look darker. If comparing two or more images, it is helpful to set the brightness and contrast for each image to be equivalent. Without doing so, it will be more difficult to make any comparisons between the images.

Most networked DICOM viewers, such as the Picture Archiving and Communication System (PACS), provide a scale from black to white with a series of grayscale steps useful in calibrating a particular monitor's contrast and brightness level. This is especially useful for networked systems in which the images may be viewed on many different monitors (CRT and LCD) distributed around a facility.

Comparing Scans Acquired on Different Occasions

Comparison between images obtained on different occasions is becoming more common, especially as the availability of serial scanning has increased. Given the dynamic nature of many neurological conditions, follow-up brain imaging has become a valuable tool in monitoring illness progression or the effects of a specific treatment regimen. To assist the clinician in comparing images obtained on two or more occasions, DICOM viewers often have the ability to load multiple scans in order to provide simultaneous displays using a window-based system. Some viewers also allow one to synchronize the scans so that as you scroll through one, the other will scroll at the same rate. Synchronization of scrolling allows one to quickly review scans taken on different occasions without having to switch back and forth between them to set the specific image slice.

When comparing images obtained during different sessions, spend extra time analyzing the images to determine whether the differences are due to changes in pathology or are related to the angle of the head, relative position of the slices, or the thickness of the slices.

When different imaging sequences are obtained during the same session, the patient's head remains in the same position for all sequences. However, when images are obtained from different sessions, the patient's head may be positioned in the scanner at a slightly different position or angle, resulting in slices being acquired at a different angle or level. This is especially true if the images are acquired with thick slices of approximately 5 mm or more. In these cases, smaller brain structures or pathological findings may be evident on one occasion but not on the next, owing to the structures or pathology falling between the relatively thick image slices. Comparison of such images may suggest a change in anatomy or pathology, when the difference is actually an artifact of the technology. Similar errors are possible when the acquisition angle is different between sessions, resulting in the images having a different appearance because of the different image plane angle, not any pathological process. Being aware of such possibilities will minimize the chances that you will make mistakes in your interpretations.

Presentation of Simultaneous Images

Computer rendering software allows the viewer to simultaneously present all three orientations on one or more screens (Figure 2-46). As one scrolls through a particular slice, reference lines appear on images from other orientations, providing a reference to the primary slice position. The ability to view all image planes simultaneously allows for pseudo-3D viewing; one can appreciate the area from different angles by visualizing a variety of acquisition planes.

At times, it is beneficial to put several images of the same orientation on a screen. With many imaging protocols producing a variety of sequences from a single orientation, DICOM viewers allow one to compare similar slices and areas of interest using different sequence parameters. Figure 2-47 is a screen shot showing simultaneous presentation of axial slices produced using T2, T1, DTI-FA, and color DTI-FA sequences.

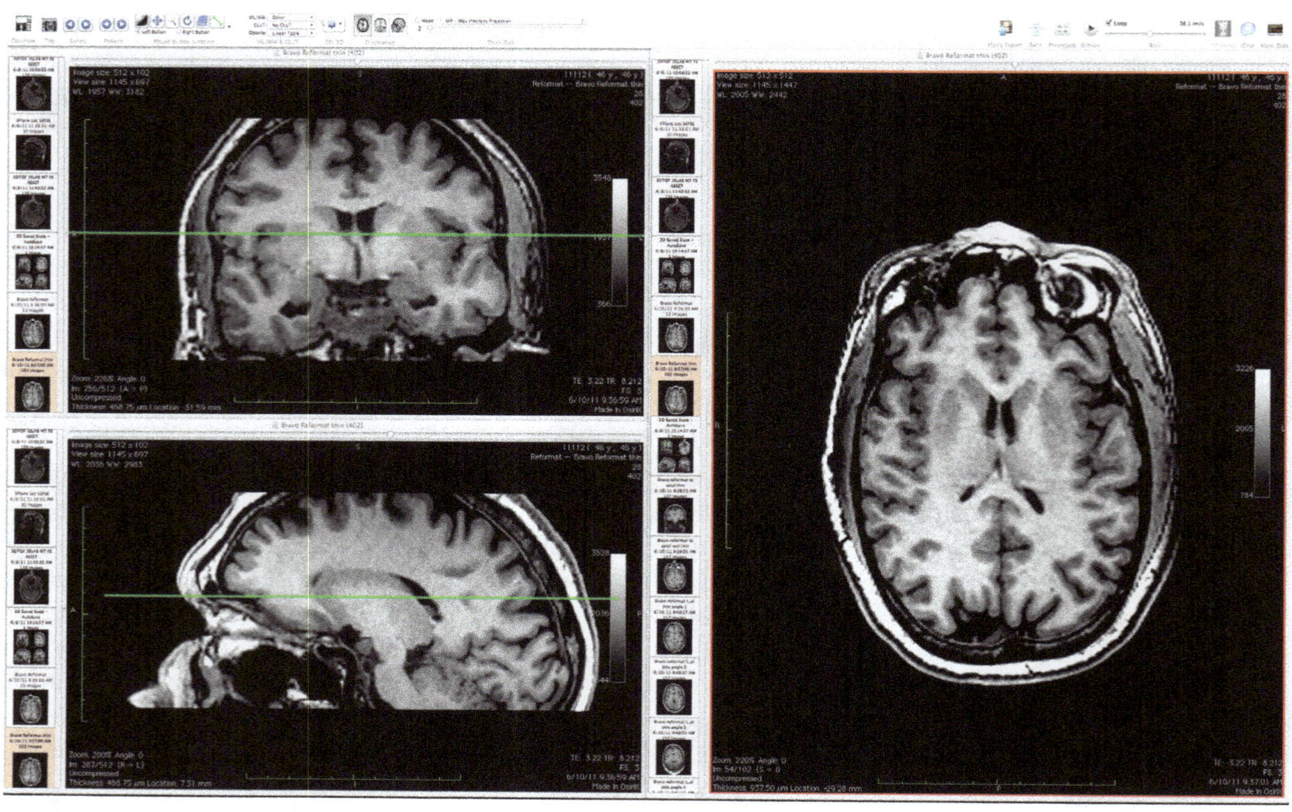

Figure 2-46 OsiriX screen capture.

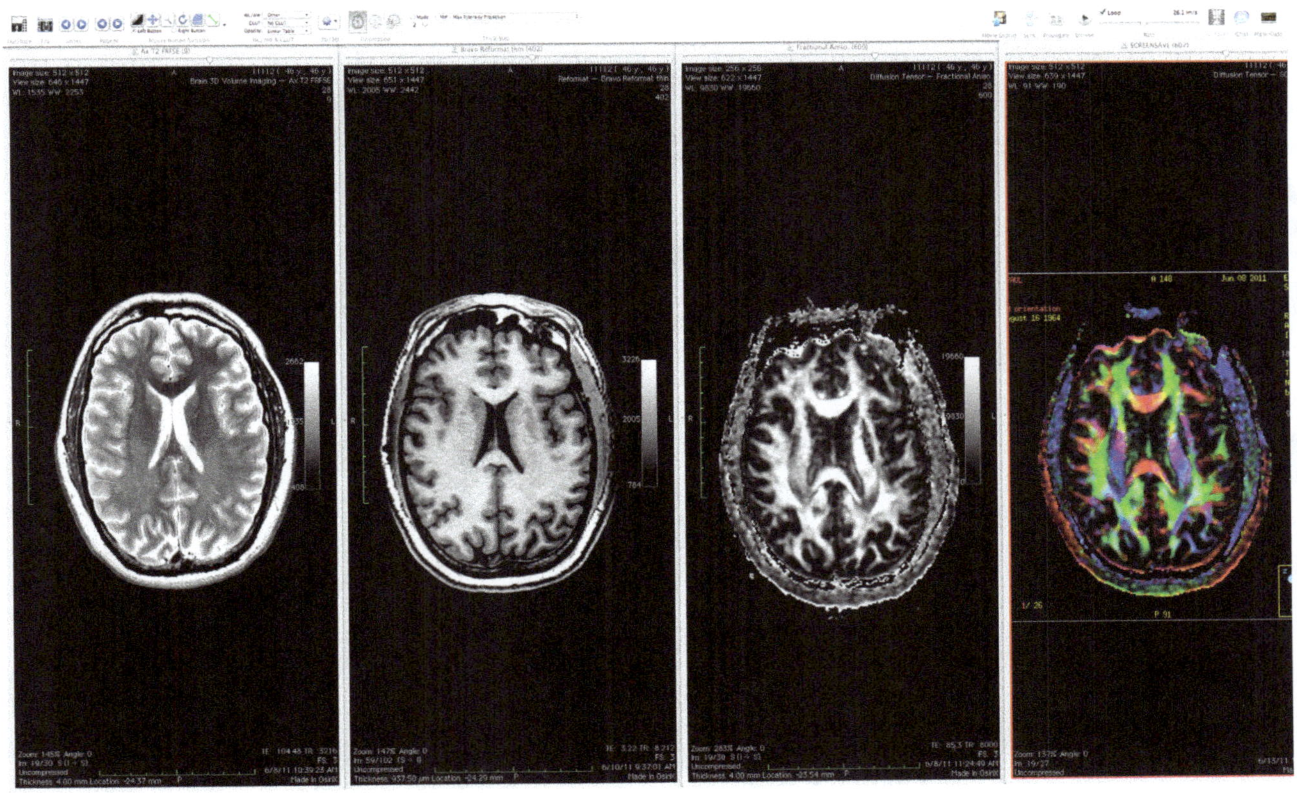

Figure 2-47 OsiriX screen capture of axial slices produced using T2, T1, DWI-FA, and color DWI-FA sequences.

When viewing brain scans, the ability to assess multiple images simultaneously can make interpretation much easier and should be your standard practice. It may take some time to become familiar with a particular DICOM viewer, but the time will be well spent, as the advantages of simultaneous viewing are profound, especially when first developing your skills.

Recognizing that the appearance of an area suggests pathology is only one component of using brain scans clinically. It is important for you to gain a basic understanding of how to interpret different types of brain scans and determine whether there is pathology in a particular area. Just as important to you clinically is the ability to easily identify key neuroanatomical structures using brain images in order to determine how the pathology may affect your patient's functioning. Chapter 3 will present imaging-based neuroanatomy using a format similar to that available with DICOM viewers. For example, anatomical areas will be presented in multiple orientations, with reference lines to assist you in determining the source position of a particular slice. A color-coded system will be used that is not currently available on DICOM viewers but was incorporated into this text to assist you in developing your ability to identify various key structures or regions on brain scans.

3

IMAGING-BASED NEUROANATOMY

Knowledge about the primary anatomical landmarks visible on brain scans is critical to accurate interpretation. Neuroanatomy courses or textbooks often present brain structures in multicolored diagrams or pictures with obvious margins between structures or cortical regions. On an actual brain, structures are much more difficult to differentiate, and cortical regions may have no identifiable margins. This is most evident with the regions of cortex at the back of the brain and close to the parietal, occipital, and temporal lobes. Other areas of the brain are more easily identified, though still not as easily as suggested by many anatomy texts. Presenting the brain as a series of two-dimensional black and white slices makes structure identification even more difficult, especially for the clinician without specific training or years of experience reading and interpreting brain imaging.

When using brain scans, limitations in technology can result in poor visual resolution between neighboring structures or regions of the brain. This is most evident on CT scans, as density or absorption of the ionizing radiation dictates how a specific area will be displayed on the final image. Areas with similar absorption profiles will look the same on the scan, making it difficult to accurately identify transitions between structures or regions. Sometimes the use of different types of images or different image sequences can assist in differentiating structures of the brain, as various technologies or image-rendering techniques highlight tissue in different ways.

The use of multiple orientations can also assist in identifying many structures of the brain. Often, an area may be more easily visualized using one particular axis (axial, coronal or sagittal) than with another. Knowledge of the primary anatomical landmarks and brain structures can assist in identifying less obvious structures or regions. Once these landmarks are recognized, knowledge of the spatial relationship between subtle brain structures and the landmarks allows one to easily find them on the scans. General guidelines can also be helpful in identifying areas of the brain depicted on an image.

This chapter will highlight the primary anatomical areas of the brain using brain images taken from all three primary axes, along with three-dimensional graphics, anatomical dissection views, and pictures from a brain model. General guidelines will be introduced to assist the reader in identifying primary brain structures that are often of clinical importance.

Many image examples in this chapter use MRI T1 spoiled gradient echo sequences using 3D FSPGR, BRAVO or MPRAGE protocols for high-contrast resolution between gray and white matter. T1 3D FSPGR, BRAVO and MPRAGE sequences are acquired using imaging parameters designed to emphasize the contrast between gray and white matter, with square voxels of equal length sides to allow three-dimensional reconstruction and re-slicing using different angles and slice thinknesses.

Reference Lines

Throughout the remainder of this text, color-coded borders and reference lines are included in many examples. To maintain consistency and assist the reader, axial images have a green border, coronal images have a red border and sagittal images have a blue border. Figure 3-1 provides

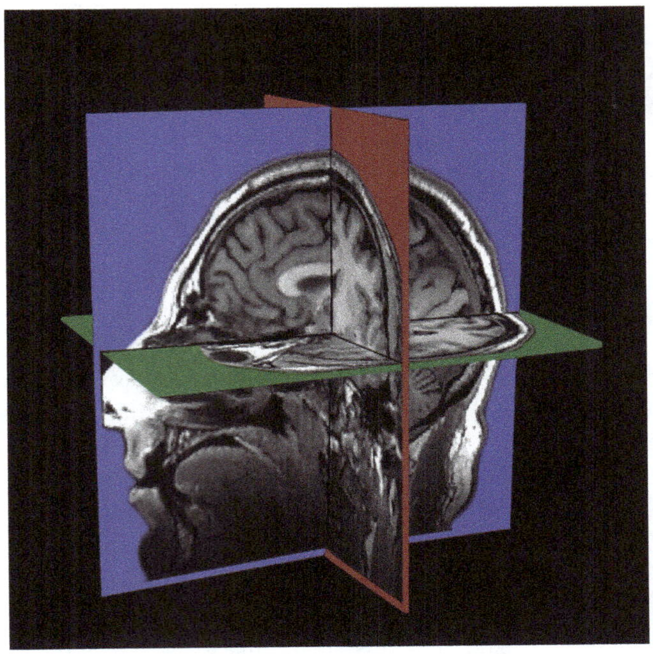

Figure 3-1 Green: Horizontal/lateral cut, or the axial plane. Red: vertical/lateral cut, or coronal plane. Blue: longitudinal cut, or sagittal plane.

a three-dimensional example of the colors used for the primary slice orientations. In addition, all of the reference lines used throughout this book will have the same color-coded format. For an axial image with a green border, the source location will be indicated on coronal and sagittal images by a green line. For coronal images with a red border, the source location will be indicated on axial and sagittal images as a red line. For sagittal images with a blue border, the source location will be indicated on axial and coronal images as a blue line. Regions of interest (ROI) are often identified by the intersection of the colored reference lines. For most examples, the axial, coronal, and sagittal slices were chosen because they intersect at a particular ROI. For images containing more than one ROI, the one identified by the intersecting lines was chosen as an exemplar, or the primary ROI. For example, on a coronal image showing the hippocampi, only one hippocampus is identified by the intersection of the lines. In this case, the ROI is an example and should not be interpreted as the only structure or lesion referenced in the text.

Anatomy texts often introduce brain structures using a logical progression from the outer cortical layers to the deeper nuclei or vice versa. Or structures are introduced according to functional units, with sections dedicated to motor, sensory, emotional, intellectual, or other functional domains. Sometimes anatomy texts introduce structures in the order of development, beginning with embryological divisions and progressing to adult divisions. This guide will use a relatively unusual approach to neuroanatomy, in that the order of presentation for different brain structures will not follow a standard anatomical or developmental approach. When viewing brain scans, it is helpful to first identify primary landmarks and then use the landmarks to identify other structures on the basis of their relative positions. For example, when attempting to identify the head of the caudate nuclei on a brain scan, the easiest approach is to first locate the body of the lateral ventricles and then identify the small area of gray matter on the lateral wall of the ventricle, just medial to the white matter tract of the internal capsule. Accordingly, this chapter will first introduce structures and tissues that make up the primary landmarks. It will then cover the other regions of the brain in a more standard anatomical approach.

PRIMARY ANATOMICAL LANDMARKS

When identifying neuroanatomical structures on brain images, it is helpful to have a basic understanding of the location in relation to primary landmarks. The landmarks used here were chosen because of their ease of viewing on brain scans and their locations in the brain. The ventricles

Neuroanatomy often elicits apprehension and anxiety in many students. With advances in technology and the use of three-dimensional graphics the study of neuroanatomy has become less arduous and even pleasurable for many more students. In the past, radiology-based neuroanatomy required the study of two-dimensional images along with an ability to form three-dimensional internal mental representations of brain space, something that many found challenging. Today, three-dimensional rendering is available on many imaging workstations, desktop or laptop computers, or even portable devices such as smartphones, tablet computers, or other devices. In addition, the use of three-dimensional brain models enables visual and tactile learning of brain structures and organization, especially if the model is produced to represent the same proportions as on an average human brain.

To assist you in learning basic neuroanatomy, this guide includes screenshots from a three-dimensional brain atlas[1] available on a desktop computer or iPad or iPhone, color photographs of a brain model[2], color photographs of coronal brain sections, and black and white photographs of brain and skull sections from a dissection guide[3]. Such multimodal learning allows for a level of anatomical understanding not possible with two-dimensional drawings or brain scans. It is hoped that the use of the different types of illustrations will assist you in this endeavor.

[1] Permission was kindly granted to publish three-dimensional images from the 3D brain atlas originally created by AXS Biomedical Animation Studio, Incorporated, as part of the 3D Brain, an interactive atlas of the human brain created for Cold Spring Harbor's Dolan DNA Learning Center. The 3D Brain is available as a free iPhone or iPad App and online at Genes to Cognition (G2C) Online. Images © 2005–2009, Cold Spring Harbor Laboratory. All rights reserved.

[2] Permission was kindly granted by Somso, Inc., to use pictures of their brain model BS 25.

[3] Black and white dissection images were adapted with permission from Bruni & Montemurro (2009). *Human Neuroanatomy, A Text, Brain Atlas, and Laboratory Dissection Guide*. New York: Oxford University Press.

and cisterns are useful as landmarks because they are located throughout the brain and are filled with cerebral spinal fluid (CSF), which shows up easily on all major types of brain imaging. Other structures that are located throughout the brain and are relatively easy to differentiate on brain scans are the axon pathways that run across the brain from one side to the other, down the brain from the cortical regions to the spinal cord, or between the front and brain of the back.

Ventricles

The ventricles provide the clearest landmarks on a brain scan and simplify the task of identifying many other brain structures on the images. The ventricles located throughout most of the brain and the CSF contained within the structures are readily visible on a variety of brain imaging sequences. Areas most easily located using the ventricles include the structures of the basal ganglia, the hypothalamic region, the brain stem structures, and many white-matter pathways, such as the corpus callosum and optic radiations. As you progress through this chapter, consider the relationship of the many structures presented to key regions of the ventricular system, or the primary cisterns. For example, after reading this chapter you should be able to quickly locate the head of the caudate nucleus on any brain slice (axial, coronal, or sagittal). The head of the caudate is identified as a gray-matter structure that makes up the outside wall of the frontal horns of the lateral ventricles. Similarly, locating the optic radiations is simple given that they make up the lateral wall of the occipital horns of the ventricular system.

The body makes approximately 500–600 milliliters of CSF each day—about the same amount of fluid as contained in a 16-ounce water bottle. Most CSF is made by the choroid plexus, a collection of epithelial and vascular tissue located in the ventricles. Of note, choroid plexus is not located within the frontal horns of the lateral ventricles nor in the cerebral aqueduct of Sylvius. Because the choroid plexus is highly vascular, on brain imaging it can have the appearance of blood (Figures 3-2A–C arrows).

CSF flows under pressure from the lateral ventricles to the third ventricle located in the center of the brain. From the third ventricle, the fluid flows down a small tube-like structure called the cerebral aqueduct of Sylvius to the fourth ventricle. Eventually the CSF flows to the outside of the brain and spinal cord into the arachnoid layer and to various other cavities called cisterns. Ultimately, the CSF is reabsorbed into the venous blood supply via the arachnoid granulations located within the superior sagittal sinus.

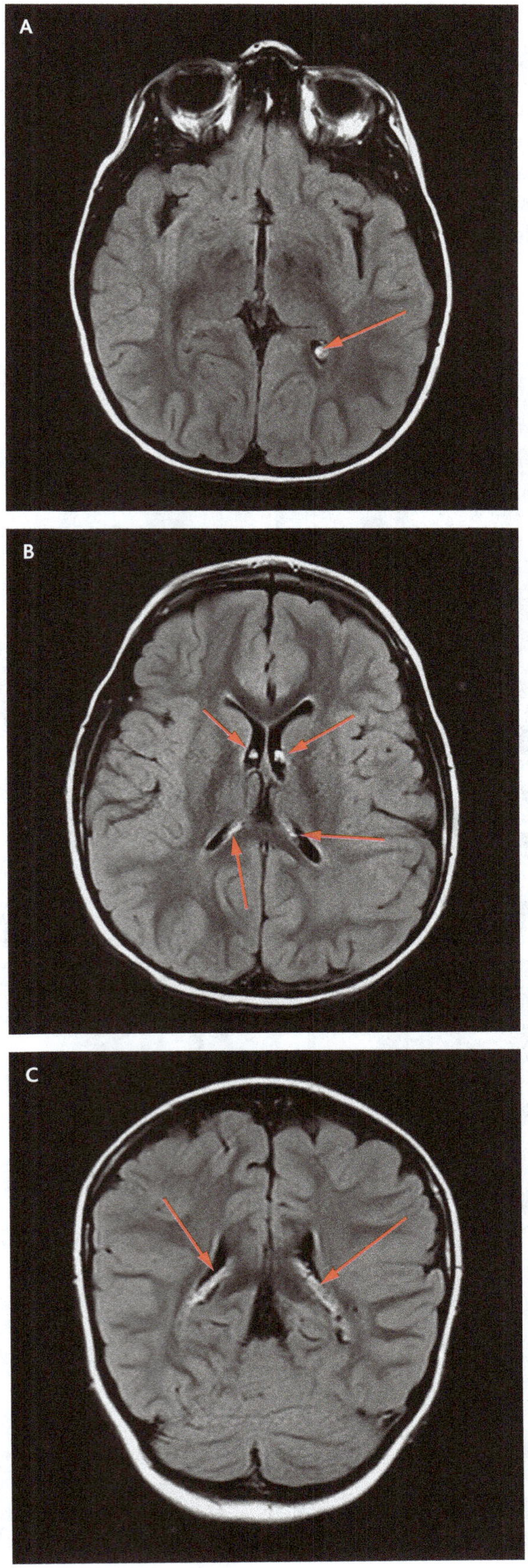

Figures 3-2A–C Choroid plexus. Note the bright appearance of the choroid plexus within the ventricles.

The various segments of the ventricles are shown within the three-dimensional illustration of the brain from an anterior, lateral and superior perspective (Figures 3-3A–C). The ventricles are also illustrated using brain sections, with the slices being acquired from an anterior location (Figure 3-4A) to a more central location (Figures 3-4B and C) and also a posterior location (Figure 3-4D). Figures 3-5A and B provide a graphical reference to the slice locations used to show the ventricles on cornal image sections (Figures 3-5C–F) with the slices being acquired from anteriorally (c) to posteriorally (f). Figures 3-6A and 3-6B provide a graphical reference to the slice locations used to show the ventricles on axial image sections (Figures 3-6C-F) with the slices being acquired from an inferior level (c) to a superior level (f). Figures 3-7A–C provide examples of sagittal images slices cutting through various segments of the ventricular system, with figure 3-7A being acquired from a mid-sagittal location, and Figures 3-7B–C being acquired more laterally.

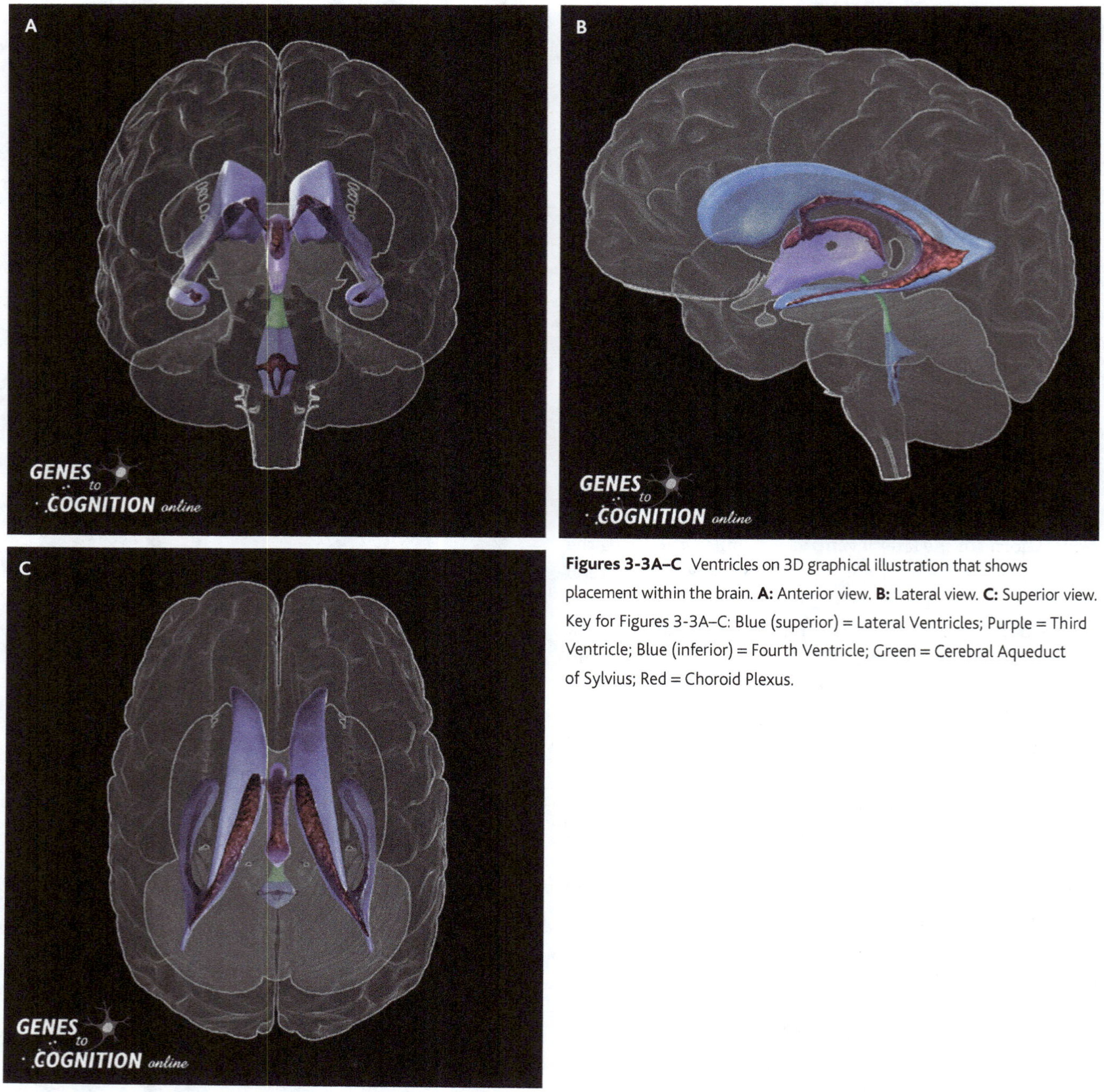

Figures 3-3A–C Ventricles on 3D graphical illustration that shows placement within the brain. **A:** Anterior view. **B:** Lateral view. **C:** Superior view. Key for Figures 3-3A–C: Blue (superior) = Lateral Ventricles; Purple = Third Ventricle; Blue (inferior) = Fourth Ventricle; Green = Cerebral Aqueduct of Sylvius; Red = Choroid Plexus.

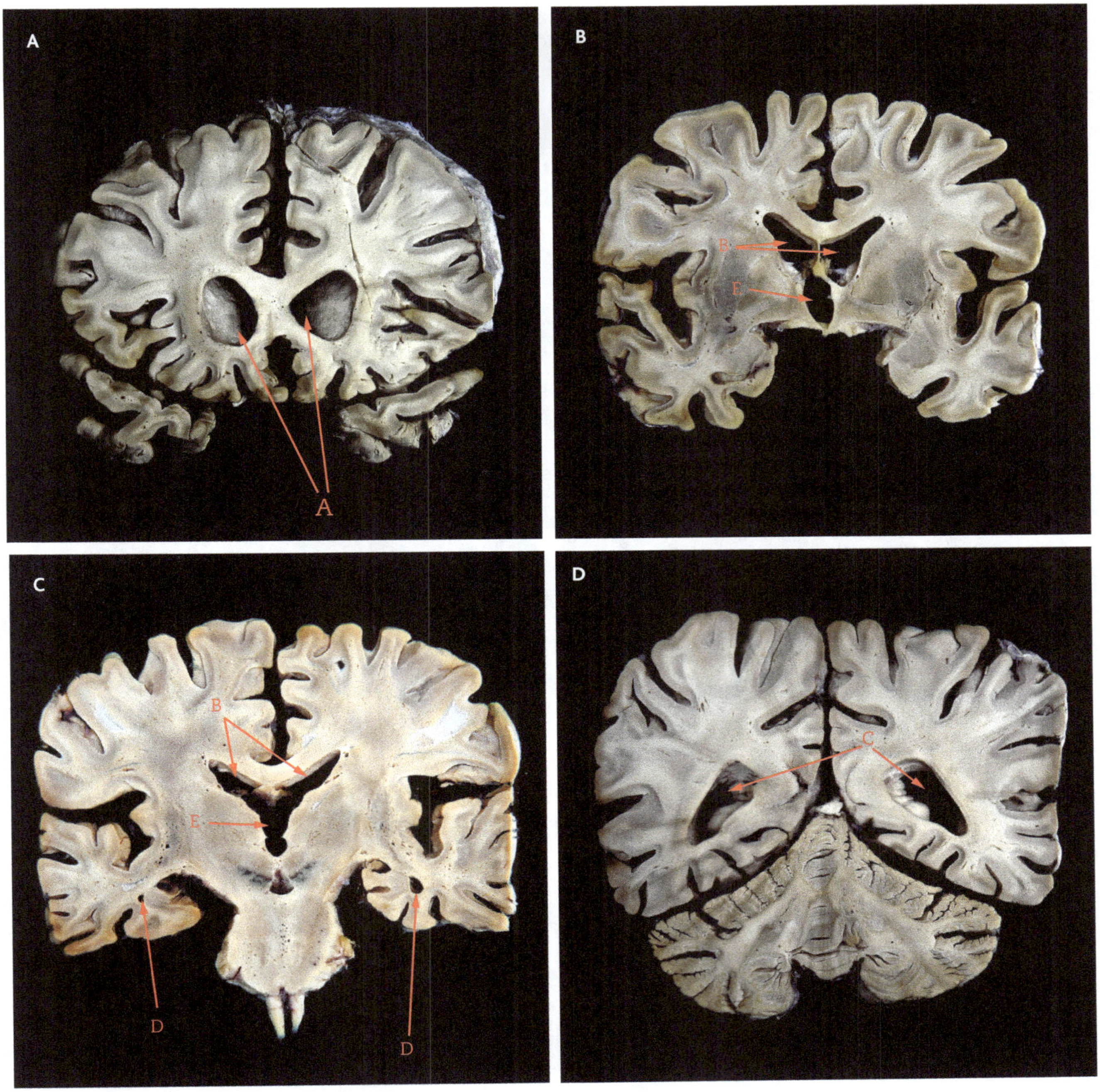

Figures 3-4A–D Ventricles on coronal brain sections. **A:** Anterior. **B:** Central. **C:** Central. **D:** Posterior. Key provided below.

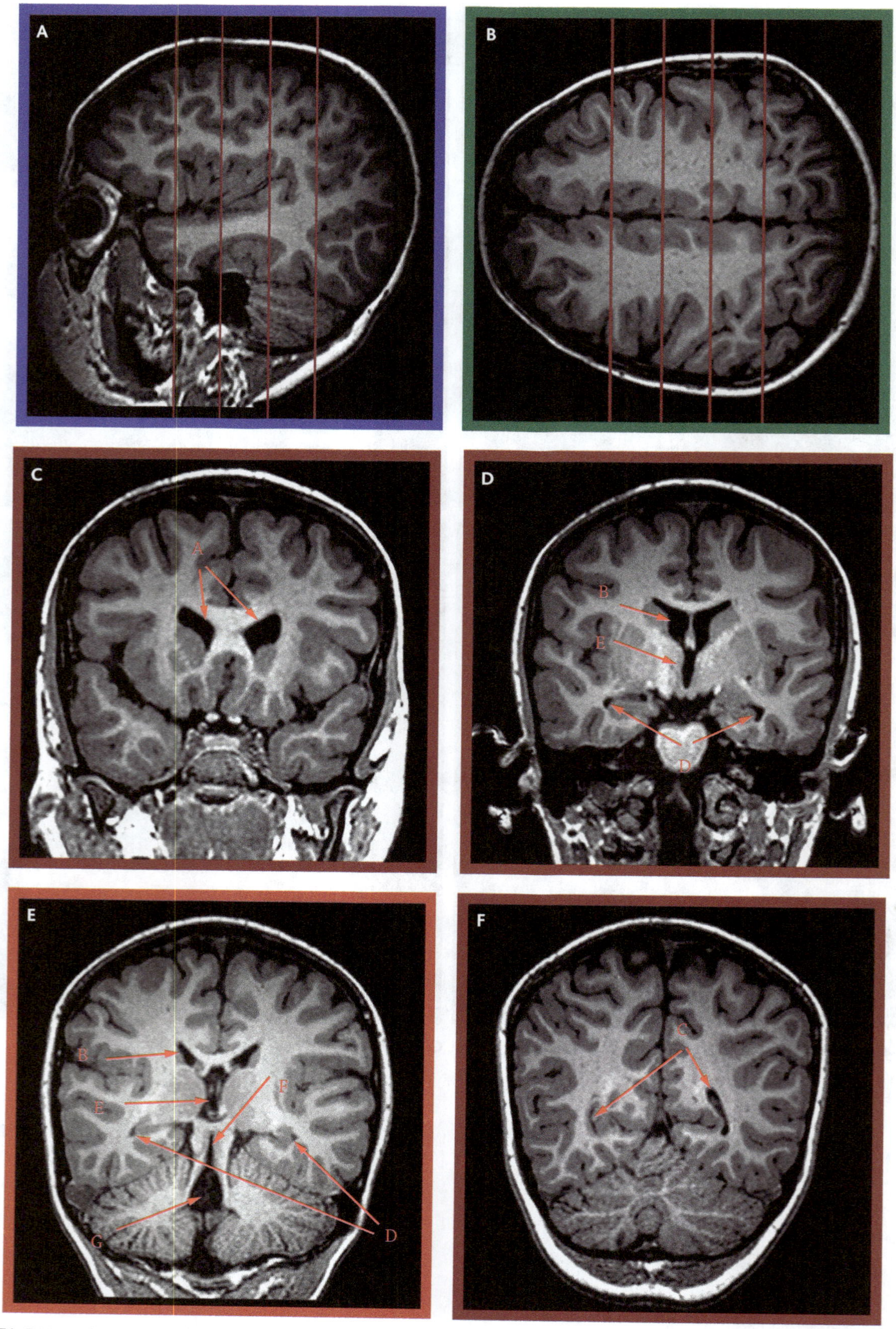

Figures 3-5A–F Ventricles on coronal MRI. The red reference lines on the sagittal and axial slices correspond to the locations of the coronal images, with 3-5C being most anterior and 3-5F most posterior. Key provided below.

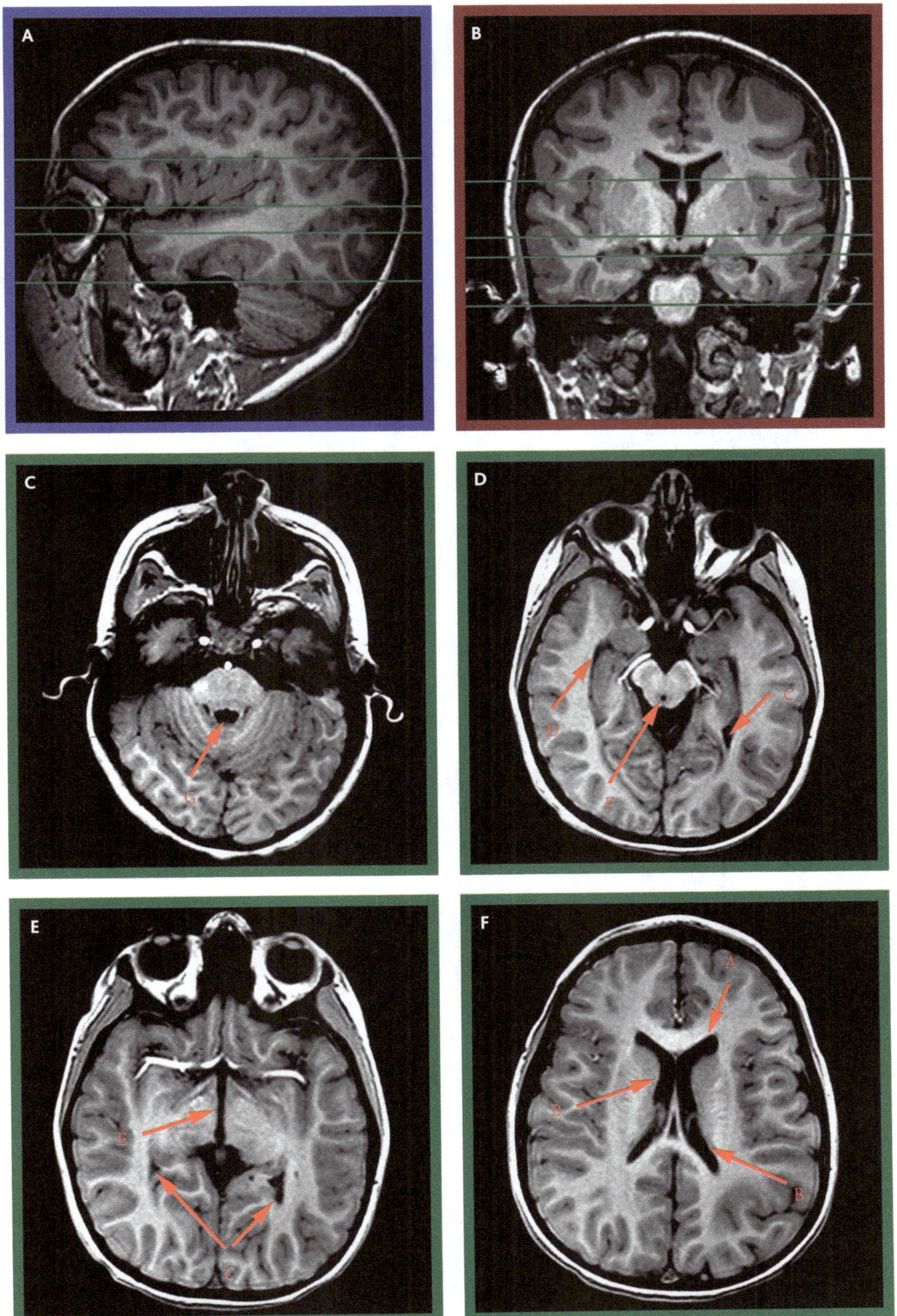

Figures 3-6A–F Ventricles on axial MRI. The green reference lines on the sagittal and coronal slices correspond to the locations of the axial images, with 3-6C being most inferior and 3-6F most superior. Key provided below.

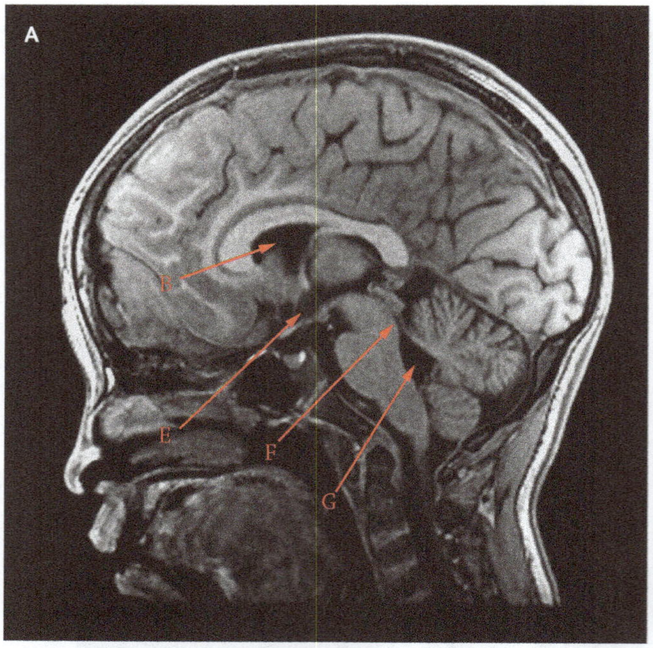

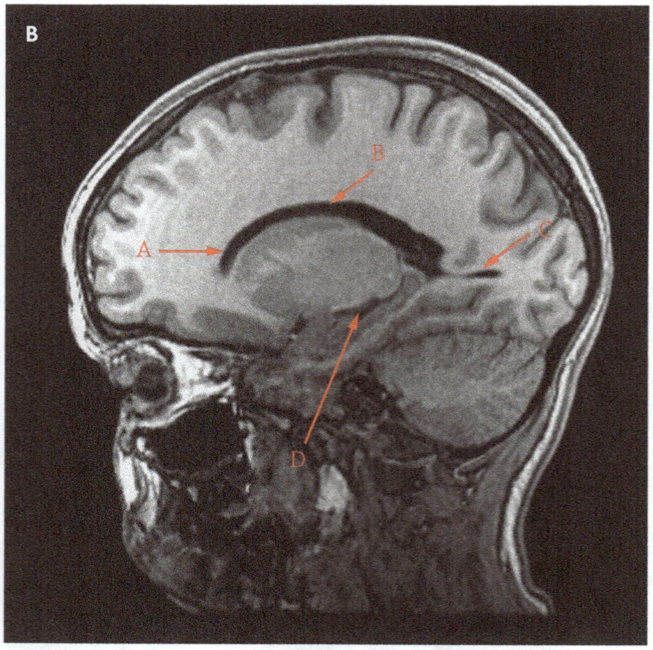

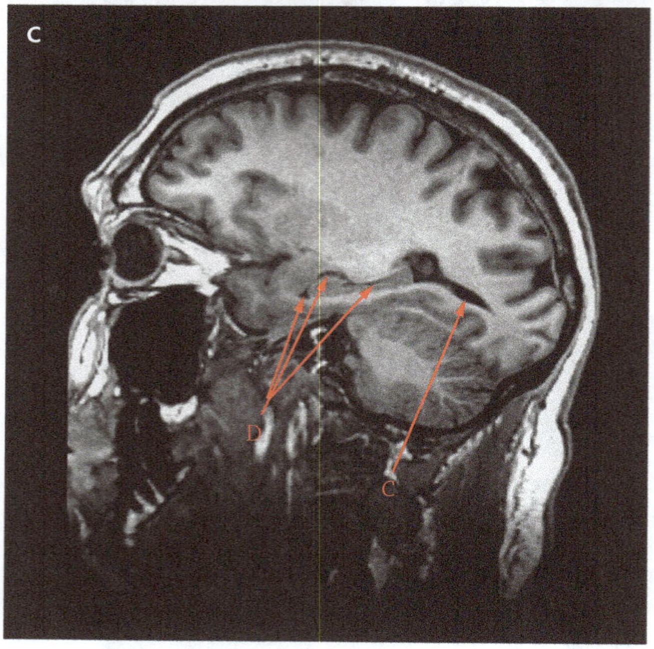

Figures 3-7A–C Ventricles on sagittal MRI.

Key for Figures 3-4A to 3-7C: A = Lateral Ventricles - Frontal Horn/s; B = Lateral Ventricles - Body; C = Lateral Ventricles - Atrium/Trigone to Posterior (occipital) Horn/s; D = Lateral Ventricles - Inferior (temporal) Horn/s; E = Third Ventricle; F = Cerebral Aqueduct of Sylvius; G = Fourth Ventricle.

PEARL Axial and coronal images are produced using a variety of acquisition angles. This results in the ventricles having a different appearance depending on the angle used (Figures 3-8A and B). When using the ventricles as anatomical landmarks or when interpreting pathology based on the appearance of the ventricles, it is helpful to consider the three-dimensional structure and not memorize the two-dimensional appearance on a particular brain slice. Once you have a good understanding of the three-dimensional shape of the ventricles, variations in image plane angle becomes less problematic and ventricles can be useful landmarks no matter what the acquisition angle.

PERIL When comparing axial CT with axial MRI, there is a tendency to expect that the ventricles will appear similar on the two images. However, acquisition angles for CT and MRI scans are frequently different, making direct comparison difficult. Try to get out of the habit of assessing the ventricular system using a predetermined mental image of how it should look on a particular brain slice. The more you consider the three-dimensional nature of the ventricles, the easier it is to compare images acquired using different technologies, on different occasions, or with different acquisition angles.

To illustrate the effects of various axial slice angles on the appearance of the ventricles, the sequences in Figures 3-8A and 3-8B are shown with different axial acquisition angles. The yellow lines on the sagittal images provide a reference showing the location of the axial slice and angle used to produce the axial images. For comparison purposes, the axial-image slices were set so that both pass through the genu of the corpus callosum. Because of the different slice angles, the axial images provide very different views of the ventricles.

In Figure 3-8A, the slice passes through almost the entire body of the lateral ventricle, with no other segments of the ventricular system being visible. In Figure 3-8B, the slice passes through the frontal or anterior horns of the lateral ventricles, the third ventricle, and the posterior horns of the lateral ventricles close to the atrium or trigone.

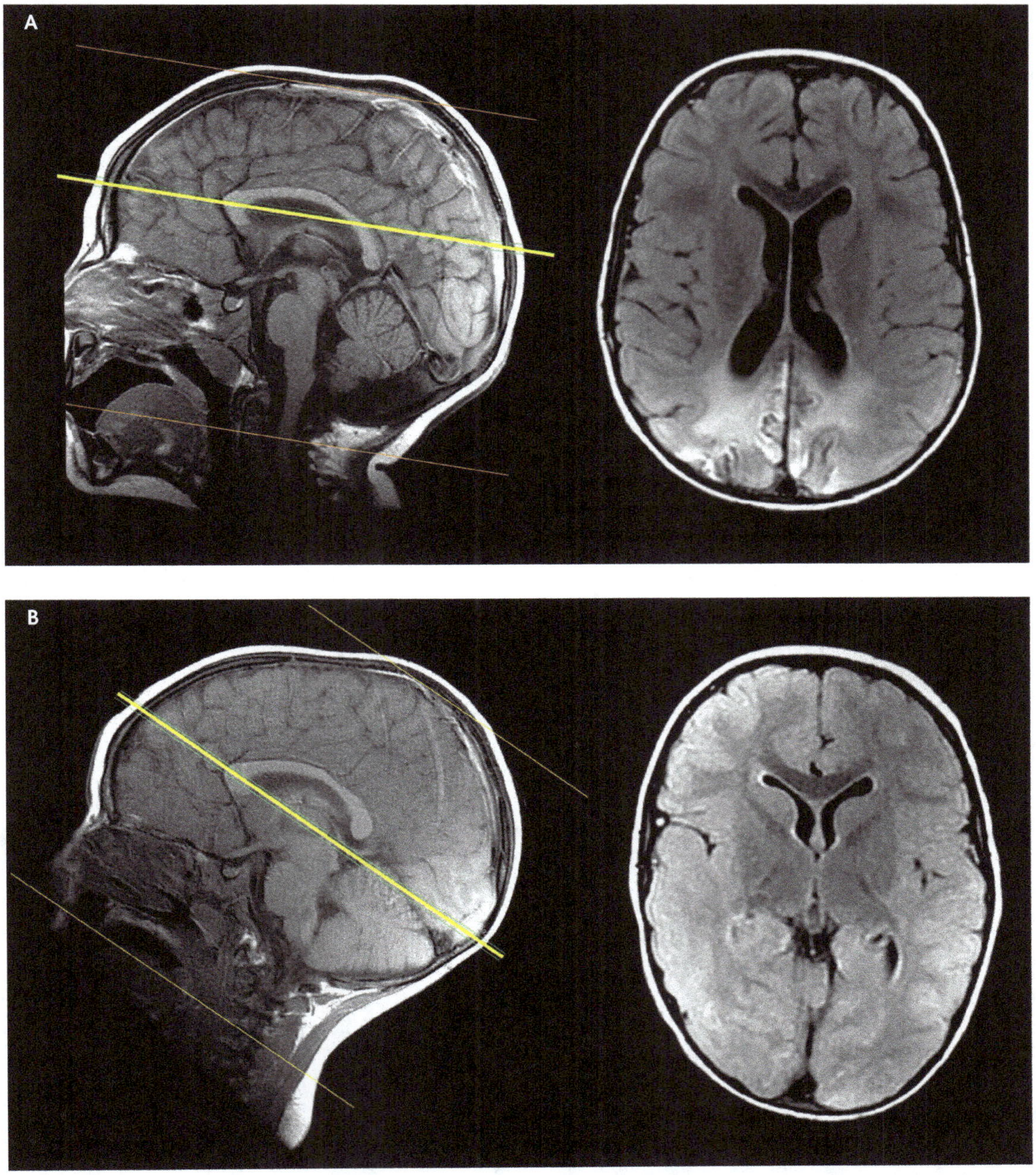

Figures 3-8A and B Sequence with different axial acquisition angles. The yellow lines represent the locations and respective acquisition angles used for the axial slices.

Meningeal Layers

The meninges provide protection and nourishment to the brain and form cavities through which fluids can flow (arachnoid spaces and cisterns for CSF, and sinuses for venous blood). The meninges are formed from three epithelial layers—the dura mater, arachnoid layer, and the pia mater. The dura mater is also referred to as the pachymeninges. The arachnoid layer and the pia mater are collectively referred to as the leptomeninges.

The meningeal layers can be used as primary anatomical landmarks when viewing brain scans. The layers separate many primary areas of the brain and are often easily identifiable on brain scans owing to the CSF within the arachnoid layer and also the fibrous tissue of the dura mater. The meningeal layers are used by radiologists as references to divisions between discrete regions of the brain. As such, a solid understanding of their anatomy can assist in one's understanding of radiology reports. For example, supra- and infratentorial are terms that describe the location of findings, such as brain tumors. *Supratentorial* refers to findings above the tentorium, and *infratentorial* refers to findings below the tentorium, usually within the posterior fossa. See section on tentorium cerebelli for information on its location. Similarly, hemorrhages are frequently described on the basis of their relationship to the dura. The blood vessels on the surface of the brain travel through the leptomeninges (pia and arachnoid layers) and can cause subdural or subarchnoid hemorrhages. Bleeds between the dura and the skull are called epidural hematomas.

Inflammation of the meningeal layers is called meningitis and may be most visible on MRI T2 FLAIR or post-contrast MRI or CT images (Figures 3-9A–C).

Dura and Dural Reflections (Folds)

The dura mater (Latin: *dura* = tough/durable; *mater* = mother) is a relatively thick, fibrous layer of tissue that surrounds the brain, divides regions of the brain, and forms the dural venous sinuses. Dura mater surrounding the brain is generally referred to simply as "dura." The dura splits into two dural folds, also called dural reflections, the falx cerebri and the tentorium cerebelli.

Falx Cerebri

The falx cerebri, or "falx," (Latin: *falx* = sickle-shaped) separates the two hemispheres and is located within the longitudinal or interhemispheric fissure.

The falx is best viewed on axial or coronal slices (Figures 3-10A–C arrows). Viewing the falx on axial or coronal images can provide useful information regarding mass effect, as the falx acts as a midline reference for the brain. Sagittal slices are generally too thick to allow a full appreciation of the falx.

Tentorium Cerebelli

The tentorium cerebelli, or "tentorium," (Latin: *tentorium* = tent/covering; *cerebelli* = cerebellum) sits above the cerebellum. The tentorium separates the cerebellum and brain stem structures from the occipital and temporal lobes. *Infratentorial* is used to describe structures or damage below the tentorium, and *supratentorial* refers to structures or damage above the tentorium. On brain scans, the tentorium is best visualized on sagittal or coronal slices (Figures 3-11A–C arrows).

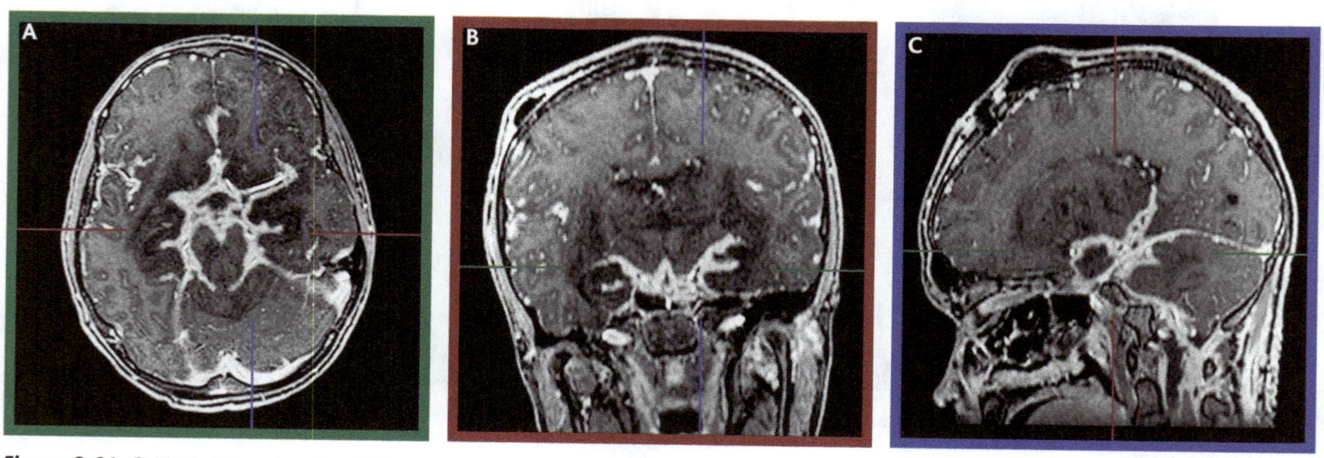

Figures 3-9A–C Meningitis and arachnoiditis on post-contrast T1 FSPGR MRI images.

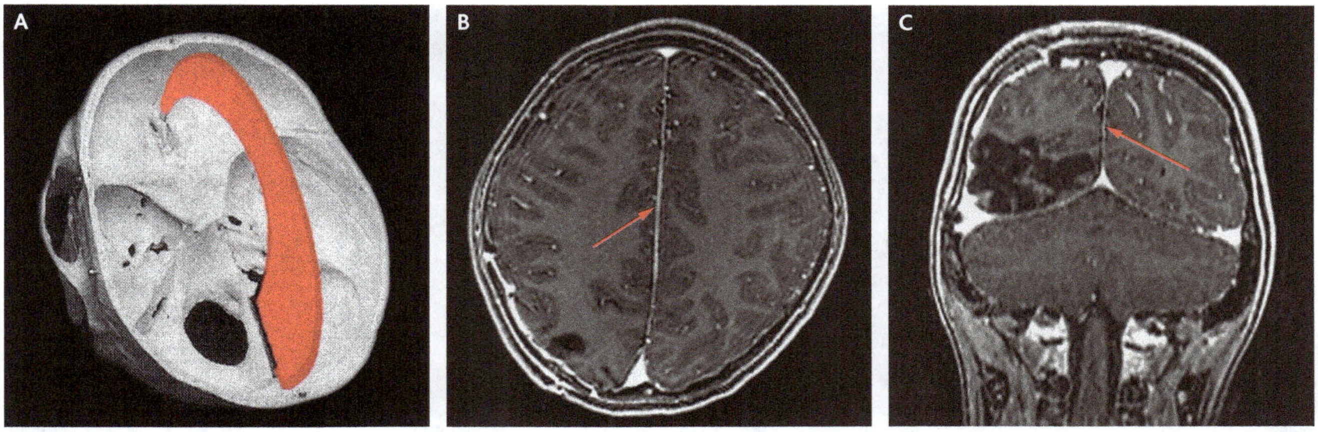

Figures 3-10A–C Falx cerebri shown in the appropriate location on a skull model (red), and on axial (B) and coronal (C) brain images.

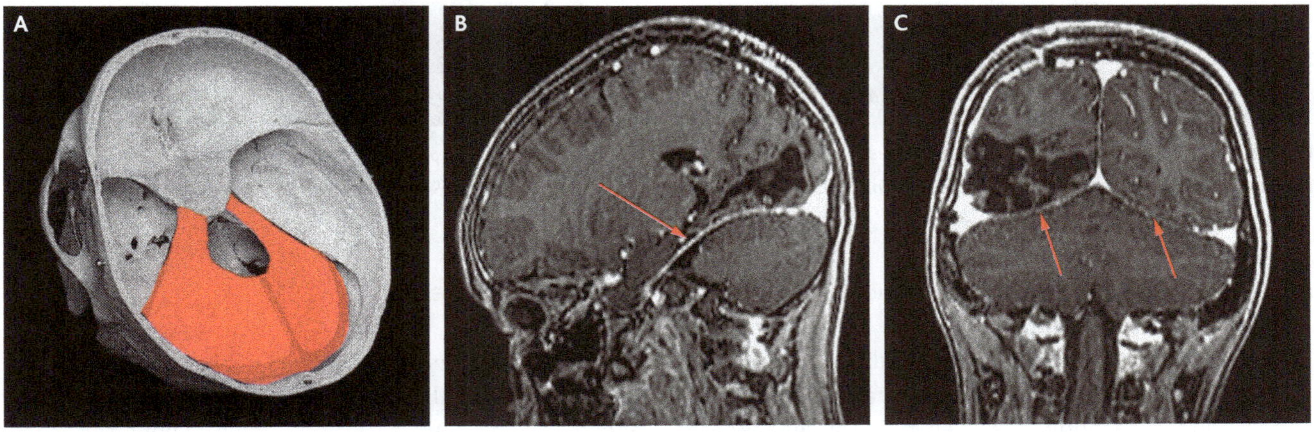

Figures 3-11A–C Tentorium cerebelli shown in the appropriate location on a skull model (red), and on sagittal (B) and coronal (C) brain images.

Dural Venous Sinuses

Blood exits the brain by draining into veins distributed around and within the brain and then into the venous sinuses. The venous sinuses are cavities within the dura through which venous blood flows to the jugular veins. The superior surface of the falx forms the inferior surface of the superior sagittal sinus. The inferior margin of the falx forms the inferior sagittal sinus that is located above the corpus callosum. The lower edge of the falx at the back of the brain forms the straight sinus as it meets the inner edge of the tentorium on each side. The back of the tentorium forms the transverse sinuses on each side of the brain. The location where the superior sagittal, transverse, and straight sinuses meet is called the confluence.

Venous sinuses are best viewed using magnetic resonance venography (Figures 3-12A and B), which is an MRI scan acquired during the introduction of a contrast agent into the venous system.

Arachnoid Layer

The arachnoid layer, sometimes called the subarachnoid space, is a channel running between the dura mater and the pia mater. The arachnoid space is mostly hollow but contains a web-like structure (Greek: *arachnid* = spider + *eidos* = web). Cerebral spinal fluid flows through the arachnoid layer after exiting the ventricular system via the foremena of **M**agendie (**M**edian aperture) and **L**uschka (**L**ateral aperture).

The arachnoid layer contains arachnoid granulations that absorb CSF into the venous sinuses, allowing it to exit the brain and re-enter the blood supply through the venous sinuses.

Small blood vessels travel through the arachnoid layer and can be torn during physical injuries to the brain. Tearing of the blood vessels within this meningeal layer results in subarachnoid hemorrhages.

As CSF flows through the arachnoid space, it is best visualized on scans that highlight CSF, such as T2 MRI. Inflammation of the arachnoid space causes

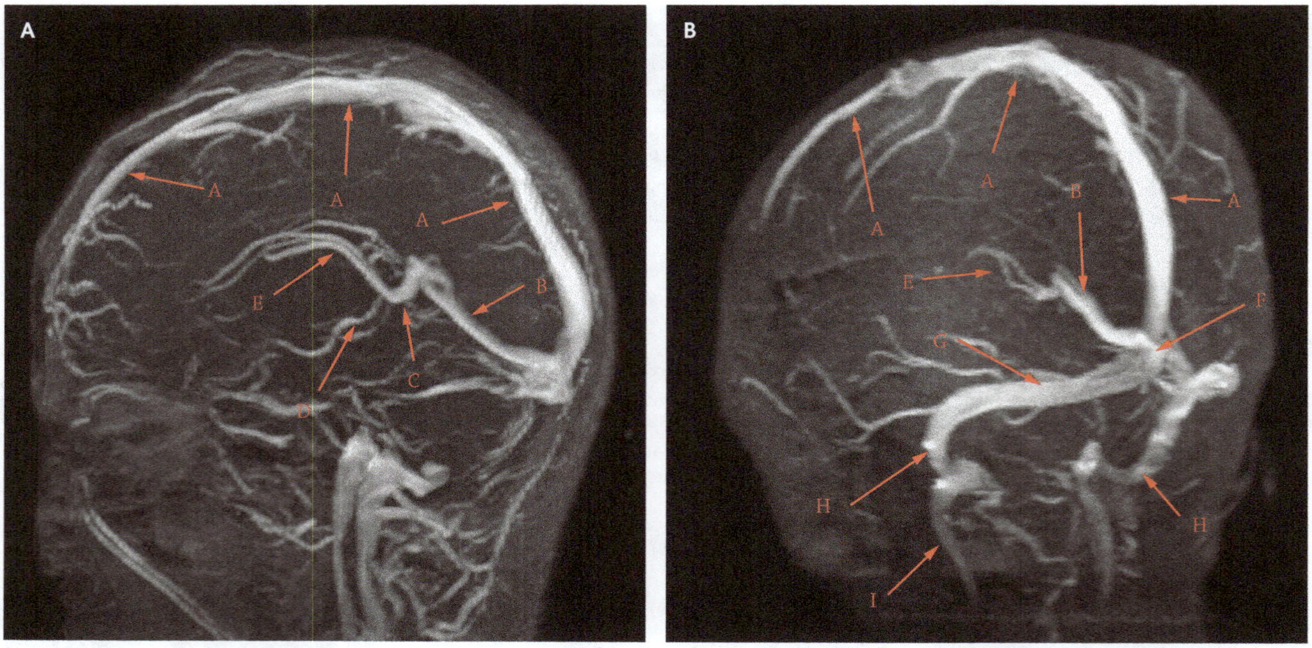

Figures 3-12A and B Venous sinus on magnetic resonance venography. *A = Superior Sagittal Sinus; B = Straight Sinus; C = Great Cerebral Vein of Galen; D = Basal Vein of Rosenthal; E = Internal Cerebral Veins; F = Confluence; G = Transverse Sinus; H = Sigmoid Sinus; I = Internal Jugular Vein.*

a condition called arachnoiditis. Pre- and post-contrast T2 and post-contrast T2 FLAIR images are useful to visualize the arachnoid layer in cases of arachnoiditis.

Traumatic damage to the brain can cause bleeds within and around the arachnoid layer. Depending on the age of the hemorrhage, these are readily visible on a variety of brain scans, especially CT. Blood from arachnoid hemorrhages resulting from physical trauma is seen above the corpus callosum on axial CT (Figure 3-13A arrow). Coronal and sagittal CT images show several areas of arachnoid hemorrhage around the corpus callosum, inferior temporal lobes and close to the optic chiasm (Figures 3-13B–C arrows).

Arachnoid Cisterns

The meninges follow the contours of the cortical and subcortical surfaces. Although the pia mater (see below) closely adheres to the brain surface, in some regions the arachnoid layer is separated from the surface of the brain. The wide separation of the arachnoid and pia layers results in an enlarged subarachnoid space, called an arachnoid cistern. The cisterns are filled with CSF and are contiguous with each other and the ventricular system via the pathways of the fourth ventricle (foramina of Magendie and Luschka). Owing to the cortical organization, most cisterns

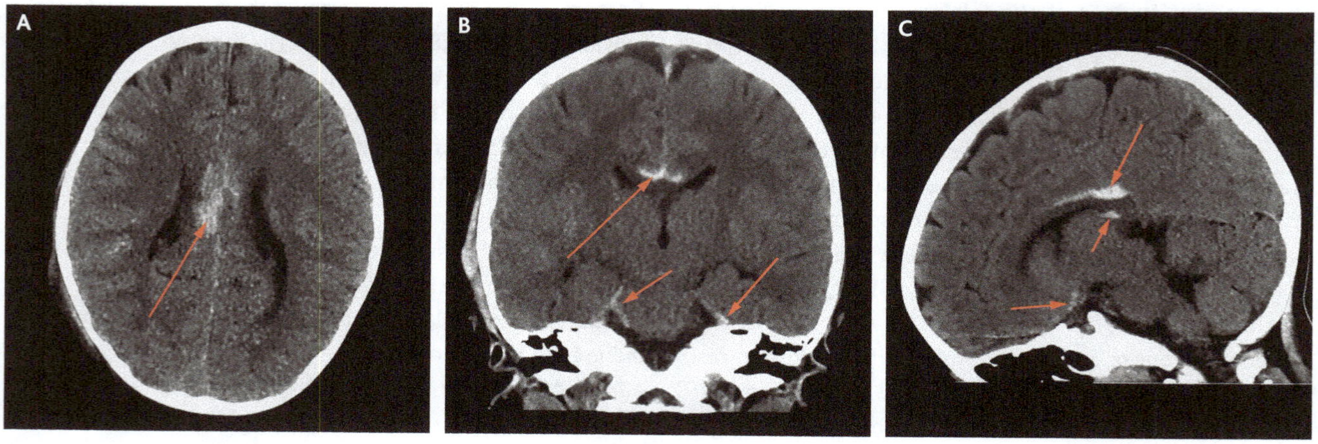

Figure 3-13A–C Hemorrhages within and around the arachnoid layer caused by a traumatic brain injury.

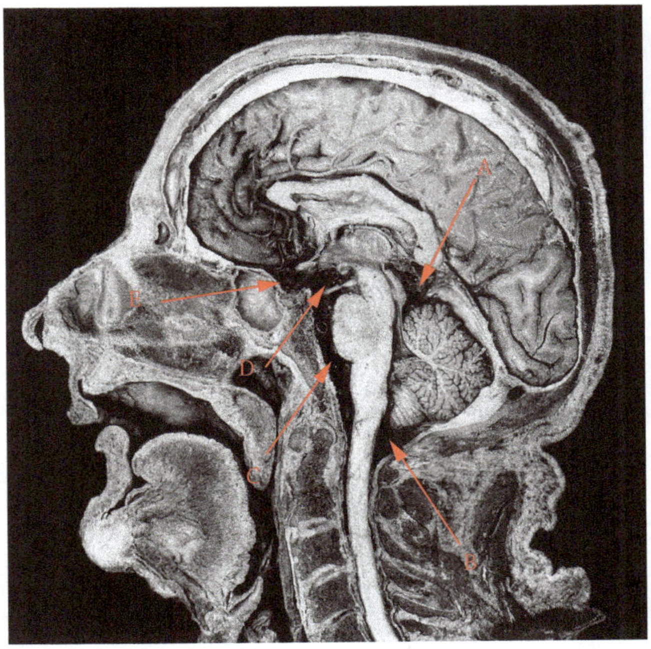

Figure 3-14 The CSF-filled arachnoid cisterns provide anatomical landmarks for many critical regions of the brain, such as the midbrain (superior, perimesencephalic or quadrigeminal cistern), pons (pontine cistern), and the medulla (cisterna magna).
Key for Figure 3-14: A = Superior/perimesencephalic/quadrigeminal Cistern; B = Cisterna Magna; C = Pontine Cistern; D = Interpeduncular/basal Cistern; E = Chiasmatic Cistern.

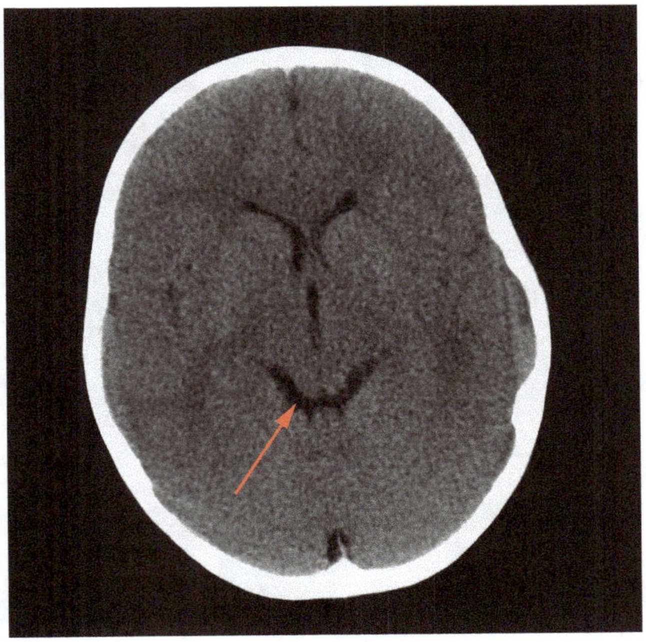

Figure 3-15 Superior cistern, also called the perimesencephalic or quadrigeminal cistern.

are located around the base of the brain and the subcortical structures (Figure 3-14).

Many of the cisterns have more than one label, adding confusion to their use in radiology reports. For example, the superior cistern is also called the perimesencephalic or quadrigeminal cistern, and the interpeduncular cistern is also called the basal cistern. For the sake of clarity, more than one label may be used in this section to describe a single cistern.

Changes in cistern volume apparent on brain scans can be used to assess for a variety of conditions. Compression of the superior cistern, also called the perimesencephalic or quadrigeminal cistern, can be indicative of diffuse swelling to the brain parenchyma. As brain tissue swells, the cistern becomes compressed and is less visible on imaging. Ongoing swelling can result in herniation of the brain stem through the foramen magnum. If this occurs, the cisterna magna will decrease in size as the brain parenchyma fills the cavity usually filled with CSF.

Superior cistern

The superior cistern is also referred to as the perimesencephalic or quadrigeminal cistern because it is located just posterior to the mesencephalic structures of the corpora quadrigemini. On CT axial images, the cistern forms what can appear to be the smiling mouth (arrow) of a smiley face formed from the lateral ventricles as the eyes and third ventricle as the nose (Figures 3-15). Figures 3-16A–C show axial, coronal and sagittal views of a normal or patent (open) superior cistern on MRI T1 imaging. Figures 3-17A–C provide CT examples of a compressed superior cistern, resulting from diffuse cerebral edema and increased intracranial pressure.

Interpeduncular or basal cistern

Located anterior and superior to the pons and between the cerebral peduncles is a cavity called the interpeduncular or basal cistern. Critical vascular structures such as the circle of Willis are located within this cistern. Following traumatic brain injury, subarachnoid hemorrhages within the cistern may be the only evidence of injury, especially on CT. Figures 3-18A–C show the general location of the basal cistern at the intersection of the reference lines, using T1 MRI sequences.

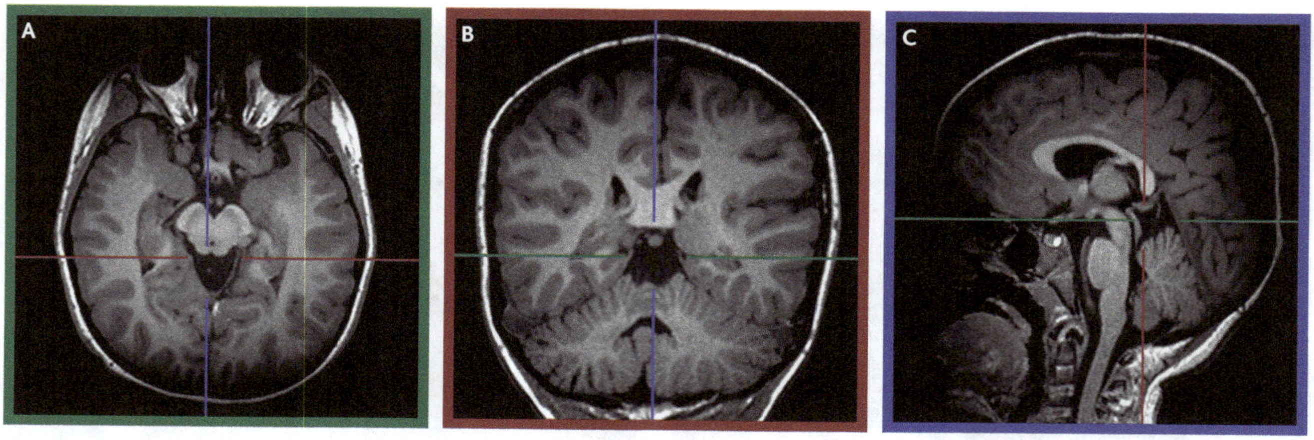

Figures 3-16A–C Axial, coronal, and sagittal MRI at the level of the superior cistern.

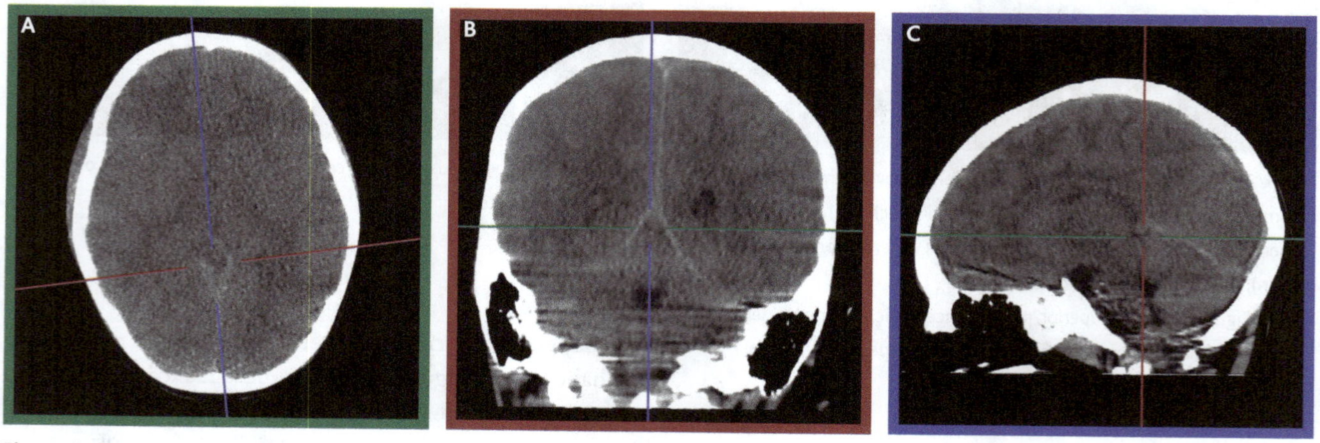

Figures 3-17A–C Compressed superior/perimesencephalic/quadrigeminal cistern on CT.

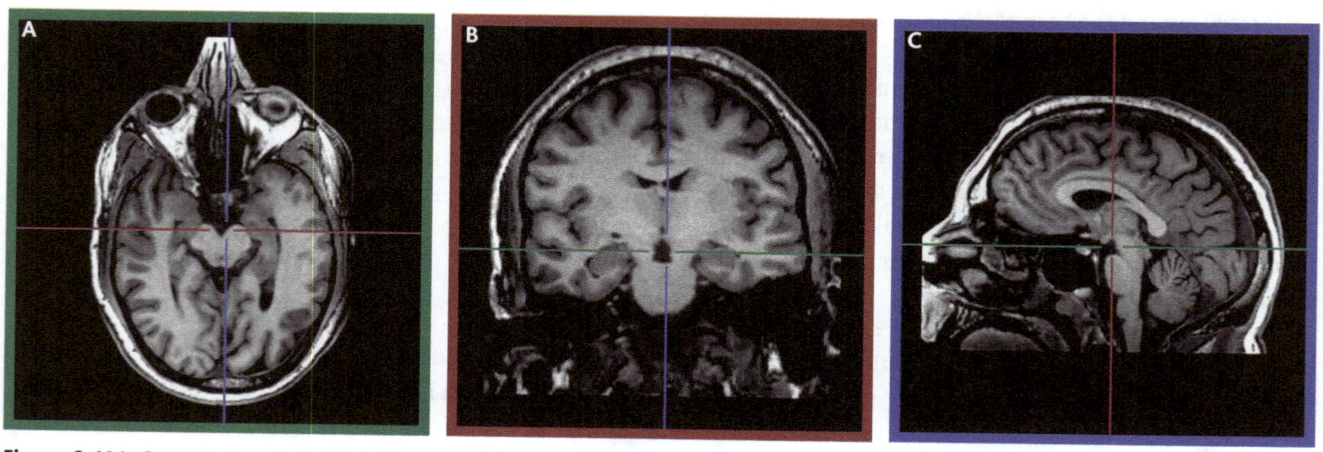

Figures 3-18A–C Interpeduncular or basal cistern on axial, coronal and sagittal MRI.

Pia Mater

The pia mater (Latin: *pia* = tender/soft; *mater* = mother) is located below the arachnoid layer. Pia is a delicate layer of tissue that sits on the surface of the brain. Within the pia is a matrix of tiny blood vessels supplying the cortical surface. Pia also forms the choroid plexus that produces CSF and which is found within the ventricular system. In Figure 3-19A, the pia has been peeled from part of the brain, shown in the top half of the figure. Note the many blood vessels located between the pia and the brain, and the arachnoid granulations close to the interhemispheric or longitudinal fissure, in the center and lower half of the picture. Figure 3-19B shows the delicate nature of this tissue as it is being peeled from the surface of the brain.

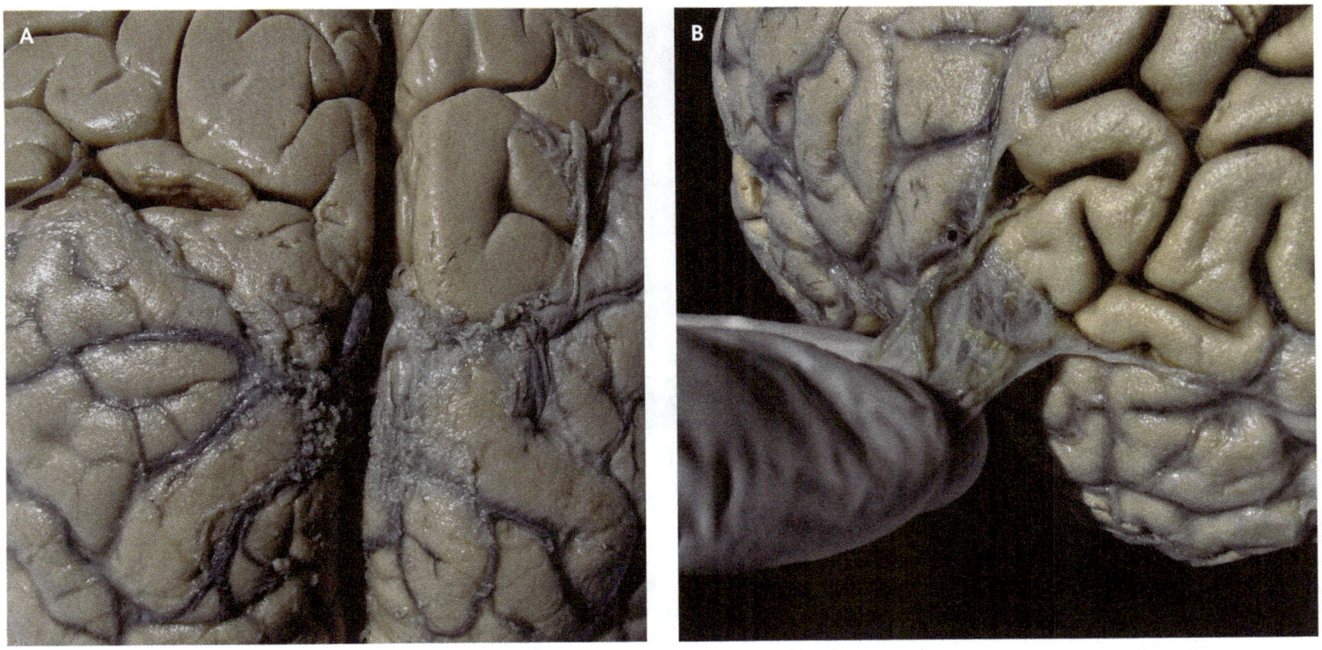

Figure 3-19 **A:** Pia peeled from part of the brain. **B:** Pia and blood vessels being removed from the surface of the brain to show the delicate nature of the pial layer.

White-Matter Pathways

The communication fibers of the brain are surrounded by a lipid layer called myelin. Myelin appears white because of the fat content, resulting in axon pathways appearing white on brain specimens and during surgery. As such, the axon pathways are collectively called the "white matter" of the brain.

With advances in brain imaging, it has become easier to display white-matter tracts or nerves within the brain. T1 images allow for reasonable differentiation of gray matter from white matter. Using specialized T1 sequences such as spoiled gradient echo BRAVO, FSPGR or MPRAGE, visualization of white-matter areas has become even easier (Figures 3-20A–C).

Diffusion tensor imaging (DTI) can highlight axon pathways without showing other tissue, by producing structural fractional anisotropy (FA) maps. DTI structural FA mapping has the advantage of allowing color-coding of the pathways based on their orientation. Superior–inferior pathways are coded blue, anterior–posterior pathways are coded green, and lateral fibers are coded red. DTI structural FA mapping is generally produced using an axial plane (Figure 3-21A), although it can also be acquired in the coronal (Figure 3-21B) and sagittal (Figure 3-21C) planes.

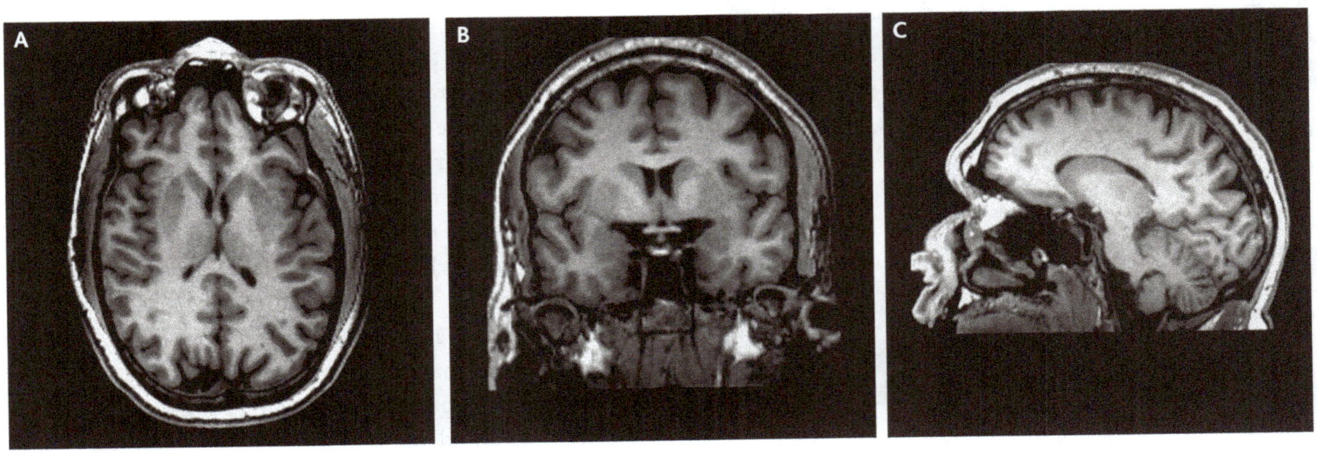

Figures 3-20A–C T1 images of white-matter pathways.

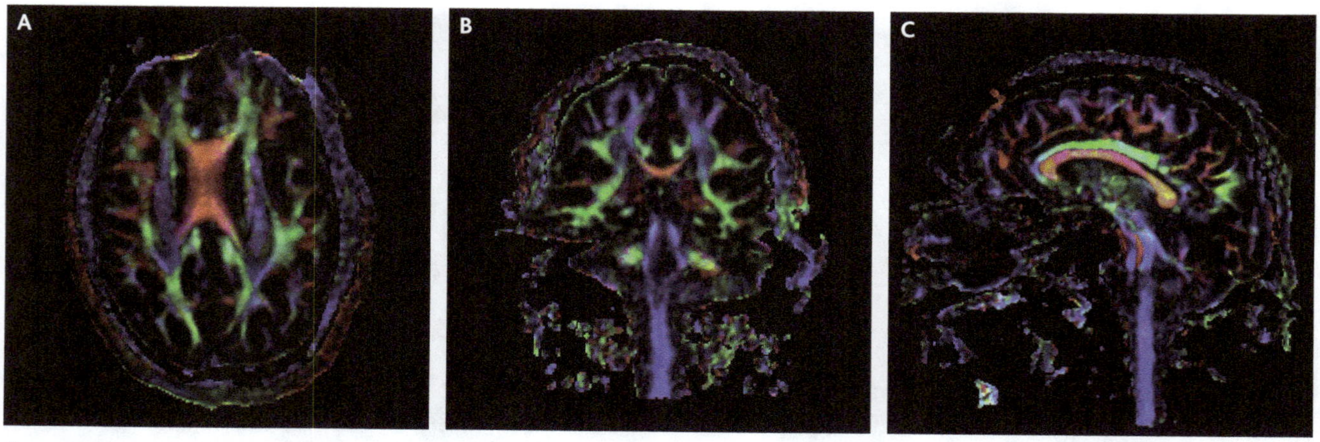

Figure 3-21A–C DTI structural FA images acquired in the axial (A), coronal (B) and sagittal (C) planes.

DTI can also be used to produce three-dimensional graphic renderings (tractography) illustrating the white-matter pathways of the brain. Selection or "seeding" of particular brain regions will result in the identification of pathways on the basis of restricted (anisotropic) directional diffusion only found in axons (Figure 3-22).

Just as the various ventricles can be used as anatomical landmarks, so too can the fiber pathways.

There are many pathways within the brain, and a detailed discussion of each pathway is beyond the scope of this text. This chapter will focus on the pathways that are most useful as landmarks for imaging-based anatomy. For example, the corpus callosum and internal capsule are useful when identifying different basal ganglia structures, and areas of the corpus callosum provide a useful reference when identifying areas of cortex.

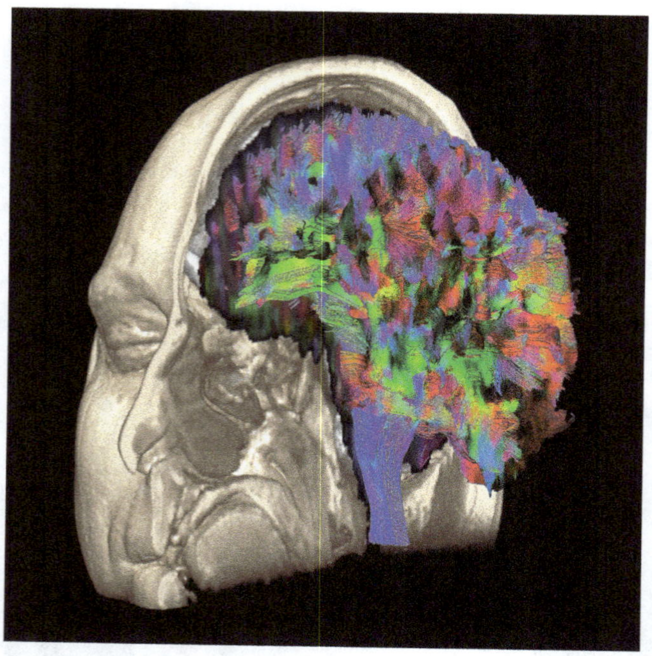

Figure 3-22 DTI tractography set to illustrate most fiber tracts in the brain.

Centrum Semiovale

The largest area of white matter that connects the cortex to the subcortical nuclei and spinal pathways is called the centrum semiovale, or the "semi-oval center" of each hemisphere. When viewing this area on brain scans, it is important to consider that different types of brain scans or sequences may present white and gray matter using different shades of gray. For example, white matter appears light on T1-weighted images but dark on T2-weighted sequences.

Figures 3-23A–C show the centrum semiovale on three different scans: a post-contrast CT, a T1 MRI, and a T2 MRI. The patient has edema within the left occipital-parietal region, shown on the right side of the figures. On CT (Figure 2-23A), both the white matter and edema appear darker than the gray matter of the cortex. Because of this, edema within the white matter of the centrum semiovale becomes difficult to appreciate on CT, even with adjustments to exaggerate the contrast between lighter and darker areas. Note that the large area of white matter on the CT scan appears relatively similar for the right and left hemispheres. The edema is evident in the slightly darker appearance of the centrum semiovale on the right side of the picture, or left hemisphere. When assessing for edema within the white matter of the brain, MRI imaging is more useful. On T1 images (Figure 3-23B), edema appears darker than normal tissue or hypointense and is evident within the left parietal lobe. On T2-weighted images (Figure 3-23C), edema appears brighter than normal, or hyperintense, as noted in the left parietal region.

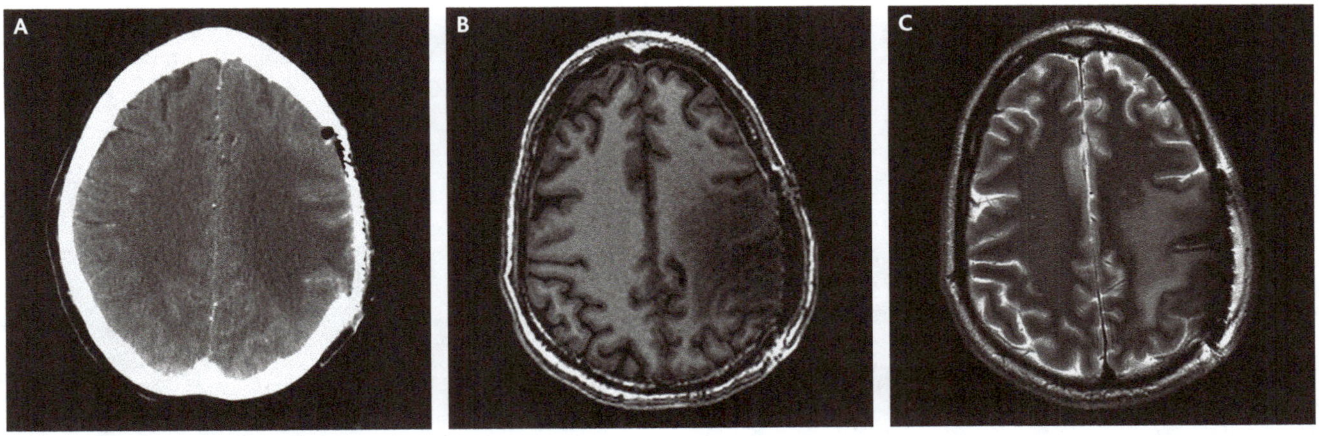

Figure 3-23A–C Images showing edema in the left occipital-parietal region of the centrum semiovale on post-contrast CT (A), T1 MRI (B) and T2 MRI (C).

Corpus Callosum

The corpus callosum is a large band of fibers that connects the right and left hemispheres. When viewed from the side (midsagittal view), several regions can be appreciated. The thickness of the primary areas of the corpus callosum correspond to the number of fibers that cross at that specific location. A larger number of fibers cross between the frontal lobes (genu) and occipital lobes (splenium), areas of relative corpus callosum thickness. Fewer fibers cross in the area below and slightly posterior to the central sulcus (isthmus), giving the corpus callosum a thinner appearance. The fewest fibers cross at the very front, below the genu, an area called the rostrum.

From the superior surface, the corpus callosum connects the right and left hemispheres in a region directly above the subcortical nuclei of the basal ganglia, thalamus, and limbic system. The corpus callosum is shorter than the length of the hemispheres and makes a butterfly shape when seen from above (Figure 3-24).

The inferior surface of the corpus callosum forms the roof of the lateral ventricles (Figure 3-25, arrow). On midsagittal images, the lateral ventricle is located directly below the body of the corpus callosum, also evident on Figure 3-25.

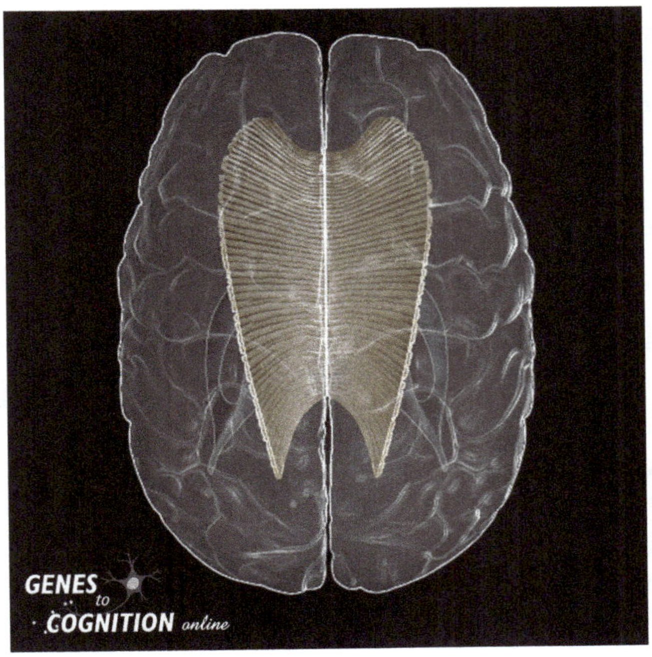

Figure 3-24 Illustration of the corpus callosum viewed from above.

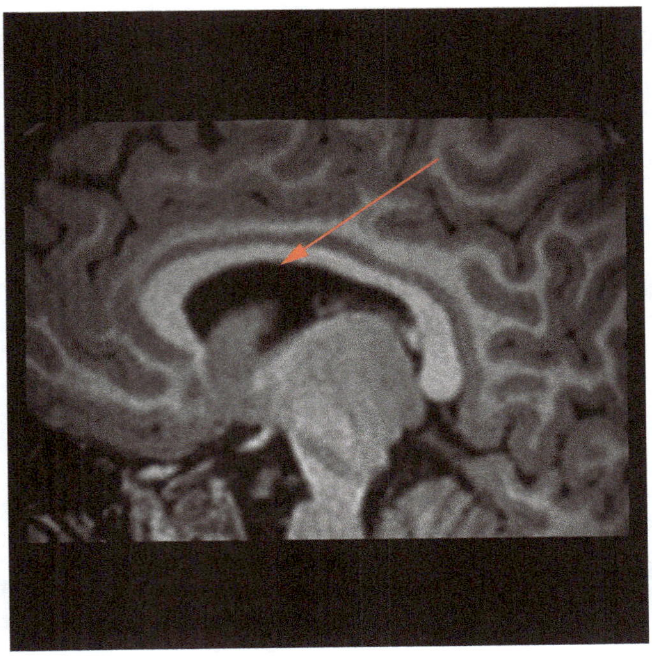

Figure 3-25 Midsaggital view of the corpus callosum.

Coronal Orientation

On coronal images, the body of the corpus callosum is most easily located as the roof or superior surface of the body of the lateral ventricles (Figure 3-26A and B arrows). The basic structure of the corpus callosum viewed from the front is illustrated within a translucent three dimensional brain in Figure 3-26C).

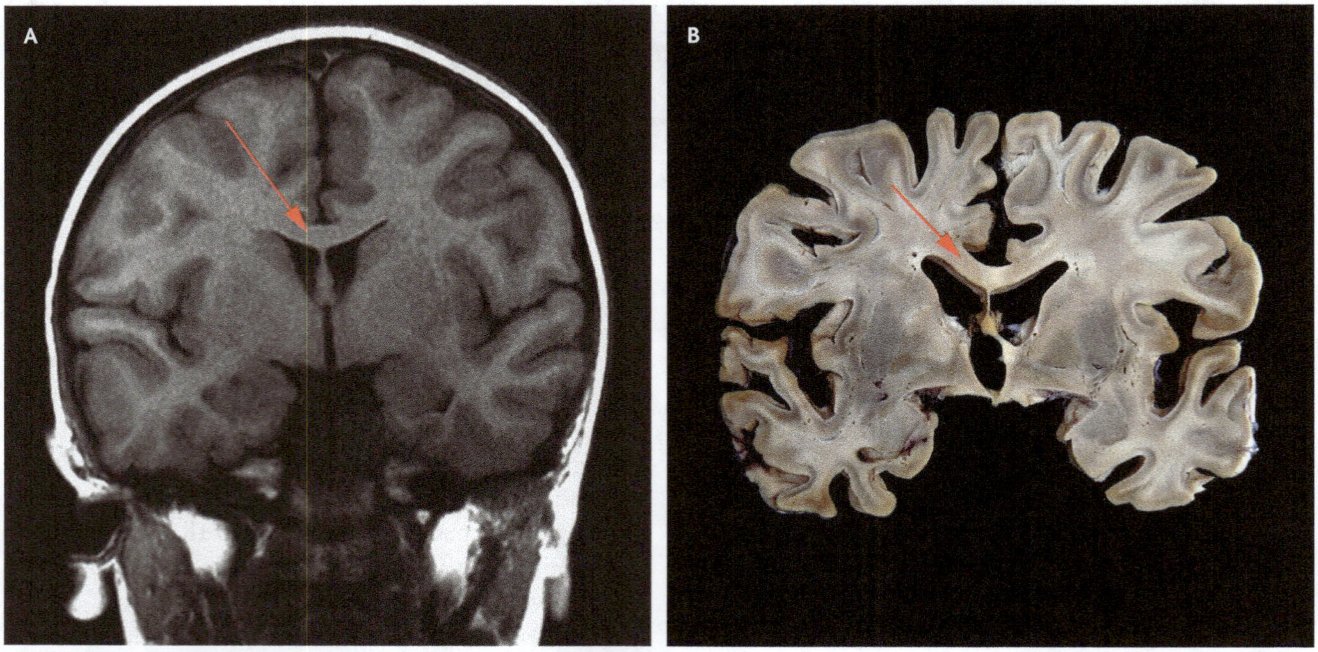

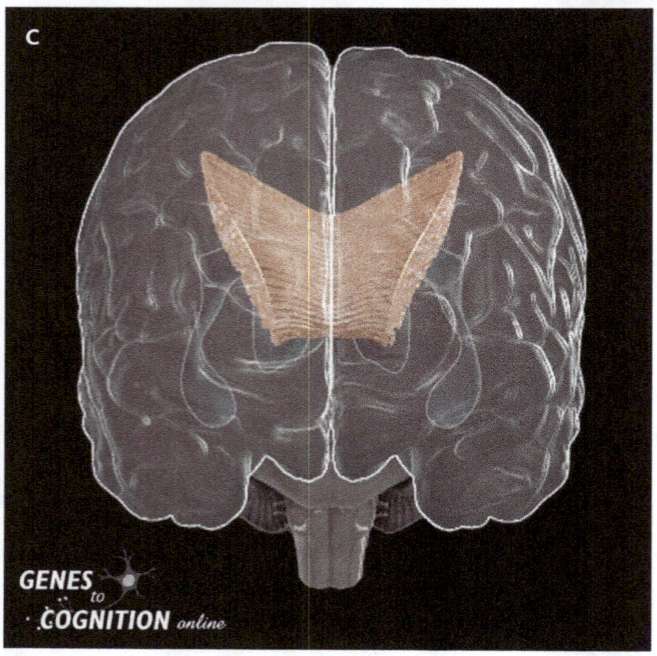

Figures 3-26A and B Coronal images of the corpus callosum, on brain imaging (A) and brain section (B). **C:** Illustration of the corpus callosum viewed from the front.

Sagittal Orientation

When viewing the corpus callosum on brain scans, variation between patients is the norm, not the exception. Although the structure maintains the same general shape, differences between individuals can be quite profound. Figure 3-27 shows silhouettes of normal corpus callosum structures taken from a series of sagittal images acquired from different individuals.

Because of the normal variation in shape and size, interpretation of colossal thinning post-injury is difficult without serial scans showing changes in thickness over time.

It is important to consider the general shape of the corpus callosum when considering damage or atrophy. One specific area of the corpus callosum, the isthmus, can appear relatively thin compared to the remaining regions, even without pathology.

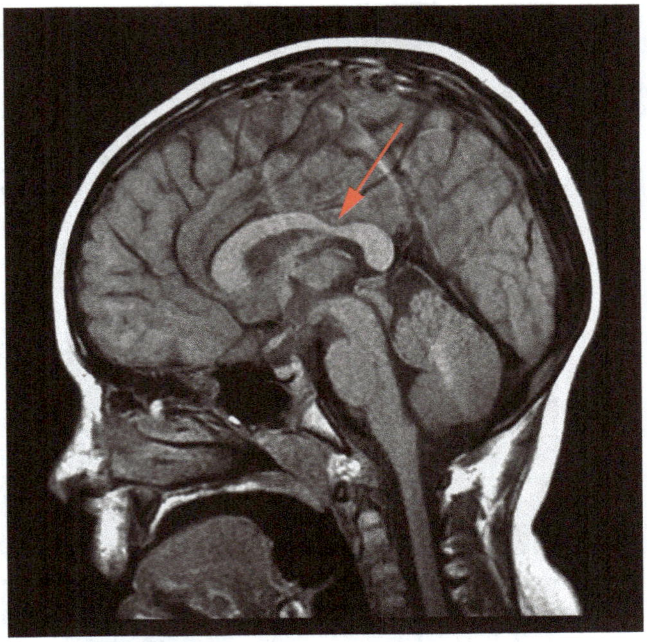

Figure 3-28 Isthmus of the corpus callosum.

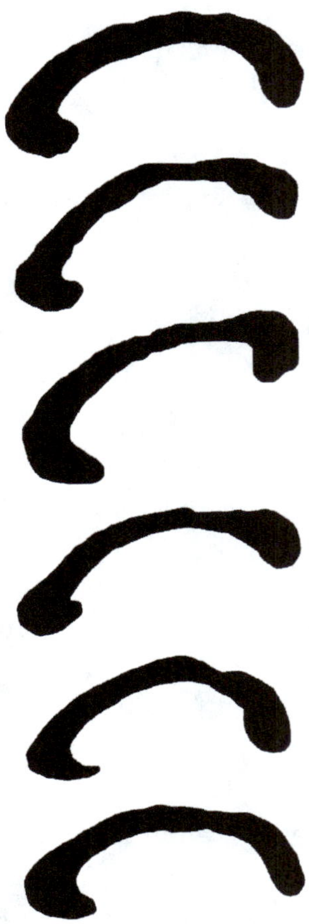

Figure 3-27 Silhouettes of normal corpus callosum structures imaged from a sagittal orientation.

The isthmus, which translates from the Latin "narrow passage," is the region just anterior to the splenium (between the splenium and the body of the corpus callosum). The isthmus is located between the parietal lobes and connects fibers from the parietal and superior temporal cortices of the two hemispheres. The region is narrower than other areas of the corpus callosum and can appear atrophied on many normal scans. The thin appearance can be accentuated by the normal gyri patterning around this area (Figure 3-28 arrow). Caution is required before assuming that this region is abnormally thin.

Axial Orientation

Viewing the body of the corpus callosum using axial slices is relatively difficult because the structure is arched. Axial cuts slice horizontally through only a small portion of the corpus callosum body (Figures 3-29A and C). If the image slices are approximately 5 mm or greater in thickness, the body will only show up on one or two slices. Images that are acquired below the level of the corpus callosum body highlight the genu and splenium, thicker areas that project inferiorally (Figures 3-29B and D). Figure 3-29E illustrates the entire corpus callosum using DTI tractography. Only the genu at the front of the corpus callosum and the splenium at the back of the corpus callosum are highlight using DTI tractography in Figure 3-29F.

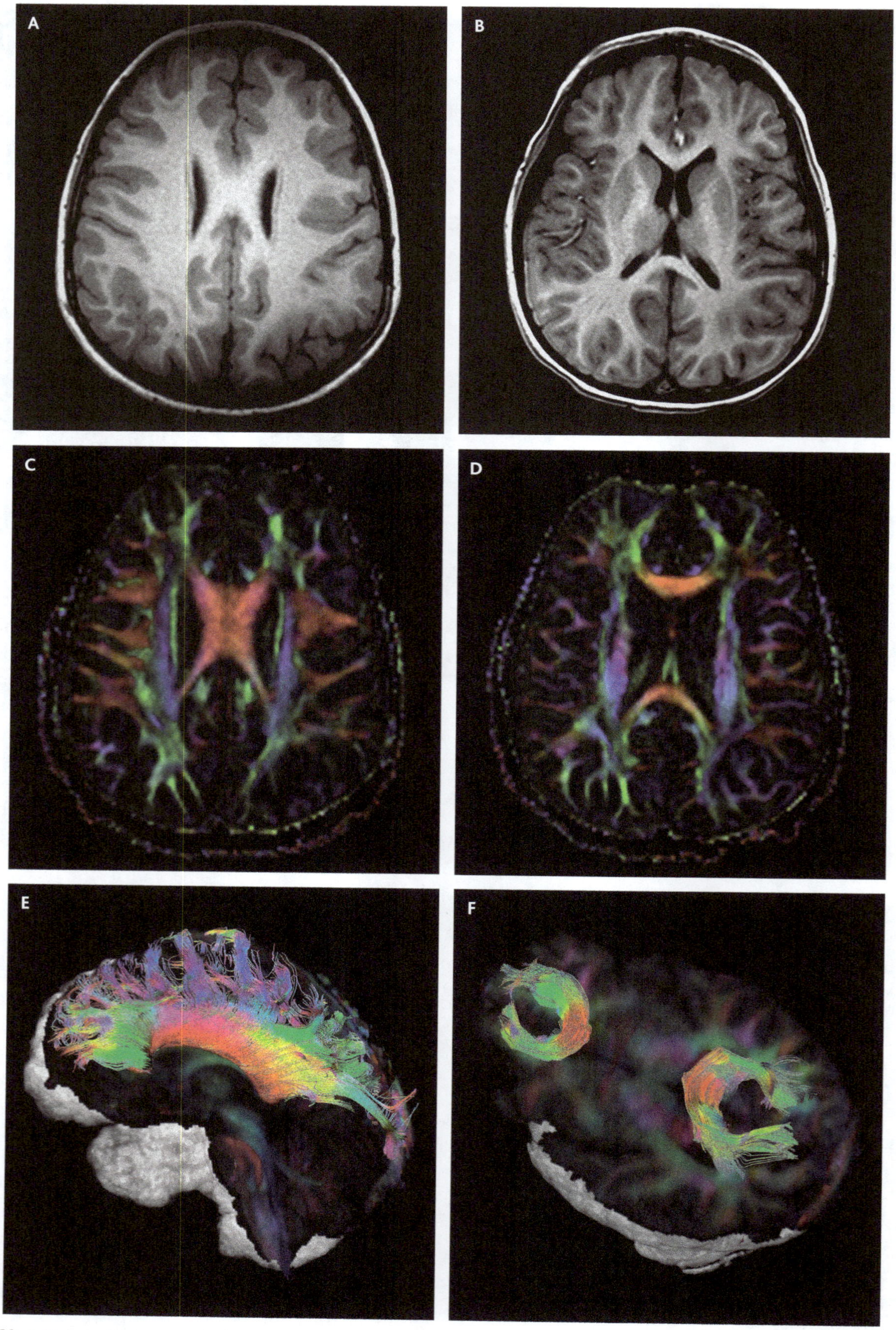

Figure 3-29 **A:** T1: body. **B:** T1: genu and splenium. **C:** DTI: body (red). **D:** DTI: genu and splenium (red). **E:** Tractography: body. **F:** Tractography: genu and splenium.

Pathology to the Corpus Callosum

Damage to the corpus callosum is best appreciated using a series of image planes and types. Correlation between sagittal, coronal, and axial planes on T1 or T2 FLAIR may be most helpful for determining the severity and extent of corpus callosum damage. Although small areas of damage to the body of the corpus callosum may not be visible on axial images, larger areas of damage can be quite evident.

CLINICAL EXAMPLE

James: Traumatic Brain Injury

James was involved in a high-speed motor vehicle accident as an unrestrained passenger. He sustained severe axonal tearing of the callosal fibers from the splenium to the body (Figures 3-30A–C). Although James also sustained some diffuse injury to the brain, his symptoms were predominantly related to the corpus callosum injury. With the corpus callosum being involved in the integration of information between the two hemispheres, James' symptoms were predominately related to higher-order cognitive abilities requiring the integration and manipulation of information. His basic cognitive abilities and general intellect were intact for his age as long as he was given adequate time to complete tasks and respond to questions. However, he exhibited notable deficits involving executive functioning. James was unable to divide his attention, multitask, rapidly switch between different tasks while maintaining focus, or complete tasks in a reasonable time because of his slowed processing speed.

Damage to the corpus callosum may involve the primary structure, as was the case with James, or the radiations that lead to and from it. Another patient, Jolie, was severely beaten and sustained injury to the body of the corpus callosum (Figure 3-31A), in addition to the callosal radiations (Figure 3-31B). The damaged tissue is identified in Figure 3-31 by the bright hyperdense areas of blood on the CT scans.

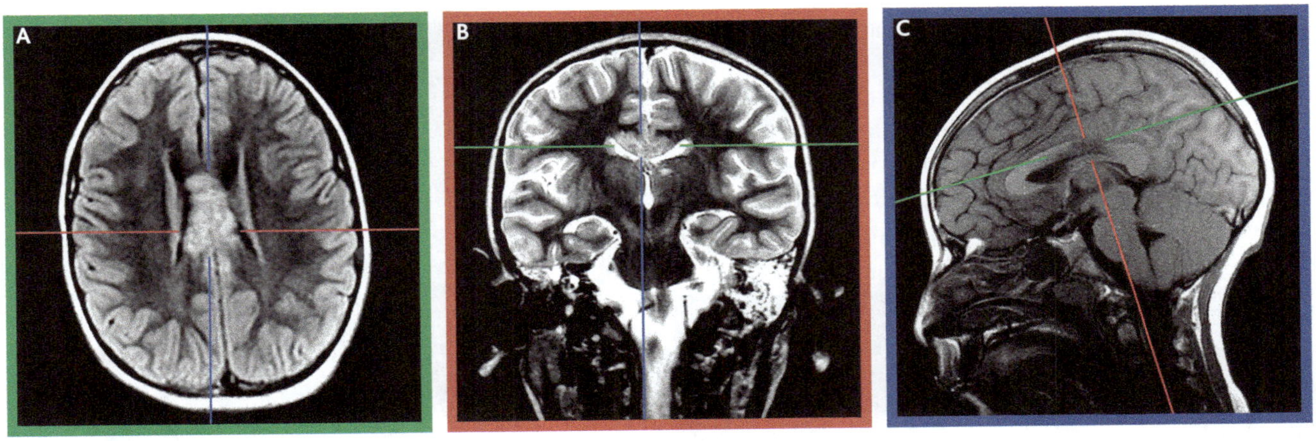

Figure 3-30A–C Corpus callosum damage on T2 FLAIR MRI (A), T2 MRI (B) and T1 MRI (C).

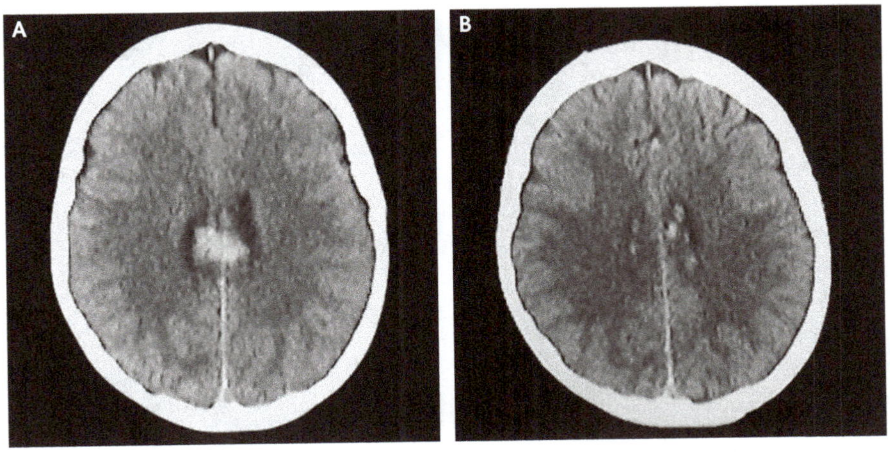

Figure 3-31 A: Jolie's injury to body of corpus callosum on CT as a hyperdense region of hemorrhage. **B:** Jolie's injury to the callosal radiations on CT as multiple hypersense punctate hemorrhages.

Cingulum

The cingulum is a bundle of axon fibers that surrounds the superior surface of the corpus callosum (Figure 3-32). The term *cingulum* was once used in ancient Rome to describe a belt or sash worn by soldiers or clerics, or by women for support. In the same way, the anatomical structure of the cingulum appears as a beltlike structure formed from a band of myelinated axons that extends from the front to the back of the corpus callosum.

The cingulum is formed from the reciprocal association fibers that connect the medial frontal and parietal lobes with the limbic structures and temporal lobes of the same hemisphere. The functions of the cingulum and cingulate gyri are numerous with marked heterogeneity. Some of the functions of this area include modulation of the prefrontal and limbic systems, integration of sensory information with emotional responses, and attentional functioning.

On axial images, the cingulum and cingulate gyri are best visualized on either side of the longitudinal or interhemispheric fissue, using a slice acquired just superior to the corpus callosum (Figures 3-33A). The cingulum is more easily viewed using a coronal section that cuts through the body of the corpus callosum, given its location on either side of the interhemispheric fissure above the corpus callosum (Figure 3-33B). On sagittal sections, the cingulum is readily identified as a band of white matter directly above the corpus callosum (Figure 3-33C). The MRI T2 FLAIR images shown in Figures 3-33D–F were obtained from a patient who contracted viral encephalitis, resulting in damage to his bilateral cingulate gyri and cingulum. Note the T2 hyperintensity within the medial gyri directly anterior to the genu of the corpus callosum (Figure 3-33D) and along most of the length of the cingulum (Figure 3-33E and F).

Using DTI, the cingulum can be identified on an FA map as the green pathway running anterior–posterior on either

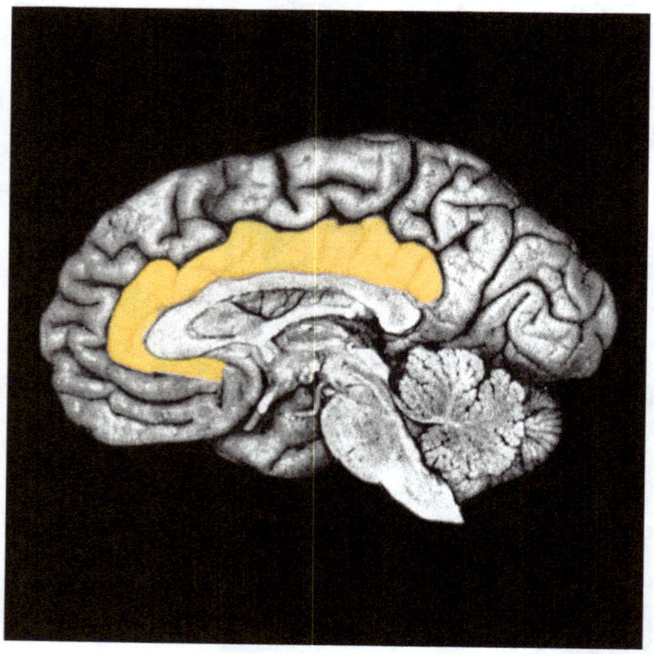

Figure 3-32 The cingulum fibers are located within the cingulate gyrus (yellow) and lie above the corpus callosum, on the most medial surface of each hemisphere.

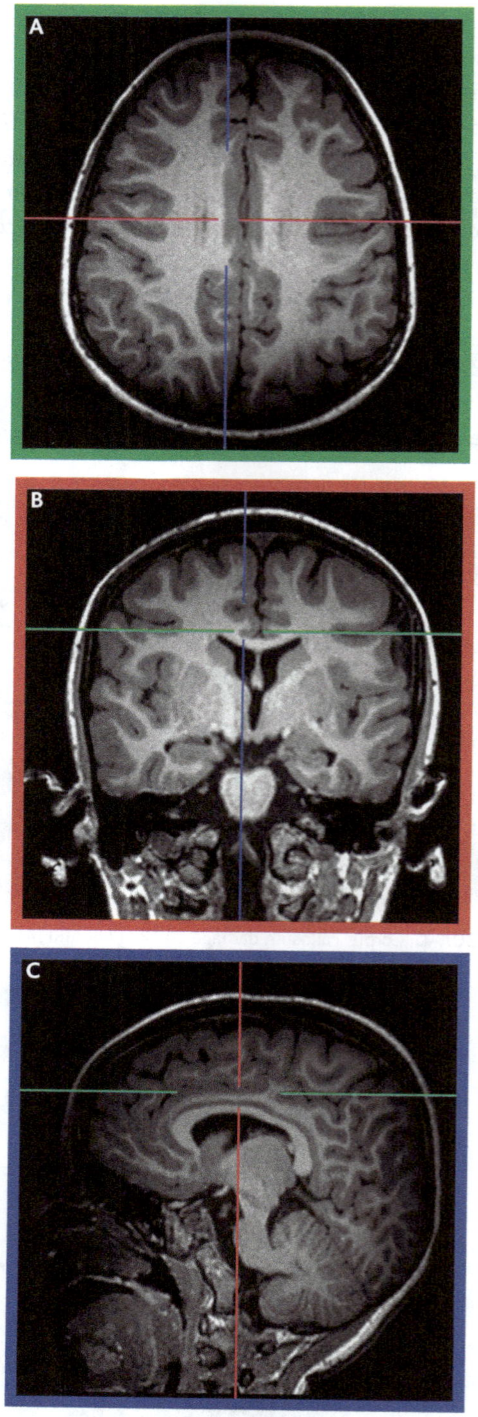

Figures 3-33A–C The cingulum and cingulate gyrus are identified on a variety of image orientations as the most medial gyrus of each hemisphere, beside the longitudinal fissure, and directly above the corpus callosum.

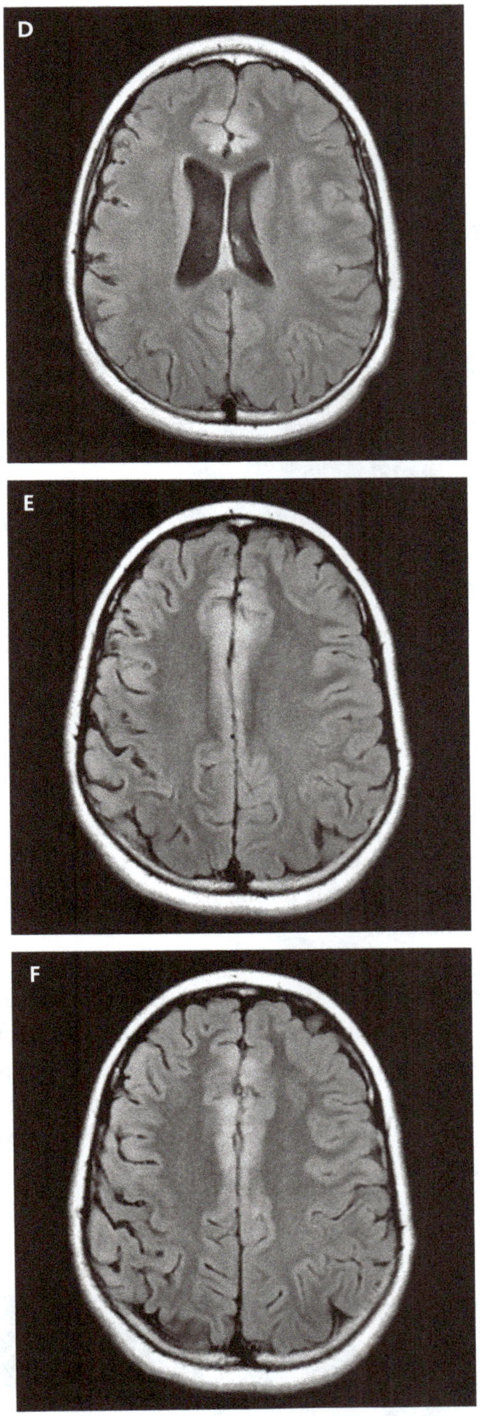

Figures 3-33D–F MRI T2 FLAIR images showing areas of hypoxic ischemic injury to the cingulate gyrus shown as brighter regions along the medial gyrus of each hemisphere, lateral to the longitudinal fissure.

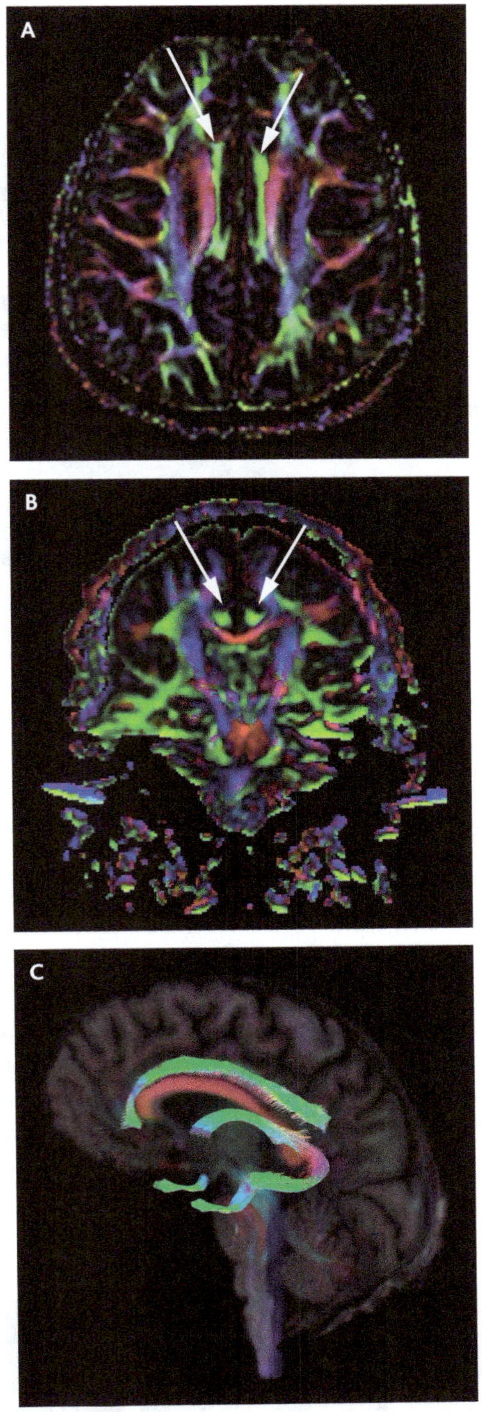

Figures 3-34A and B Axial and coronal DTI structural FA maps: cingulum shown in green. **C:** Cingulum on tractography with the fornix and hippocampi for reference.

side of the longitudinal fissure and above the corpus callosum (Figures 3-34A and B). Using tractography, the cingulum can be isolated relatively easily (Figure 3-34C: the fornix and hippocampi are included below the cingulum for reference).

Corona Radiata

The corona radiata is formed from the axon pathways connecting the higher cortex with the subcortical structures, the brain stem and spinal cord. On a dissected view, the

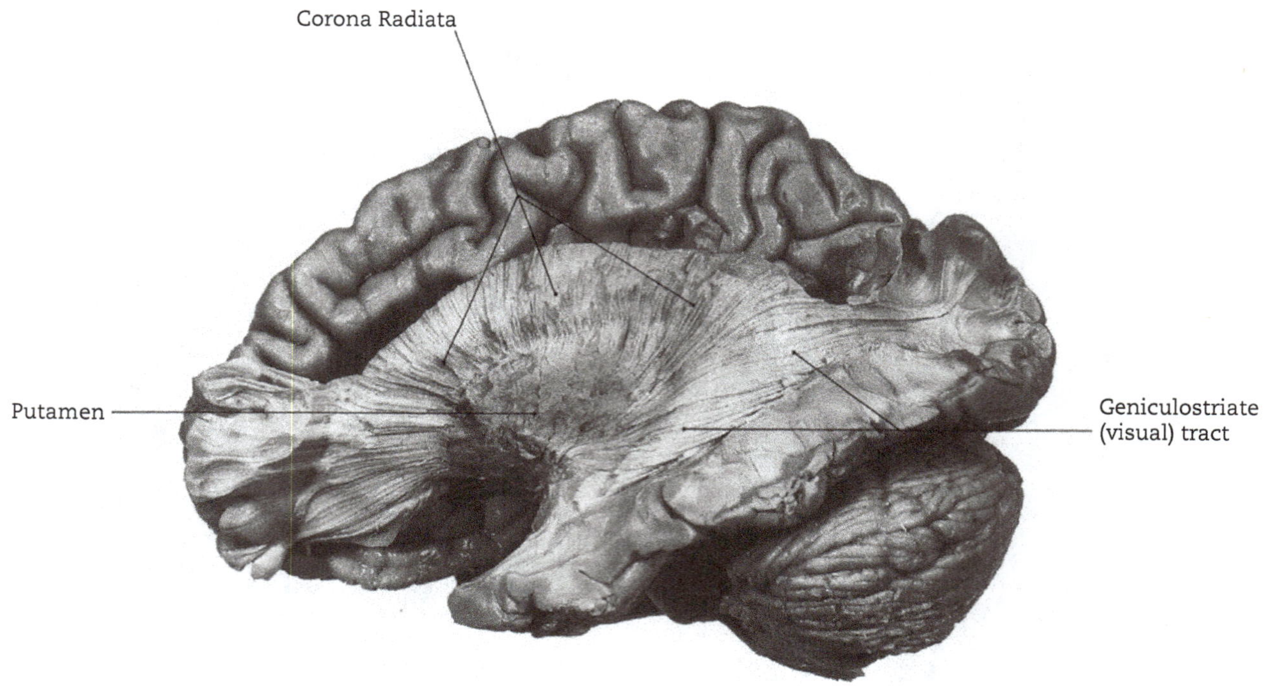

Figure 3-35 Corona radiata on dissected view.

pathways take on the appearance of a radiating crown, thus the term *corona radiata* (Figure 3-35).

On a brain scan, the corona radiata is most easily viewed on an axial image, although correlation with coronal or sagittal images may be helpful (Figures 3-36A–C). The pathways of the corona radiata border the outside edges of the lateral ventricles, at the level close to the top of the ventricles.

When assessing for damage to the corona radiata, axial and coronal image slices tend to be most useful. Often damage to the corona radiata is caused by diffuse axonal shear injury and, as such, is bilateral. Look for damage on each side of the brain just above the corpus callosum. Symptoms from corona radiata damage depend on the specific pathways involved and can mimic those of cortical or corpus callosum damage.

Using DTI, the corona radiata can be identified on a structural FA map as the blue pathway running superior–inferior and located either side of and lateral to the body of the lateral ventricles, at the superior aspect of the corpus callosum (Figure 3-37A). Using tractography, the corona radiata can be isolated and visualized relatively easily (Figure 3-37B).

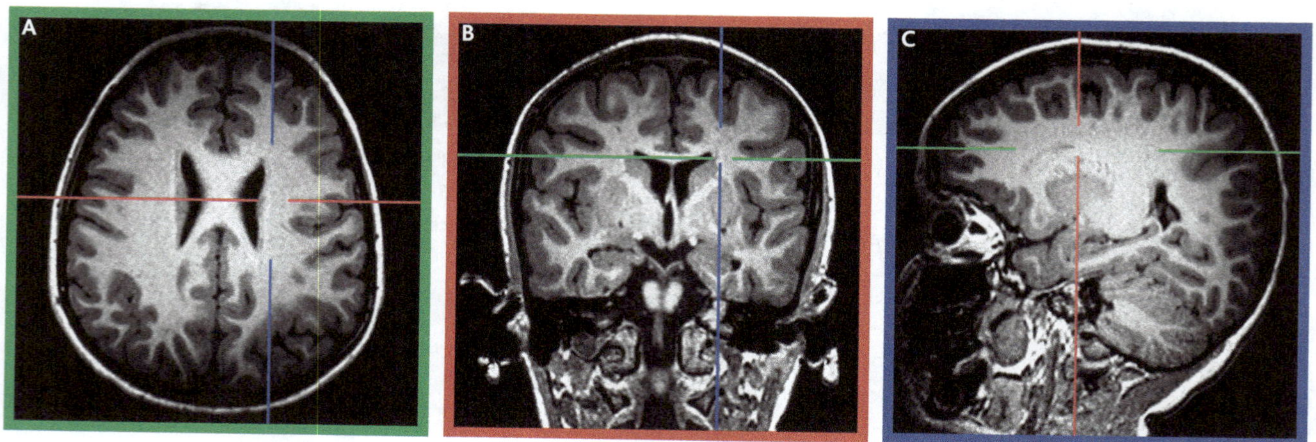

Figures 3-36A–C Corona radiata on axial (A), coronal (B) and sagittal (C) MRI images.

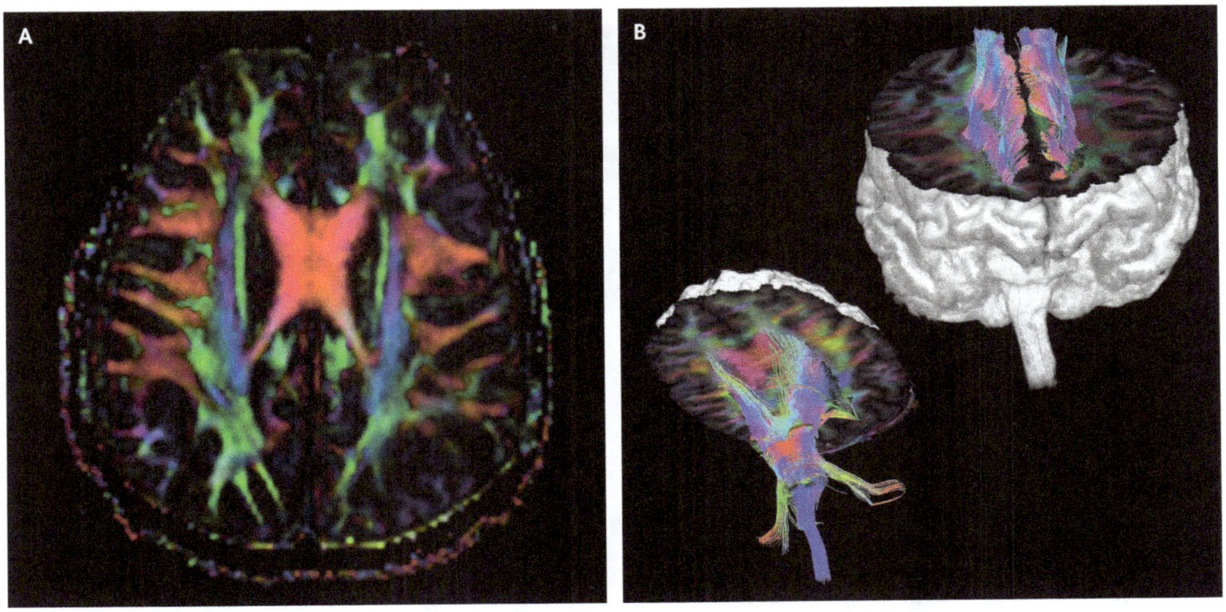

Figure 3-37 **A:** DTI structural FA map of corona radiata shown in blue. **B:** DTI-tractography of corona radiata.

Internal Capsule

The internal capsule is formed from the reciprocal fibers that make up the corona radiata, and is composed of three primary sections; the anterior limb, the genu and the posterior limb (Figure 3-38). Many of the fiber pathways that connect the higher cortical regions of the frontal and parietal lobes to the spinal cord travel via the corona radiata and internal capsule.

Anterior Limb of the Internal Capsule

The anterior limb of the internal capsule contains the corticofugal (corticopontine) fibers that connect the frontal cortex with the pons. Thalamocortical fibers connecting the thalamus with the frontal lobes also form part of the anterior limb of the internal capsule.

Genu of the Internal Capsule

The genu, or middle part, of the internal capsule is formed primarily from corticobulbar fibers connecting the cortex to the brain stem nuclei.

Posterior Limb of the Internal Capsule

The posterior limb contains the corticospinal or pyramidal tract that connects the cerebral cortex with the spinal cord.

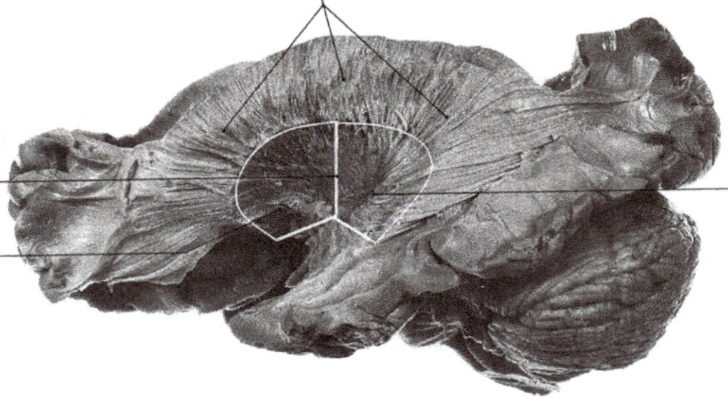

Figure 3-38 Internal capsule on dissected view.

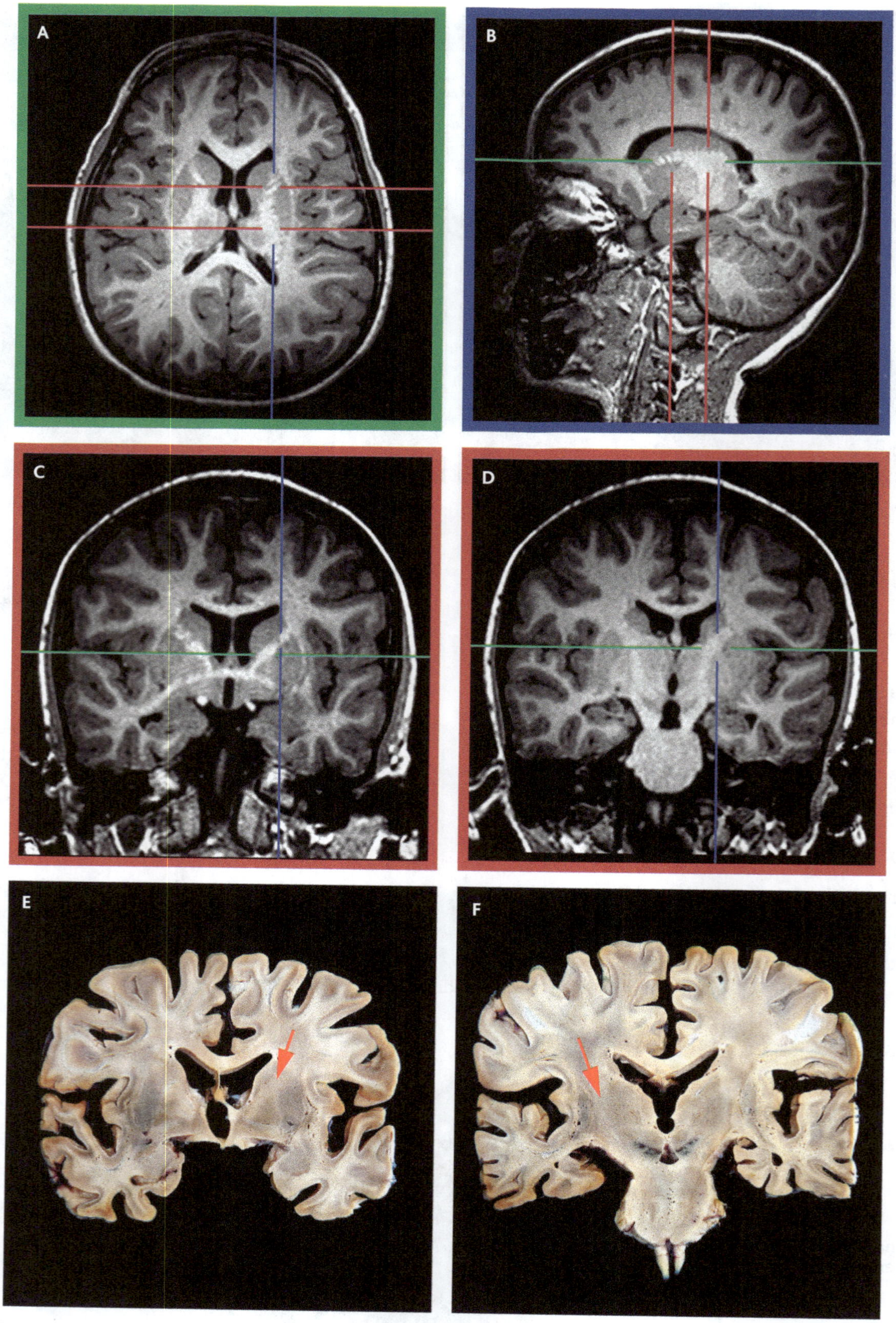

Figures 3-39A to 3-39F The red reference lines in 3-39A and 3-39B correspond to the coronal image slices in 3-39C and 3-39D. The anterior reference line cuts through the anterior limb of the internal capsule shown in 3-29C. The posterior reference line cuts through the posterior limb of the internal capsule shown in 3-39D. Anatomical brain sections are provided, with 3-29E being cut at the level of the anterior limb and 3-39F at a level to show the posterior limb of the internal capsule. **C:** Anterior limb. **D:** Posterior limb. **E:** Anterior limb. **F:** Posterior limb.

The pyramidal tract is primarily formed from motor neurons that travel to the spinal cord and are responsible for voluntary motor functioning. Other motor neurons within the pyramidal tract travel to the cranial nerve nuclei and are considered part of the corticobulbar tract. The posterior limb of the internal capsule also contains sensory fibers from the body.

The most posterior part of the internal capsule, behind the lenticular nuclei (retrolenticular), is formed from fibers connecting the lateral geniculate nucleus of the thalamus with the optic radiations. The areas of the internal capsule below the lenticular nuclei contain auditory fibers from the medial geniculate nucleus to the auditory radiations leading to the temporal lobe.

The internal capsule is best viewed on axial and coronal sequences, as the axons pass by the subcortical structures of the basal ganglia and thalami (Figures 3-39A–F).

On axial images, the fibers form an angular-shaped structure (shallow *V*) as they pass through the level of the basal ganglia. The base of the shallow *V* separates the anterior limb from the posterior limb and is called the genu of the internal capsule.

On coronal images, the internal capsule is easily identified as the white-matter tract that runs diagonally and superior–inferior, between the various basal ganglia structures.

On sagittal images, the internal capsule is visible below the elongated structure of the caudate nucleus and above the lentiform nuclei and thalamus. It forms a white-matter tract between the caudate (above) and the lentiform nucleus (below/anterior), and thalamus (below/posterior).

CLINICAL EXAMPLE
Yoshi: Internal Capsule Injury

Yoshi had a small left internal capsule stroke most clearly evident on T2 FLAIR (Figure 3-40). Few other areas were affected by the stroke, although there was some disruption of her left basal ganglia region. Yoshi's symptoms were primarily related to disruption of the pathways traveling through her left internal capsule and the structures of the left basal ganglia. Long-term recovery was excellent except for some residual motor deficits on her right side.

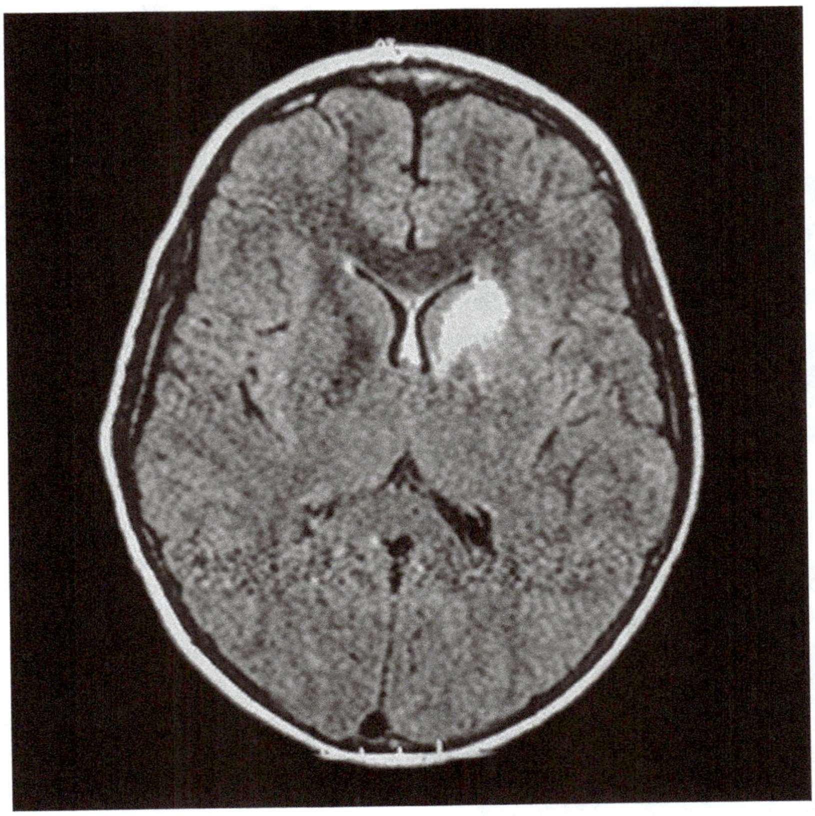

Figure 3-40 Case example Yoshi: internal capsule injury.

Optic Tract and Radiations

The optic nerves from each retina are referred to as the optic tract once becoming part of the central nervous system. Above the pituitary gland, the optic nerves from each eye combine to form a structure shaped like an *X* or the letter *chi* in the Greek alphabet; this structure is accordingly called the optic chiasm.

Optic Chiasm

The optic chiasm shown at the intersection of the reference lines in Figures 3-41A–C is where information from the nasal hemiretina from the right eye crosses to the left hemisphere and the nasal hemiretina from the left eye crosses to the right hemisphere. The information from the temporal hemiretinas stays ipsilateral (on the same side of the brain), with fibers from the temporal hemiretina of the right eye going to the right hemisphere and fibers from the temporal hemiretina from the left eye being projected to the left hemisphere.

Optic Radiations (Geniculostriate Tract)

The optic radiations that form the geniculostriate tract connect the lateral geniculate nucleus of the right or left hemisphere with the corresponding occipital cortex, also called striate cortex (Figure 3-42). The lateral geniculate nuclei are components of the thalamic complex and are located at the posterior and inferior parts of the thalami.

The optic radiations are relatively simple to find on a brain scan as they form the lateral or outside wall of the posterior horns of the lateral ventricles (Figures 3-43A–C). The fibers that make up the radiations are arranged with the same organization as the retina (retinotopic); damage to a specific region of fibers will correspond to a specific area of visual space (visual field).

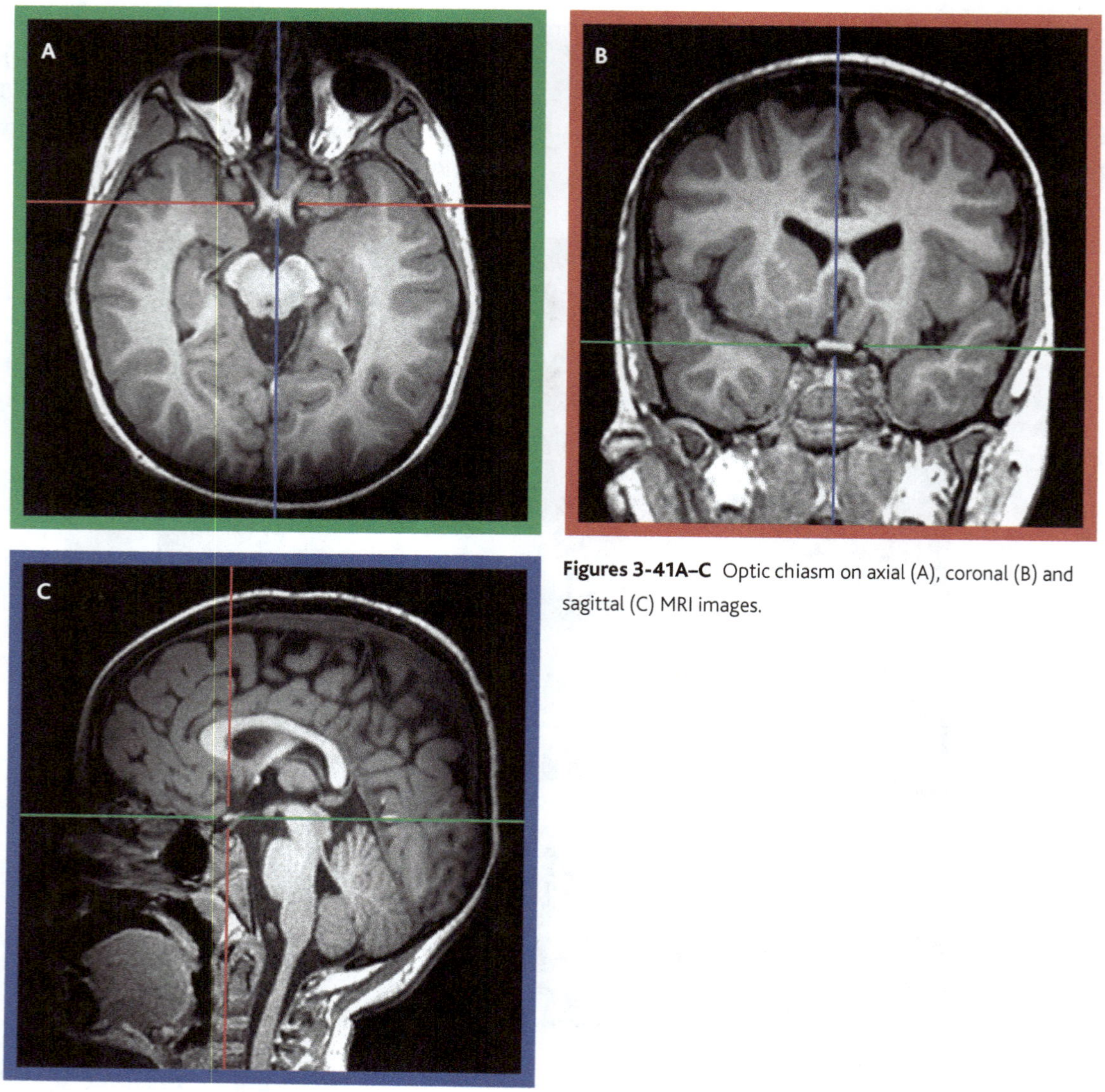

Figures 3-41A–C Optic chiasm on axial (A), coronal (B) and sagittal (C) MRI images.

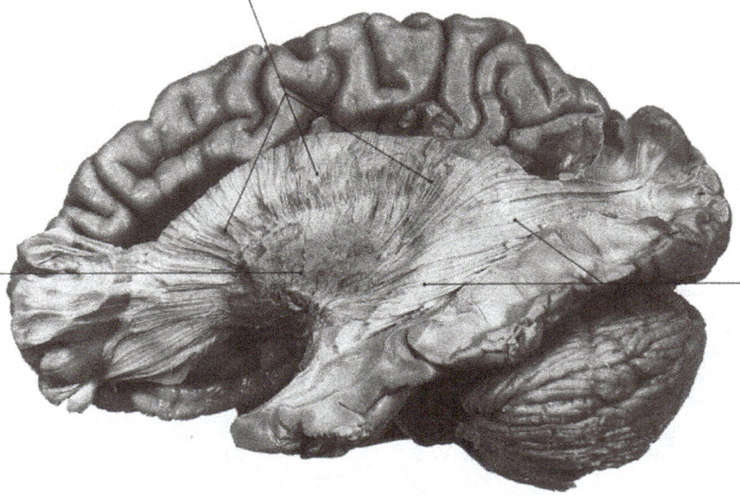

Figure 3-42 Optic radiations on dissected view.

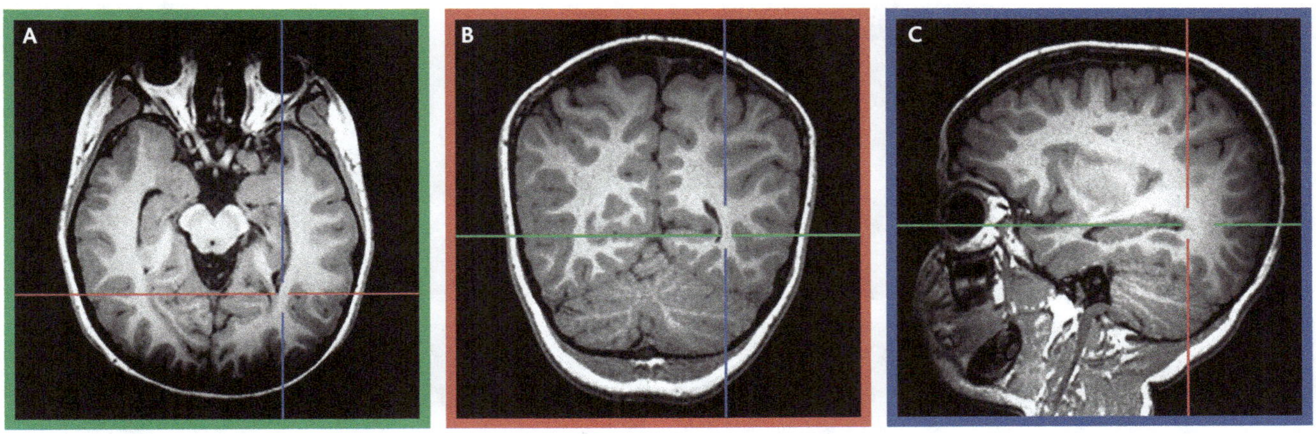

Figures 3-43A–C Optic radiations form the lateral or outside wall of the posterior horns of the lateral ventricles.

Information from the left side of where someone is looking is referred to as the left visual field, and information from the right side of visual fixation is referred to as the right visual field. The left and right visual fields map directly onto the visual cortex via the optic tract and, ultimately, the optic radiations. The relationship between the visual fields, visual pathways, and cortex can be summarized as follows:

- Information from the left side of visual space (left visual field) is sent to the right hemisphere.
- Information from the right side of visual space (right visual field) is sent to the left hemisphere.
- Information from above the fixation point is sent to the visual cortex below the calcarine fissure.
- Information from below the fixation point is sent to the visual cortex above the calcarine fissure.
- Information from where the eyes are fixated (foveal vision) is sent to the occipital poles.
- Information from the periphery of the visual fields is sent to the cortex away (medial and anterior) from the occipital poles.

Damage to a specific location within the optic radiations or occipital lobe will result in loss of vision within the corresponding area of the visual field.

Examples of visual-field impairments

Homonymous right hemianopia

Damage to the pathways within the left hemisphere, or left occipital cortex, will result in loss of visual perception for information from the right visual field, called a homonymous right visual field hemianopia (Figures 3-44A–D).

Homonymous left hemianopia

Damage to the pathways within the right hemisphere, or right occipital cortex, will result in loss of visual perception for information from the left visual field, called a homonymous left visual field hemianopia (Figure 3-45A).

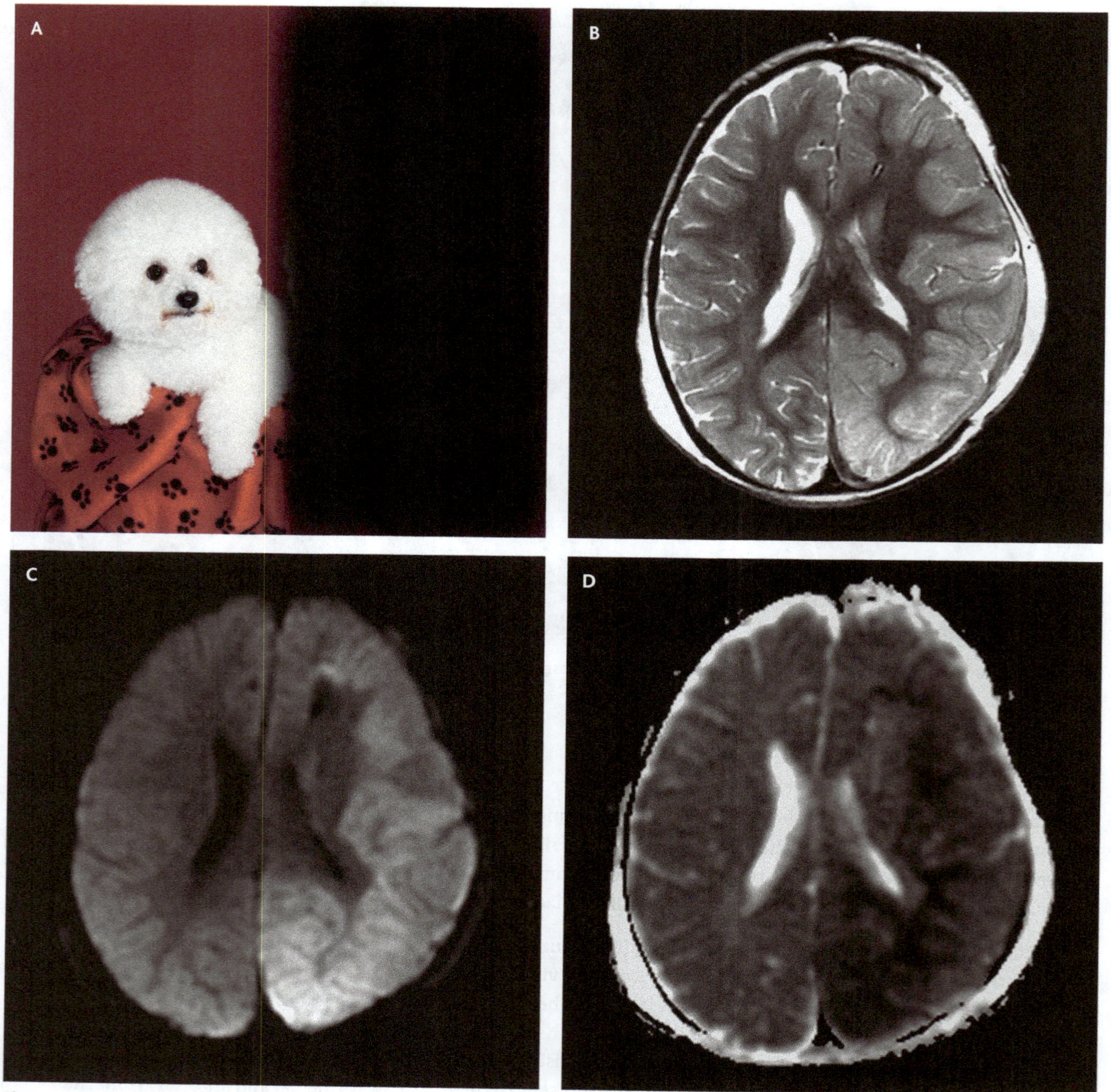

Figures 3-44A–D Nonaccidental trauma (shaken baby) with left occipital lobe injury. Because the injury involved the pathways and cortex in the left hemisphere, vision was lost for the right side of space. The injury is evident as slight hyperintensity on T2, more prominent hyperintensity on DWI and hypointensity on ADC. **A:** right homonymous hemianopia. **B:** T2. **C:** DWI. **D:** ADC.

Meili was hospitalized with rapidly deteriorating neurological status following an overdose of ecstasy and amphetamines. Initial workup suggested multiple strokes, the largest involving the right posterior parietal and occipital lobes. The smaller strokes involved the deeper subcortical structures, midbrain, and brain stem. After waking, Meili was unable to perceive visual information from the left side of space within her left visual field (Figure 3-45A), as expected given imaging findings of damage to her right occipital cortex and optic radiations. On imaging studies, the primary stroke is evident as an area of hypodensity on CT within the right occipital lobe or visual cortex (Figure 3-45B). The damage appears as an area of hyperintensity on T2 FLAIR imaging (Figure 3-45C), and "lightbulb bright" on DWI sequences (Figure 3-45D). No ADC sequences were acquired for this patient, although restricted diffusion is suggested by the

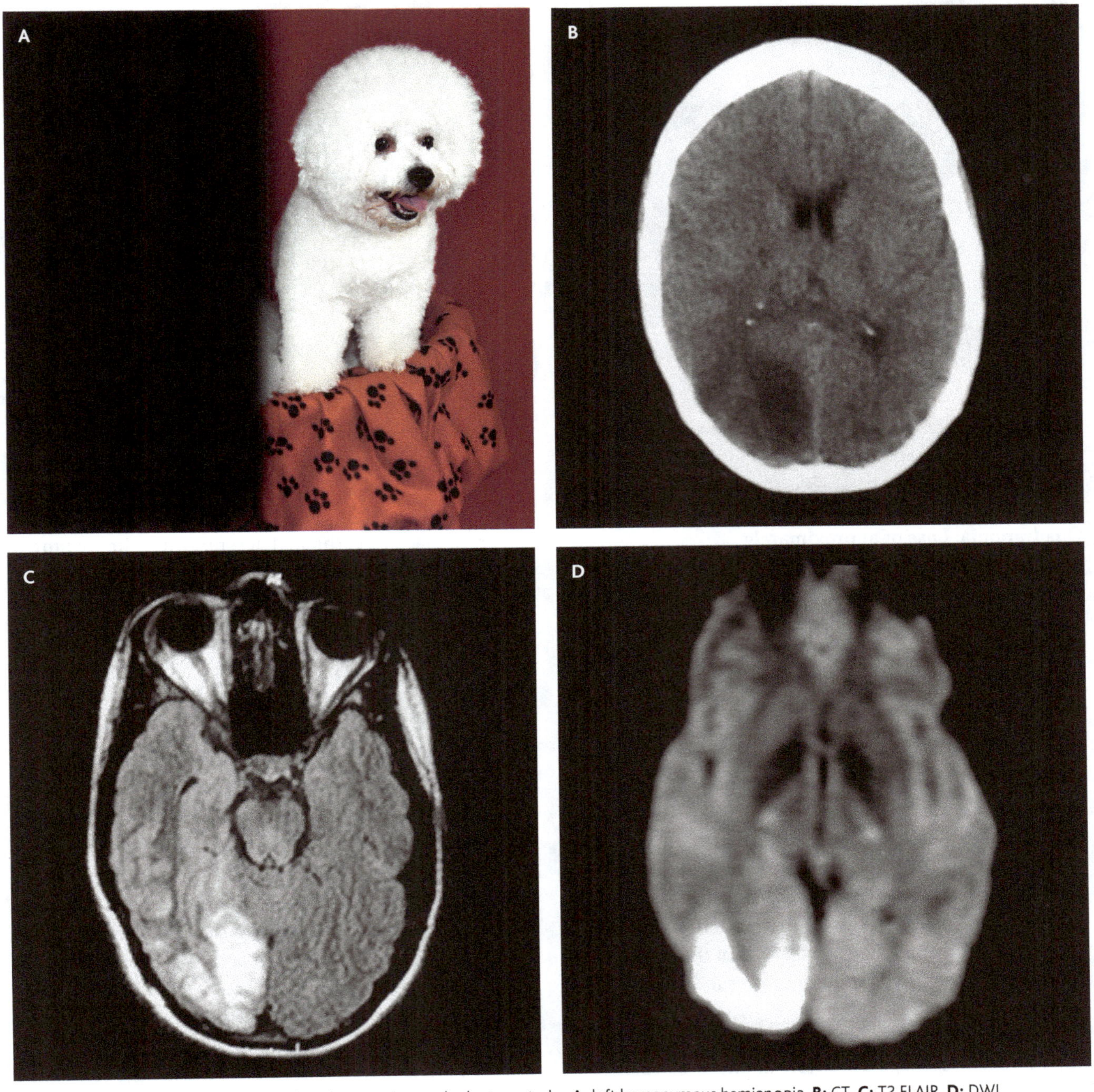

Figures 3-45A–D Clinical example Meili: right posterior cerebral artery stroke. **A:** left homonymous hemianopia. **B:** CT. **C:** T2 FLAIR. **D:** DWI.

excessive brightness on DWI, greater than would be expected with T2 shine-through alone. Meili's case was especially interesting in that she also experienced Charles Bonnet syndrome with constant hallucinations in her "blind" left visual field. Meili was able to describe shapes, lines, and colors in her impaired visual field, with some of her hallucinations being complex and involving the perception of rooms with furniture, or natural scenes. Unfortunately, a few days after being hospitalized, Meili began to experience respiratory distress and loss of central nervous system arousal. It is believed that she may have experienced vascular compromise due to the smaller strokes involving her brain stem. Deterioration continued until she died only a couple of weeks following her initial hospitalization.

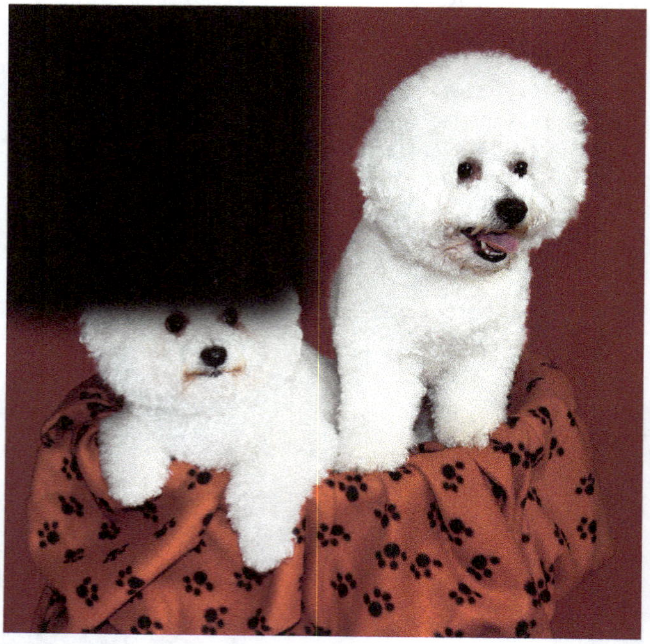

Figure 3-46 Quadranopia.

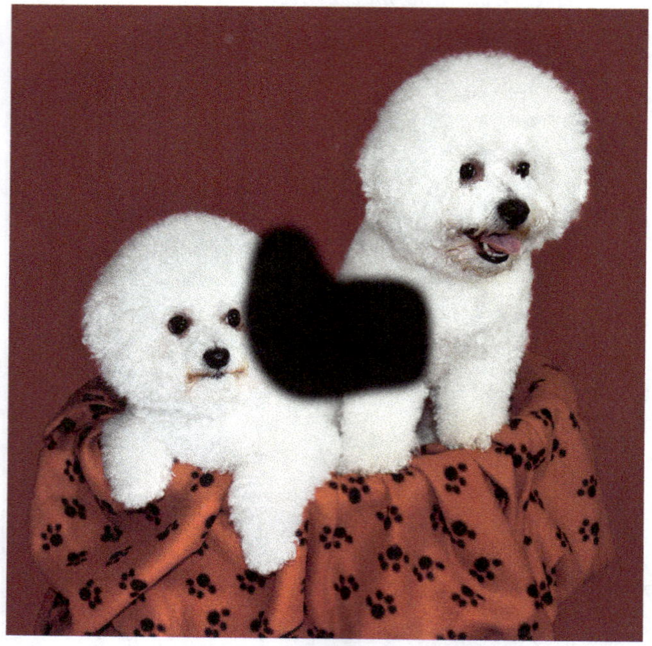

Figure 3-47 Central-field scotoma.

Quadranopia: Loss of approximately one quarter visual field

Damage to the lower part of the visual cortex (below the calcarine fissure) in the right hemisphere will result in visual loss to the upper quadrant of the left visual field (upper-left quadranopia), as illustrated in Figure 3-46. Quadranopias can be in any of the four quadrants, depending on the specific location of damage.

Scotoma: Visual-field loss other than half or one quarter

Damage to the pathways or cortex that does not correspond to a specific half or quarter visual field (hemianopia or quadranopia) is called a scotoma. A small area of damage to the occipital poles can result in a central field scotoma, as illustrated in Figure 3-47. Damage within the visual cortex but lateral to the occipital poles can result in a peripheral scotoma.

Patients with visual field loss due to visual pathway or cortex damage are often unaware of their deficits and may not realize that they have a hemianopia, quadranopia, or scotoma. Therefore, it is important to do a thorough visual-field assessment following review of any brain scan suggesting damage to the visual pathways or cortex.

CLINICAL EXAMPLE

Julia: Left Visual Field Hemianopia

Julia suffered a gunshot wound to her right hemisphere. The bullet traveled from her right frontal lobe, through the soft tissue of the brain, and exited through the parietal lobe. The bright white on the CT scan (Figure 3-48) represents bone, and the lighter areas or light gray represent blood. Note the piece of bone located within the optic radiations of the right hemisphere, just lateral to the posterior horn (arrow). Julia was fortunate that her language was localized to her left hemisphere, resulting in no language deficits.

Julia's primary symptoms involved a dense left-sided hemiparesis and a left visual-field hemianopia. Because the injury

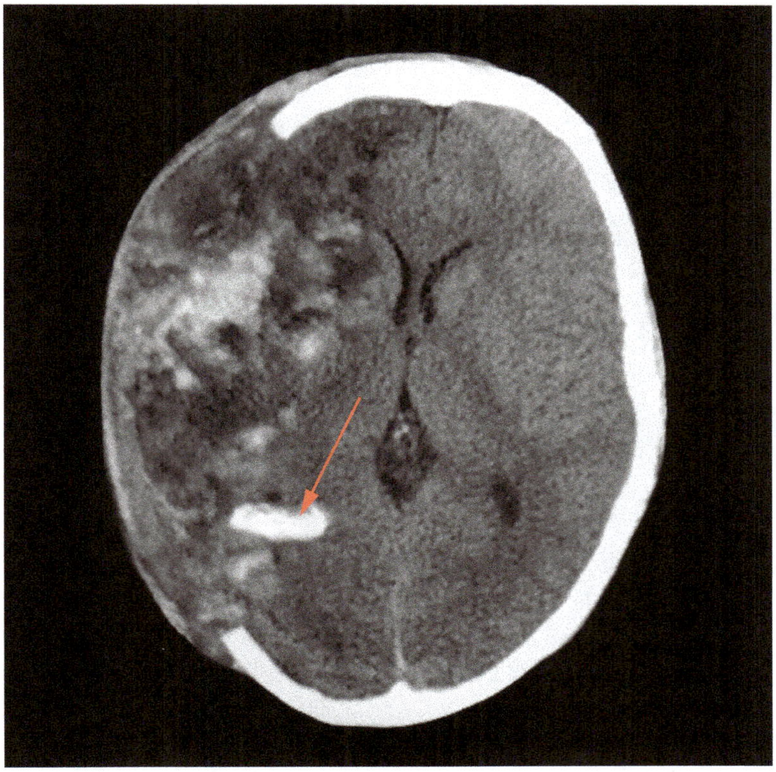

Figure 3-48 Clinical Case Julia: bone in the optic radiations of the right hemisphere.

included her right parietal lobe, she experienced both a hemianopia and a left-sided hemineglect. Julia's neglect syndrome meant that she did not spontaneously pay attention to the left side of her body, often failing to attend to her left arm. To help her pay more attention to her left arm, she named it "Amelia" and made a point of checking in with "Amelia" when moving or changing positions. Julia also neglected to pay attention to information on the left side of her attentional field. Even though she only perceived information from the right visual field, her left neglect meant that she did not pay attention to the left side of her right visual field, making visual tasks even more difficult.

BASIC ANATOMICAL AREAS OF THE BRAIN

The primary areas of the brain are organized in a hierarchy (Figure 3-49). The structures are named using two protocols, one from embryology and the other from adult anatomy. Radiologists may use both embryologic and adult anatomical terms within the same report, which can become confusing. This section will use the most common terms for the various structures and, where appropriate, provide more than one label for a particular brain structure. The primary functional areas of the brain will be discussed in this

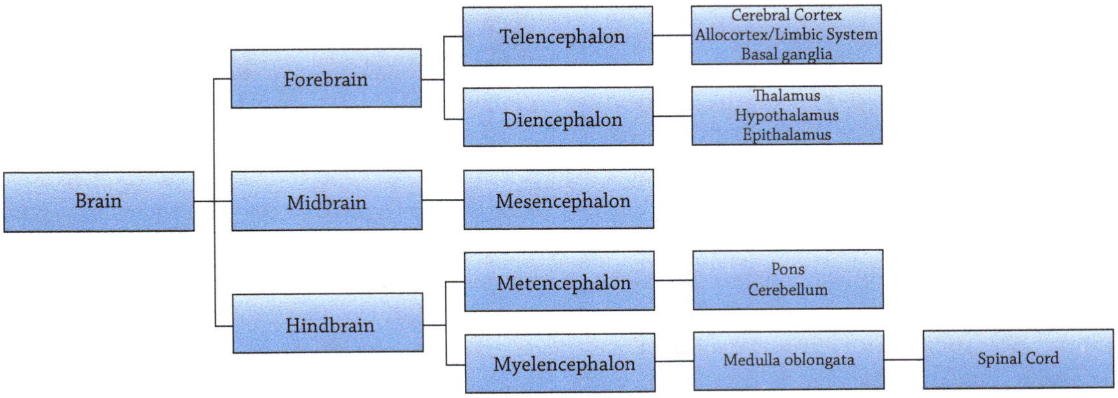

Figure 3-49 Primary areas of the brain.

section. Appendix 3-1 provides a summary of the general functions for many of the areas described below.

Forebrain

The forebrain consists of two primary areas. The largest component of the forebrain is the telencephalon, which makes up the cerebral cortex, allocortex or limbic system, and the basal ganglia. The other part of the forebrain is the diencephalon, primarily made up of the thalamus and hypothalamus.

Telencephalon

The most common name for the telencephalon is the *cerebrum*. The telencephalon is primarily responsible for cognition and intellect, personality, social and emotional control, sensory processing, and voluntary movement. The largest parts of the telencephalon form the cerebral cortex, the outside surface of the brain, and the white-matter tracts below the cortex. The telencephalon includes the allocortex, also called the limbic system or Papez circuit, a group of structures and pathways located deep within the brain. Close to the limbic structures are the nuclei that make up the basal ganglia, also considered part of the telencephalon.

Cerebral Cortex

The outer layer of the brain forms the cerebral cortex, often called "gray matter," owing to the dark appearance of the layer on brain slices. The cortex (Latin = bark or rind) is formed from six layers of neurons. The lamina organization was first described by Santiago Ramon y Cajal. Figure 3-50 depicts a Nissl-stained adult cortex (left) and motor cortex (middle) showing the cell bodies and neurons. The right picture shows a Golgi-stained infant cortex, highlighting the dendrites and axons.

On a brain slice, the cortex is visible as the approximately 2- to 3-mm thick convoluted layer around the periphery of the brain (Figure 3-51). The small grooves within the cortical surface are called sulci (singular sulcus), and the bulges are called gyri (singular gyrus). The larger divisions between areas of cortex are called fissures.

Given the folding of the brain during development, there are areas of cortex within each hemisphere that are covered and not visible from the outside. The insular (Latin: = island) cortices are covered by the temporal lobes and the frontal and parietal operculum, or overhang (Latin: *operculum* = little lid or cover) (Figures 3-52A–C).

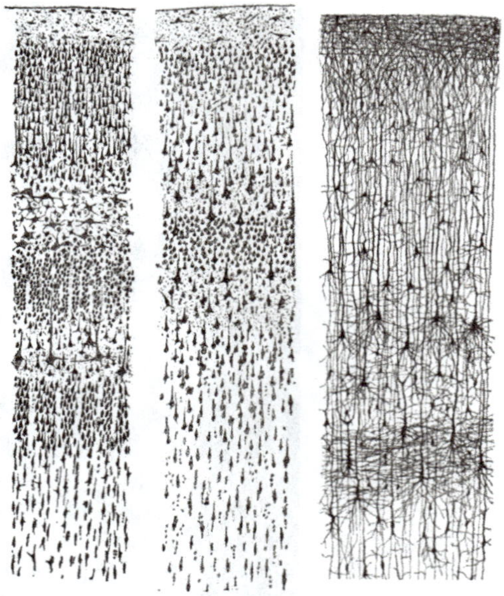

Figure 3-50 Cerebral cortex. Nissl-stained adult cortex (left) and motor cortex (middle). Golgi-stained infant cortex (right). Images from Finger, S. (1994). *Origins of neuroscience*. New York: Oxford University Press.

Damage to the cortex can result in a variety of symptoms, depending on the specific area or areas affected.

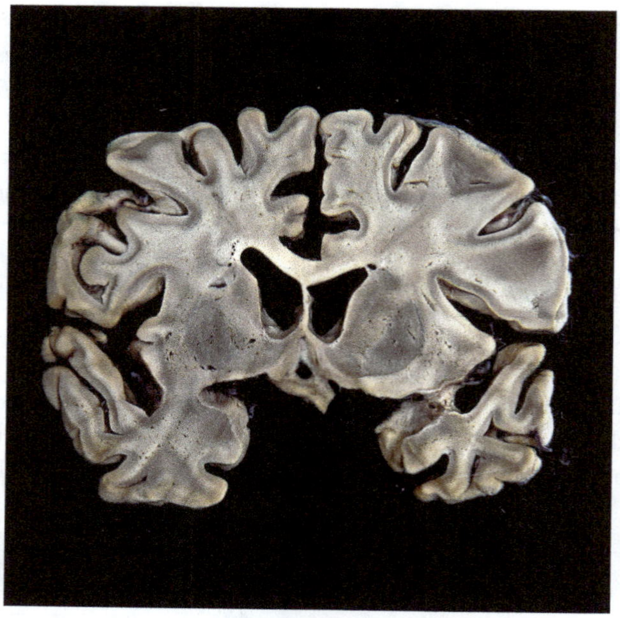

Figure 3-51 Brain slice showing cerebral cortex as the outer most layer of dark tissue.

Aaron was injured during a motor vehicle accident. Most of his brain injury was within the medial and lateral right frontal lobe and medial occipital lobe. Over time, breakdown of his cortical lamina became increasingly apparent on brain imaging. Cortical lamina necrosis may be difficult to appreciate on CT and appears as a hypodense rim following the contours of the sulci and gyri (Figure 5-53a).

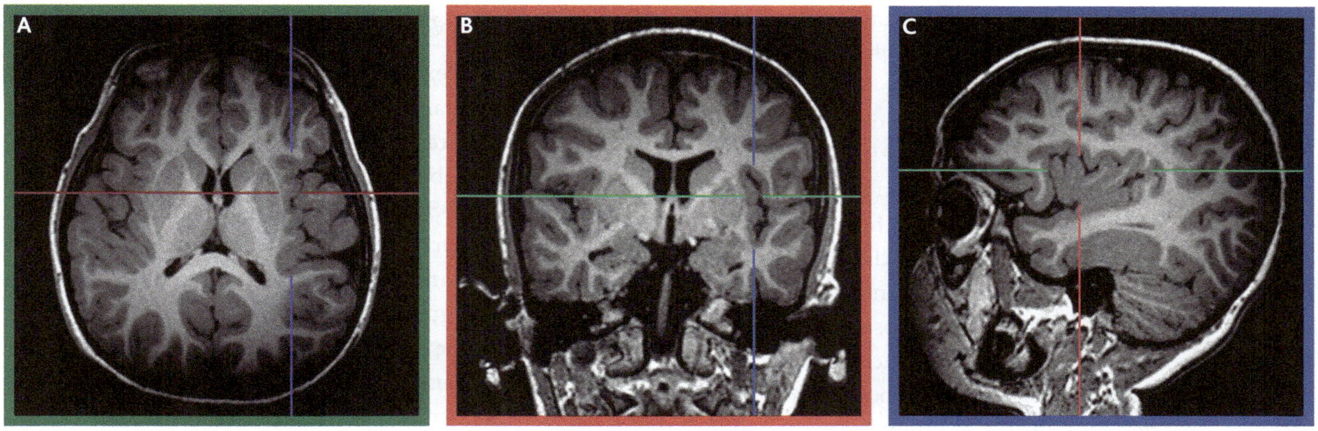

Figures 3-52A–C Insular cortex on axial (A), coronal (B) and sagittal (C) views.

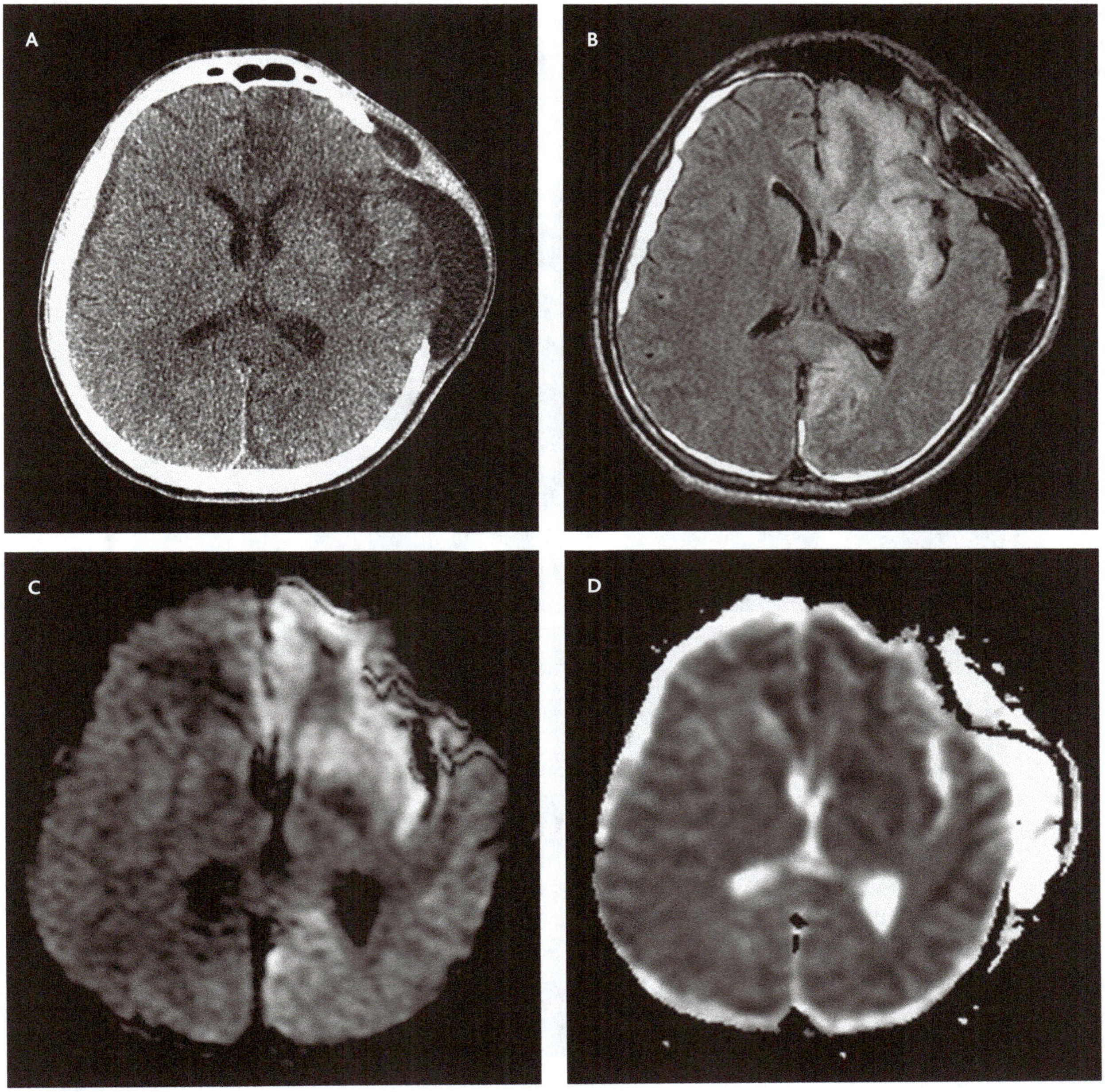

Figures 3-53A–D Clinical example Aaron: damage to the cortex—lamina necrosis. **A:** CT. **B:** T2 FLAIR. **C:** DWI. **D:** ADC.

Cortical lamina necrosis is more readily evident on T2 FLAIR and DWI/ADC MRI sequences, with hyperintensity on T2 (Figure 3-53b) and DWI (Figure 3-53c) sequences and hypointensity on ADC (Figure 3-53d) images.

Although cortical laminar necrosis can be relatively simple to visualize on a variety of brain scans, more subtle damage to the cortical layers is much more difficult to appreciate on brain imaging. The identification of minor cortical malformations is often critical in medical management of the patient, especially for those with refractory epilepsy. Once an identifiable lesion such as cortical dysplasia is identified and found to have a location concordant with ictal data derived from electroencephalography (EEG) or magnetoencephalography and magnetic source imaging (MEG-MSI), surgical treatment options may become available to the pateint. As MRI magnet strength increases, the ability to visualize small areas of cortical dysplasia or damage not currently visible on lower-strength imaging systems will increase.

Lobes of the brain

The cerebral cortex is divided into four primary lobes: the frontal, parietal, temporal, and occipital lobes of each hemisphere. Colored pictures in anatomy texts make it appear that the lobes have discrete divisions on the brain surface (Figures 3-54a–d). In reality, the divisions between the lobes are often difficult to appreciate when looking at the brain surface and even harder to differentiate on brain images. Sulci and gyri patterns are not equal across persons and may make lobe identification even more complex.

Although systematic localization of cortical functioning dates back over 100 years, it is still important to consider that there is some normal variability across persons. Two individuals may have significant functional differences related to the same cortical area. This is especially true for those who suffer a brain injury at an early age, where neural plasticity and reorganization are a component of recovery. Children with neurodevelopmental disorders may also have

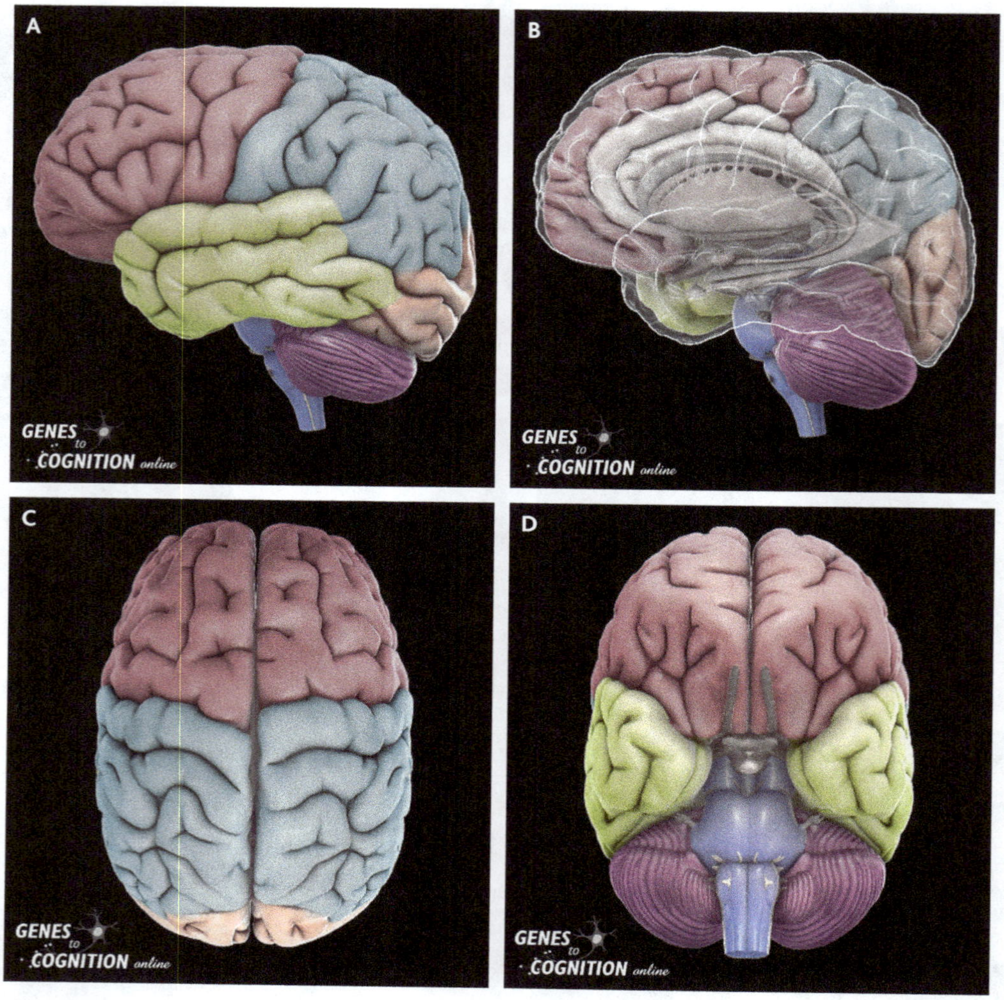

Figure 3-54A–D Lobes of the brain on three dimensional illustration. **A:** Lateral view. **B:** Medial view. **C:** View from above. **D:** View from below. *Red/Rust = Frontal; Light Blue = Parietal; Yellow = Temporal; Orange = Occipital; Purple = Cerebellum; Dark Blue = Hind Brain*

functional brain organization that is different from that of a normally developed child.

Functional localization and mapping via fMRI, Wada evaluation, intrasurgical electrical stimulation during awake craniotomies, or via neuropsychological procedures are critical in assisting surgeons in determining areas of eloquent functional cortex. Through such procedures, it becomes readily apparent that small differences between patients is the norm, and at times large differences can be evident. The most obvious differences between patients involve the localization of language functions. As a general rule, approximately 70% of persons have language localized to their left peri-sylvian region. However, approximately 27% of the population have some language functioning located in their right hemisphere, with approximately 3% of the population having all of their language abilities located in the right peri-sylvian region.

When considering functional neuroanatomy from the perspective of brain imaging, it is critical to take into account the normal variation between patients, even when there is no brain injury. As such, it is not uncommon to review a brain scan and formulate an opinion of expected symptoms or deficits from the areas involved, only to discover that the patient does not exhibit such difficulties.

CLINICAL EXAMPLE
Connor: Destruction of the Left Peri-Sylvian Region

Connor sustained a gunshot wound to his left hemisphere. Review of his brain scans revealed almost complete destruction of the left peri-sylvian region, a condition that would be expected to result in global aphasia (Figure 3-55). However, upon entering his room, he looked over and began to introduce himself with clear and fluent speech. He noted that he was bored and wanted to get out of bed. Connor was lucky in that he was one of the few individuals who have their language lateralized to the right hemisphere.

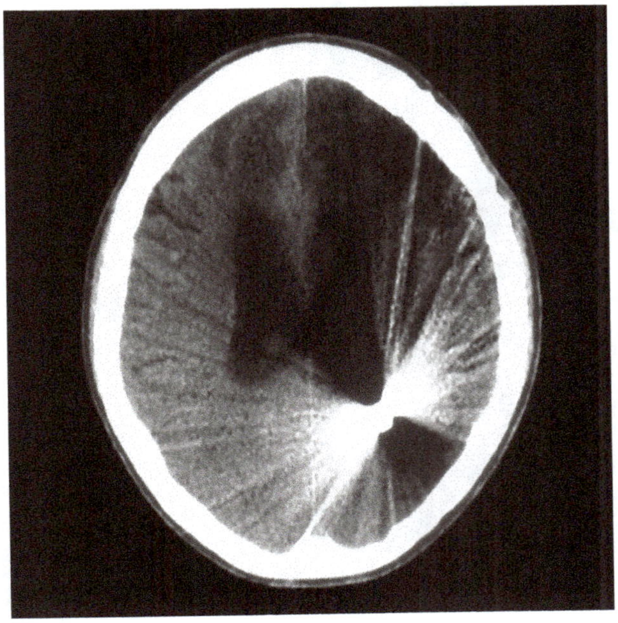

Figure 3-55 Clinical case Connor: gunshot injury to the left peri-sylvian region.

Brain mapping and functional brain imaging have consistently shown that functional areas of the brain may not precisely follow the anatomical regions thought to serve such functions. For example, it is not unusual during functional imaging or intrasurgical brain mapping to discover motor activation in areas of the parietal lobe, anatomically considered to be part of the sensory cortex. As a general rule, when mapping a brain using either functional imaging or electrically during awake surgeries, it is helpful to keep an open mind as to where functions may reside. Although the functional regions of cortex map very closely to anatomical regions, there is some variability. It is as if the functional area were distributed over the anatomical area with a small amount of variability, or "standard deviation." Over the anatomical region there is a very high probability of localizing the respective function, with the probability of localizing the function decreasing as you move away from the area. Given the variability of cortical localization, it is often better to be driven by your clinical examination than by findings on a brain scan. For example, if your patient presents with motor deficits but the brain scan appears to show damage only within the sensory cortex, do not become concerned about the discrepancy; just treat the patient as if you had never seen the scans. The patient still has a motor deficit, irrespective of the neuroimaging findings.

CLINICAL EXAMPLE
Kathy: Cavernoma

Kathy was experiencing new-onset seizures. Her brain imaging revealed a small cavernoma close to the central sulcus of her left hemisphere. She was right-handed, and damage to the cortex around the lesion could result in a right upper-extremity paralysis, something to be avoided if at all possible. fMRI and intrasurgical motor mapping of the region was performed before resection.

Findings from motor-based fMRI suggested that primary motor functioning for the right hand was located medial and superior to the cavernoma. In addition, the motor cortex for the right hand was localized to the postcentral gyrus, generally considered to be sensory cortex. In Figures 3-56A–D the cavernoma is identified by the arrows, and the area of greatest fMRI activation is identified by the orange and yellow regions.

During surgery, areas producing a clear motor, language, or sensory response were marked using small, square labels placed on the surface of the cortex (Figures 3-57A and B). The labels shown in green in Figure 3-57B cover the cortical regions found to map onto the patient's right hand and which were medial and superior to the cavernoma within the postcentral gyrus. Although it is difficult to appreciate given the view of the brain without clear references, the green areas are the same regions activated during right-hand movement using fMRI, as described above. Interestingly, stimulation around the cavernoma also produced speech arrest similar to that seen when Broca's area is electrically stimulated. This may seem unusual given the location of the cavernoma to the parietal lobe, although it is somewhat expected. The arcuate fasciculus is located directly medial and inferior to the cavernoma, a pathway leading directly to Broca's area. It is likely that the electrical stimulation around the cavernoma was communicated via this pathway to Broca's area, producing a response similar to that expected with direct stimulation of Broca's gyrus.

On the basis of fMRI and intrasurgical motor mapping, the surgery was performed in a manner to spare the region functionally identified as eloquent motor cortex. Kathy experienced no motor or sensory deficits after surgery.

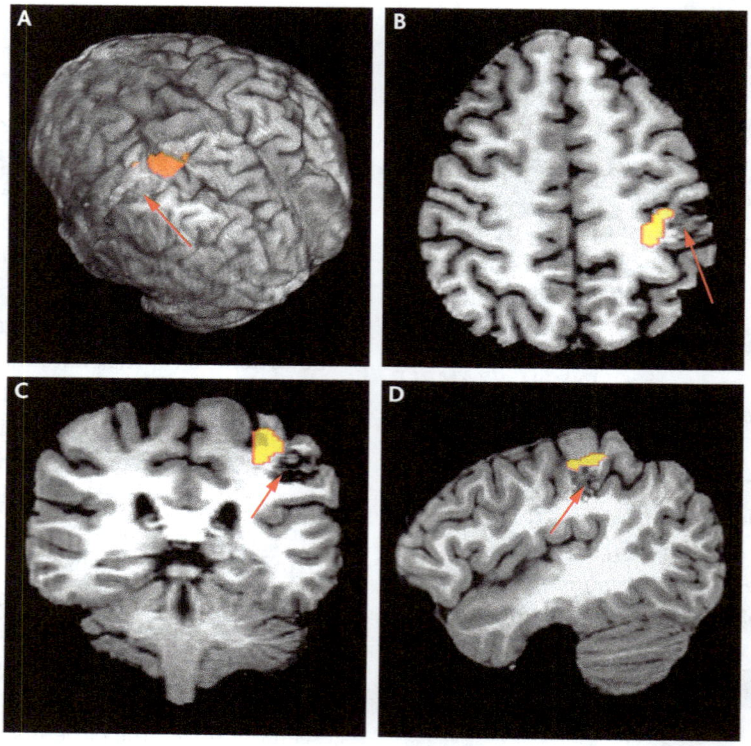

Figures 3-56A–D Clinical example Kathy: cavernoma. fMRI motor mapping of the right hand. Activation from her right hand is shown in orange/yellow, and the cavernoma is identified by the arrows.

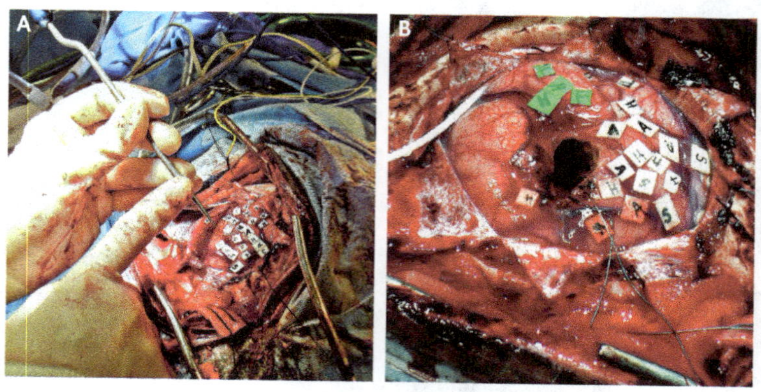

Figures 3-57A and B Clinical example Kathy: intrasurgical electrical stimulation with cortical motor mapping. **A:** Mapping before resection. **B:** Post-resection cavity. *Images courtesy of Margaret Verrees, M.D.*

As a general guide to functional neuroanatomy, clinicians have used the nomenclature of Korbinian Brodmann (1868–1918) for over a hundred years. Brodmann mapped the human cortex on the basis of cell structure, organization, and staining properties, but not according to function (Figure 3-58). However, over the past century, it has become clear that these areas match very closely the functional areas of cortex and are now used to describe both an anatomical structure and a functional region. For example, Area 17 is considered both the anatomical area and the primary functional area for visual processing.

Areas 1, 2, & 3 Primary somatosensory cortex

Area 4 Primary motor cortex

Areas 5 Somatosensory association cortex

Area 6 Supplementary/pre-motor cortex

Area 7 Somatosensory association cortex—pre-cuneus

Area 8 Frontal eye fields

Area 9, 46 Dorsolateral frontal cortex

Area 10 Frontal pole

Areas 11, 12 Orbital-frontal lobe

Areas 13, 14 Insular cortex

Area 15, 38 Anterior temporal lobe

Area 16 Insular—association cortex

Area 17 Primary visual cortex (V1)

Area 18 Secondary visual association cortex (V2)

Area 19 Tertiary visual association cortex (V3)

Area 20 Temporal lobe—inferior gyrus

Area 21 Temporal lobe—middle gyrus

Area 22 Temporal lobe—superior gyrus (close to Wernicke's area)

Areas 23, 24, 29, 31, 32, 33 Cingulate gyrus

Area 25 Subgenual cortex

Area 26, 30 Retrosplenial cortex

Area 27 Amygdala—medial temporal lobe

Areas 28, 34 Entorhinal cortex—medial temporal lobe

Area 35 Perirhinal cortex—medial temporal lobe

Area 36 Parahippocampal cortex—medial temporal lobe

Area 37 Fusiform gyrus

Area 39 Area close to the angular gyrus

Area 40 Supramarginal gyrus

Area 41 Superior temporal gyrus—primary auditory cortex

Area 42 Superior temporal gyrus—secondary auditory association cortex

Area 43 Subcentral area (at the base of the somatosensory gyrus)

Area 44 Subfrontal pars opercularis (Broca's area)

Area 45 Subfrontal pars triangularis

Area 47 Inferior orbital frontal gyrus

Area 48 Retrosubicular area of the temporal lobe

Area 49 Parasubicular area (between the presubiculum and entorhinal cortex)

Area 50 Band of cortex located on the frontoparietal operculum

Area 51 Piriform and the periamygdaloid cortices

Area 52 Parainsular area (between the temporal lobe and the insular)

Note: Not all areas are visible on brain diagrams or present in humans.

From Lebby, P.C., & Asbell, S. J. (2007). *The source for TBI: Children and adolescents.* East Moline, IL: LinguiSystems, Inc.

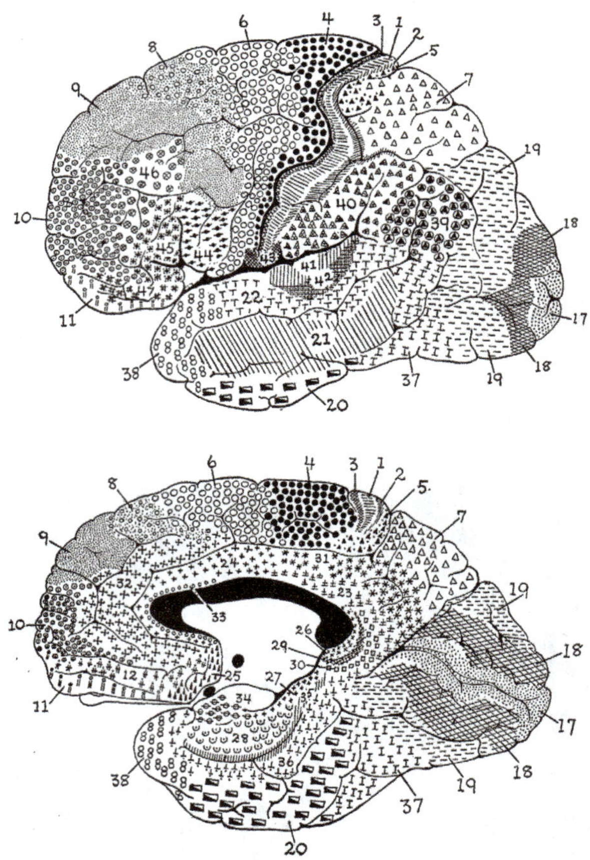

Figure 3-58 Brodmann map of human cortex. Brodmann, K. (1909). Reproduced with permission from: Finger, S. (1994). ***Origins of neuroscience***. New York: Oxford University Press.

Identifying areas of cortex on brain images

It is difficult to identify lobe margins on the lateral surface of a brain (Figure 3-59). Determination of lobe location or divisions between lobes using two-dimensional brain scans is even more challenging.

This section will present anatomical landmarks that are helpful in identifying the margins between the various cortical lobes when viewing two-dimensional brain images. See Appendix 3-1 for a general description of functions attributed to the various lobes.

PEARL Because of the lack of clear margins between the parietal, temporal, and occipital lobes on the lateral surface of the brain, it is best to describe structures or damage within these regions using two or more labels. For example, at the border between the parietal and occipital lobe, the term *parietal-occipital* is more appropriate than one or the other. Similarly, within the region between the parietal, temporal, and occipital lobes, the use of all three labels is appropriate, such as the *parieto-temporo-occipital junction*. Most traumas to the brain, whether caused by physical forces, infections, hypoxia, or other etiologies, affect relatively large regions of cortex and white matter. As such, it is not uncommon for descriptions of affected areas to involve more than one lobe. For example, damage can be described as predominantly frontotemporal, with some parietal involvement.

PERIL Do not become overly focused on margins between cortical regions, especially when considering the clinical effects of damage or a lesion. Often the functional margins are less clear than the anatomical margins presented in anatomy books. In addition, the sulci–gyri pattern differs a small degree between patients, making it difficult to determine the exact anatomical location of cortical tissue on brain images.

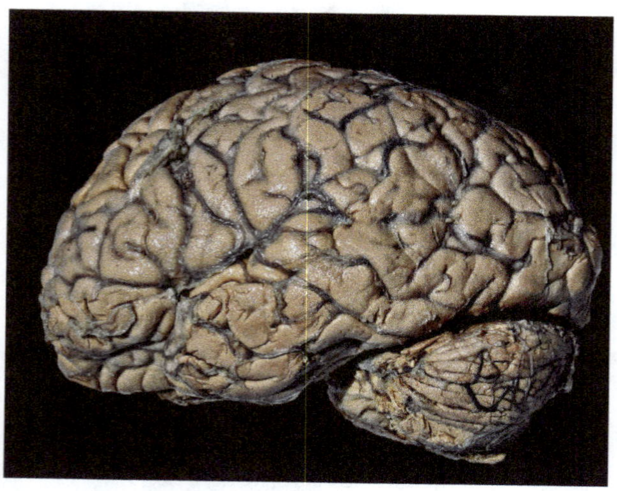

Figure 3-59 Lateral surface of brain shown on brain section.

Frontal and parietal lobes

When viewing the brain from the outside or lateral surface, the frontal lobes are identified by the direction of the gyri. From the front of the brain the gyri are organized horizontally (front to back). The lowest gyrus is the inferior frontal gyrus; above, there is the middle frontal gyrus; and at the top, the superior frontal gyrus. Broca's area, responsible for speech expression, is located at the most posterior aspect of the inferior frontal gyrus. When moving from front to back, the first gyrus oriented somewhat vertically is the precentral gyrus or primary motor cortex.

The frontal lobes extend from the frontal pole to the back of the precentral gyrus, or motor strip. At the back of the precentral gyrus, or motor strip, is a groove called the central sulcus. The central sulcus, also called the Rolandic sulcus, acts as a visual divider between the frontal and parietal lobes. Behind the central sulcus is another gyrus organized somewhat vertically, called the postcentral gyrus, or primary sensory cortex. The primary sensory cortex is considered part of the parietal lobe. Because the motor cortex is within the frontal lobe and the sensory cortex is within the parietal lobe, from a clinical standpoint, cortical damage that causes motor deficits is considered frontal, and that which causes sensory deficits is considered parietal. When dealing with pathways or subcortical structures, this becomes more complex.

It is important to understand that the precentral (motor cortex) and postcentral (sensory cortex) gyri are not organized completely vertical when the head is in its normal position. The precentral and postcentral cortices are angled diagonally backward, with the bottom of the gyri being more anterior than the top. This makes determination of frontal from parietal lobe structures on two-dimensional brain imaging difficult, especially if the central sulcus is not clearly evident on the particular slice being viewed.

On brain scans, locating the central sulcus is more difficult than when viewing the lateral surface of the brain, as it is difficult to appreciate the location of the gyri, sulci, and fissures.

Central sulcus—inferior margin

It is sometimes best to start with a sagittal paramedian image, with the slice close to the lateral edge of the brain (Figure 3-64). As long as the image slice is close to the edge

As an example of the variation in sulci–gyri patterning across patients, the following images were acquired from three different brains using axial, coronal, or sagittal slices acquired at similar slice locations and angles (3-60A–C, 3-61A–C, 3-62A–C). Note the gross similarities between the three brains, but also the differences in sulci–gyri patterning over most of the cortical surfaces.

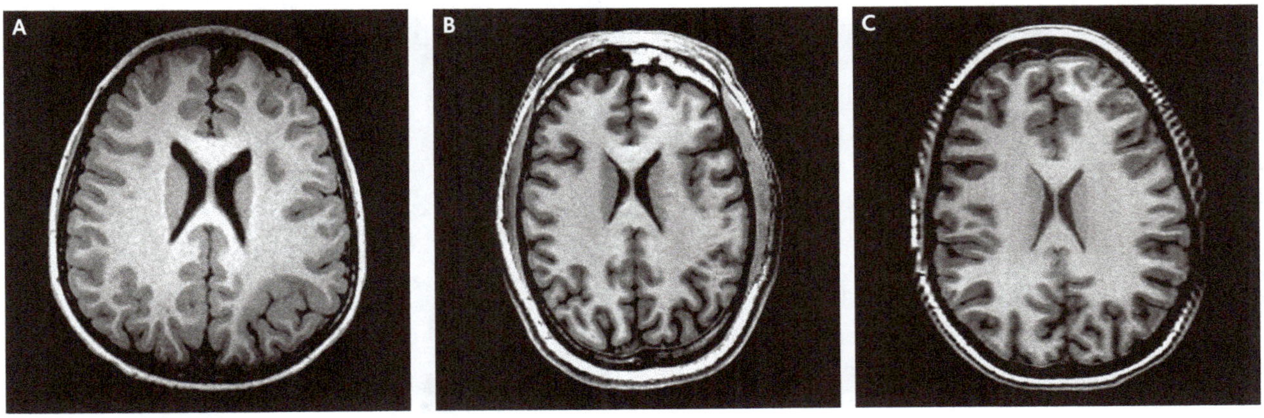

Figure 3-60 A: Brain A. **B:** Brain B. **C:** Brain C.

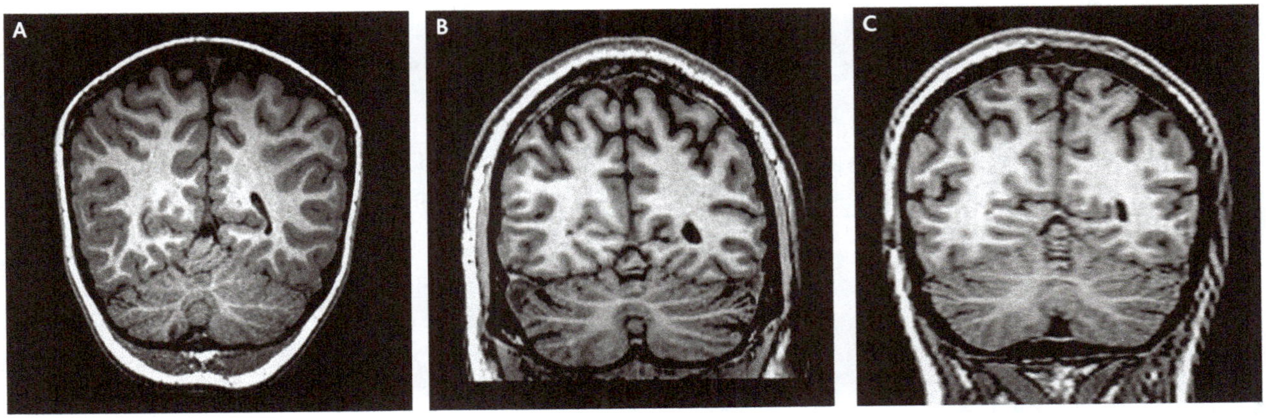

Figure 3-61 A: Brain A. **B:** Brain B. **C:** Brain C.

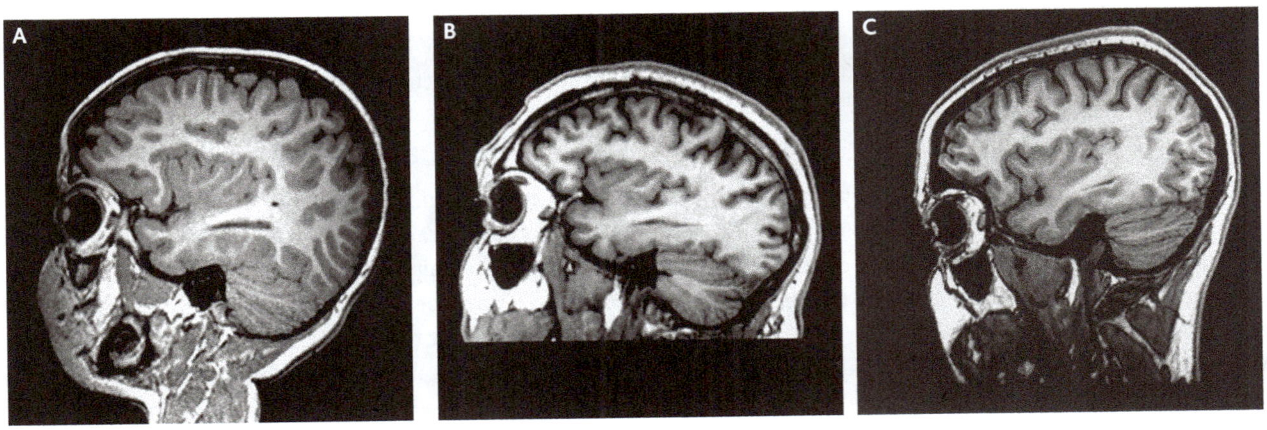

Figure 3-62 A: Brain A. **B:** Brain B. **C:** Brain C.

When attempting to identify the margin between the frontal and parietal lobes of the brain, it is helpful to know the general location of the central sulcus. On the outside of the brain, the easiest way to find the central sulcus is to scan the brain from the front to the back. The frontal gyri are oriented parallel to the horizontal axis of the brain until the precentral gyrus, or motor cortex. The precentral gyrus is the first gyrus to be organized more vertically, although it is actually at approximately a 30-degree angle. Working backward, the sulcus behind the motor cortex is the central sulcus, with the postcentral gyrus or sensory cortex directly behind.

In Figure 3-63, the frontal lobe is colored red, and the parietal lobe blue. The precentral gyrus forms the back margin of the frontal lobe. The central sulcus is represented by the diagonal line that splits the red and blue areas, or the frontal and parietal lobes.

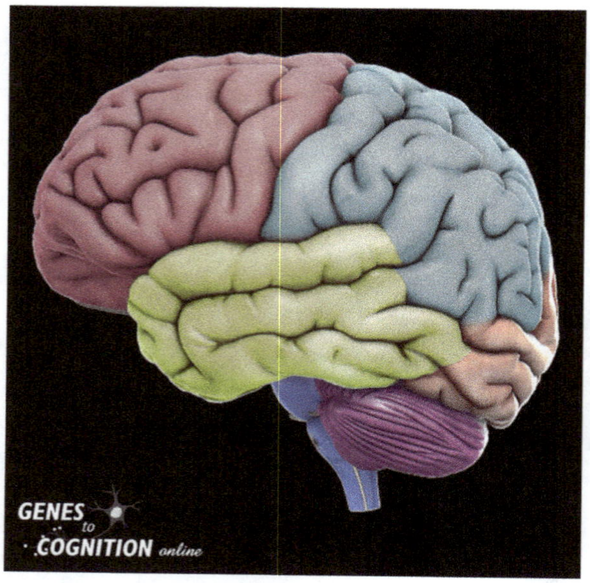

Figure 3-63 Frontal lobe (red) and parietal lobe (blue).

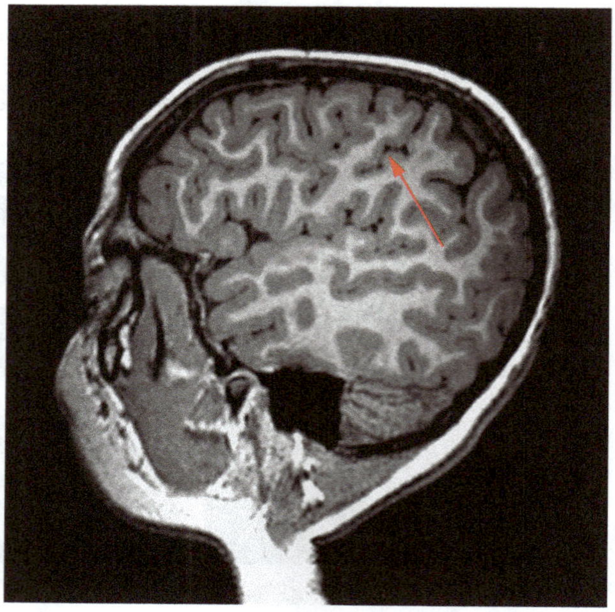

Figure 3-64 Central sulcus—inferior margin. Arrow shows central sulcus behind motor cortex.

of the brain, the direction of gyri can be appreciated. On the sagittal image, look for the horizontal gyri of the frontal lobe. Then follow the gyri moving more posteriorly until you see the mostly vertical or diagonal gyrus of the motor cortex. The sulcus behind the motor cortex is the central sulcus (Figure 3-64, arrow).

When viewing axial or coronal images, the assessment of gyri orientation is much more difficult. When using axial or coronal images, it is helpful to identify some key features evident on all image planes. At the base of the motor strip, or precentral gyrus, sits Broca's area, usually in the left hemisphere, although there is an analogous gyrus in the right hemisphere. Broca's area is located just anterior to the inferior motor cortex. With practice, this region is relatively simple to locate on all image planes.

- On axial view (Figure 3-65A), Broca's area can be identified as the curled gyrus just anterior to the insular and temporal poles.
- On coronal view (Figure 3-65B), Broca's area is identified as the tissue directly above the temporal poles on a slice just forward of where the temporal poles become separated from the rest of the brain.
- On sagittal view (Figure 3-65C), Broca's area is identified as the lobular gyrus above the temporal poles and just above the most anterior part of the Sylvian fissure.

Central sulcus—middle section

Locating the central sulcus on a more superior cut is made simple by choosing a sagittal slice close to the outside of the brain. The most common mistake is to assume that the sulcus should be at the front of the brain, as it separates the frontal and parietal lobes. However, as the sulcus moves more superior, it also moves back owing to the diagonal angle of the sulcus. At the level of the body of the lateral ventricles, look for the central sulcus a little more than half

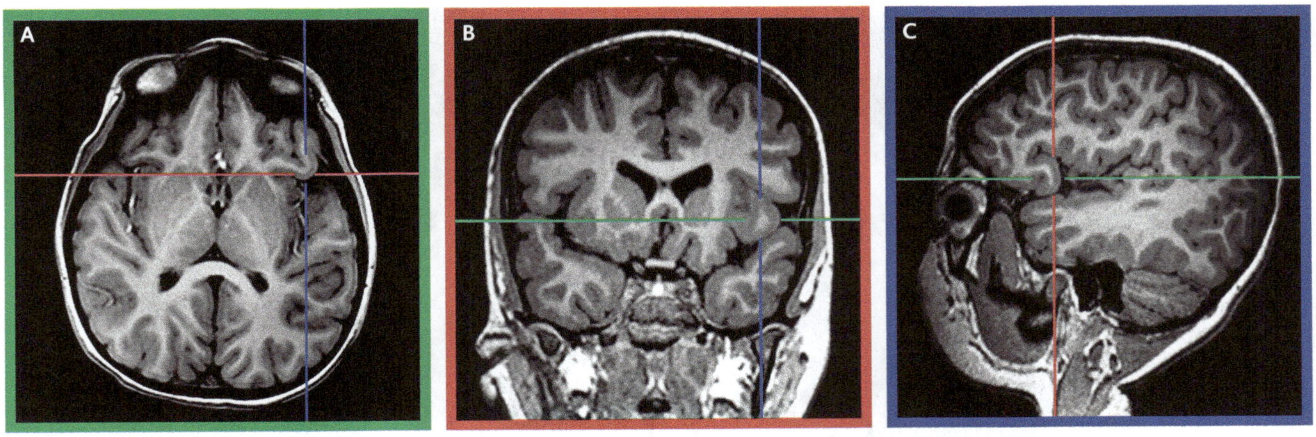

Figure 3-65 **A:** Axial image identifying the location of Broca's area. **B:** Coronal image identifying the location of Broca's area. **C:** Saggital image identifying the location of Broca's area.

way back from the front of the brain and above the Sylvian fissure.

- On axial images (Figure 3-66A), the middle of the central sulcus is located across from the splenium of the corpus callosum at a level often showing the complete lateral ventricles.
- On coronal images (Figure 3-66B), the central sulcus is located just above the superior temporal gyrus and Sylvian fissure.
- On sagittal images (Figure 3-66C), the central sulcus is located above and just forward of the most posterior part of the Sylvian fissure.

Central sulcus—superior margin

On the superior aspect of the brain, the division between the frontal and parietal lobes is further back than expected, given the diagonal angle of the central sulcus. The sulcus is evident along the edges of the lateral cortex and below the surface at the top of the brain (Figure 3-67, red-shaded sulcus).

- On axial images at the top or most superior aspect of the brain (Figure 3-68A), the central sulcus is identified between the first and second gyri clearly oriented laterally, but also angled diagnonally, approximately two thirds of the distance from the front to back.
- On coronal images at the top or most superior aspect of the brain (Figure 3-68B), the central sulcus is difficult to differentiate and such distinctions are best performed via reference to other image planes.
- On sagittal images at the top or most superior aspect of the brain (Figure 3-68C), the central sulcus is best viewed on a midsagittal slice with the central sulcus generally being located directly above the region between the isthmus and the splenium of the corpus callosum.

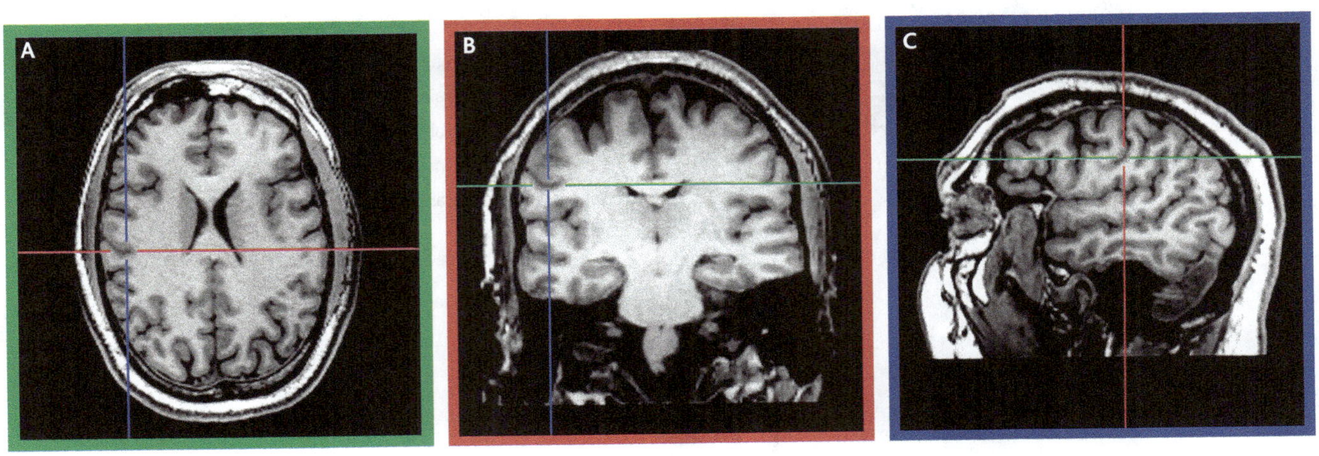

Figure 3-66 **A:** Axial view of central sulcus. **B:** Coronal view of central sulcus. **C:** Sagittal view of central sulcus.

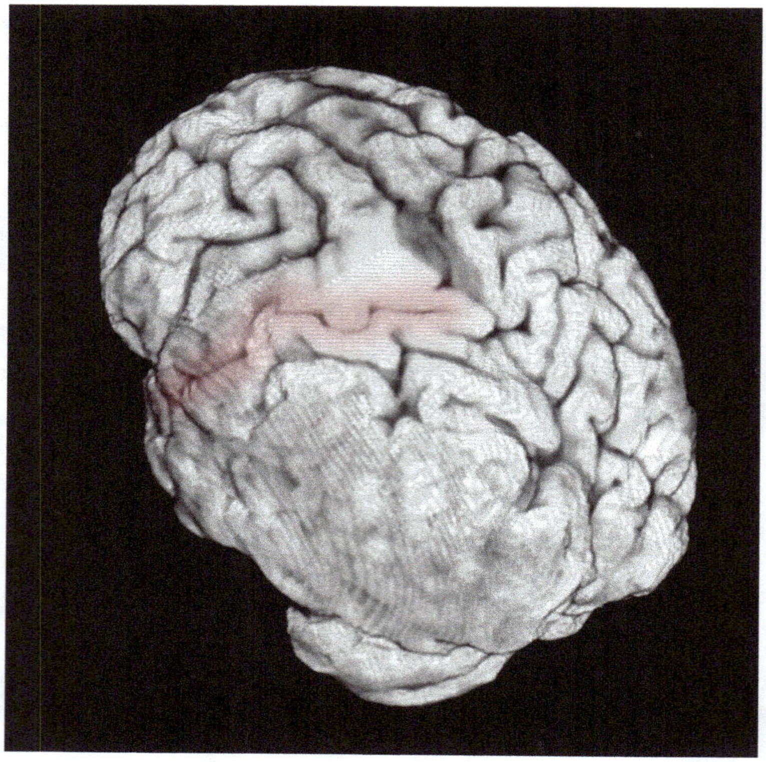

Figure 3-67 Central sulcus is shown by the red shading on 3D MRI.

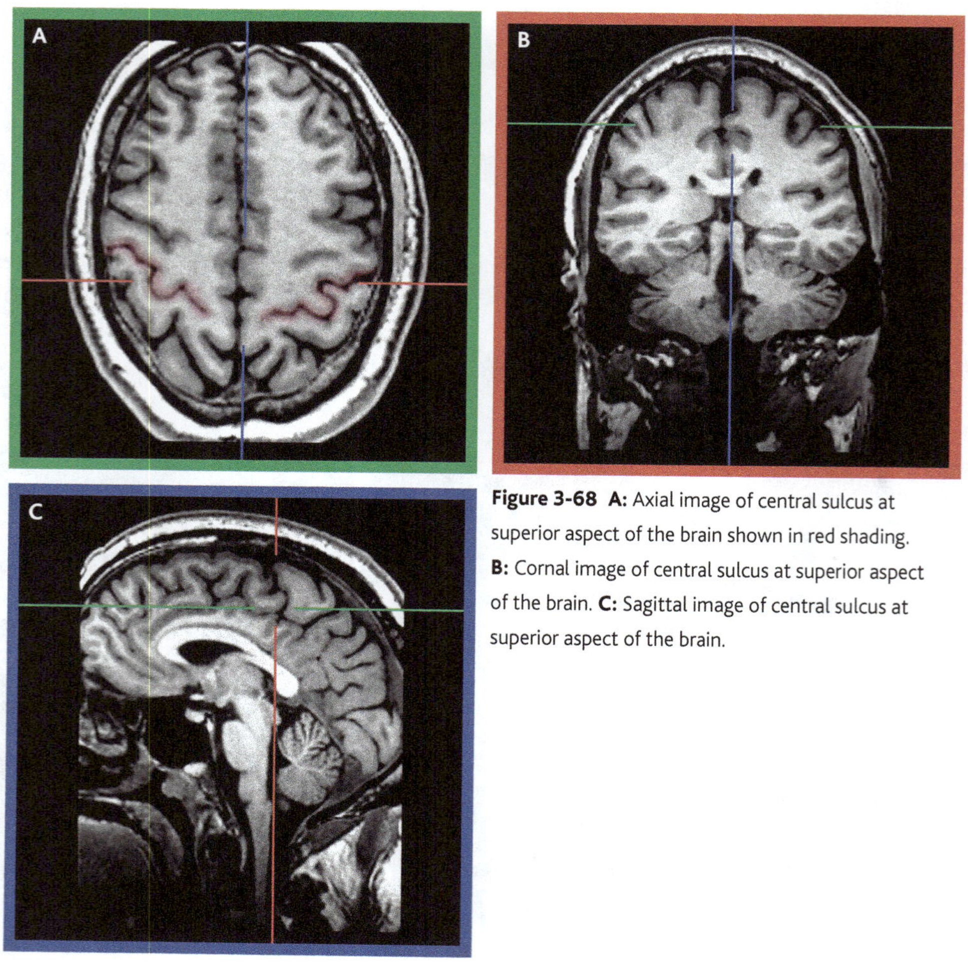

Figure 3-68 **A:** Axial image of central sulcus at superior aspect of the brain shown in red shading. **B:** Cornal image of central sulcus at superior aspect of the brain. **C:** Sagittal image of central sulcus at superior aspect of the brain.

When Front Is Actually Back

One of the more difficult concepts to appreciate when viewing brain scans is the impression that the superior motor cortex is located at the back of the brain. This is most evident on axial image slices acquired with an angle that cuts perpendicular to the spinal cord axis. What makes this even more confusing is that the motor cortex is part of the frontal lobe, and one would assume that it should appear at the front of the brain scan.

When laying on one's back, the head and brain position results in superior axial slices cutting through most of the frontal and just a small section of the parietal lobes. Most of the parietal lobe and all of the occipital lobe may fall outside of the image "window" and not be evident on the scan. As is clear from Figures 3-69a–d, the top of the motor cortex is actually at the back of an axial image that cuts through the superior part of the brain. Although it can seem to contradict the understanding that the motor cortex is within the frontal lobe, and the frontal lobe is at the front of the brain, the posterior margin of the frontal lobe can be located at the back of many axial images.

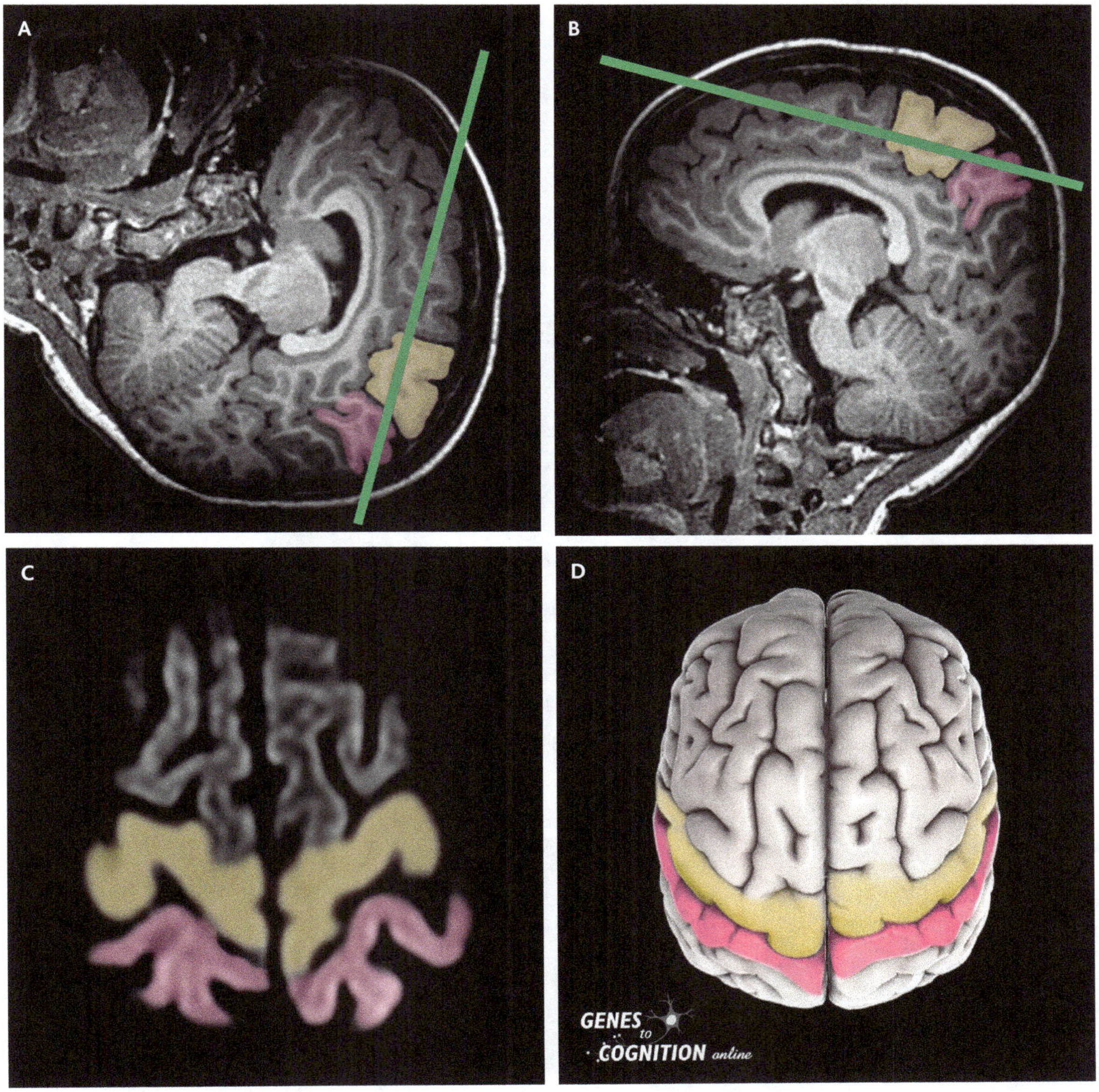

Figure 3-69 **A:** Patient lying on back. **B:** Standard orientation. **C:** Axial scan. **D:** Brain graphic. Note how far back the yellow gyrus appears on Figures 3-69C and 3-69D, even though it is still within the frontal lobe of the brain. *Green = Image slice; Yellow = Pre-central gyrus, part of the frontal lobe; Pink = Post-central gyrus, part of the parietal lobe.*

Temporal lobes

The temporal lobes sit below the frontal lobes (temporal pole) and parietal lobes (posterior temporal region). At the most anterior aspect, the temporal lobes are completely separated from the rest of the brain, although the middle and back of the temporal lobes are connected to the rest of the brain by both white-matter tracts and cortical tissue (Figures 3-70A–C). The anterior and middle sections of the temporal lobes are relatively simple to locate on any image plane as they are separated from the main brain structures by the Sylvian fissure, sometimes called the lateral sulcus or lateral fissure. Because of the lack of definitive margin between the posterior temporal and anterior occipital lobes, the margin is usually unclear on brain imaging (Figure 3-70C).

Occipital lobes

The occipital lobes are located at the back of the brain, above the cerebellum (Figure 3-71A–C). There is no definitive margin between the occipital lobes and the parietal lobes on the lateral surface of the brain. However, on the medial surface, the two lobes are divided at the parieto-occipital sulcus, generally only visible on midsagittal image sections (Figure 3-72 green shaded sulcus). On sagittal slices that do not transect the longitudinal fissure or on axial and coronal image views, it is difficult to clearly define the borders between the parietal, temporal, and occipital lobes. One way to locate the primary visual cortex on an axial or coronal slice is to follow the optic radiations that run lateral to the posterior horns of the lateral ventricles to the back of the brain where they terminate in the primary visual cortex.

Within the occipital lobe, there is a sulcus that divides the superior part of the cortex from the more anterior cortical tissue, called the calcarine fissure (Figure 3-72 red shaded fissure). Information from above the point of visual fixation is projected to the cortex below the calcarine fissure, and information from below the point of fixation is projected to the cortex above the calcarine fissure.

Information from the right visual field is projected to the left hemisphere, and information from the left visual field

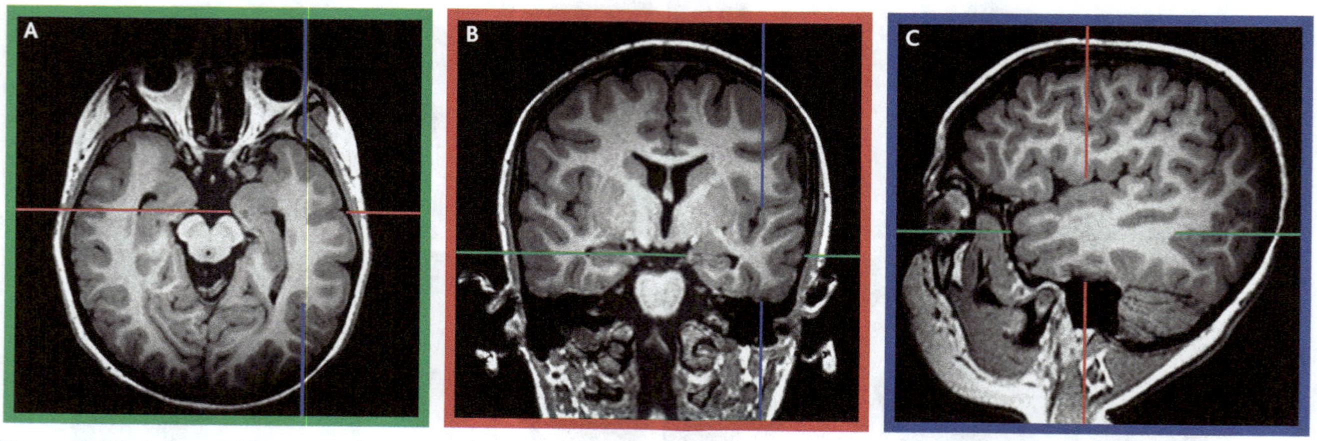

Figures 3-70A–C Temporal lobes presented on axial (A), coronal (B) and sagittal (C) MRI images.

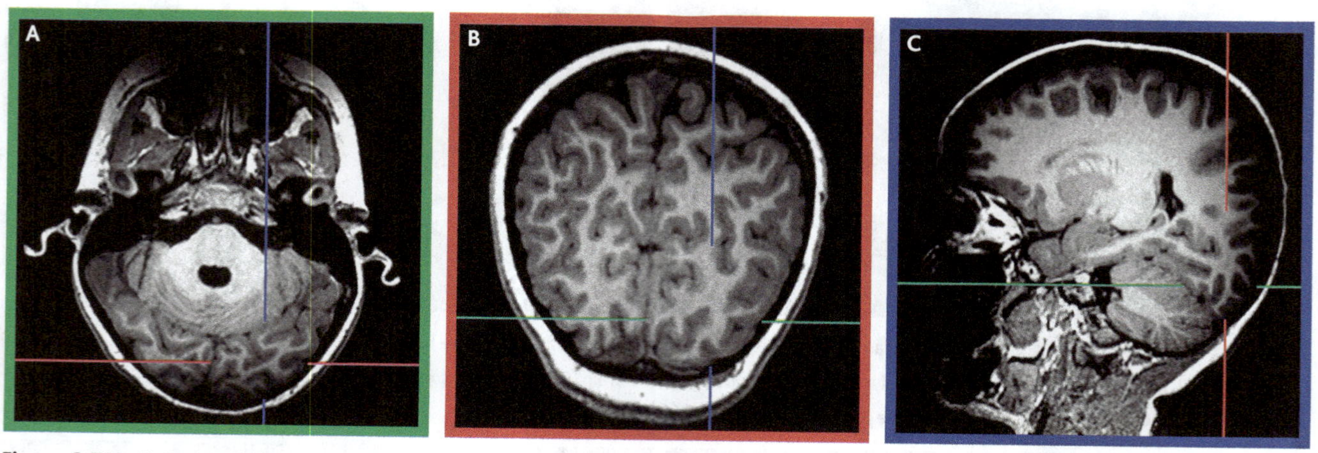

Figures 3-71A–C Occipital lobes presented on axial (A), coronal (B) and sagittal (C) MRI images.

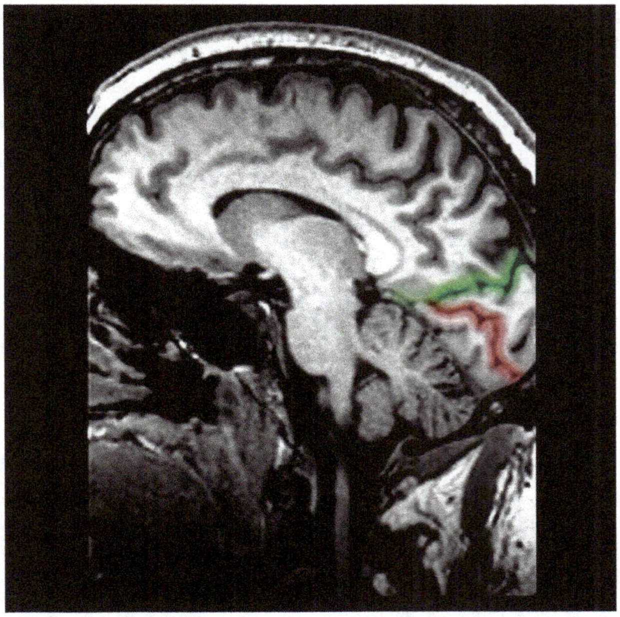

Figure 3-72 Midsagittal image of occipital lobes illustrating the location of the parieto-occipital sulcus (green) and the calcarine fissure (red).
Key for Figure 3-72: Green = Parieto-occipital sulcus; Red = Calcarine fissure

to the right hemisphere. Damage to the visual cortex follows the same basic rules as described in the white-matter pathway section earlier.

The occipital lobes are organized so that the primary or initial processing of visual information takes place at the most posterior part of the cortex. Within primary visual cortex, basic information relating to lines, contrast, color, and movement is processed, before being relayed to other areas of the occipital lobes for more complex and integrated processing. Increasingly complex and integrated visual functioning takes place deeper within the brain, in an area called visual association cortex. Visual association cortex is located between the occipital lobes and the temporal and parietal lobes. As a general rule, processing related to location in space takes place between the occipital and parietal lobes, and processing related to visual recognition takes place between the occipital and temporal lobes.

Limbic System or Lobe (Allocortex)

The limbic system, also called allocortex, is located below the primary areas of cortex described above and, as such, is considered part of the subcortical systems of the brain. The structures of the limbic system form a hypothetical circuit of nuclei and white-matter tracts, sometimes called the Papez circuit. The allocortex is tightly connected to the frontal lobes via white-matter pathways such as the uncinate fasciculus. These connections allow the frontal lobes to keep the primitive emotions and drives associated with the limbic system "in check" (e.g., aggression, rage, sexual behavior, predation, and fear), thus giving people the ability to behave appropriately in various social situations.

Areas of the limbic system include, but are not restricted to, the mammillary bodies, fornix, hippocampi, and amygdala bodies. The fornix is an arched white-matter pathway that connects the mammillary bodies to the hippocampi. Because much of the limbic system is formed from small groups of cells and thin white-matter tracts, it is difficult to differentiate many of the structures on MRI, and even less so using CT. The exception is the identification of the hippocampus, which is located within the medial surface of the temporal lobe and can be seen relatively easily on all image planes.

Hippocampi

The hippocampi (Latin: *hippocampus* = seahorse) are critical for memory consolidation and retrieval. Loss of both hippocampi and surrounding tissue generally results in severe anterograde amnesia or the inability to store new explicit memories.

The hippocampi are located within the medial, inferior surface of the temporal lobes. The hippocampi sit below and slightly medial to the inferior horns of the lateral ventricles. The fornix (Latin: arch) is located between the two bodies of the lateral ventricles and below the corpus callosum. The fornix bifurcates below the splenium of the corpus callosum as it connects to the hippocampal structures in each hemisphere (Figure 3-73).

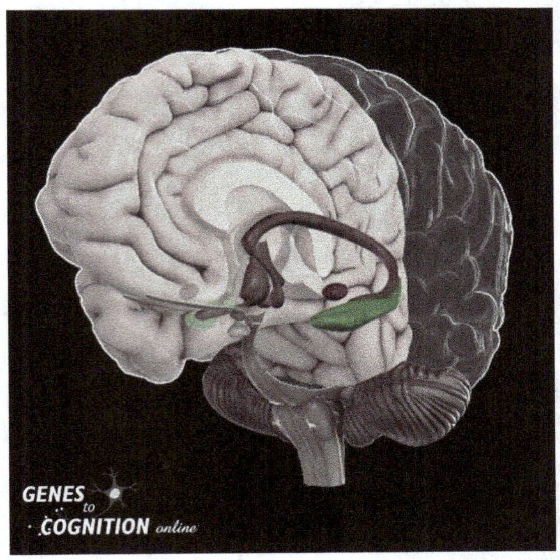

Figure 3-73 Hippocampi shown on a three dimensional brain illustration in green, with the posterior pathways forming the fornix shown in brown. The round, almond-shaped structure directly above the hippocampus in the left hemisphere is the amygdala. The brown lobular structures at the anterior section of the fornix are the mammillary bodies and hypothalamus.

Locating the hippocampi on brain scans

Axial

To locate the hippocampi on axial images (Figure 3-74A), use a slice that transects the temporal lobes between the middle and the poles. Look for the inferior or temporal horns of the lateral ventricles. The hippocampal structures form the inside wall of the inferior horns of the lateral ventricles, making them relatively simple to locate.

Coronal

On coronal images (Figure 3-74B), the hippocampi can be located on the medial edge of the inferior horns of the lateral ventricles. They also form the most medial gyri of the temporal lobes, sitting close to the cerebral peduncles as they form below the internal capsule. On coronal images, the hippocampi appear as curled structures, owing to the folded layers of cortical tissue that make up the structures.

Sagittal

On sagittal images (Figure 3-74C), the hippocampal structures can be located as a strip of gray matter deep within the temporal lobe and bordering the inferior horns of the lateral ventricles.

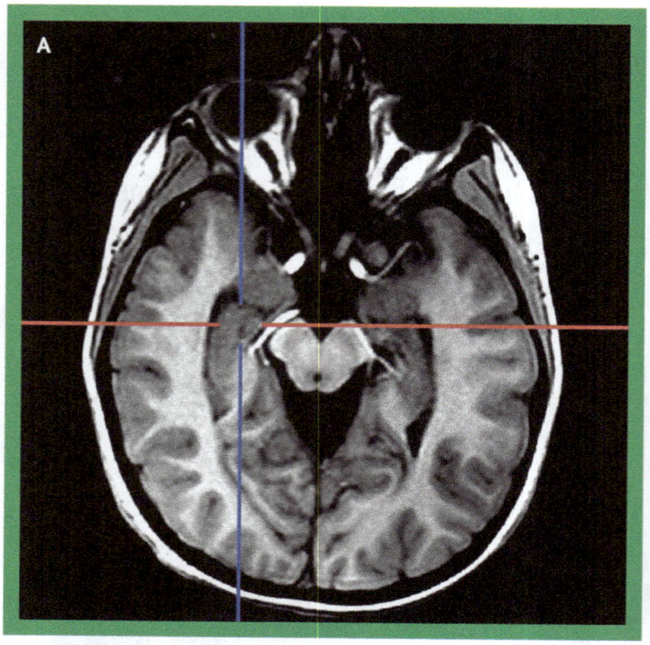

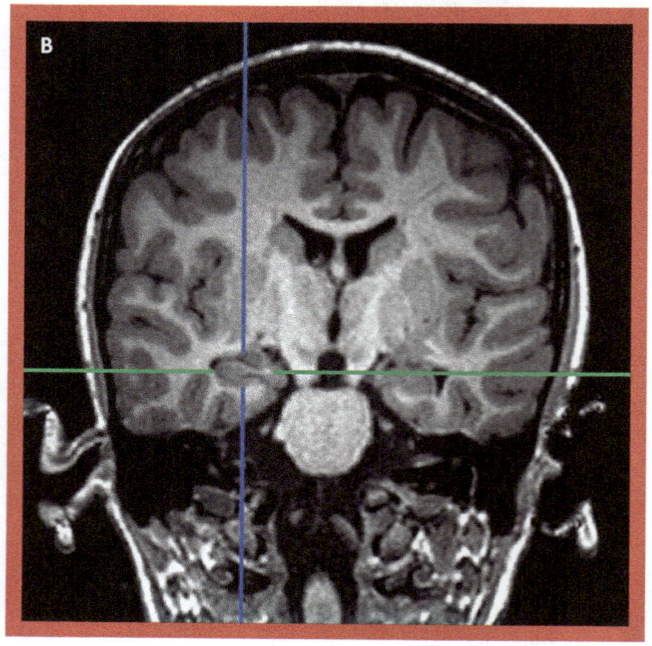

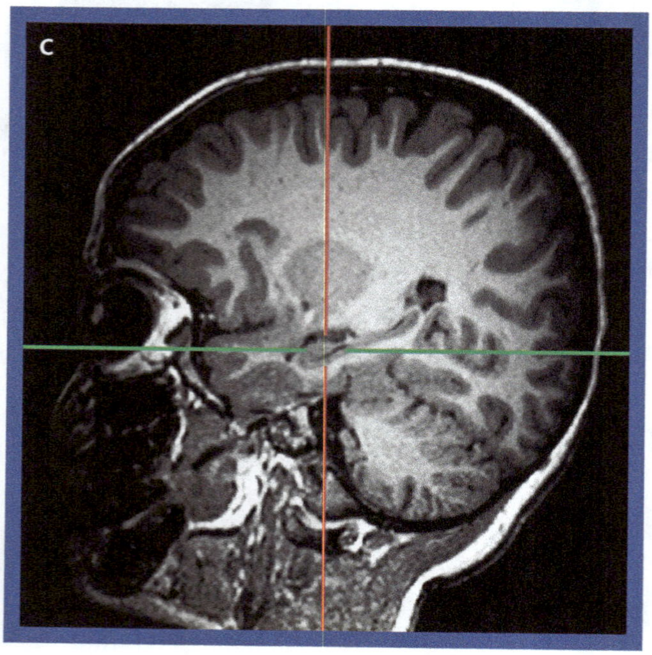

Figure 3-74 **A:** Hippocampi on axial image. **B:** Hippocampi on coronal image. **C:** Hippocampi on sagittal image.

Jack sustained notable damage to both of his hippocampi due to herpes encephalitis. When one hippocampus is damaged but the other remains intact, functional learning and memory is often preserved. However, when both hippocampi become damaged, the patient's ability to consolidate new memories becomes severely compromised, and anterograde amnesia is often the result. Jack's brain scans suggested bilateral damage to the hippocampi, the right hippocampus sustaining greater damage than the left (Figures 3-75A–C). In the hospital, Jack was unable to store new memories and forgot information after only a few seconds. When asked about his location, he would look around the room and guess on the basis of the type of furniture that he observed. When asked how long he had been in the hospital, he reported, "I didn't know I was in a hospital." Jack would introduce himself to the staff each time he met them, even if it had only been a few minutes between meetings. It was as if he were meeting them for the first time. When told that he had been in the hospital for several months, his response was, "Are you serious?"

As is often the case with patients who have anterograde amnesia from bilateral hippocampal damage, Jack failed to store new explicit memories but did develop implicit memories, such as a sense that he knew someone when asked, and a familiarity with his routine and equipment used during rehabilitation. It was hoped that Jack would recover the ability to store new memories with ongoing recovery. Unfortunately, even several years after discharge from the hospital, Jack was still unable to store new memories. When asked about his age, he reported an age consistent with that at the time of his illness. When told his actual age, he again responded, "Are you serious?"

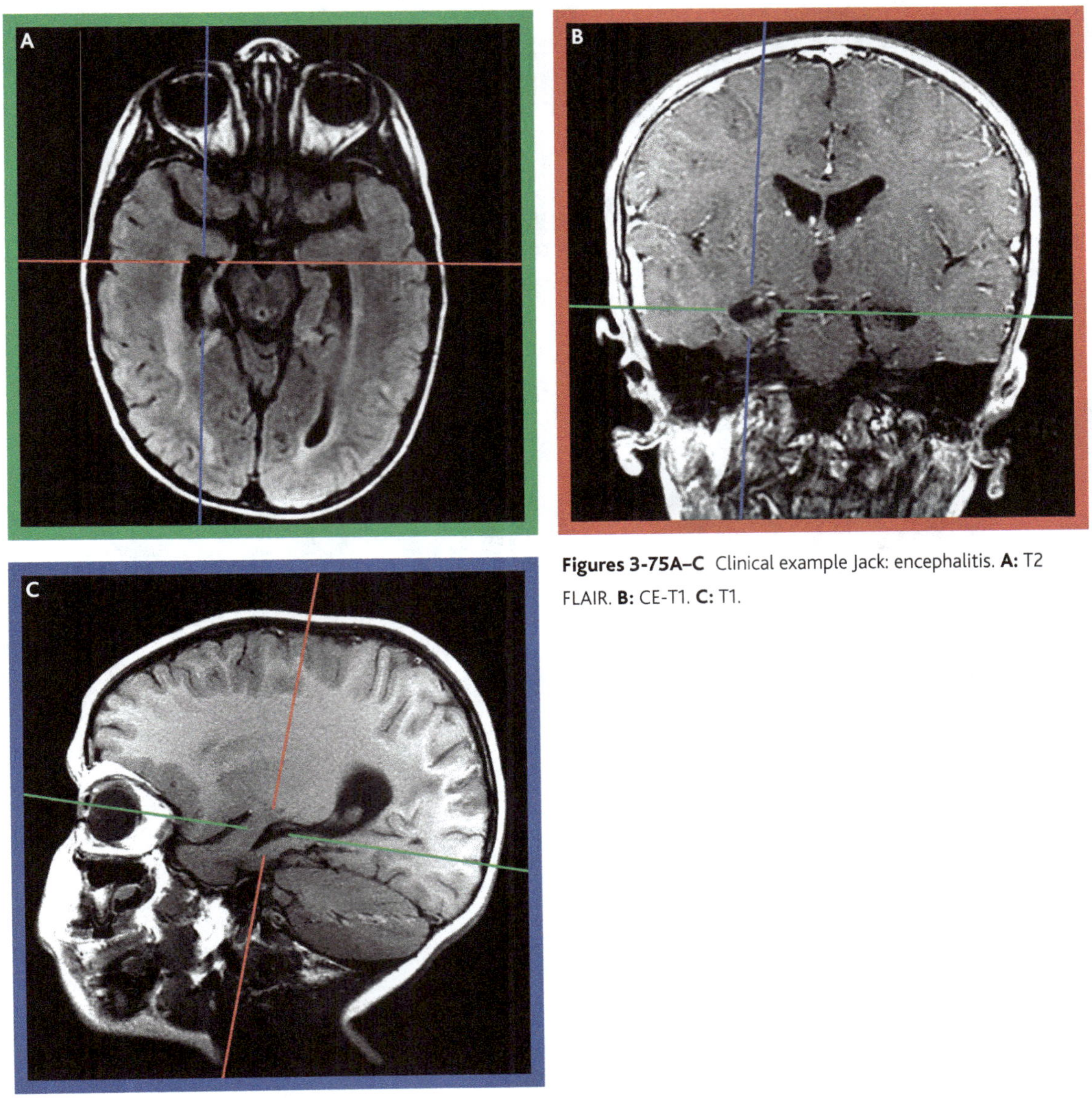

Figures 3-75A–C Clinical example Jack: encephalitis. **A:** T2 FLAIR. **B:** CE-T1. **C:** T1.

Microscopic damage to the hippocampi is a common cause of partial seizures. Until recently, MRI systems have been able to image the general structure of the hippocampi but have not had the resolution to produce adequate images of the microscopic layers, or mild mesial temporal sclerosis (MTS), a common cause of refractory epilepsy. With advances in MRI technology, MRI systems using 3 Tesla and higher magnet strengths can now produce images of adequate hippocampal resolution to enable improved medical management. When the MRI demonstrates increased hippocampal T2 signal or evidence of hippocampal atrophy suggestive of MTS ipsilateral to EEG localization, 95% of the patients who undergo temporal lobectomies became seizure free. In contrast, less than 50% of patients with normal or discordant MRIs became seizure free (Garcia et al., 1994). Unfortunately, patients with partial epilepsy are often denied surgical procedures to treat the condition because there is no localizing lesion on MRI concordant with EEG data. For many of these cases, the lack of MRI finding may be a type I error, or the failure to identify a signal (lesion) when one actually exists. The use of higher-resolution MRI imaging may enable better identification of lesions responsible for partial-seizure disorders. Normal hippocampal structures are showin in Figure 3-76A, with evidence of right mesial temporal sclerosis being illustrated in Figure 3-76B (arrow). The examples shown in Figures 3-76A and 3-76B were produced with a 4 Tesla MRI magnet providing adequate clarity and resolution of the medial temporal lobe structures to allow for improved diagnostic utility.

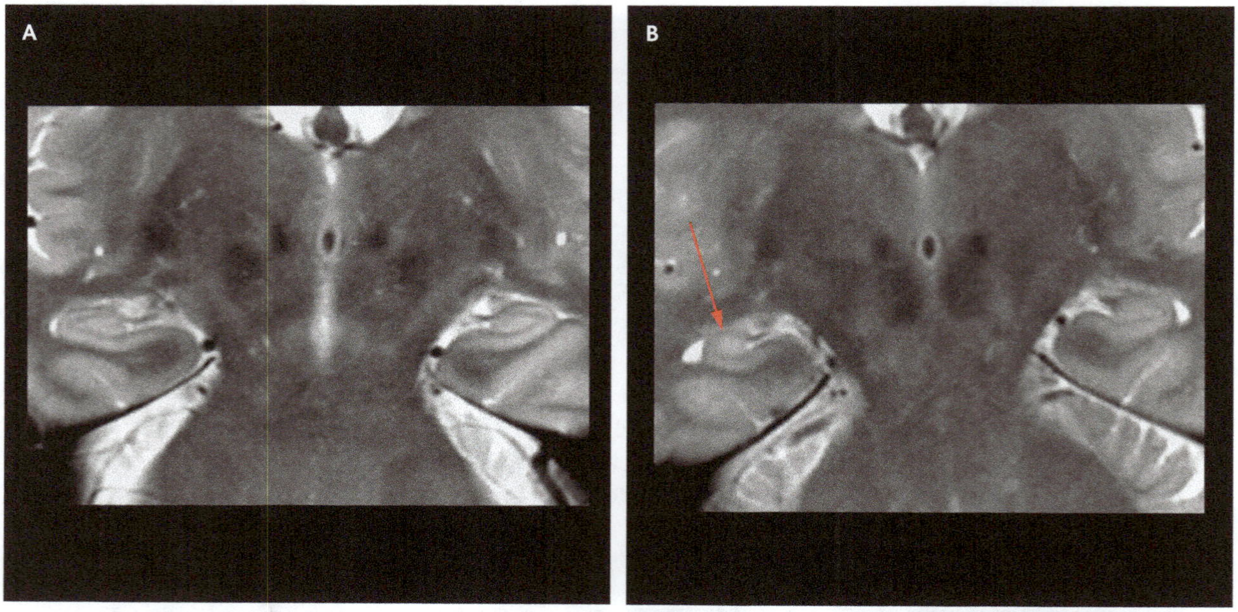

Figure 3-76 **A:** Normal patient. **B:** MTS of the right hippocampus (arrow). Images 3-76A and 3-76B courtesy of Kenneth D. Laxer, M.D. *Garcia, P. A., Laxer, K. D., Barbaro, N. M., & Dillon, W.P. (1994). Prognostic value of qualitative magnetic resonance imaging hippocampal abnormalities in patients undergoing temporal lobectomy for medically refractory seizures. Epilepsia, 35, 520–524.*

Amygdala

The amygdala (Latin: almond) bodies are located just anterior and superior to the hippocampi, within the medial temporal poles. The right and left amygdala nuclei have extensive connections with other areas of the limbic system and brain. They are responsible for instinctive fear responses and the modulation of the hypothalamic–midbrain mechanisms involving primitive sexual behavior, aggression, defensive responses, and hormonal control of behavior. On Figure 3-77, the right and left amygdala bodies are shown in blue.

Axial

On axial images (Figure 3-78A), the amygdala bodies are located just anterior and superior to the hippocampi within the medial temporal poles. A relatively simple method of locating them is to follow the inferior or temporal horn

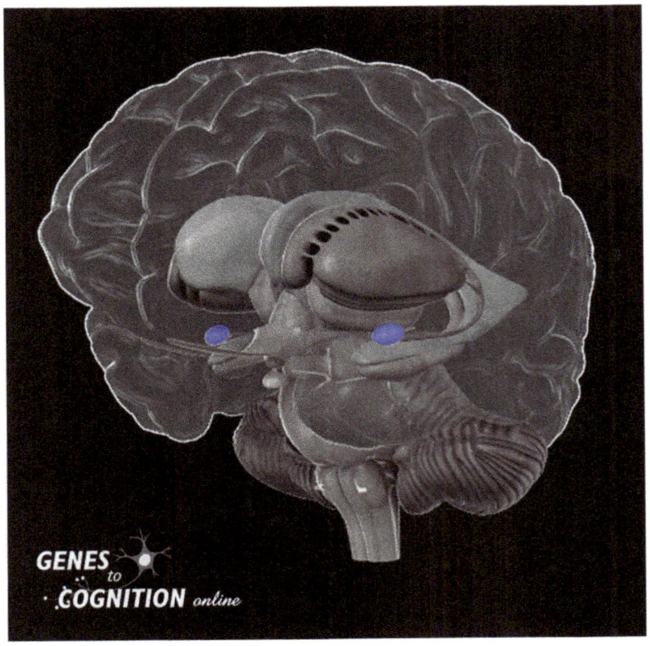

Figure 3-77 Amygdala bodies shown on a three dimensional brain illustration as the two blue structures.

of the lateral ventricles forward until it ends close to the amygdala.

Coronal

On coronal images (Figure 3-78B), the amygdala bodies are located below the optic tract on the medial surface of the temporal lobes, just anterior to the hippocampi. The anterior tip of the inferior or temporal horns of the lateral ventricles is often seen inferior and lateral to the amygdala.

Sagittal

On sagittal images (Figure 3-78C), the amygdala bodies are located just in front of and superior to the hippocampi at the most anterior end of the temporal horn of the lateral ventricles.

Mammillary bodies

Although the mammillary bodies are considered to be part of the posterior hypothalamus, given their connections and functioning, they are more often described as a component of the limbic system. The mammillary bodies are located at the anterior end of the fornix, with the hippocampi being located at the posterior–inferior end of the fiber path.

As expected, given their location at the end of the fornix, they receive their primary input from the hippocampi. Output from the mammillary bodies communicates with the anterior thalami via the mammillothalamic tract and the midbrain and pons via the mamillotegmental tract. Damage to the structures due to thiamine deficiency is a component of Wernicke-Korsakoff syndrome, with patients experiencing impaired memory, with confabulations.

The mammillary nuclei form two small, round structures that protrude into the interpeduncular fossa. On anatomical specimen or brain model, they are best viewed from an inferior, or bottom-up, perspective (Figures 3-79A and B, arrows).

On CT imaging it is difficult to appreciate the mammillary bodies because of their small size and the limited resolution of the images. In addition, if relatively thick slices are used, the bodies can fall between slices, preventing them from showing on the scan.

On MRI, the mammillary bodies are most clearly appreciated when using high-resolution, thin-slice T1 sequences, with reformatting to a variety of slice angles (Figures 3-80A–C).

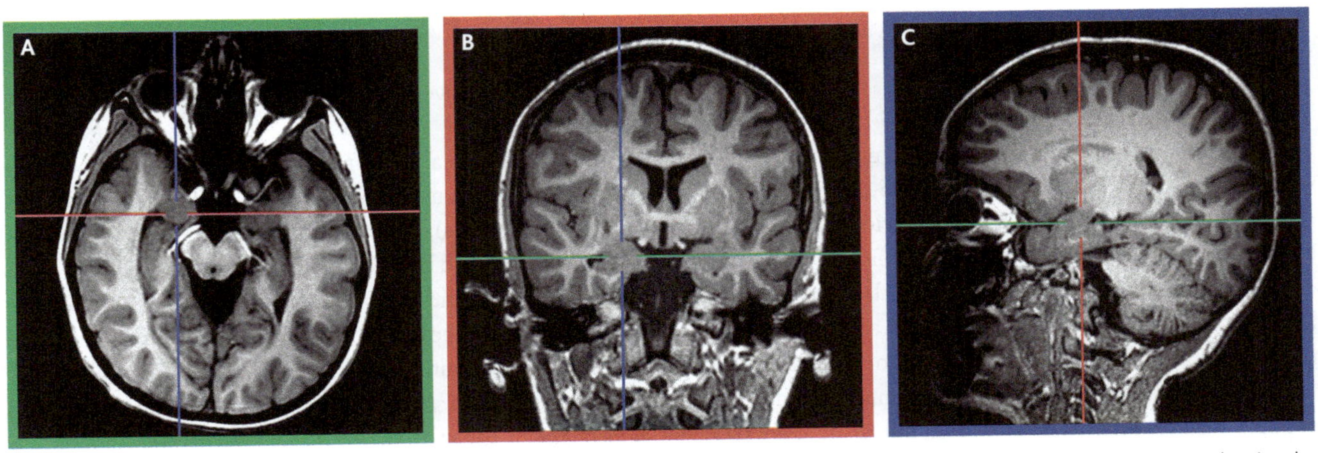

Figure 3-78 **A:** Axial image showing the location of the amygdala. **B:** Coronal image showing the location of the amygdala. **C:** Sagittal image showing the location of the amygdala.

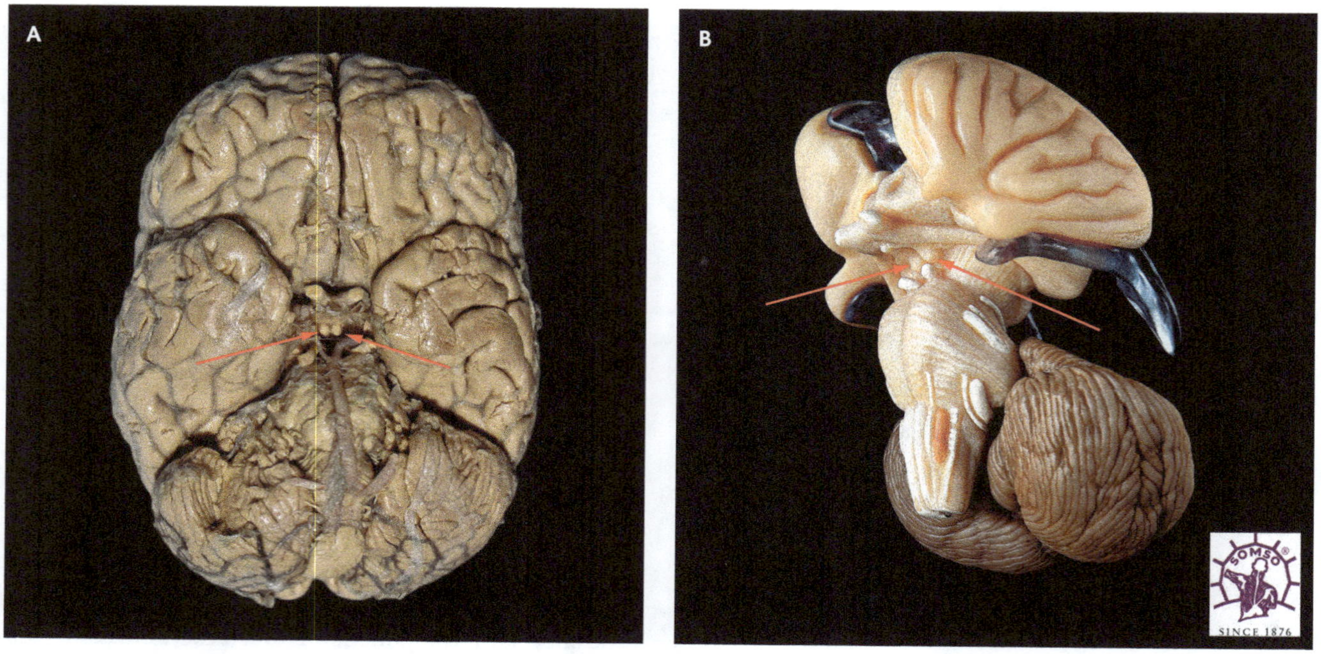

Figure 3-79 **A:** Inferior view of the brain showing the mammillary bodies. **B**: Mammillary bodies shown on brain model of the subcortical structures.

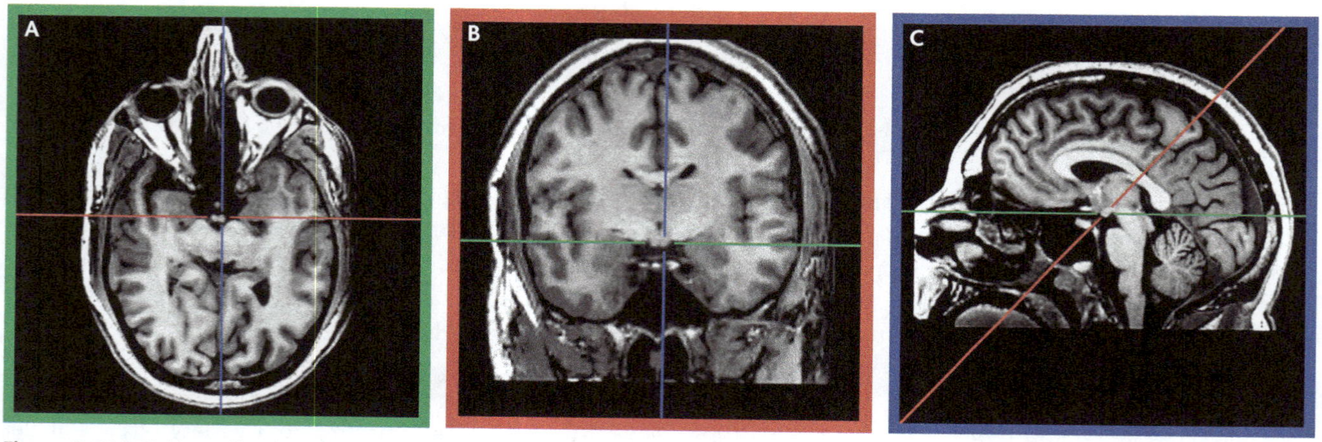

Figures 3-80A–C Mammillary bodies shown on axial (A), coronal (B) and sagittal (C) MRI images.

Basal Ganglia

The basal ganglia are a group of nuclei located below the level of the cortex and within an area with extensive white-matter pathways. These white-matter pathways can assist you in identifying the various basal ganglia structures. Because of the white-matter and gray-matter complexity of this subcortical region, damage within the location of the basal ganglia can cause a variety of symptoms and functional deficits. In addition, the structures of the basal ganglia are responsible for multiple motor and cognitive functions, including but not restricted to the modulation of movement and the automaticity of routines and behaviors.

The basal ganglia are formed from three main structures: the caudate nucleus (Latin: *cauda* = tail), global pallidus (Latin: light globe), and putamen (Latin: to prune—dark appearance like old bark, shell, husk) (Figures 3-81a–c). The caudate nucleus and the putamen collectively are called the corpus striatum because of the striated appearance of these structures. The putamen and globus pallidus collectively are called the lenticular or lentiform nucleus because of the lens shape of the structures.

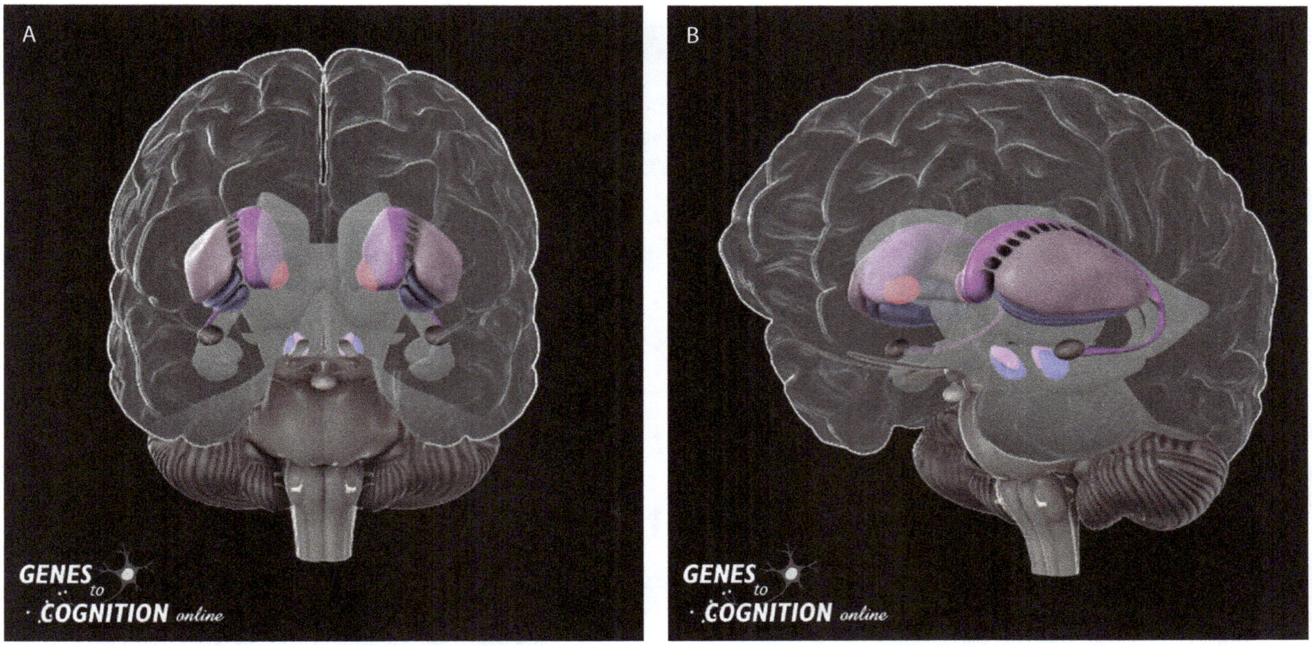

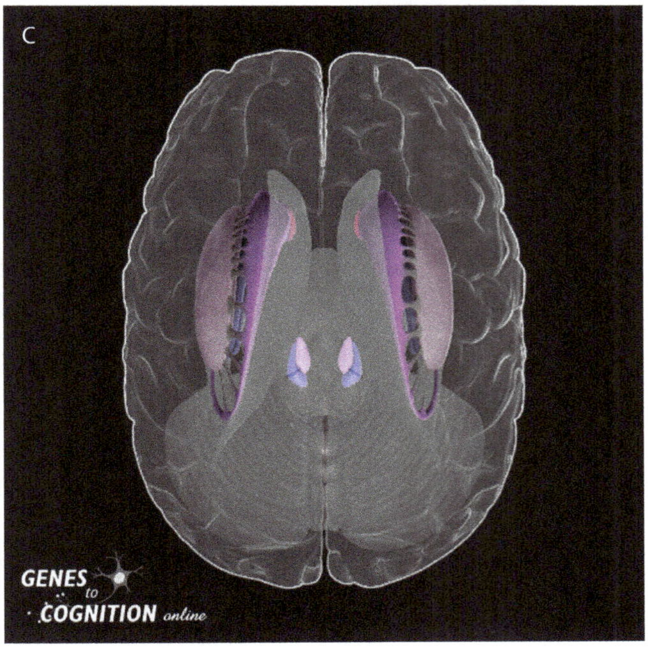

Figures 3-81A–C Basal ganglia structures shown on three dimensional brain illustration. *Dark Blue = Globus Pallidus; Mauve = Putamen; Dark Purple = Caudate Nucleus; Light Blue = Substantia Nigra; Light Purple = Subthalamic Nucleus; Bright Pink = Nucleus Accumbens.*

Other areas considered part of the basal ganglia include the nucleus accumbens, substantia nigra, and the subthalamic nuclei. The caudate nucleus is formed from a larger head and thin tail. The head is more visible on brain imaging and is relatively simple to locate. The putamen nuclei are the most lateral structures within the constellation of basal ganglia. They are located between the internal capsule and the external capsule, making them relatively simple to identify on most high-resolution MRI sequences. The globus pallidus is located on the inside edge (medial) and slightly below the putamen, and is bordered by the internal capsule. The three primary basal ganglia structures of the caudate, putamen and globus pallidus are readily visible on coronal brain sections just lateral and slightly inferior to the body of the lateral ventricles (Figures 3-82A and B). The section shown in Figure 3-82A was acquired from a location slightly more anterior than the section shown in Figure 3-82B.

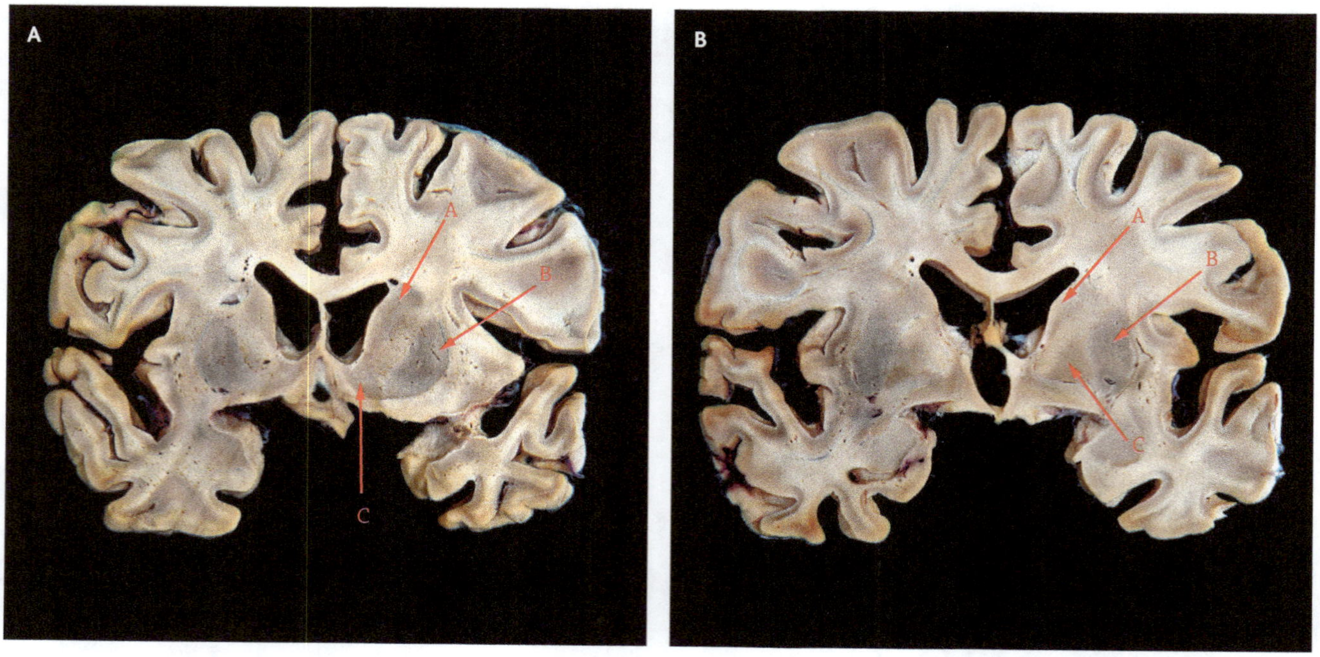

Figures 3-82A and B Basal ganglia on axial brain sections, with slice 3-82A being more anterior than slice 3-82B. Arrow A = Caudate Head; Arrow B = Putamen; Arrow C = Globus Pallidus.

Basal ganglia on brain imaging

When locating the basal ganglia structures on two-dimensional brain scans, it is helpful to view all three orientations in order to fully appreciate their locations. Use the lateral ventricles and white-matter tracts, such as the internal and external capsules, as guides. The use of white matter tracts is especially helpful when viewing low-resolution images with poor contrast, such as CT scans.

Given the shape and organization of the basal ganglia, the appearance of the various nuclei will differ depending on the level of an axial slice. To assist you in visualizing the basal ganglia from different levels, the structures presented here are at the level of the body of the lateral ventricles, the foramen of Monro, and the third ventricle, using an acquisition angle orthogonal to the vertical axis of the brain. Many axial slices that you will encounter in the clinic will be taken using different acquisition angles, thus slight variations in appearance will be apparent at each level.

Level: Body of the lateral ventricles

- On axial images (Figure 3-83A), only the head of the caudate is visible lateral to the ventricles.
- On coronal images (Figure 3-83B), the right and left heads of the caudate are seen adjacent to the lateral ventricles, on the lateral wall. Inferior and lateral to the head of the caudate sits the internal capsule, which runs diagonally between the basal ganglia structures. The putamen and globus pallidus structures are located inferior and lateral to the internal capsule, between the internal capsule and the insula. The globus pallidus structures are located inferior and medial to the putamen.
- On sagittal images (Figure 3-83c), the head of the caudate is easily identified as the large elongated region of gray matter located at the base of the lateral ventricles. Inferior to the head of the caudate sits the internal capsule. The globus pallidus is located below the internal capsule anteriorly, and the thalamus is located below the internal capsule posteriorly.

Level: Foramen of Monro

- On axial images (Figure 3-84A), the caudate nuclei are most easily identified as bulging structures that make up the lateral wall of the body of the lateral ventricles. The head of the caudate is separated from the other basal ganglia structures by the internal capsule. The anterior limb of the internal capsule separates the caudate from the putamen, which is located lateral to the head of the caudate. The putamen is the most lateral nuclei within the basal ganglia and is located beside the insula.

- On coronal images (Figure 3-84B), the arrangement of structures appears almost identical to that on axial images, with the head of the caudate being adjacent to the lateral ventricle, and the putamen being the most lateral nuclei, separated from the caudate by the internal capsule. The globus pallidus structures are located medial and slightly inferior to the putamen.
- On sagittal images (Figure 3-83C), the head of the caudate is located adjacent to the lateral ventricle and the putamen is located below, separated by the internal capsule. The globus pallidus is located just inferior and posterior to the putamen.

Level: Third ventricle

- On axial images (Figure 3-85A), the caudate is viewed as the most anterior and medial structure of the subcortical nuclei. The putamen is located just posterior and lateral to the caudate head separated by the anterior limb of the internal capsule. The globus pallidus is located in an area surrounded on the outside by the putmen and medially by the posterior limb of the internal capsule. Medial and slightly posterior to the globas pallidus is the thalamus, separated by the posterior limb of the internal capsule.
- On coronal images (Figure 3-85B), the arrangement of structures appears similar to that on axial images, with the head of the caudate being adjacent to the lateral ventricle, the putamen being the most lateral nuclei and divided from the caudate by the internal capsule, and the globus pallidus being inferior and medial to the putamen, adjacent to the posterior limb of the internal capsule.
- On sagittal images (Figure 3-85C), the caudate appears as an elongated area of gray matter at the base of the lateral ventricle, with the putamen below (anteriorally) and the globas pallidus below (middle). The thalamus is seen below the head of the caudate at the most posterior aspect.

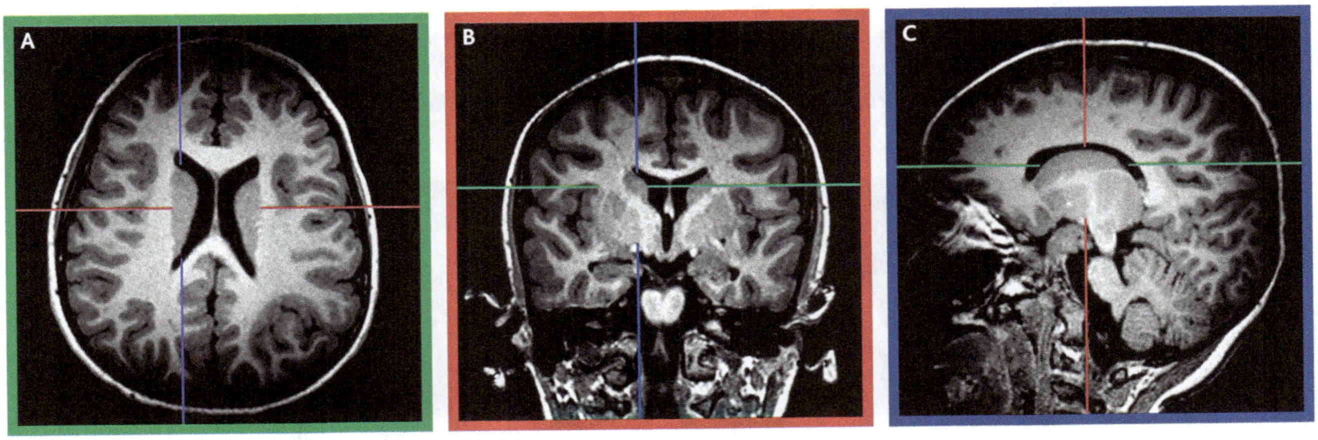

Figure 3-83A–C Basal ganglia structures imaged at the level of the lateral ventricles on axial (A), coronal (B) and sagittal (C) MRI images.

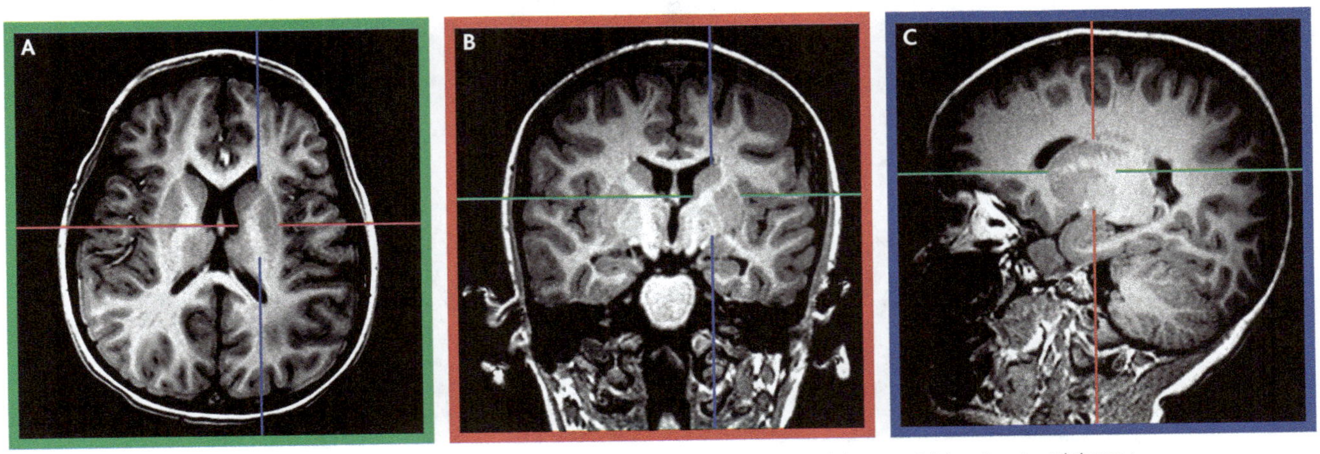

Figure 3-84A–C Basal ganglia structures imaged at the level of the foramen of Monro, on axial (A), coronal (B) and sagittal (C) MRI images.

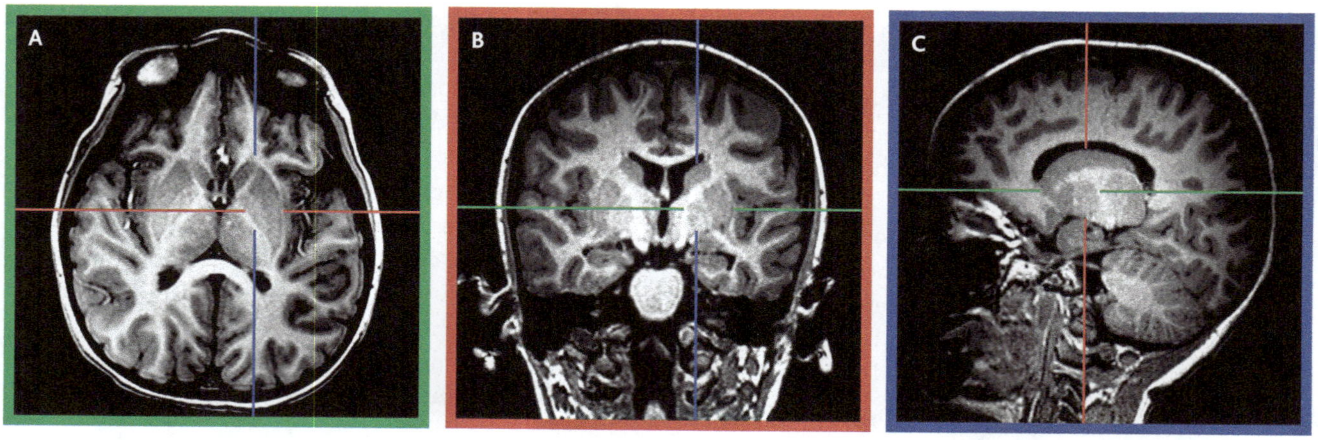

Figure 3-85A–C Basal ganglia structures imaged at the level of the third ventricle, on axial (A), coronal (B) and sagittal (C) MRI images.

CLINICAL EXAMPLE
Jennifer: Basal Ganglia Inflammation

Jennifer contracted a severe case of acute disseminated encephalomyelitis (ADEM). Imaging suggested significant inflammation within both the subcortical white matter and the basal ganglia structures. Consistent with these findings, Jennifer presented with significant symptoms relating to basal ganglia disruption, including a bilateral extrapyramidal movement disorder. Several weeks later, follow-up imaging revealed significant improvement to the white matter and basal ganglia inflammation, with hyperintensities being mostly resolved exception for the bilateral putamina (Figure 3-86, arrows).

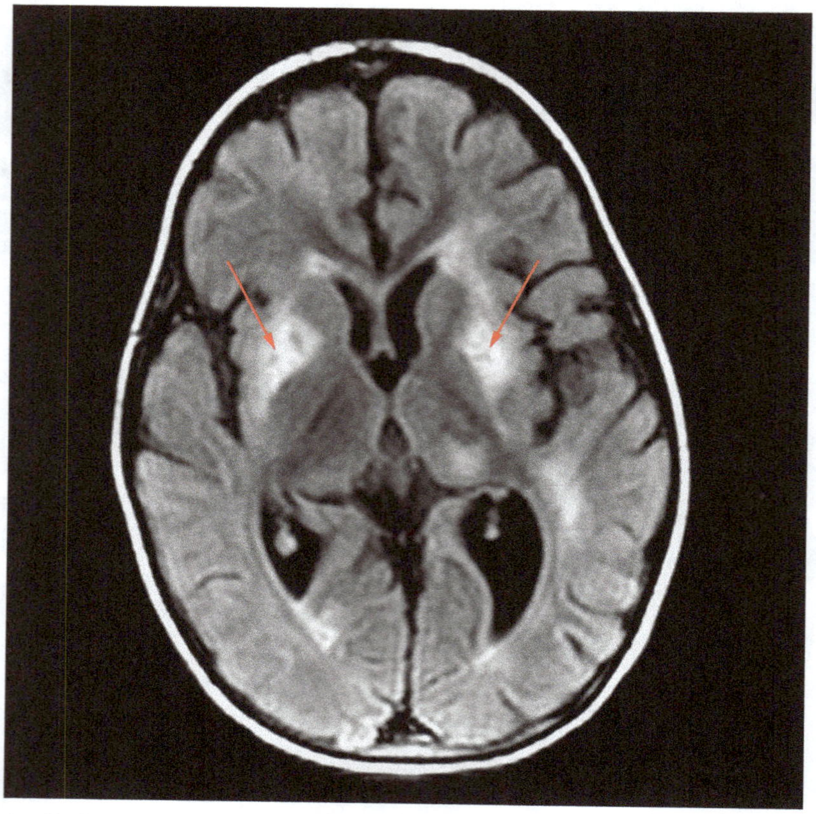

Figure 3-86 Clinical example Jennifer: basal ganglia inflammation. Inflammation is most marked in the bilateral putamen nuclei (arrows), the only structures to show residual injury following resolution of Jennifer's condition.

Tyler was not as fortunate as Jennifer. While Jennifer demonstrated improvements in her condition and basal ganglia symptoms, Tyler experienced gradual deterioration of his condition. Tyler's disseminated cocci meningoencephalitis caused infarction of his basal ganglia structures. Approximately 1 month after admission, CT (Figure 3-87A) and T2 FLAIR imaging (Figure 3-87B) revealed areas of primary damage to the right caudate and putamen, and left globus pallidus (arrows). Approximately 1 month later, with progression of his illness, it was clear that lacuna infarctions were becoming evident in his left caudate and putamen and bilaterally in the globus pallidi (Figure 3-87C arrows).

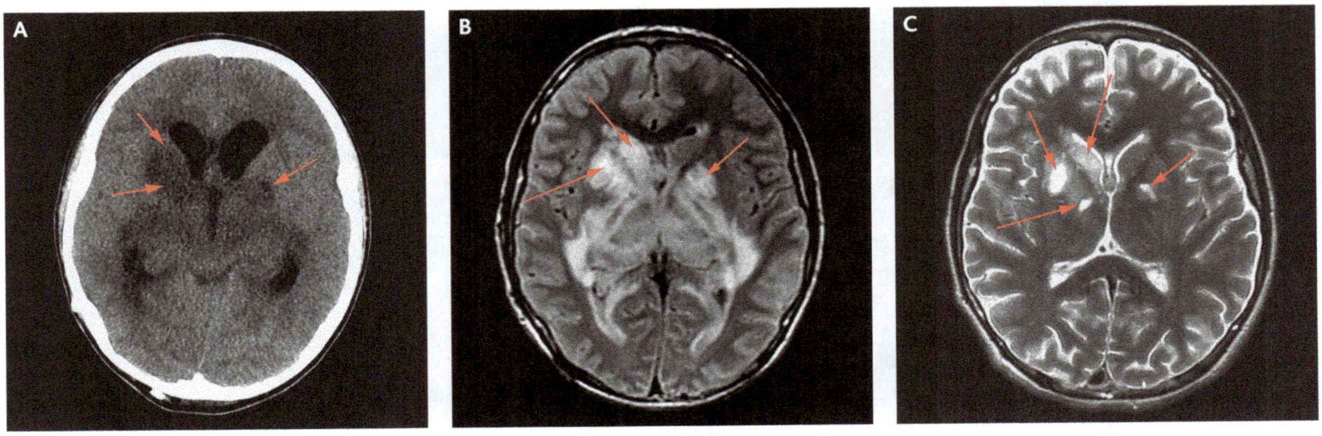

Figures 3-87A–C Clinical example Tyler: 1 month post-hospitalization for meningoencephalitis. **A:** CT. **B:** T2 FLAIR. **C:** T2 at 2 months.

Diencephalon

The diencephalon (Latin = between brains) is located between the upper cortex and the midbrain and brain stem structures. The diencephalon is composed of two primary structures, the thalamus and hypothalamus (Latin = below thalamus).

Thalamus

The thalamus can be considered a complex relay and processing station for information that passes to and from the cortex and subcortical nuclei. Pathways from the thalamus connect to most other areas of the brain, including but not restricted to the frontal, parietal, temporal, and occipital lobes. Not only does information pass through the thalamus, but it also becomes processed at a high level of complexity. For example, the thalamus is responsible for the processing of various types of sensory information, determining what is salient and what should be ignored. An example is when you put on clothing, after a short time you stop sensing the tactile feel of the clothing on your body as the thalamus attenuates the signals from your skin to the higher areas of cortex.

The thalami are relatively large, lobed masses of gray-matter and white-matter pathways within each of the hemispheres. They are located above the midbrain close to the center of the brain at the level of the third ventricle (Figures 3-88A–C). On a brain model, the thalami are best viewed from the back as lobulated structures inferior and medial the to lateral ventricles (Figure 3-89A arrows). On an axial brain section, the thalami are best viewed on a slice cutting through the posterior aspect of the temporal lobes and the anterior aspect of the pons and midbrain. The thalami are identified as gray matter globe shaped structures lateral to the posterior portion of the third ventricle (Figure 3-89B arrows).

Thalami on brain imaging

- On axial images (Figure 3-90A), the thalami form the inferior-lateral walls of the third ventricle, at the posterior aspect of the ventricle.
- On coronal images (Figure 3-90B), the thalami are best viewed on a section showing the body and foramen of Monro of the lateral ventricles. The thalami form the lateral walls of the third ventricle, just below the foramena of Monro.
- On sagittal images (Figure 3-90c), the thalamus is best viewed on a slice close to midline and is the lobular structure below the isthmus or thinnest part of the corpus callosum (toward the back).

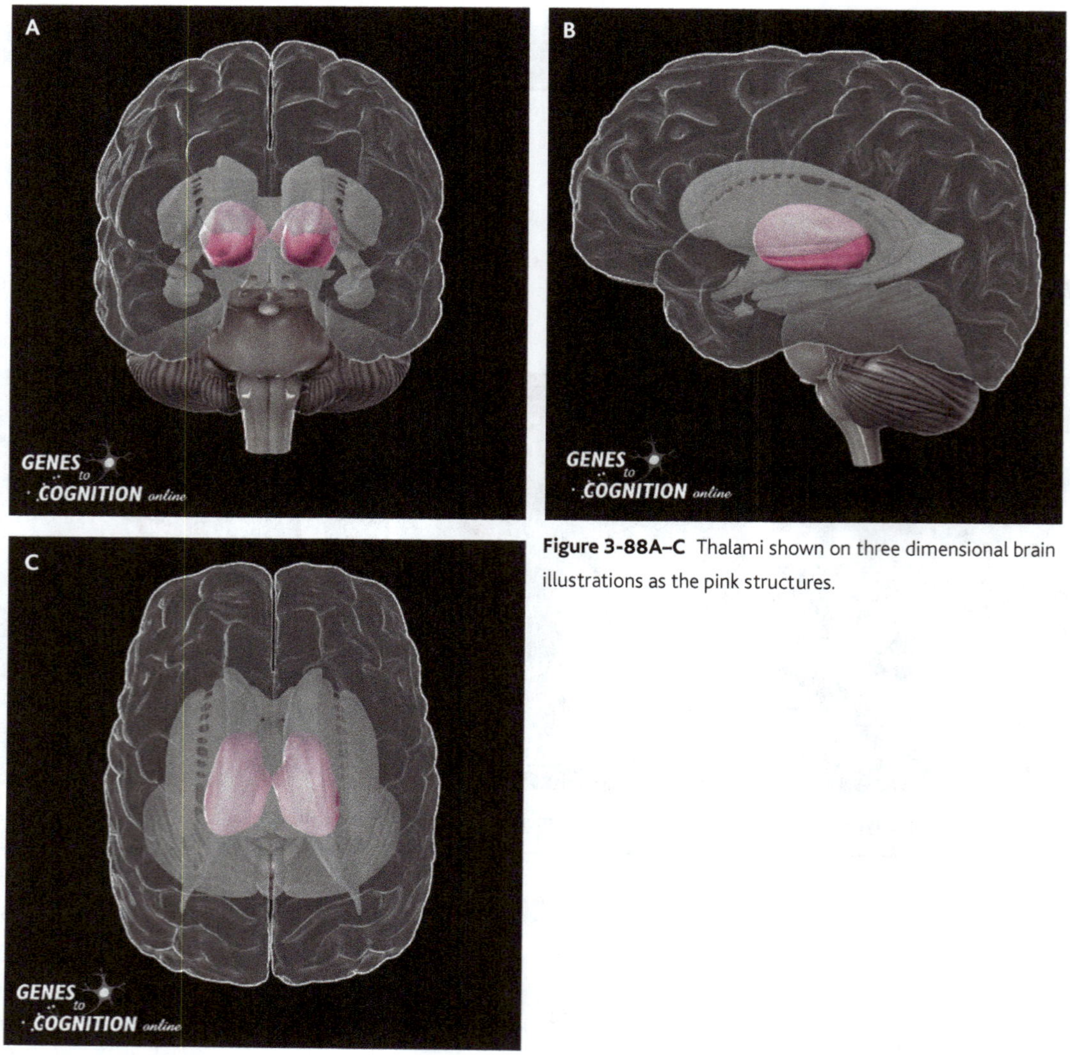

Figure 3-88A–C Thalami shown on three dimensional brain illustrations as the pink structures.

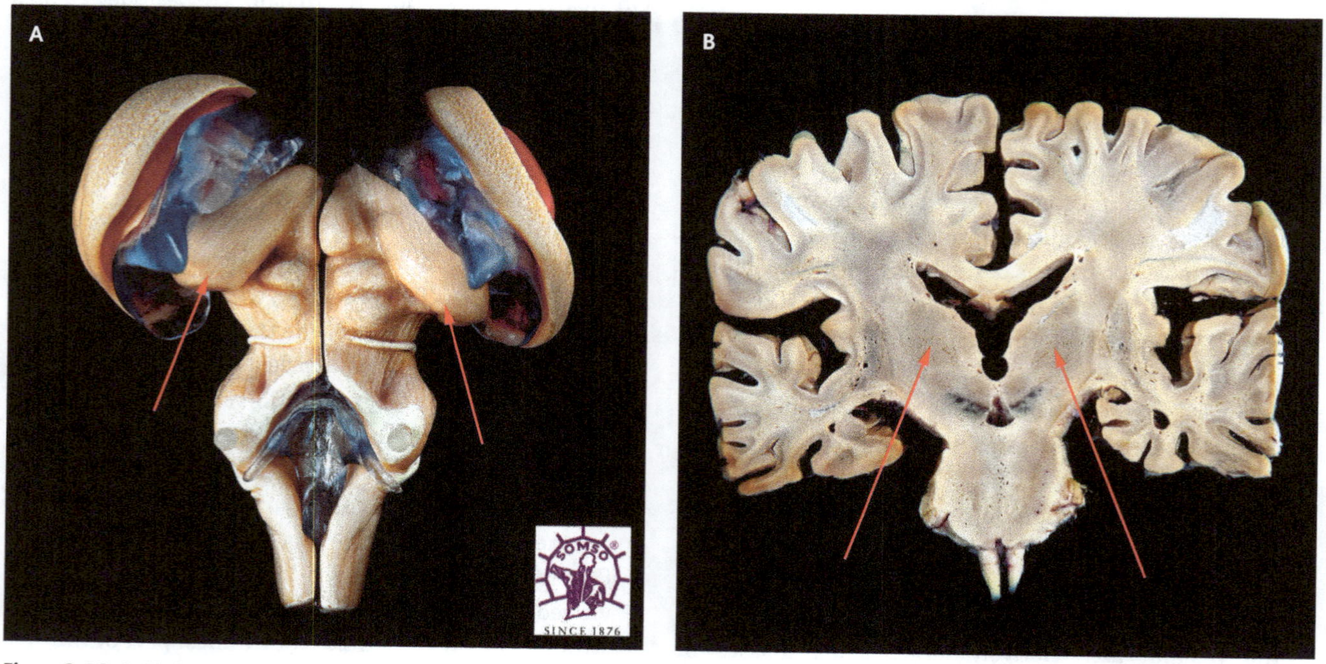

Figure 3-89 **A:** Thalami on brain model, posterior view (arrows). **B:** Thalami on brain slice (arrows).

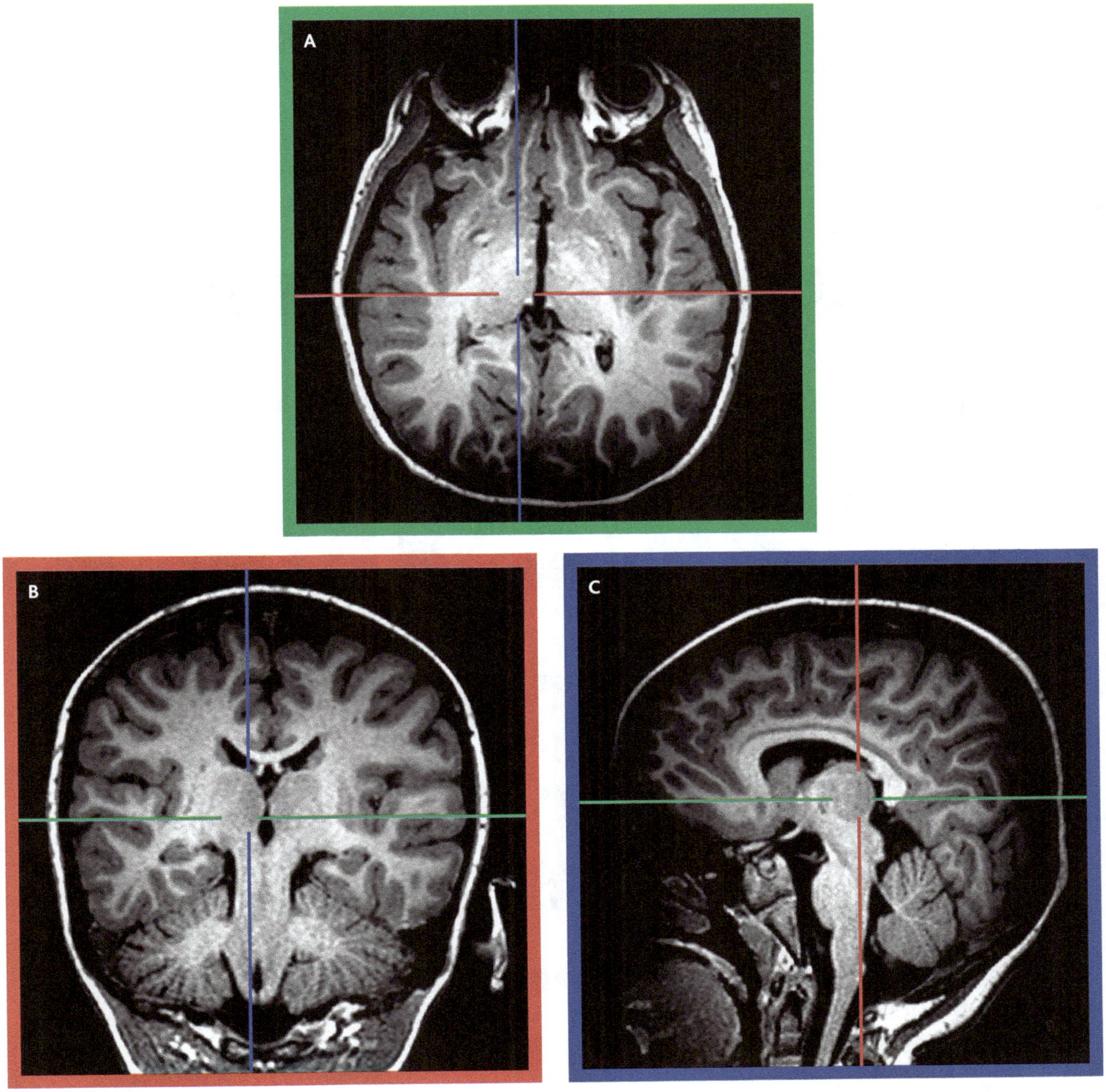

Figure 3-90 A: Axial image of thalami. **B:** Coronal image of thalami. **C:** Sagittal image of thalami.

Annette: Acute Necrotizing Encephalopathy of Childhood

Annette contracted acute necrotizing encephalopathy of childhood (ANEC), a rare condition that produces a somewhat unique profile on brain imaging (Figures 3-91A–I). ANEC generally results in symmetrical lesions involving the right and left thalamic structures. It can also involve the bilateral basal ganglia structures, brain stem, cerebellum, and periventricular white matter. Because the thalami are critical to many brain functions and the lesions can often include other subcortical structures, prognosis is poor, with a high rate of mortality or severe functional compromise.

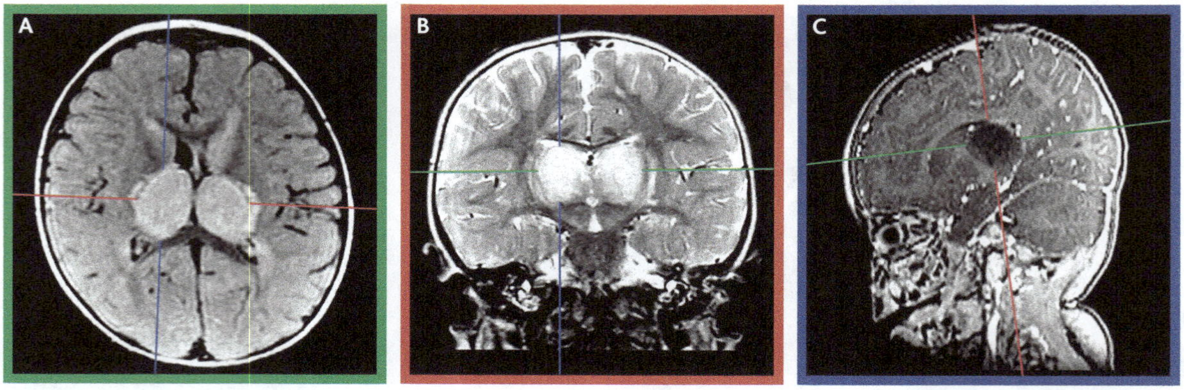

Figures 3-91A–C *Clinical Example Annette: acute necrotizing encephalopathy of childhood.* MRI series at 1 week post-hospitalization. Note the T2 and T2 FLAIR hyperintensities of the right and left thalamic bodies and T1 hypointensity of the thalami. **A:** T2 FLAIR. **B:** T2. **C:** T1 FSPGR.

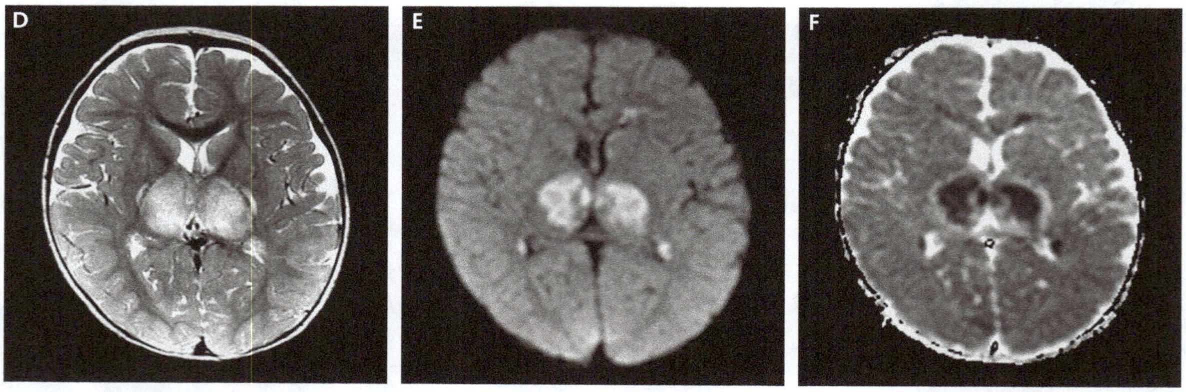

Figures 3-91D–F *Clinical Example Annette: acute necrotizing encephalopathy of childhood.* Diffusion series suggests infarction with a bright appearance on T2 and DWI, and a dark appearance on ADC. **D:** T2. **E:** DWI. **F:** ADC.

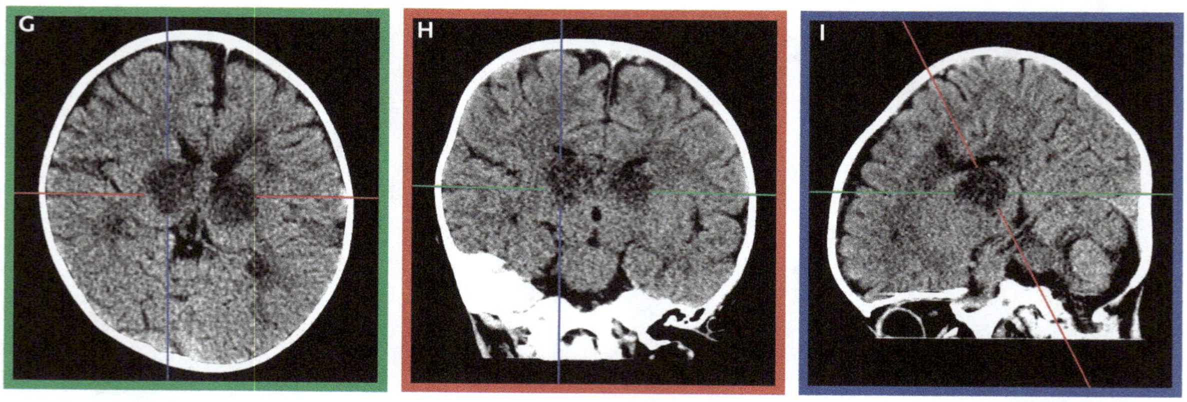

Figures 3-91G–I *Clinical Example Annette: acute necrotizing encephalopathy of childhood.* CT series at 2 weeks post-hospitalization. Note the low-density appearance of the thalami, suggesting encephalomalacia and loss of tissue density. **G:** CT. **H:** CT. **I:** CT.

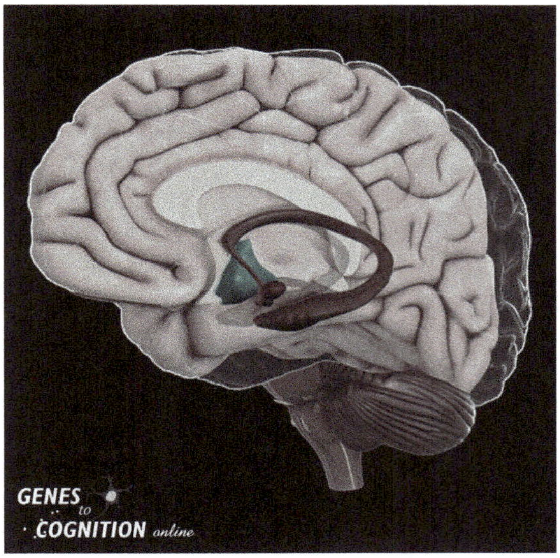

Figure 3-92 Hypothalamus shown on three dimensional brain illustration as the green structure.

Hypothalamus

The hypothalamus is located just anterior and inferior to the thalamus and forms part of the lateral wall of the third ventricle (Figure 3-92). The hypothalamus is formed from many different nuclei, although on brain images, these are not readily discernable. The nuclei of the hypothalamus are important in the regulation of internal bodily states, the control of the autonomic nervous system, and the hormonal system via the pituitary gland. The pituitary gland is connected to the hypothalamus via the pituitary stalk, or infundibulum, and is located below the optic chiasm and the hypothalamus.

Hypothalamus on brain imaging

- On axial images (Figure 3-93A), the hypothalamus is best viewed at a horizontal height that cuts through the bottom of the third ventricle.
- On coronal images (Figure 3-93B), the hypothalamus is difficult to differentiate, owing to the small size of the structure and location. The hypothalamus is best viewed on a slice at the very front of the third ventricle, just above the pituitary and below the anterior commissure. On high resolution imaging, the optic pathways are often visible inferior and lateral to the hypothalamic structures.
- On sagittal images (Figure 3-93C), the hypothalamus is best viewed on a midsagittal slice or a sagittal slice just lateral to the third ventricle. The anterior-lateral walls of the third ventricle are formed from the hypothalamic structures.

Epithalamus

The epithalamus is formed from the dorsal (posterior) region of the diencephalon. The primary structure within the epithalamus is the pineal body, a structure with notable historical significance.

Pineal body—"epiphysis"

The pineal body or gland is located between the thalami, just superior to the mesencephalon (Figure 3-94 arrow). As a single structure located along the centerline of the brain, and surrounded by CSF, historically the pineal body was believed to be the location of information integration and where the body interacts with the soul. René Descartes (1596–1650) proposed the pineal gland as being the solution to the mind–body problem and a location that unifies the views from the two eyes, or the sounds from the two ears to one percept. Because the pineal was seen as the only structure in the brain that was not replicated in both hemispheres and was centrally located and surrounded by animal spirits (CSF), it was considered the one place where sensations, the body, and the soul could be unified.

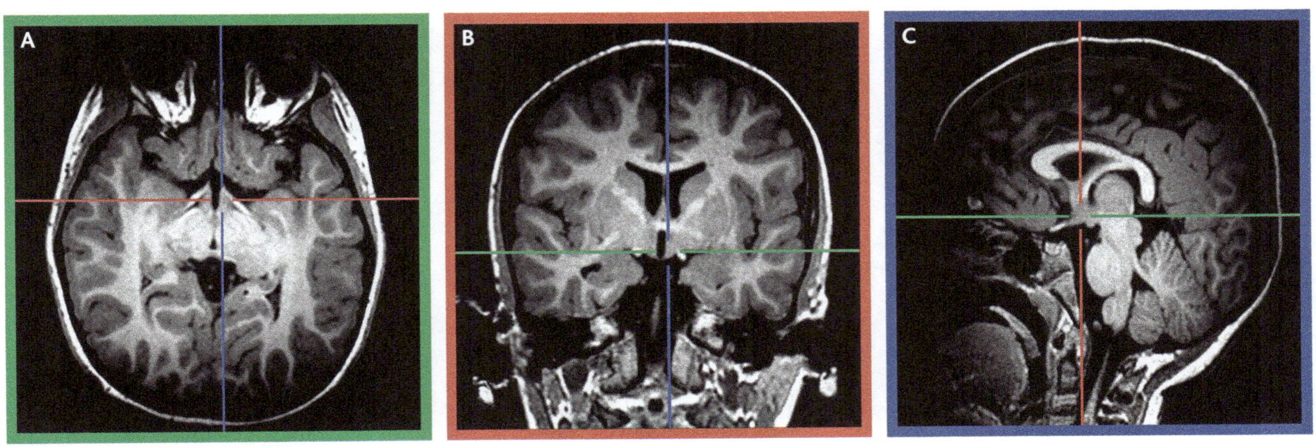

Figure 3-93 **A:** Axial image of hypothalamus. **B:** Coronal image of hypothalamus. **C:** Sagittal image of hypothalamus.

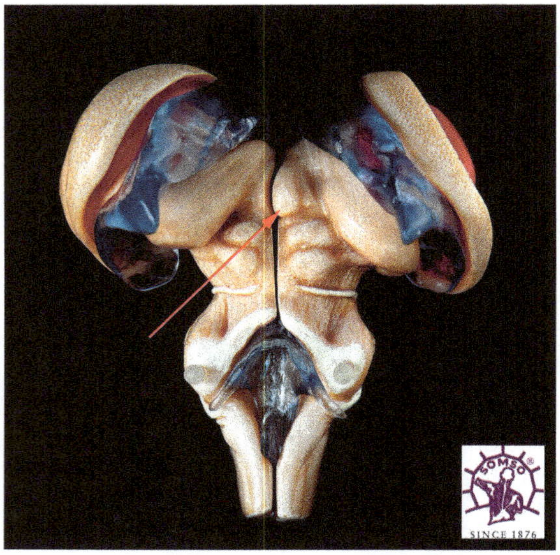

Figure 3-94 The pineal is shown between the thalami on a brain model viewed from the back to show the posterior aspect of the midbrain.

It is now known that the pineal body is primarily responsible for the synthesis and secretion of melatonin, a hormone that is involved in biological rhythms. The response of the pineal to light and dark cycles is the reason why it is sometimes referred to as the "third eye." The pineal body receives information regarding light and dark indirectly from the retina via the suprachiasmatic nucleus of the hypothalamus, descending pathways to the spinal cord sympathetic ganglia, and, ultimately, the postganglionic ascending pathways to the pineal.

Pineal body on brain imaging

- On axial images (Figure 3-95A), the pineal body is located by choosing a slice that passes through the thalami and third ventricle. The pineal is located posterior to the third ventricle within the perimesencephalic or quadrigeminal cistern.
- On coronal images (Figure 3-95B), the pineal body is most easily located by choosing a slice that cuts through the thalami at the level of the perimesencephalic or quadrigeminal cistern. On some slice angles, the pineal can be seen above the corpora quadrigemini.
- On sagittal images (Figure 3-95C), the pineal body is located below the splenium, most posterior aspect of the corpus callosum, above the corpora quadrigeminal structures at the back of the midbrain. Midsagittal slices are usually best to visualize the pineal, which sits within the perimesencephalic or quadrigeminal cistern.

Given the location of the pineal body, tumors of the pineal often result in disrupted CSF flow and subsequent hydrocephalus. Early symptoms are consistent with increased ventricular pressure, producing headache, nausea, vomiting, and possibly mild disruption of cognition and motor or sensory functioning.

Pituitary Gland—Hypophysis

Below the hypothalamus is a small, pea-sized structured called the pituitary gland or hypophysis. The pituitary is attached to the hypothalamus by a small pathway called the infundibulum or pituitary stalk. The pituitary gland sits in a bony cavity called the sella turcica, which literally translates to "turkey chair" but has since been translated to the "Turkish chair," or "Turkish saddle."

The pituitary gland is sometimes called the "master gland," as it controls other endocrine glands. The pituitary can be thought of as the part of the central nervous system that integrates neuronal activity (from the hypothalamus) with hormonal activity. The pituitary has two primary lobes, the anterior lobe and the posterior lobe, with a smaller intermediate zone. The pituitary gland produces a

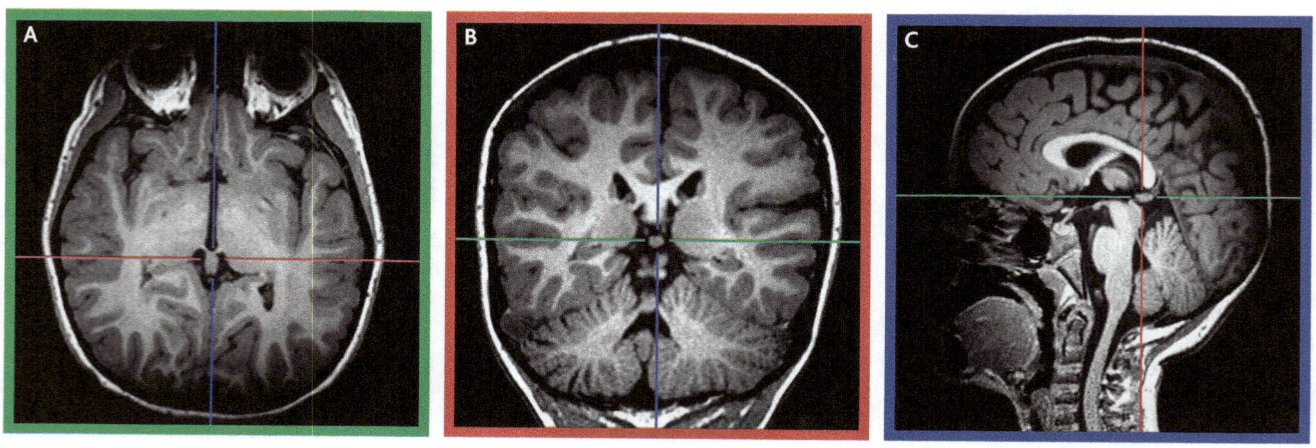

Figure 3-95 **A:** Axial image of pineal body. **B:** Coronal image of pineal body. **C:** Sagittal image of pineal body.

Natasha presented with a pineal tumor that was restricting CSF flow and causing mild diffuse disruption of her cognitive abilities (Figures 3-96A–C). On examination, her intellectual abilities were intact, although Natasha had difficulty with higher-order tasks requiring active or complex attention (ability to manipulate information mentally), executive functioning involving multitasking and divided attention, and cognitive processing speed. Problem solving was inefficient and inflexible, with Natasha having difficulty thinking of alternate solutions to reasoning problems. Natasha was fortunate to have no functional limitations following resection of her pineal tumor. After surgery, her performance returned to premorbid levels, with the only residual deficits relating to an oculomotor cranial nerve palsy, likely due to the pressure effects of the space-occupying tumor or the hydrocephalus. Long-term prognosis is guarded for Natasha, as hers was a high grade malignant tumor, and treatment had only just begun.

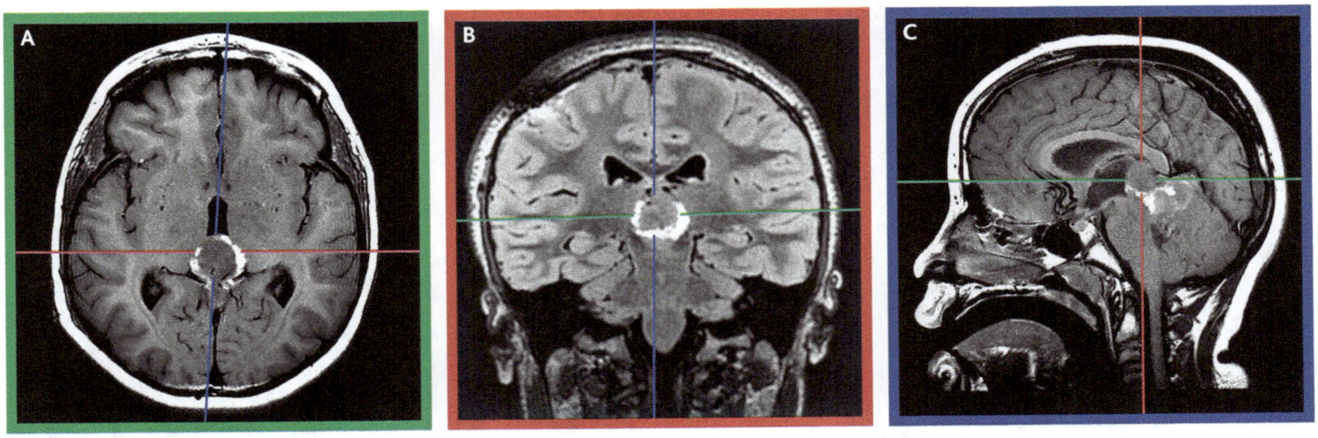

Figure 3-96A–C Clinical example Natasha: pineal tumor. **A:** Axial T1. **B:** Coronal CE-T2. **C:** Sagittal T1.

number of hormones, such as growth hormone, prolactin, adrenocorticotropic hormone (ACTH), thyroid-stimulating hormone (TSH), follicle-stimulating hormone (FSH), luteinizing hormone (LH), antidiuretic hormone (ADH), and oxytocin.

> It is important to consider that the pituitary gland can appear "abnormally bright" on T1 sequences, even without pathology. The bright appearance in both the anterior and posterior lobes is most pronounced in babies and infants, with the brightness of the anterior lobe normalizing in children and the bright appearance of the posterior lobe remaining in many children and adults. The so-called posterior pituitary bright spot is thought to be due to the high neurophysin content in the posterior pituitary, but not the anterior lobe.

Pituitary gland on brain imaging

- On axial images (Figure 3-97A), the pituitary gland is located at a level just below the optic chiasm between the poles of the temporal lobes. If the image slice it too thick, the pituitary may not be visible on the scan.
- On coronal images (Figure 3-97B), the pituitary gland is best located below the optic chiasm and between the temporal poles. Choose a cut showing the anterior temporal lobes without the hippocampi, as the pituitary is anterior to the hippocampal structures.
- On sagittal images (Figure 3-97C), the pituitary gland is best viewed using a midsagittal slice running through the longitudinal fissure. Follow the third ventricle forward and down until you reach the pituitary. You can also look below the genu of the corpus callosum, with the pituitary gland being just below the bottom of the frontal cortex.

Adenomas—suprasellar craniopharyngioma

Adenomas, another name for tumors of the pituitary, invariably result in disruption to a patient's hormonal

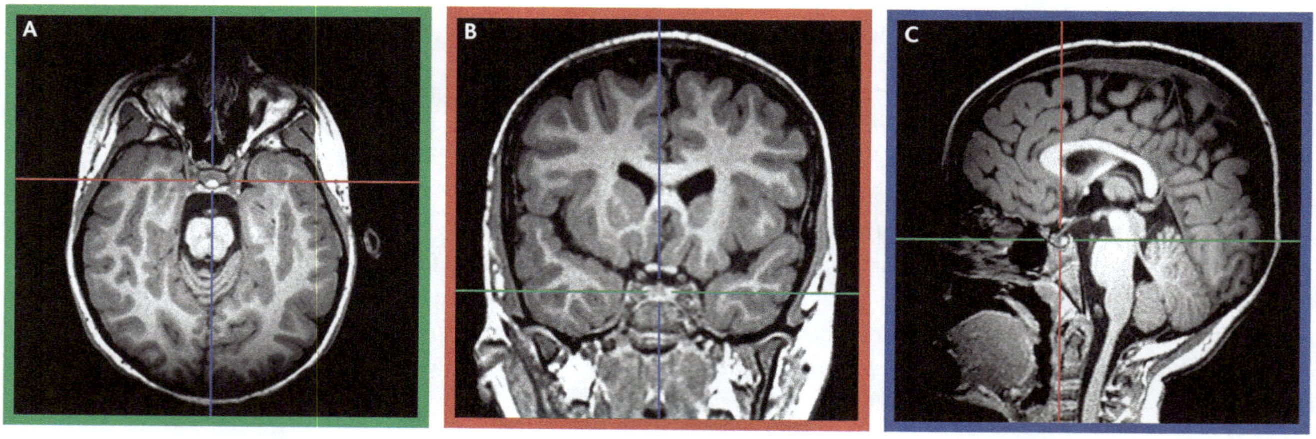

Figure 3-97 **A:** Axial image of pituitary gland. **B:** Coronal image of pituitary gland. **C:** Sagittal image of pituitary gland.

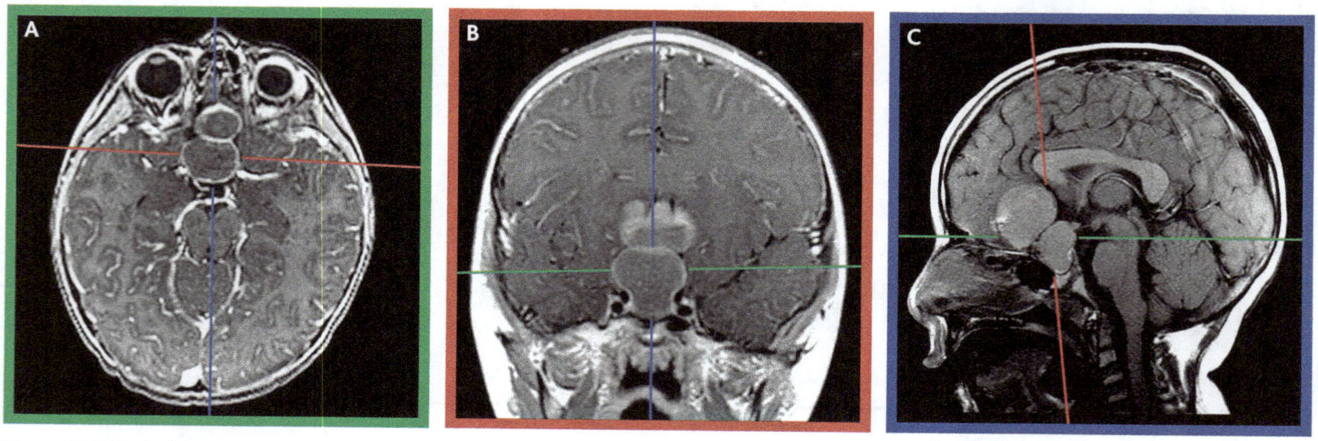

Figures 3-98A–C Adenoma-suprasellar craniopharyngioma shown on axial (A), coronal (B) and sagittal (C) MRI images.

system. Pituitary tumors can also result in visual impairment if they are large enough to put pressure on the optic chiasm. As such, unexplained new-onset changes in emotion, behavior, or other hormone-related conditions, such as puberty, should clue you into also testing visual-field functioning. Adenomas that grow out of the sella turcica and push onto the optic pathways can result in very specific visual impairments. Note the proximity of the suprasellar craniopharyngioma to where the optic tract and chiasm are located (Figures 3-98A–C).

Mesencephalon

The midbrain is the only primary component of the mesencephalon. The midbrain is formed from a number of smaller areas and is located directly below the thalamus, making it relatively simple to locate on brain scans.

Midbrain

The midbrain contains nuclei and white-matter tracts that control a variety of functions such as sleep, arousal, attention, muscle tone and motor function, pain, instinctive drives, and the processing of visual and auditory information at the unconscious level.

Red Nuclei

This nuclei is involved with the control of movement.

Substantia Nigra

The substantia nigra (Latin: black substance) is involved in the production of the neurotransmitter dopamine and communication to and from the basal ganglia structures.

Pressure from a pituitary tumor can result in a very specific visual-field loss due to partial disruption of the optic pathways passing through the chiasm. Damage to the optic chiasm can result in bitemporal visual-field loss. Tumors compressing the optic chiasm from above result in inferior heteronymous bitemporal quadranopias (Figure 3-99A). Tumors compressing the optic chiasm from below result in superior heteronymous bitemporal quadranopias (Figure 3-99B), and tumors that infiltrate the optic chiasm can result in bitemporal or peripheral hemianopias (Figure 3-99C).

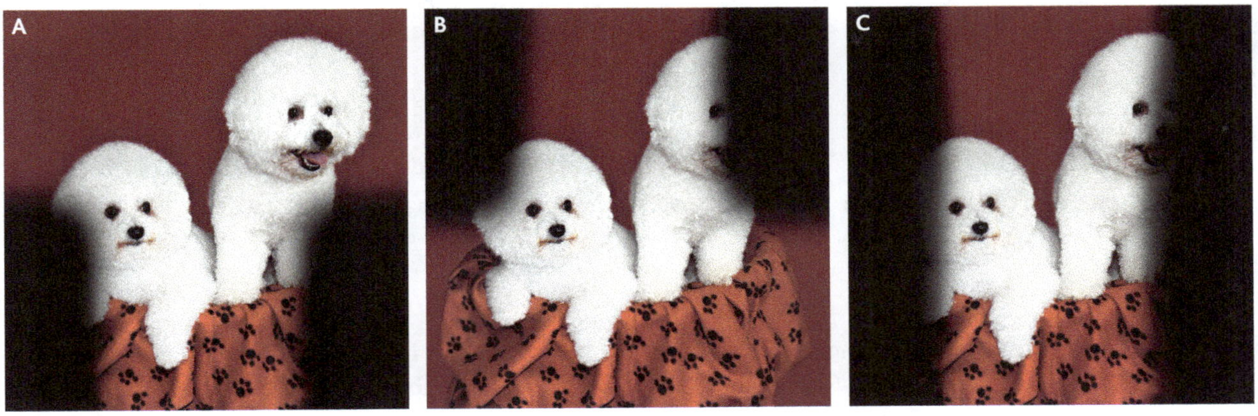

Figure 3-99 **A:** Inferior heteronymous bitemoral quadranopia. **B:** Superior heteronymous bitemporal quadranopia. **C:** Peripheral hemianopia.

The substantia nigra is relatively simple to locate on a brain section because of the presence of neuromelanin (Figure 3-100 arrows).

It is more difficult to locate on brain scans as the neuromelanin often does not appear any differently than the surrounding tissue. On spoiled gradient echo T1 images using BRAVO, FSPGR or MPRAGE protocols, the area may be visible as a dark region within the midbrain.

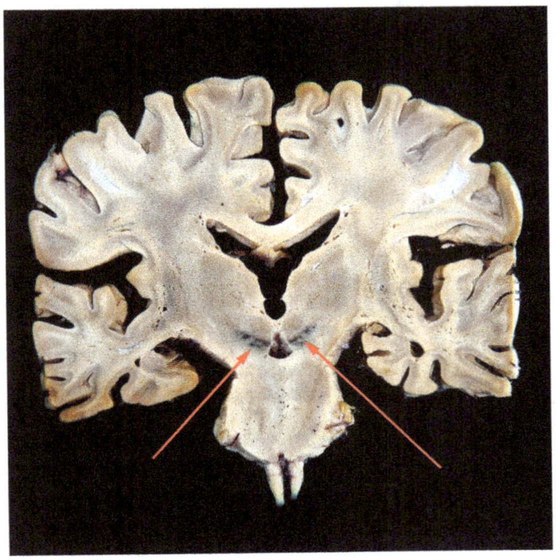

Figure 3-100 Substantia nigra shown on brain slice as the dark substance within the midbrain (arrows).

Substantia nigra on brain imaging

- On axial images (Figure 3-101A), the substantia nigra is most easily visualized on a slice that cuts through the top of the midbrain where the midbrain takes on the appearance of the cross section of a V8 engine. The substantia nigra appears as darker bands on either side and anterior to the cerebral aqueduct, or using the V8 engine analogy, just below the rocker cover on each of the cylinder heads.
- On coronal images (Figure 3-101B), the substantia nigra is best visualized on a slice that runs through the anterior portion of the midbrain. The substantia nigra is located medial to the posterior limb of the internal capsule.
- On sagittal images (Figure 3-101C), it is often difficult to visualize the substantia nigra, which is oriented superior–inferior at the front of the midbrain, just above the top of the pons.

Reticular Formation

The reticular formation is involved with sleep, arousal, attention, muscle tone, and sensory functioning.

Central Gray/Periaqueductal Gray

The central gray is involved in species-typical behavior, such as mating, fighting, and innate behaviors. This is also the site of primary opiate activation and analgesic effects.

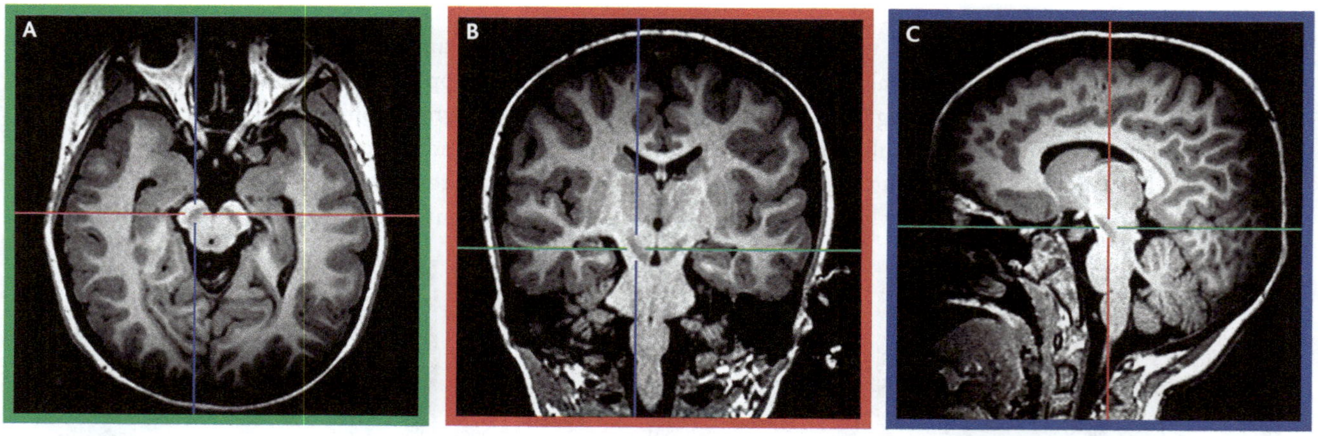

Figure 3-101 **A:** Axial image of substantia nigra. **B:** Coronal image of substantia nigra. **C:** Sagittal image of substantia nigra.

Corpora Quadrigemini

As the name implies, the corpora quadrigemini (Latin: quadruplet bodies) are made up of four bodies, two from the superior colliculus and two from the inferior colliculus.

The corpora quadrigemini are located at the back of the midbrain and appear as four "bumps" directly below the pineal and medial-inferior to the thalami (Figure 3-102).

The two upper bodies are the superior colliculi, and the two lower bodies are the inferior colliculi. The superior colliculi are involved in visually based spatial localization and awareness. The inferior colliculi are involved in auditory-based spatial localization and awareness.

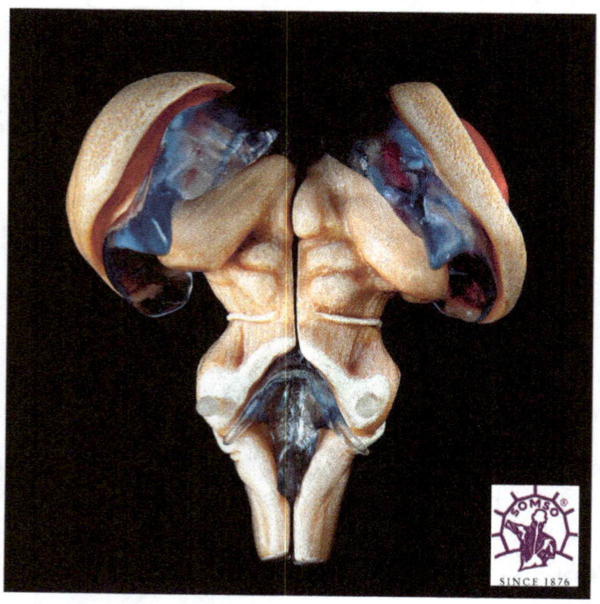

Figure 3-102 Posterior view of a brain model showing the midbrain structures of the corpora quadrigemini, as four bumps located directly below the pineal body.

Corpora quadrigemini on brain imaging

- The colliculi may be difficult to visualize on brain imaging. The ability to appreciate the structures is dependent on the slice angle and thickness. Because these structures are small, thick slices may not capture them, with the structures falling between slices.
- On axial images (Figure 3-103A), the colliculi appear as two horizontally oriented bumps on the back of the midbrain, just posterior to the cerebral aqueduct.
- On coronal images (Figure 3-103B), the colliculi appear as four bumps within the perimesencephalic or quadrigeminal cistern, just below the thalami.
- On sagittal scans (Figure 3-103C), the colliculi appear as two vertically oriented bumps on the back of the midbrain and protruding into the perimesencephalic or quadrigeminal cistern.

General Location of the Midbrain Structures

- On axial images (Figure 3-104A), the midbrain is located medial to the hippocampi and takes on the shape of the cross section of a V8 engine. The "cylinder heads" of the V8 engine are formed from the posterior limb of the internal capsule as it becomes the cerebral peduncles. The darker layer below the capsule is the substantia nigra. The posterior part of the midbrain is formed from the corpora quadrigemini. The cerebral aqueduct of Sylvius is visible running down the center of the midbrain.
- On coronal images (Figure 3-104B), the midbrain is located between the white-matter tracts of the cerebral peduncles and directly above the pons. At the most anterior aspect of the mesencephalon, the posterior limb of the internal capsules makes up the lateral walls, with the substantia nigra being medial.

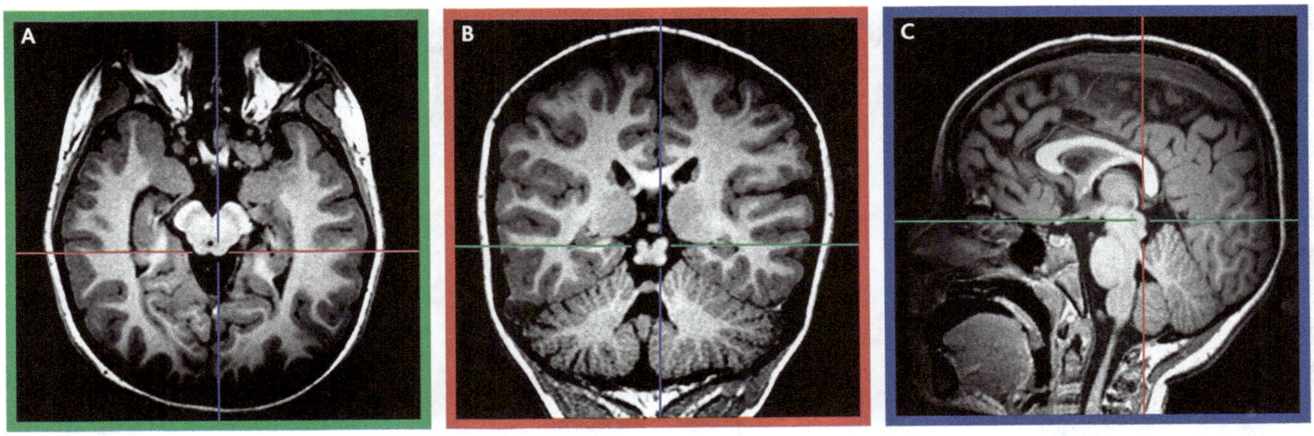

Figure 3-103 **A:** Axial image of corpora quadrigemini, with the slice cutting through the superior colliculi. **B:** Coronal image of corpora quadrigemini. **C:** Sagittal image of corpora quadrigemini.

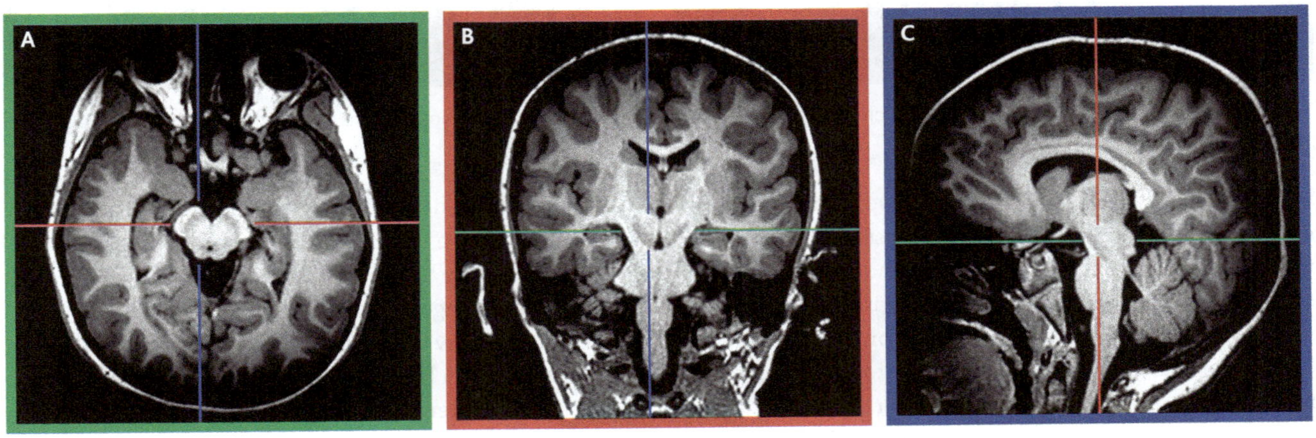

Figure 3-104 **A:** Axial image of midbrain structures. **B:** Coronal image of midbrain structures. **C:** Sagittal image of midbrain structures.

- On sagittal images (Figure 3-104C), the midbrain is located below the thalamus and above the pons. On the anterior aspect of the midbrain, the pathways of the posterior limb of the internal capsule are visible with the substantia nigra being just posterior to the internal capsule. On the posterior aspect of the mesencephalon, the superior and inferior colliculi are often visible. The cistern just behind the colliculi is the peri-mesencephalic or quadrigeminal cistern, named because the midbrain is part of the mesencephalon, and it sits posterior to the corpora quadrigemini.

Hindbrain

The hindbrain is located directly below the midbrain, and there is no clear boundary between the two regions. The various parts of the hindbrain function to support vital bodily functions relating to motor activity, postural control, sleep and arousal, internal equilibrium, breathing, and blood circulation. The hindbrain has two primary divisions, the metencephalon with the pons and cerebellum and the myelencephalon, which contains the medulla oblongata and connections to the spinal cord.

Metencephalon

The metencephalon is composed of the pons and the cerebellum. The pons is located directly below the midbrain, and the cerebellum is located behind the pons and inferior to the occipital lobes.

Pons

The pons (Latin = bridge) contains both gray-matter nuclei and white-matter tracts. The pons is illustrated on a three dimensional diagram as the purple structure (Figure 3-105A), and on a brain model by the arrow (Figure 3-105B). The nuclei of the pons are responsible for relaying information to and from the cerebellum, the

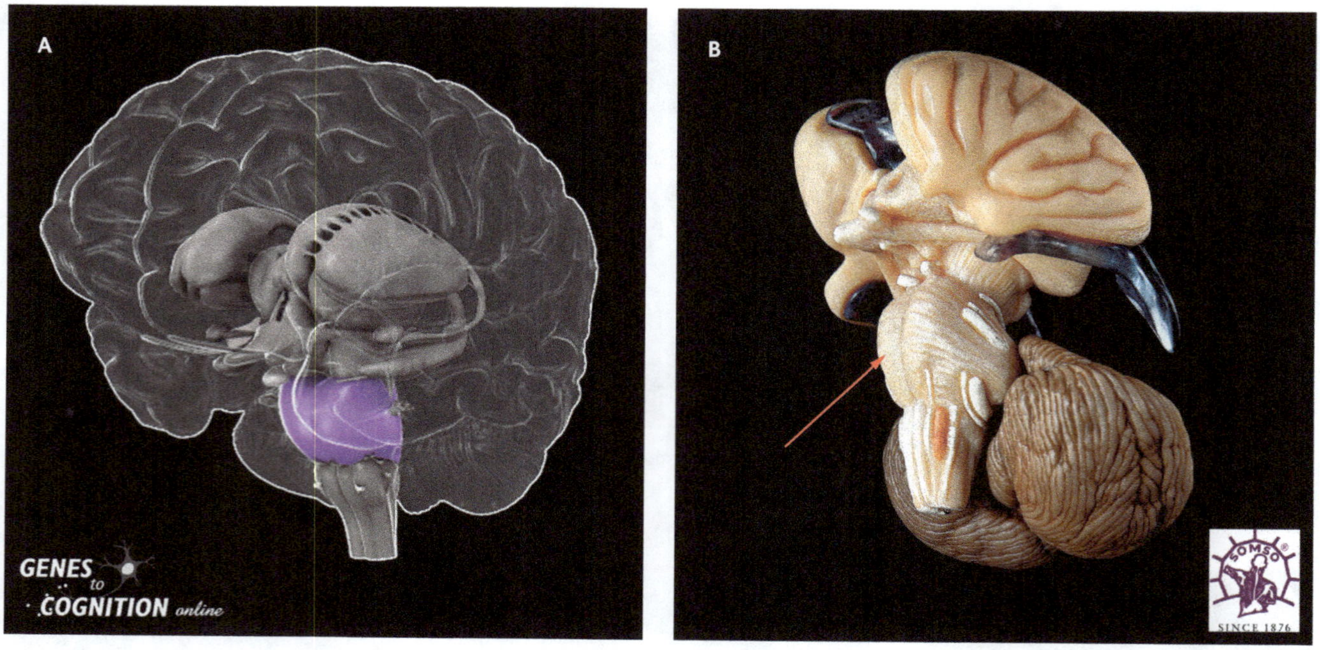

Figure 3-105 **A:** Three dimensional brain illustration showing the pons in purple. **B:** Brain model showing the pons (arrow) viewed from the front.

modulation of sleep and arousal, respiratory function, swallowing, bladder control, hearing, taste, eye movement, facial expressions, postural control, and general internal equilibrium. The white-matter tracts within the pons are responsible for transmitting information to and from the higher cortical and subcortical areas to the cerebellum, medulla, and spinal cord. At the posterior aspect of the pons there are two large white-matter tracts called the cerebellar peduncles, that connect the pons to the cerebellum.

Pons on brain imaging

- On axial images (Figure 3-106A), the pons is best visualized at the level where the slice transects the superior portion of the cerebellum and/or the inferior-posterior portion of the occipital lobe depending on the acquisition angle. The pons is identified as the primarily white matter structure located anterior to the fourth ventricle.
- On coronal images (Figure 3-106B), the pons is visualized below the midbrain and above the medulla. It is located at a level close to that of the inferior surface of the temporal lobes and is recognize by its distinctive shape. As the internal capsule meets the pons, there is a widening of the white-matter region on the scan as the cerebellar peduncles form on the lateral aspects of the structure.
- On sagittal images (Figure 3-106C), the pons is easily identified as the elongated, bulbous structure at the front of the hindbrain and anterior to the fourth ventricle.

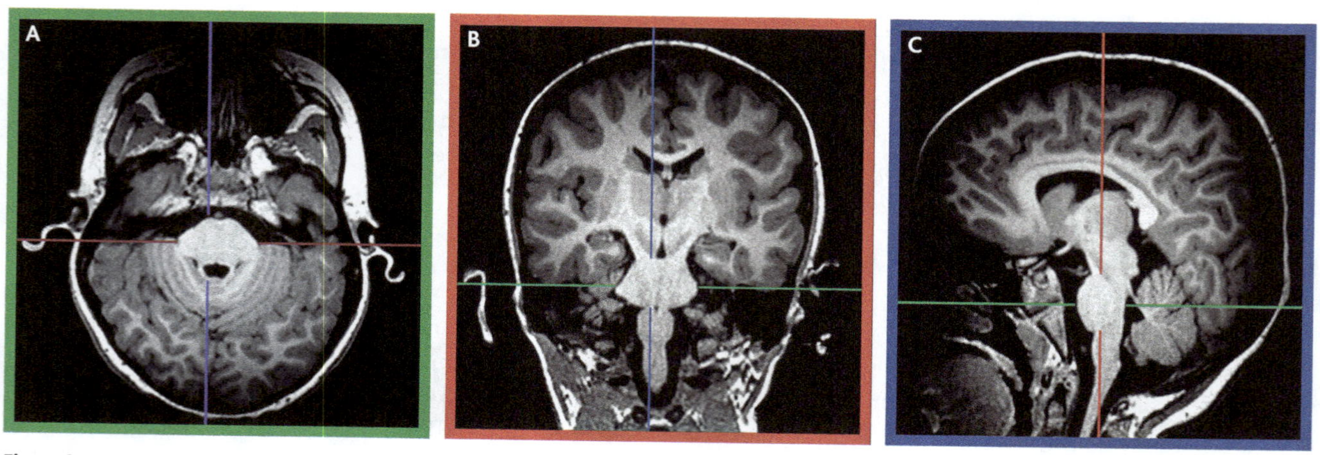

Figure 3-106 **A:** Axial image of the pons. **B:** Coronal image of the pons. **C:** Sagittal image of the pons.

Cerebellum

The cerebellum has the appearance of a small brain with cortex, white matter, sulci, and gyri, hence the name (Latin: *cerebellum* = little brain) (Figures 3-107A–D). The cerebellum plays an important role in the integration of motor and sensory systems. The primary role of the cerebellum is in the coordination of the motor system required for balance, muscle tone, posture, and fine motor movements. Nuclei within the cerebellum play a role in the sensory input from visual, auditory, vestibular, and somatosensory systems, integrating it with appropriate motor output. The cerebellum is also important in the modulation and coordination of many areas of the brain involved in cognitive processing, including attention, language, memory, social awareness, and intellect.

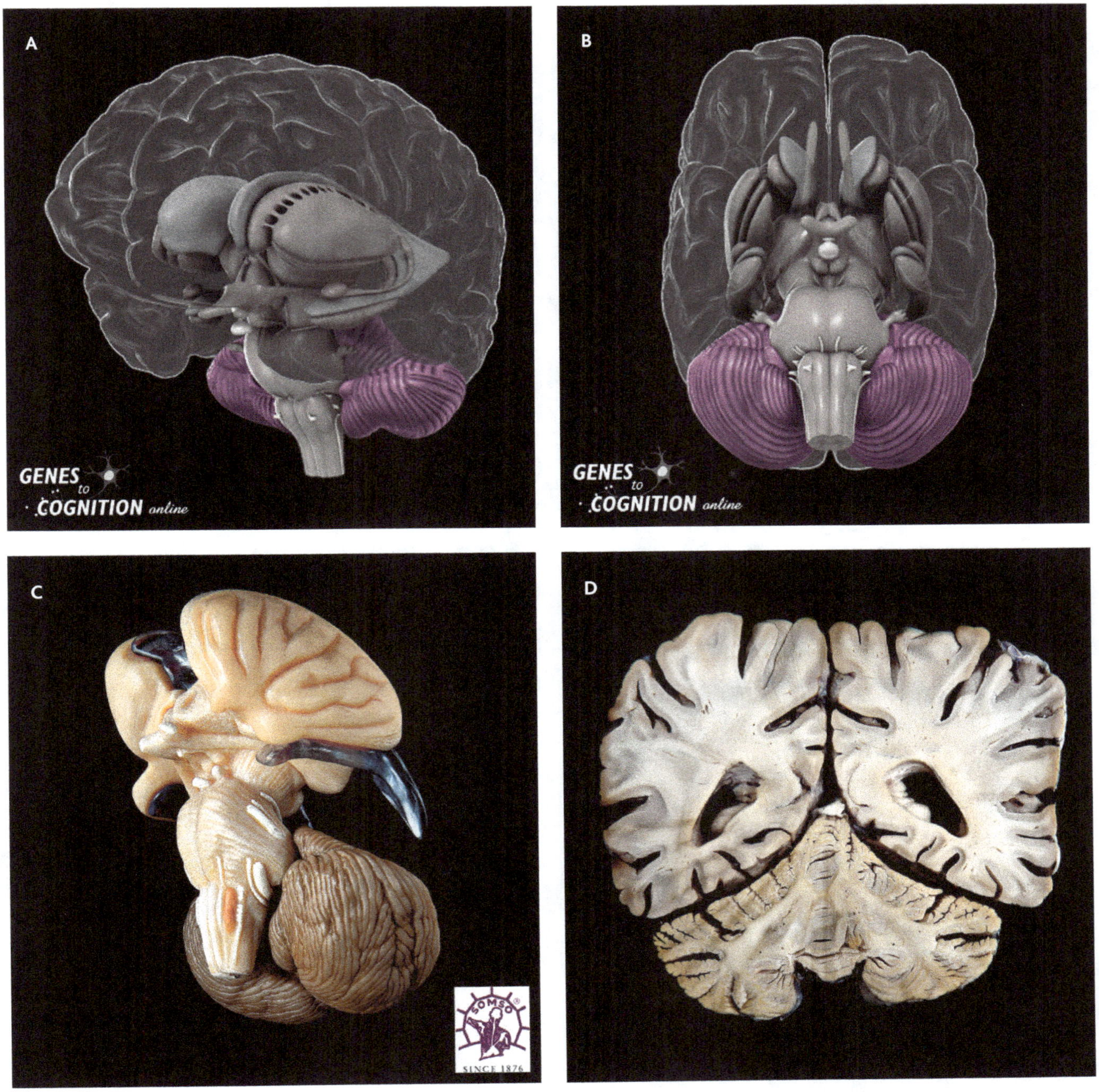

Figure 3-107A–D Illustrations showing the location of the cerebellum. On the three dimensional brain illustrations (A) and (B), the cerebellum is identified as the purple structure. On the brain model (C), the cerebellum is located behind the pons, and on coronal brain section (D), the cerebellum is identified as the triangular structure separated from, and below the parietal lobes.

Generally, visualizing the cerebellum on brain imaging is relatively simple, given its size and its relation to other brain structures. Sometimes, CT scans that slice through both the cerebellum and parts of the occipital lobe can appear confusing, as the areas can appear similar. However, with practice, differentiating the two areas becomes quite simple. On Figure 3-108A, the very back of the image has some occipital lobe showing, with the remainder of the posterior structure being cerebellum. On coronal images, the main body of the cerebellum appears as a triangular shaped structure below the temporal-occipital cortex (Figure 3-108B). Figure 3-108C illustrates why both cerebellar and occipital cortex is visible in Figure 108a. The axial slice used for Figure 108a was acquired from the location represented by the green reference line, which passes through the body of the cerebellum and the most inferior part of the occipital lobe.

The cerebellar tonsils are located on the inferior-medial aspect of the cerebellum and are normally located above the foramen magnum, or above a hypothetical line (McRae's line) drawn between the bottom of the clivus and the posterior margin of the foramen magnum. McRae's line is located across the opening of the foramen magnum. When the cerebellar tonsils are herniated more than approximately 3 to 5 mm below McRae's line, the patient is considered to have a Chiari I malformation. Chiari I malformations can result in a number of symptoms relating to disrupted CSF flow, such as hydrocephalus, a spinal cord syrinx, headaches, or other neurological signs. Sometimes, Chiari I conditions are asymptomatic and discovered during imaging for other conditions, as was the case in the clinical example shown in Figures 3-109A–C.

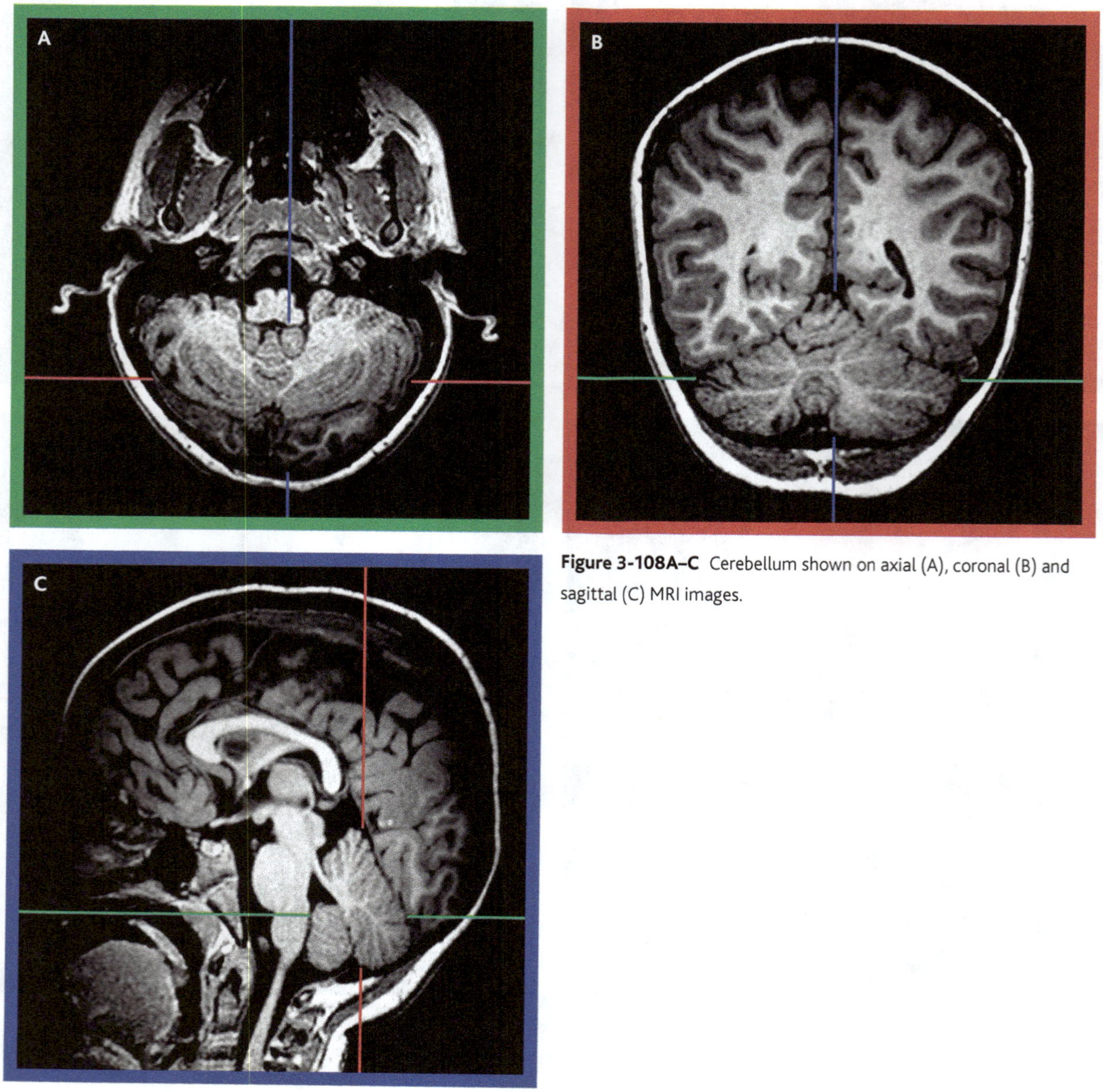

Figure 3-108A–C Cerebellum shown on axial (A), coronal (B) and sagittal (C) MRI images.

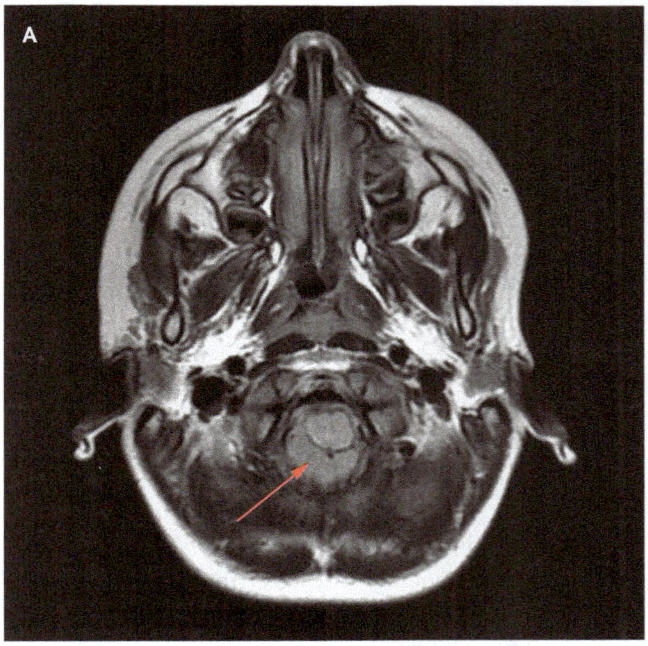

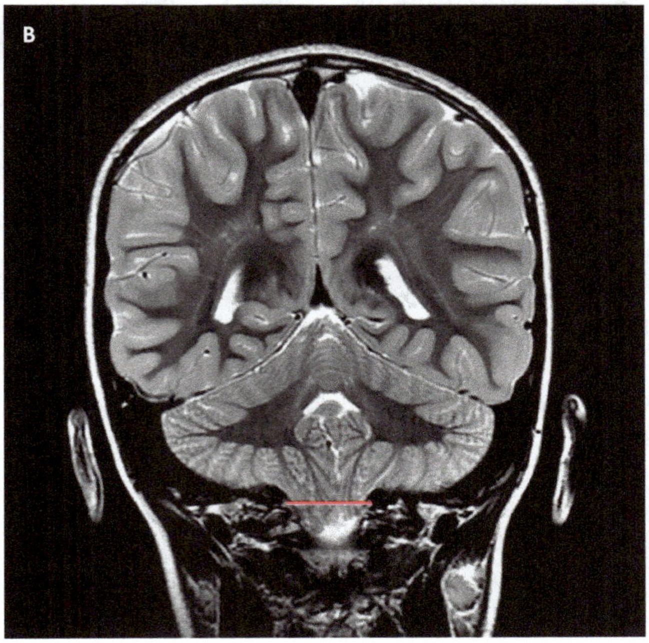

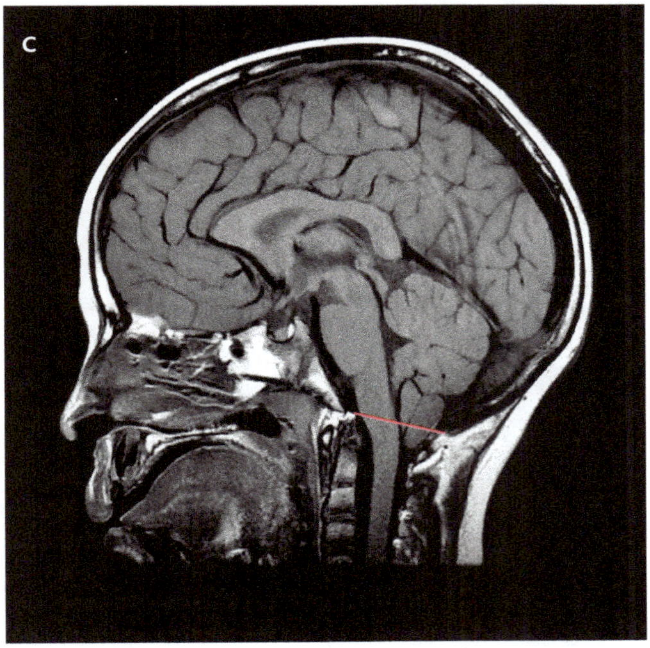

Figure 3-109A–C Clinical example: Chiari I malformation. MRI images acquired at a level close to the opening of the foramen magnum or at McRae's line. Note the cerebellar tonsils close to the spinal cord (3-109A, arrow), due to them protruding below McRae's line or level. The red line shown in 3-109B and 3-109C represents McRae's line, or the opening of the foramen magnum. Note that the cerebellar tonsils are clearly shown as protruding below McRae's line or the opening of the foramen magnum, a sign of Chiari I Malformation. **A:** Axial T2 FLAIR. **B:** Coronal T2 FLAIR. **C:** Sagittal T1.

Myelencephalon

The myelencephalon is composed of the medulla oblongata and the spinal cord and is involved in a variety of critical functions, including, but not restricted to, respiration, consciousness, cardiac function, body temperature, involuntary muscle functioning, sneezing, coughing, vomiting, and swallowing.

Medulla oblongata

The medulla oblongata, shortened to "medulla," is located between the pons and the spinal cord and acts as a pathway between the brain and body via the spinal cord. The medulla contains reticular nuclei responsible for the control of breathing, cardiac function, muscle tone, and arousal.

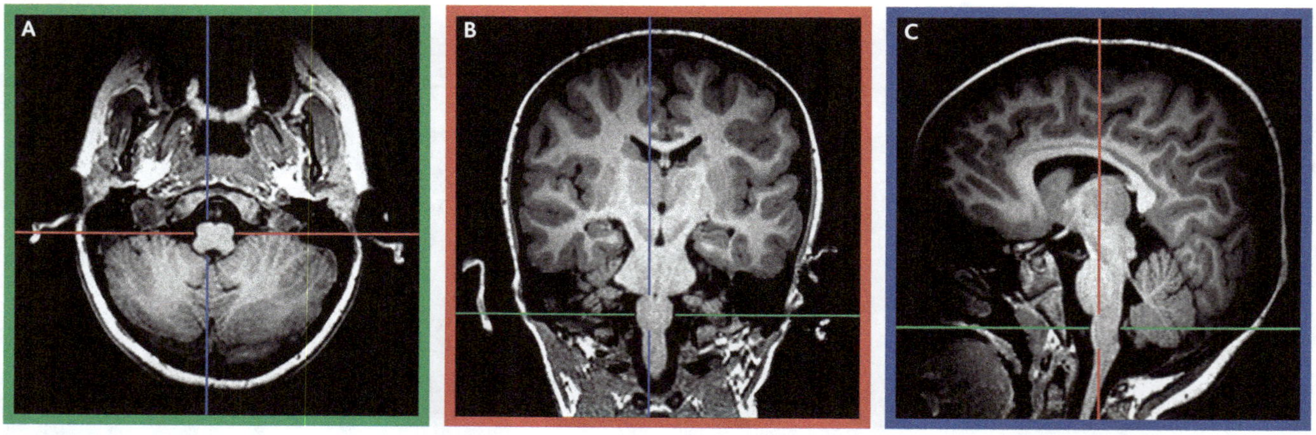

Figure 3-110A–C Medulla shown on axial (A), coronal (B) and sagittal (C) MRI images.

On brain scans, the medulla is easily identified as the structure between the hindbrain/pons and the spinal cord (Figures 3-110a–c). Behind the medulla is the basal cistern, an area of particular interest when assessing for imminent herniation of the brain stem through the foramen magnum.

Vascular System

The blood vessels in the brain have a different wall structure designed to protect the brain from pathogens. The vessel walls have smaller gaps between the cells, providing a barrier between the blood and the brain called the blood–brain barrier (BBB). The presence of the BBB allows radiological techniques to be used to image the blood vessels. The introduction of a radiopaque contrast agent for CT and paramagnetic contrast agent for MRI enables the visualization of blood within the vessels, techniques called computed tomographic angiography (CTA) and magnetic resonance angiography (MRA), respectively. Contrast agents can also be used to identify areas of BBB compromise caused by pathological processes such as rapid tumor growth, infection, or inflammation.

The blood vessels of the brain carry approximately three-fourths of a liter of oxygenated blood to the brain structures every minute. There are four main blood vessels that supply the brain: the right and left internal carotid arteries and the right and left vertebral arteries. The two vertebral arteries converge to become the basilar artery at the bottom of the pons, with the basilar artery running up the anterior surface of the pons.

Internal Carotid and Vertebral Artery Distributions to the Cortex

The internal carotid arteries supply blood to the middle cerebral arteries and the anterior cerebral arteries on each side of the brain. Figures 3-111A and B illustrate the general cortical distributions for the middle cerebral arteries (red vessels) and anterior cerebral arteries (orange vessels). The vertebral arteries form the basilar artery, which supplies blood to the posterior cerebral arteries on each side of the brain. The general cortical distribution for the posterior cerebral arteries is illustrated by the yellow vessels on Figures 3-111A and B.

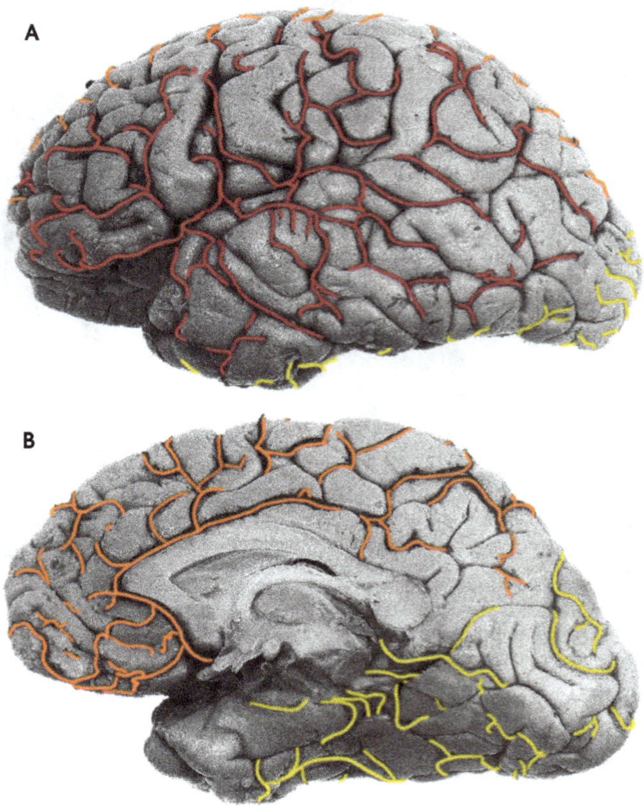

Figures 3-111A and B Internal carotid and vertebral artery distributions to the cortical surface of the brain. The middle cerebral artery vessels are shown in red, the anterior cerebral artery vessels are shown in orange, and the posterior cerebral arteries are shown in yellow.

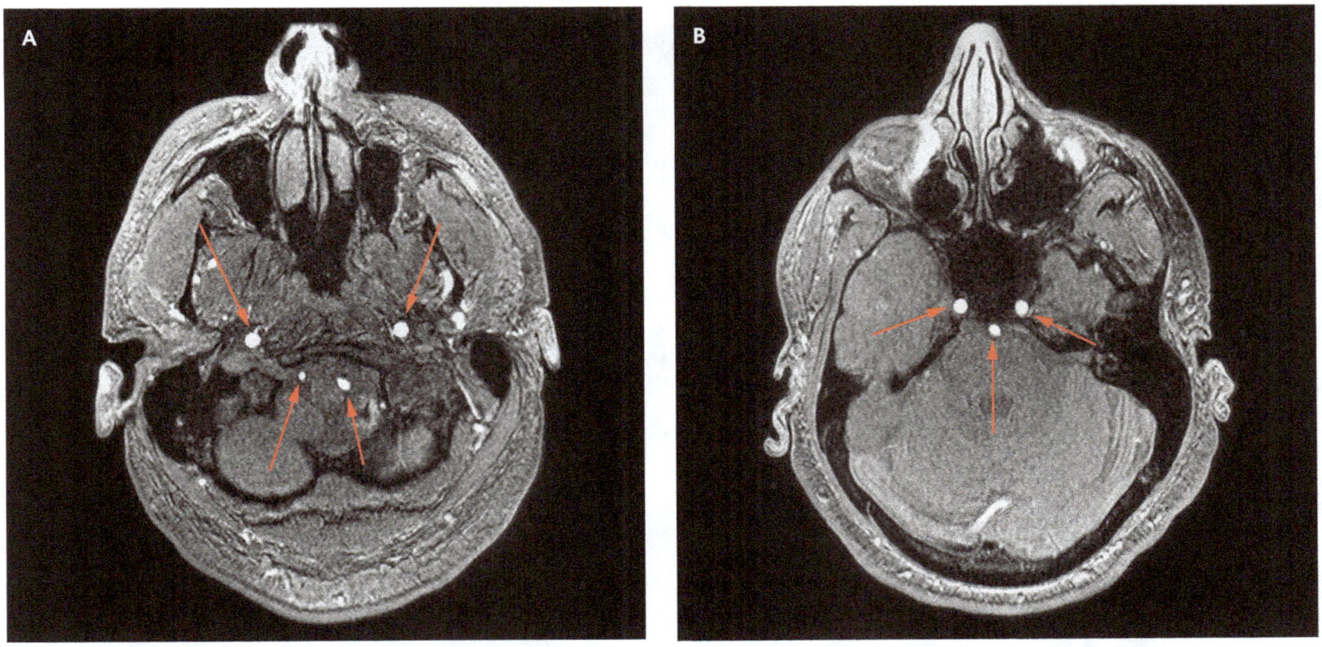

Figure 3-112 **A:** Right and left carotid arteries (anterior arrows); right and left vertebral arteries (posterior arrows). **B:** Right and left carotid arteries (anterior arrows); basilar artery (posterior arrow).

On TOF images shown on two-dimensional slices, a preferred format for radiologist, it is relatively simple to identify the vessels as long as they are patent with good flow. The internal carotid arteries are shown in Figure 3-112A as the two anterior widespread vessels (arrows). The vertebral arteries are closer and more posterior on the image (arrows). On Figure 3-112B, the right and left carotid arteries are seen closer together and just medial to the temporal lobes (arrows). Behind the carotid arteries and in the center of the picture on the anterior surface of the pons, the basilar artery is visible (arrow).

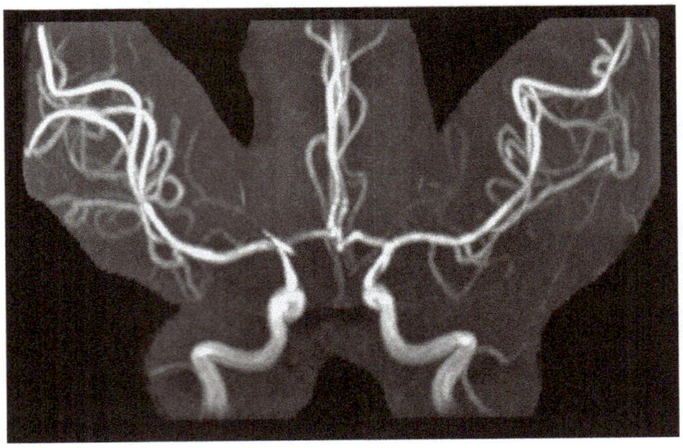

Figure 3-113 The internal carotid arteries are seen at the bottom within each hemisphere. They move superior and then laterally to become the middle cerebral arteries. The vessels along the centerline of the picture are the anterior cerebral arteries, supplying the medial surface of each hemisphere.

Right and Left Internal Carotid Distribution

Most of the blood supply to the brain passes via the right and left internal carotid arteries (Figure 3-113). After entering the brain, the internal carotid arteries turn outward and become the middle cerebral arteries for the respective hemisphere. The middle cerebral arteries send smaller branches to the subcortical structures of the basal ganglia, thalamus, hypothalamus, and limbic system. Once reaching the lateral convexity of each hemisphere, the middle cerebral arteries supply a distribution covering most of the lateral cortex. Blood from the carotid arteries also travels to the medial surface of each hemisphere via the anterior cerebral arteries seen at the center of the image and oriented vertically in Figure 3-113.

Right and Left Vertebral Artery and Basilar Distribution

The vertebral arteries combine just below the level of the pons to become the basilar artery. The basilar artery is located adjacent to the anterior pons and branches at the top of the pons to form the right and left posterior cerebral arteries (Figure 3-114). The right and left posterior cerebral

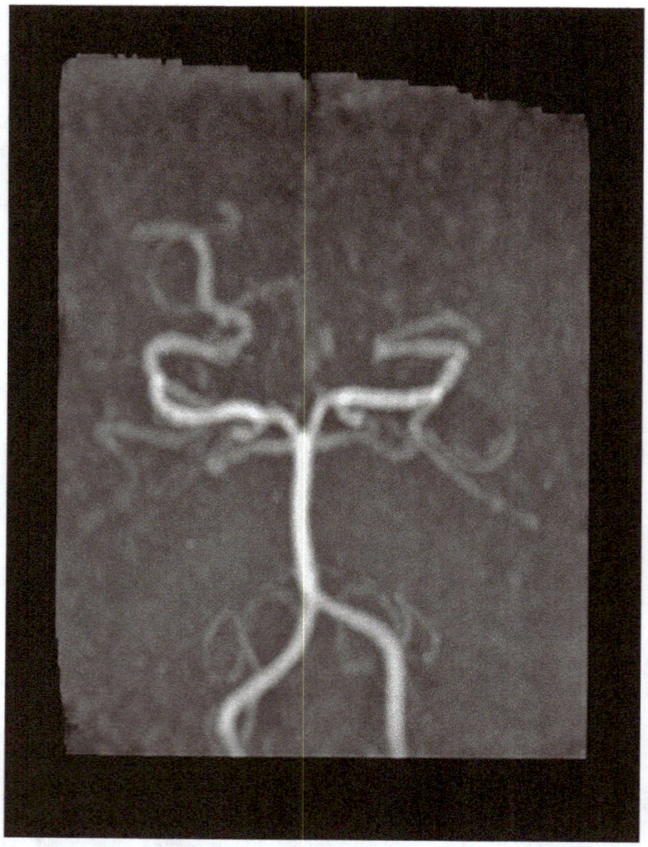

Figure 3-114 The vertebral arteries shown at the bottom of the image form the single basilar artery, which then bifurcates to the right and left posterior cerebral arteries shown at the top of the image.

arteries supply the underside of the temporal lobes and the occipital lobes. Blood also flows from the basilar artery via smaller vessels to the hindbrain, brain stem, cerebellum, and spinal cord.

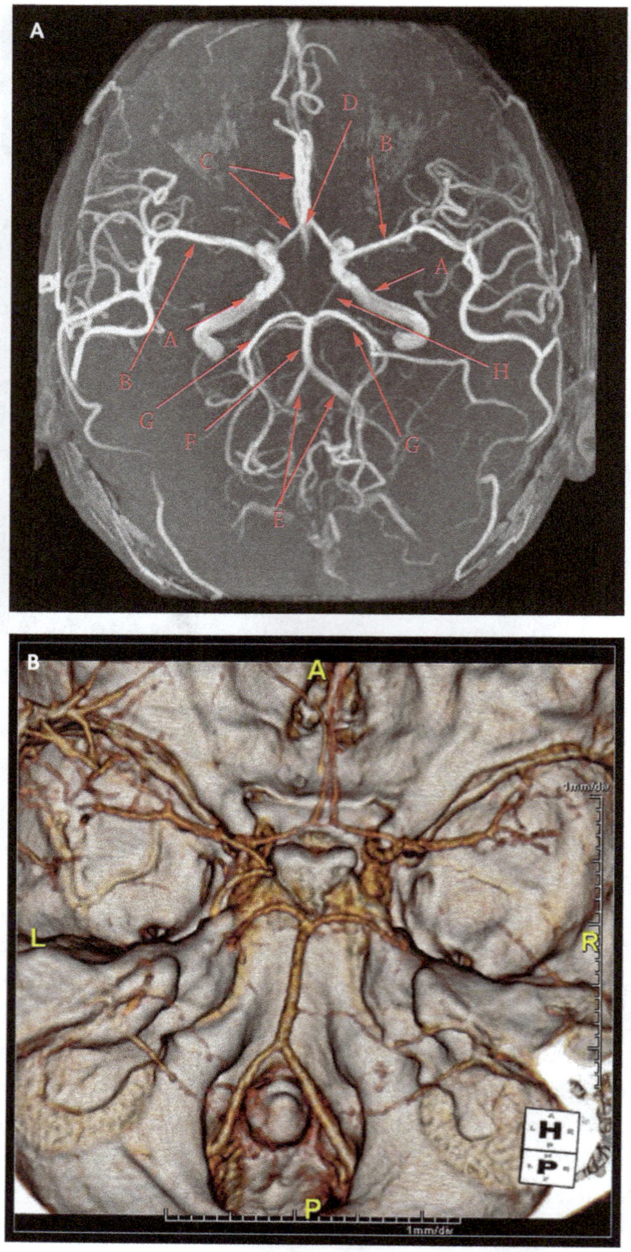

Figures 3-115A and B Circle of Willis shown using time-of-flight sequence (COW TOF) in Figure 3-115A and three dimensional CT vessel reconstruction in Figure 3-115B. *A = Internal Carotid Artery; B = Middle Cerebral Artery; C = Anterior Cerebral Artery; D = Anterior Communicating Artery; E = Vertebral Artery; F = Basilar Artery; G = Posterior Cerebral Artery; H = Posterior Communicating Artery.*

Circle of Willis

The main vessels of the internal carotid arteries and the posterior cerebral arteries are connected via communicating arteries to form a structure called the circle of Willis. The circle of Willis is a circle-like vascular structure, or anastomosis, where the blood supply from different areas is combined (Figures 3-115A and B). The circle of Willis provides some redundancy of blood supply to critical structures of the brain. If there is reduced flow in one vessel, supply can be provided via a communicating artery from another vessel. The redundancy is limited, however, as the communicating arteries are very thin and often not adequate to compensate for a significant decline in blood flow through one of the primary vessels.

Although the blood vessels from the right and left hemispheres are connected anteriorly by the anterior communicating artery and posteriorly via the basilar–posterior artery junction, blood from one side of the brain generally stays on that side. Figure 3-116 shows an angiogram of blood flow through the right internal carotid artery to the right anterior and middle cerebral arteries. Note how the blood stays on one side of the brain. Blood from the anterior supply (internal carotid arteries) and the posterior supply (vertebral arteries) will also remain within the respective distributions, without a large degree of cross-flow or mixing.

The mains distributions remain relatively isolated because, without disruption to normal flow, there is equal pressure within all vessels, reducing the probability of cross-flow from right to left or front to back. When there is disrupted blood flow or unequal pressure from one distribution, the circle of Willis can allow some cross-flow between the hemispheres or even between the anterior and posterior distributions in order to supply the area with limited flow. More often though, there is not enough compensatory flow via the communicating arteries to prevent brain damage due to restricted blood flow through one of the primary feeding arteries.

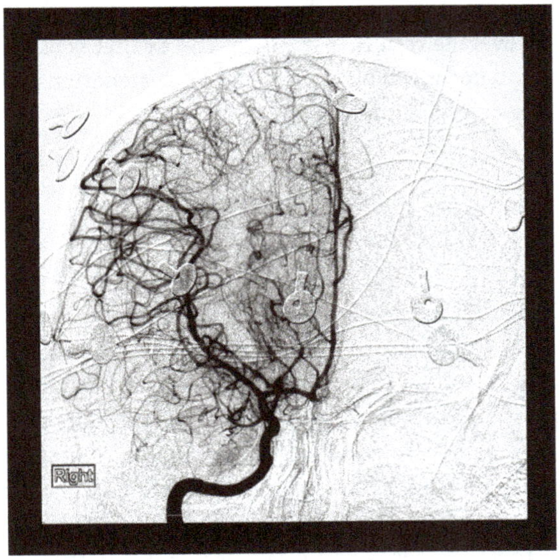

Figure 3-116 Angiogram of blood flow through right internal carotid artery to right anterior and middle cerebral arteries. Note how the blood remains within the right hemisphere without crossflow to the left hemisphere.

CLINICAL EXAMPLE

Lupita: Circle of Willis Compensation for Internal Carotid Thrombosis

Lupita had significantly reduced left internal carotid artery blood flow, but she did not present with symptoms of a stroke. Lupita's MRI was incidental to a physical injury involving her neck in a motor vehicle accident. The injury to the base of her skull had caused damage to the left internal carotid artery as it passed through the base of the cranium. The damage resulted in almost no blood flow through the left internal carotid, as evident on the axial TOF image (Figure 3-117 arrow).

In Lupita's case, she was lucky that the left middle cerebral artery distribution started to draw blood from the basilar artery via the posterior communicating artery. In Figures 3-118A and B, the middle cerebral arteries appear patent on both sides of the brain, even on the left where there is no evidence of flow through the internal carotid artery. Flow is apparent through the posterior communicating artery, a vessel that is often difficult to see on TOF imaging. Flow is also evident through the left anterior cerebral artery, likely coming from the right arterial supply via the anterior communicating artery.

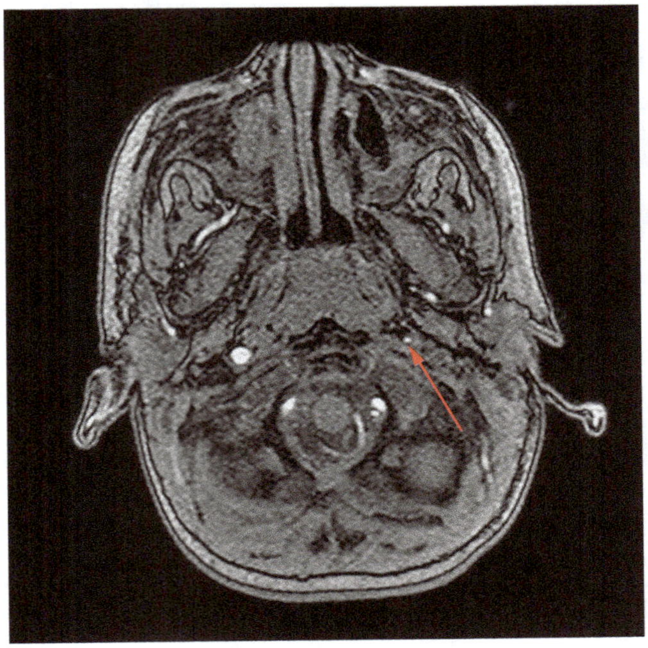

Figure 3-117 Clinical example Lupita: circle of Willis compensation for reduced flow through left internal carotid artery. TOF axial image shows almost no blood flow through left internal carotid artery (arrow).

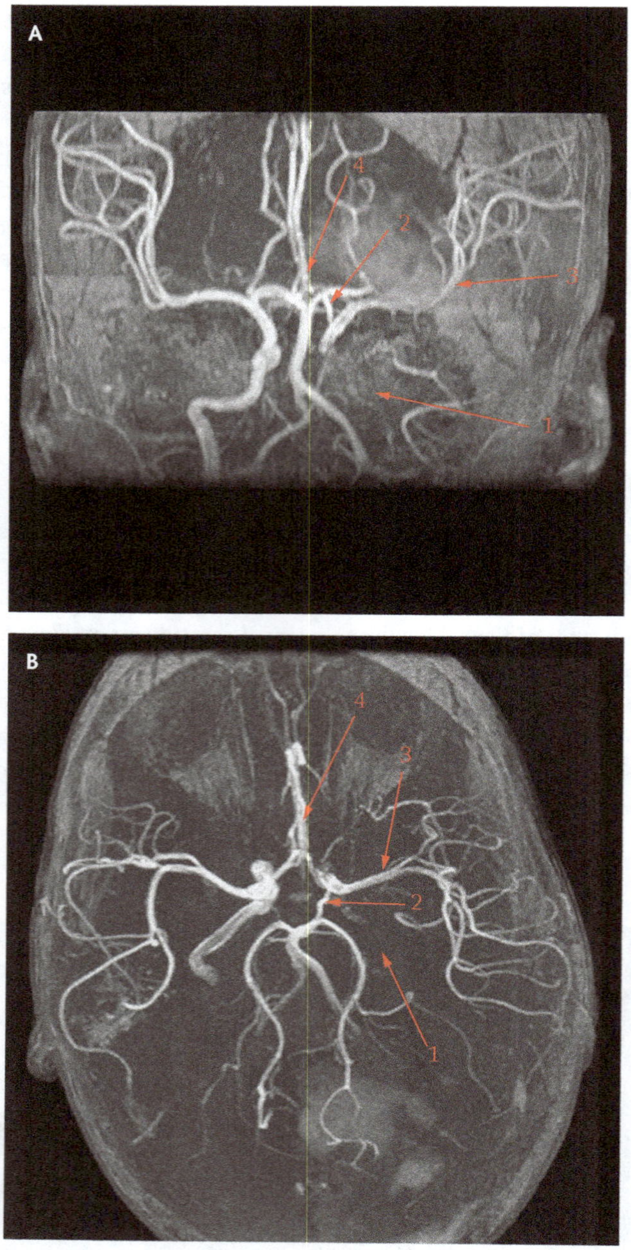

Figures 3-118A and B Clinical example Lupita: Circle of Willis compensation for internal carotid thrombosis. Left middle cerebral artery appears patent, even without flow through the left internal carotid artery. A: Anterior-Posterior (AP) view; B: Axial Circle-of-Willis (COW) view. *Arrow 1 = no flow through the left internal carotid artery; Arrow 2 = flow through the left posterior communicating artery; Arrow 3 = left middle cerebral artery flow from the posterior communicating artery; Arrow 4 = left anterior cerebral artery flow from the anterior communicating artery.*

Watershed Area

It is important to note that there are areas of cortex that receive less blood than other areas because the primary distributions fail to overlap. The watershed area is located between the fingers of the middle, anterior, and posterior cerebral arteries (Figure 3-119 purple region). The fingers of the middle cerebral artery do not cover the entire lateral surface of the brain. Even though the fingers of the anterior cerebral artery wrap over the medial surface to supply the outer rim of lateral cortex, they do not extend all the way to the fingers of the middle cerebral artery. Similarly, at the back of the brain, the fingers of the posterior cerebral artery do not meet those of the middle cerebral artery. The watershed area is located between the fingers of the three primary distributions on the surface of the cortex. The poor vessel coverage results in a ring of cortex that is especially prone to a decline in blood pressure or oxygenation and can lead to watershed infarctions.

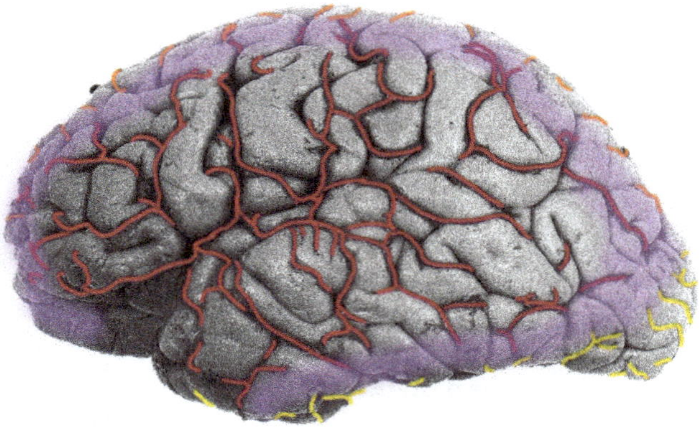

Figure 3-119 Illustration of the watershed area (purple), or the region between the fingers of the middle cerebral artery (red), anterior cerebral artery (orange) and posterior cerebral artery (yellow).

CONCLUDING REMARKS

Having a basic understanding of how to use and interpret brain images, in addition to a solid foundation of imaging-based neuroanatomy, will allow you to more efficiently and accurately integrate neuroimaging data into you clinical practice. However, up this this point, only standard technologies have been discussed. Few details have been introduced relating to how the different imaging systems work, their strengths and weakness, and also the various technologies and sequences available to you. Chapter 4 will introduce the technology behind some of the more common imaging systems, such as CT, MRI, and angiography, in addition to more advanced systems such as SPECT, PET, MEG, and even hybrid systems that combine different technologies. Within each category of technology, some of the more common sequences will be discussed, such as T1, T2, FLAIR, DWI, and ADC, with and without contrast agents. Chapter 4 will also introduce different imaging techniques to use in order to visualize various tissues, particularly techniques helpful when assessing dense material such as bone, soft tissue such as brain parenchyma, or even fluids, such as blood within the vessels.

Once you have a solid foundation of knowledge pertaining to the various imaging technologies and sequences, you will find the interpretation of brain scans much easier and useful. You will know which scans are most helpful for a particular tissue of pathological process, and you will become more efficient at comparing different scanning techniques and sequences in order to build a more comprehensive picture of the damage to the brain. No one scanning system can provide all of the information required to fully appreciate brain pathology. By viewing a combination of scans, you will find yourself much more able to fully appreciate a specific brain condition. In addition, you will be better able to determine which sequences you may wish to order, given a particular clinical presentation or question.

APPENDIX 3-1

Parts of the Brain and Their Functions

Frontal Lobes
- Executive functioning
- Expressive language (left hemisphere)
- Prosody and use of intonation (right hemisphere)
- Voluntary motor functioning
- Socially appropriate judgment and insight
- Motivation and self-drive or initiation of behavior
- Behavioral and emotional control
- Attentional vigilance and allocation
- Level of arousal

Parietal Lobes
- Sensory input from the body
- Receptive and complex language comprehension (left hemisphere)
- Reading, writing, and math processing (left hemisphere)
- Visual–spatial functioning (right hemisphere)
- Integration of sensory information (auditory, visual, and tactile)
- Directed attention to visual, auditory, or tactile space

Temporal Lobes
- Auditory processing
- Receptive language comprehension (left hemisphere)
- Prosody and intonation comprehension (right hemisphere)
- Memory storage and retrieval
- Emotional function
- Instinctive drives involving fear, aggression, sexual behavior, hunger, etc.

Occipital Lobes
- Light perception
- Perception or experience of seeing
- Visual processing from simple to complex
- Recognition of visual information (close to the temporal lobe)
- Attention to visual space (close to the parietal lobe)

Allocortex/Limbic System
- Storage and retrieval of memories
- Primitive emotional drives (e.g., aggression/defense, sexual behavior, predation/feeding)
- Instinctive and species-specific behaviors (e.g., dominance-submission, male–female, adult–infant, approach–avoidance)
- Feeling of pleasure, rage, and fear

Basal Ganglia
- Modulation of the body's motor systems
- Automaticity of functions, routines, and behaviors

Thalamus
- Relays information between different parts of the brain
- Processing and "gating" of information depending on need (i.e., even though the sensory information from the skin always goes to the brain, often we do not notice this information; the thalamus helps you ignore the feeling of your watch strap, clothing, or a hat after a few seconds or minutes)

Hypothalamus
- Controls internal bodily states such as emotion, hunger, thirst, body temperature, sexual/reproductive behavior, circadian rhythms, and the fight-or-flight response
- Autonomic nervous system and hormonal system via pituitary function

Midbrain
- Contains nuclei and pathways that control movement, arousal, sleep, attention, muscle tone, pain, and species-typical behaviors (e.g., mating, fighting); also includes areas that control visual and auditory orienting responses

Brain stem
- Connects the brain with the spinal cord
- Controls breathing, heartbeat, consciousness, and muscle tone
- Movement of the eyes and mouth
- Sensory information regarding hot, cold, pain, and hunger
- Body temperature
- Involuntary movement (e.g., sneezing, coughing, vomiting, swallowing)

Cerebellum
- Motor control involving coordination, timing, and automatic behaviors
- Muscle tone

REFERENCE

Lebby, P. C., & Asbell, S. J. (2007). *The source for TBI: Children and adolescents*. East Moline, IL: LinguiSystems, Inc.

4

BRAIN IMAGING TECHNIQUES

For thousands of years, the understanding of brain functioning relied on postmortem in vitro (Latin: in glass) anatomical studies, with retrospective correlation to the person's functioning. Experimentation with live persons increased our understanding of brain–behavior relationships following injury or illness, although this method was eventually seen as inhumane. Neurosurgical procedures, such as those involving electrical brain stimulation while the patient was awake and responding, enabled investigation of cortical influences on behavior. It was not until the 1970s, when brain imaging techniques were introduced, that in vivo (Latin: in living) assessment of brain anatomy and functioning was truly feasible. As with most technological advances, early attempts at imaging the soft tissue of the brain were crude and only viable for substantial injuries or pathological processes. Often, damage or pathological processes involving the brain parenchyma had to be indirectly inferred from the shape of the ventricles, not directly from the appearance of the tissue. Until the development of computed tomography (CT) imaging, in vivo investigation of the brain was limited to identifying the ventricles through pneumoencephalography, the blood vessels via angiography, or the effects of radioactive isotopes on brain tissue.

CT technology advanced rapidly from the 1970s and remains the mainstay of most hospital radiology departments. It has only been during the past couple of decades that magnetic resonance imaging (MRI) technology has become more common in many smaller medical institutions. MRI technology has its roots in nuclear magnetic resonance (NMR) theory, the foundation required to produce an image based on magnetic resonance. NMR dates back to 1937, when Isidor I. Rabi of Columbia University, New York, observed that atomic nuclei both absorb and emit radio frequency (RF) signals when exposed to strong magnetic fields. Rabi ultimately received the Nobel Prize for this work. It was not until the 1970s that NMR techniques were used to image human tissue and produce what is now known as a magnetic resonance image, or MRI.

More recent advances in imaging technology involve the combination of CT or MRI techniques with other assessment tools in order to produce hybrid brain imaging techniques, such as positron emission tomography (PET), single photon emission computed tomography (SPECT), magnetic encephalography (MEG), and magnetic source imaging (MSI). Even within the strictest domains of pure CT or MRI imaging, advances have resulted in hundreds of options and sequences available to the radiologist, with these assessment tools being used for an ever-expanding list of pathological conditions or investigational needs. Advances in brain imaging have been so rapid over the past few years that some of the more advanced techniques are changing yearly or even faster. As an example, only a short time ago, CT scans were considered the gold standard for visualizing blood within the brain. Then gradient echo (GRE) sequences began to be used as the primary scan for visualizing bleeds. Advanced GRE sequences using echo planar algorithms were even more sensitive to blood products. Over the past few years, SWI has proved to be yet more sensitive for showing small bleeds within the brain, especially those caused by diffuse shear injuries. With the increasing strength of magnets used for MRI, pathologies once visible only under a microscope are becoming evident on MRI, leading to new ways to evaluate and treat many conditions.

The guide presented in this chapter will introduce the basic, foundational science behind the most common brain imaging techniques. In addition, as most clinicians continue to rely on basic brain imaging techniques, most of the examples within this guide will be images from more common CT and MRI sequences, available to most clinicians.

IMAGE QUALITY

While the quality of brain images has rapidly improved over the past decade, given the limits of the current technology, most brain images still fall short of the resolution seen in photographic images taken with very basic digital cameras or even cell phone cameras. Brain images have relatively low spatial resolution of approximately 512 × 512 pixels per inch depending on the system used. A resolution of 512 × 512 pixels per inch in a digital camera or digital image scanner is considered extremely low by today's standards. In addition, when compared to photographs, brain images have lower contrast resolution and a smaller dynamic range of sensitivity. They are also much more prone to the effects of noise and artifacts. CT and MRI systems currently record data using voxels, with the data being stored as a series of slices

(CT and 2D MRI), or a full three-dimensional data matrix (3D MRI) of the brain. A *pixel* is a two-dimensional square that contains a grayscale or color value and a *voxel (**volume pixel**)* is a three-dimensional cube that contains a grayscale or color value. During image acquisition and storage, the digital data from a CT or MRI reflects a series of voxel values. During image presentation using two-dimensional graphics displays such as a computer screen, the data is converted to pixel values. As such, it is not uncommon for the terms pixel and voxel to be used interchangeably within the field of brain imaging.

Spatial Resolution

Spatial resolution is the scanner's ability to differentiate between small adjacent features with different voxel values. Spatial resolution of a brain scan is dependent on the sensitivity of the system to detect variations in signal at any particular voxel site while also minimizing noise in the system. Increasing spatial resolution by decreasing the size of the voxels results in less signal at that site. However, noise remains constant across voxels, as it is a function of the hardware. Less signal with the same amount of noise results in a lower signal-to-noise ratio and a degraded image. Low signal-to-noise ratios result in images that appear grainy and have less contrast or spatial resolution due to the random fluctuations of voxel values. Some advances in magnet strength, hardware technology, and software algorithms have improved signal-to-noise ratios for many scanners. Longer acquisition times can also increase the signal-to-noise ratio but have a clinical and practical cost. Unfortunately, simply changing the spatial resolution of an image without increasing the signal strength and decreasing noise will have negative consequences in image quality.

Contrast Resolution

Contrast resolution is determined by how well the scanner can differentiate small changes in grayscale value across an image. A scanner's *contrast resolution* is the ability of the scanner to discriminate two or more anatomical tissues or structures with very similar densities or x-ray absorption profiles (CT) or properties (MRI). Parameters can be set to increase contrast resolution for tissue with similar values, such as brain parenchyma. The trade-off is that the image will have poor resolution for hard tissues such as bone. In general, contrast resolution is dependent on the signal-to-noise ratio, with increasing noise resulting in a decrease in the scanner's ability to differentiate small differences in tissue density. Contrast agents can change image contrast within certain areas of interest. In general, the imaging objectives determine the parameters used to optimize image clarity and contrast within specific anatomic structures, types of tissue, or concentrations of substances such as water, blood, or fat.

Most brain scanners are better at imaging areas of constant value across space and are poor at differentiating borders or edges between adjacent tissues. This is especially true for adjacent tissue with large differences in voxel value, or high-contrast areas. Partial-volume averaging can blur the edges between bone and soft tissue on a brain scan because of the high contrast between these tissues. Partial-volume averaging takes place when two different tissue values fall within the same voxel. The computer averages the values from the two tissues and assigns that value, resulting in that area of the image failing to truly represent either tissue.

Noise

Noise makes an image appear grainy and is caused by the designation of a value to a voxel that does not truly represent the tissue being scanned. With CT, scanning a known substance such as water can give a measure of noise, which is any voxel value greater or less than zero, the standard value for water. With statistical averaging of massive amounts of data derived from small electrical signal fluctuations, it is not expected that all values for water would be zero. However, the degree to which the values vary above or below zero provides a measure of the noise in the system, something manufacturers strive to minimize.

Quality scanning comes down to a compromise between voxel size, time available for acquisition, and minimizing the effects of noise and artifacts. Changing scanning parameters, such as using a high-pass algorithm, can allow for more detailed examination of tissues, such as bone. Using high-pass algorithms has a trade-off and results in reduced contrast resolution for soft tissue such as brain parenchyma. For small areas of bone, targeting or zooming in on that area so that it fills the scanner's field of view can result in higher contrast and spatial resolution for the structure. Targeting of small areas results in less pixels containing multiple tissue types and thus reduces partial-volume averaging and increases the accuracy of the image. This technique is different from just magnifying the area using software, which has no effect on the partial-volume averaging and image quality. In fact, too much magnification can result in a "pixelated" appearance and reduced ability to interpret small areas of contrast difference. Zooming or targeting of tissue at the time of acquisition is like using an optical zoom on a camera, with image quality remaining high. However, post-acquisition magnification is like using a digital zoom on a camera: it magnifies the image by increasing pixel size, but by doing so, reduces image resolution and also increases noise and artifacts.

PEARL With rapid advances in technology, it is important to be flexible with your understanding of brain imaging. *What once was true, may no longer be true.*

Several years ago students were taught, "if the scan you are viewing is in the coronal or sagittal orientation, it must be an MRI; CT scans only produce axial images." As you will discover in this guide, CT scans can now produce images in all three planes— axial, coronal and sagittal—, and even produce three dimensional representations of tissue, so the rule previously taught to students no longer applies.

PERIL Avoid the temptation to rely on neuroimaging information acquired during previous training without updating your understanding over time. Neuroimaging techniques are advancing rapidly, allowing for improved precision and new clinical applications. As technology advances, your role as a clinician should also change. You should familiarize yourself with the newest systems and techniques available to you so that you can provide your patients the most benefit.

WHAT TYPE OF SCAN TO USE?

With all the advances in brain imaging, it would naturally follow that medical centers would use only the most current and advanced techniques available to them. However, each brain imaging method carries both advantages and disadvantages for the clinician. A basic CT scan can be much more valuable and clinically relevant than a more complicated MRI series or very advanced technologies such as magnetoencephalography. In the acute-care setting, especially emergency departments, the safety, speed, and ease of a brain scan can trump all other considerations. Rapid deterioration of mental and neurological status can take place over minutes or even seconds due to brain hemorrhages or diffuse swelling, making the rapid acquisition times of CT more appropriate than longer sessions in an MRI. Uncooperative patients may not be able to stay still long enough for an MRI but long enough to allow rapid CT acquisition, especially with some newer systems that produce clinically useful images in only a second or two. Although most MRI sequences require several minutes of scan time, echo-planar sequences can be performed in less than a second but require longer setup time than for CT, which is problematic in acute emergency situations. CT scanning is often the safest choice in trauma rooms; its use minimizes the potential risk associated with MRI and metallic objects, such as monitoring equipment, IV poles, piercings on or in the body, or implanted metallic devices. In emergency situations, with CT scanning the trauma team and support equipment can be brought into the scanning room, a factor critical for patients with airway compromise. CT scanning is also the preferred choice for the assessment of traumatic fractures, with high resolution of bone possible in two and three dimensions.

MRI is still considered the second choice of imaging in emergency rooms but is rapidly becoming the standard of care for hospitalized patients with more stable medical conditions and for outpatient studies. Non-emergency procedures allow enough time for full screening of the patient for ferromagnetic materials, such as piercings or pacemakers, which is critical for avoiding possible complications within the MRI suite. MRI has the advantage of not requiring exposure to ionizing radiation, something that is a concern in the use of CT, especially in small children and when multiple scans are required. CT has a resolution advantage over MRI for bone, but MRI has a resolution advantage over CT for soft tissue such as brain parenchyma. With the use of high-strength magnets, very fine anatomical details can be visualized on MRI. With MRI having greater sensitivity to detect soft tissues and subtle pathologies, abnormalities

When considering whether or not to scan a patient, it is important to consider the expected yield of the imaging versus the effects of missing a critical medical condition. It is better to scan many patients without positive findings than to not scan one patient who has a life-threatening condition evident only on imaging. For example, in a patient with a head injury producing mild mental status change, a CT may reveal a slow, evolving epidural bleed requiring emergency neurosurgical intervention. Failing to scan this patient may result in herniation and death. However, many other patients with similar symptoms may have normal CT results. Ultimately, it is the physician's decision whether to scan a patient. However, closed-head trauma, or the presentation of deteriorating mental status unexplained by medical history, should precipitate imaging to rule out a critical brain-related condition.

can be determined at an earlier stage of disease progression than with CT. This is especially important when early detection of a pathological process results in a more favorable outcome for the patient. Other conditions in which MRI may show abnormalities not evident on CT include temporal lobe epilepsy, nonhemorrhagic contusions, diffuse axonal injuries, or the early stages of some neurodegenerative conditions.

One obvious advantage of MRI over CT is that many MRI sequences can be acquired in a three-dimensional (3D) matrix, instead of a series of concentric slices as is true with CT. CT scanners produce a series of images by rotating an x-ray source around a head, with a detector located directly across from the source. Because the scanner rotates around the head, only axial or horizontal slices around the axis of rotation are produced directly from the scanner. However, axial CT data can now be reformatted to produce coronal and sagittal slices, although contrast may not be as good as on the source axial image.

Both CT and MRI are capable of producing non-contrast and contrast-enhanced images, although contrast-enhanced MRI has higher resolution than that of CT. MRI has the advantage of being less affected by bone; CT images become degraded by bone artifacts. Thus MRI is the mode of choice when scanning the pituitary within the sella turcica or in the posterior fossa region. As a general rule, soft-tissue conditions that do not enhance are more evident on MRI than on CT because of the increased spatial and contrast resolution. MRI also has the advantage of being more adaptable than CT. MRI can be used to produce standard sequences or for functional imaging (fMRI) or even as a measure of the chemical composition of tissue (magnetic resonance spectroscropy [MRS]).

> The decision of whether to use CT, MRI, or even other modalities such as ultrasound is multifaceted and often depends on factors such as availability, risk versus benefit, the patient's condition, the clinical question, and the financial cost. When you are unsure about the specific type of scan to use, often a quick call to a radiologist is all that is needed to clarify your options and, once the type of scan is determined, which sequences to acquire (non-contrast, contrast, or a specific clinical series). In general, most radiologists would rather be asked about how best to examine a patient using brain imaging than receive an order for a specific type of scan or series that is inappropriate given the clinical condition of the patient or the clinical question.

MRI is often used as a secondary procedure following initial CT evaluation. This is particularly true when initial CT imaging detects a lesion but does not provide enough information to determine the actual pathological process involved.

TYPES OF IMAGING

Brain imaging is generally partitioned into two main groups: static and functional. Within these groups, finer distinctions can be made regarding the type of scan used or the type of sequence applied. However, the classification of brain-scanning techniques as either static or functional produces several problems. The most notable issue relates to scans having features of both static and functional imaging. Such hybrid scans are used to evaluate the consequences of brain processes, not the changes to brain processes caused by a specific activity or "function." Because they are not used to measure the consequences of a specific activity, they are not referred to as "functional" scans. However, because they measure the consequences of activity in the brain, such as diffusion, perfusion, and metabolism, they are not truly static either. This chapter will thus divide brain imaging into three main groups: static, hybrid, and functional. It is important to consider the overlap between these three groups. For example, many techniques within the hybrid category may also be considered static or functional.

Static Brain Imaging

Static brain imaging can best be considered pure anatomical imaging. The images represent the static nature of the tissue being scanned. Although pathological processes such as edema or bleeding influence the appearance of static brain scans, the image is more a snapshot representation of the tissue than a recording of ongoing biological processes.

Ultrasound

Ultrasound is not often associated with brain-based conditions. However, brain ultrasound can be very useful in evaluating ventricular size, especially with ventriculomegaly, or brain atrophy following injury. Ultrasound involves the measurement of the echo profile generated from high-frequency radio signals passing through the brain. Because ultrasound is sensitive to large differences in tissue density, it is used primarily to evaluate ventricular size

Ashley suffered a severe brain injury as a result of nonaccidental trauma, or child abuse. Her injury resulted in an extended hospitalization in an intensive care unit, followed by transfer to the rehabilitation unit for family training. Ashley failed to make gains, and her treatment team became concerned that she might have hydrocephalus. Because she had undergone six previous CT scans, with known cumulative risk of exposure to ionizing radiation, it was decided that ultrasound would be used to evaluate for ventricular dilation. Ultrasound imaging suggested ventricular dilation, with significant cortical atrophy. Follow-up CT images with a similar slice angle and cut location are included here for reference; note the similar appearance between the ultrasound and the CT reference images using the coronal and sagittal planes (Figures 4-1A–D).

To determine whether the ventricular dilation was due to pressure, something that can cause herniation and be life threatening, or diffuse cortical atrophy, comparison was made between her initial CT and a follow-up series performed 4 weeks later. Comparison confirmed widespread encephalomalacia with global atrophy resulting in the hydrocephalus ex vacuo, without pressure effect or imminent risk of herniation (Figures 4-2A–F).

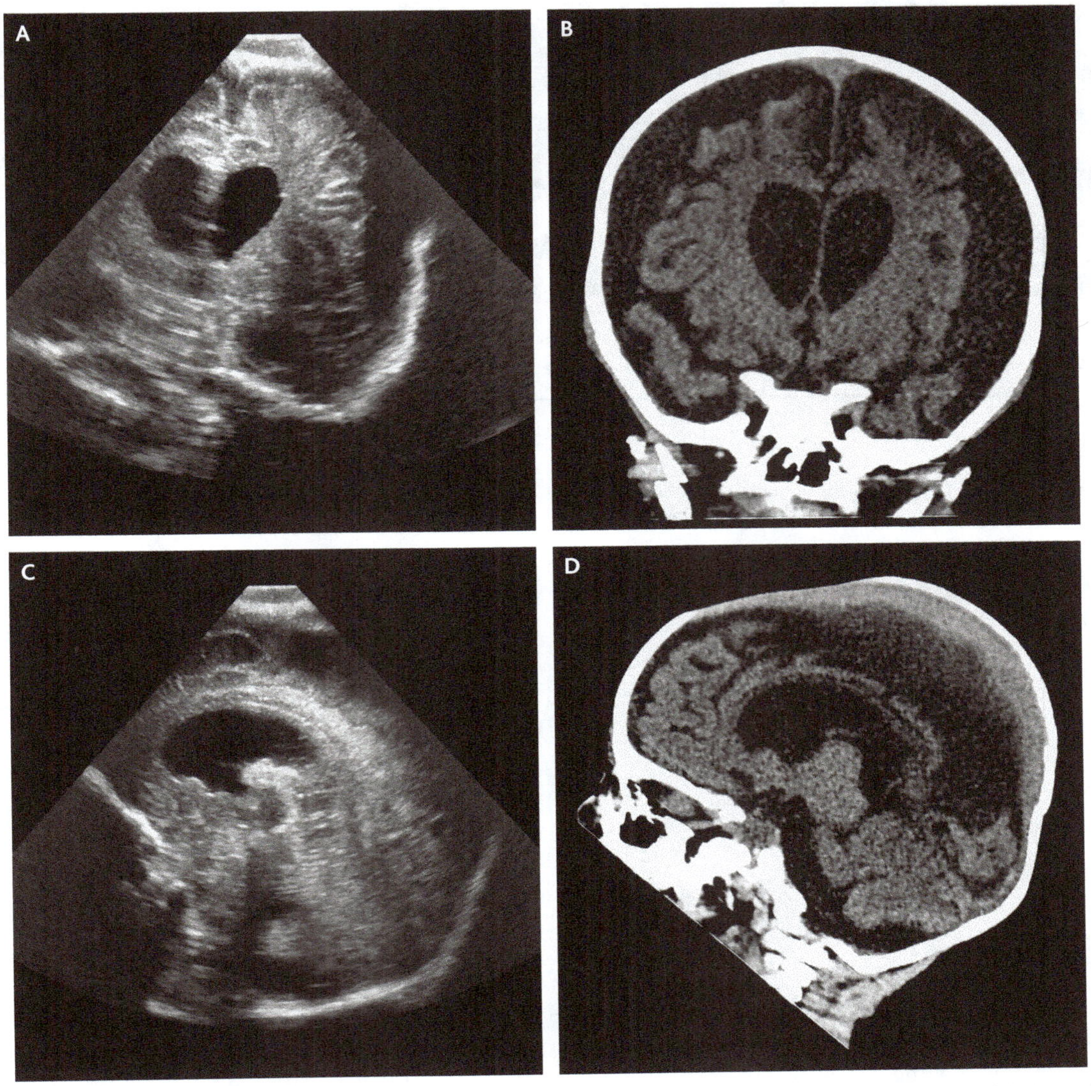

Figures 4-1A–D Clincial example Ashley: nonaccidental trauma, comparison of ultrasound and CT images. **A:** Coronal ultrasound. **B:** Coronal CT. **C:** Sagittal ultrasound. **D:** Sagittal CT

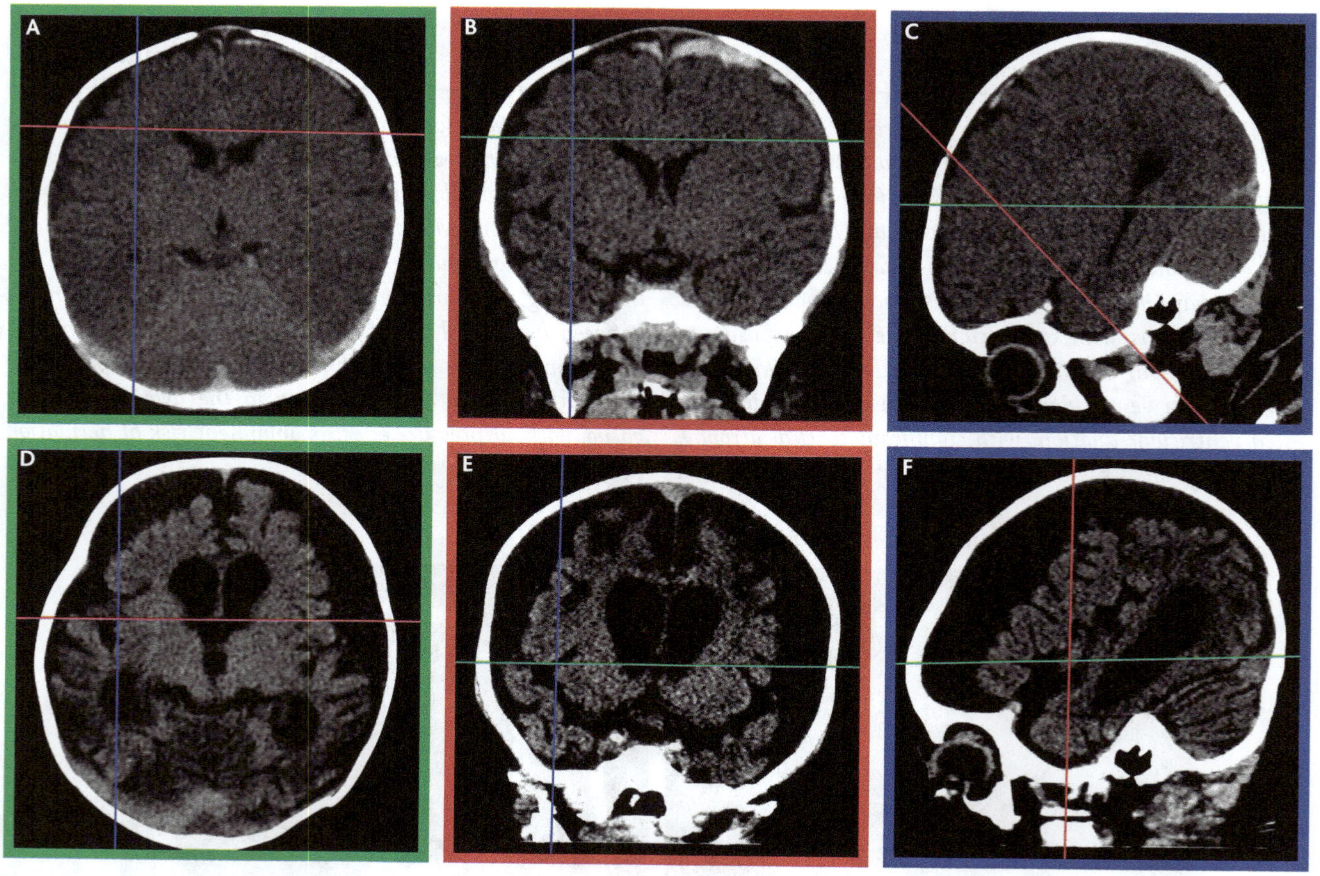

Figures 4-2A–F Clincial example Ashley: nonaccidental trauma, CT series. **A:** Acute-care axial CT. **B:** Acute-care coronal CT. **C:** Acute-care sagittal CT. **D:** Four weeks later: axial CT. **E:** Four weeks later: coronal CT. **F:** Four weeks later: sagittal CT.

when there is concern regarding hydrocephalus and risk of herniation. Ultrasound has an advantage over CT or MRI in that it is highly portable and convenient, especially for patients in the intensive acre unit (ICU) with extensive monitoring or multiple lines. In addition, unlike CT, ultrasound does not expose the patient to ionizing radiation and can be used multiple times without increased risk to the patient.

Computer Axial Tomography (CAT/CT)

The development of CT technology in the 1970s acts as a reminder of how a variety of interests can combine to produce technology previously unavailable. CT came about through the confluence of early radar physics, computer development, digital acquisition and display, x-ray science, and medicine. Having never studied at university, Godfrey Hounsfield developed an aptitude for electrical physics and mathematics while experimenting on his home farm. After a period of time in the Royal Air Force as a radar-mechanics instructor, he began a staff position at Electrical and Musical Instruments (EMI), making notable advances in computer memory, transistors, and pattern recognition. The initial idea for CT came about during a walk in the countryside: he considered if it would be possible to "determine what was in a box by taking readings at all angles through it." He experimented using finely collimated x-ray beams and used his computer and data acquisition background to develop the basics of CT technology. For the first time, CT made the quantification of tissue density within uniform slices possible, with the ability to visualize the densities as gray levels on a television monitor (Isherwood, 2005). In 1979, Sir Godfrey Hounsfield shared with Allan Cormack the Nobel Prize for physiology and medicine for their work on the development of CT technology. The Hounsfield scale is still used today to quantify radiodensities of tissue, with Hounsfield units (HU) being standardized for a variety of substances such as air (–1000), water (0), and dense bone (+1000).

REFERENCE

Isherwood, I. (2005). *Sir Godfrey Hounsfield. Radiology, 234,* 975–976.

At the time of the initial development of the CT scanner, Hounsfield was working for EMI, a company involved in the manufacture of LP music records. The Beatles were recording with EMI at the time, and it is believed that the income generated from the Beatles played a role in financially supporting the ultimate development of CT technology. The first CT scanners were called EMI scanners (Figure 4-3) because Hounsfield developed them while employed at EMI.

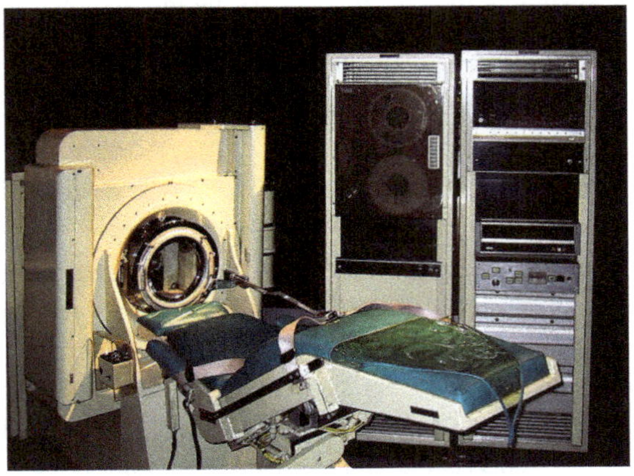

Figure 4-3 EMI scanner developed in 1971 at EMI Research Laboratories, Hayes, Middlesex, England.

Computed tomography, or CT imaging as it is now commonly called, has also been known as computer axial tomography or computer-assisted tomography, both shortened to CAT, and reconstructive tomography, or RT. At its root, a CT scanner is an x-ray machine capable of forming images of three-dimensional tissue as a series of two-dimensional slices. The x-ray tube rotates around the body, with detectors located across from an ionizing radiation source. Either the patient moves through the scanner or the scanner array moves over the patient while the narrow x-ray beam is rotated around the patient to form the thin image slices. The two main types of CT are axial (records concentric slices of tissue, one slice at a time) and helical or spiral, with continuous recording completed in a spiral fashion. All things being equal, helical/spiral CT scans expose the patient to less ionizing radiation than the older axial models. The data from the detectors are processed via computer algorithms to produce grayscale images with the brightness being inversely proportional to the transmission of the x-rays through the tissue.

Because a CT scanner involves the rotation of an x-ray source and detectors around the person's body, until recently, only axial slices were formed in the process. With improvements in computer technology and mathematical algorithms, CT technology is now able to provide images in the axial, coronal, and sagittal planes (Figures 4-4A–C). Sagittal and coronal CT images are produced via computer reconstruction or digital geometry processing, the most common technique being multiplanar reformatted

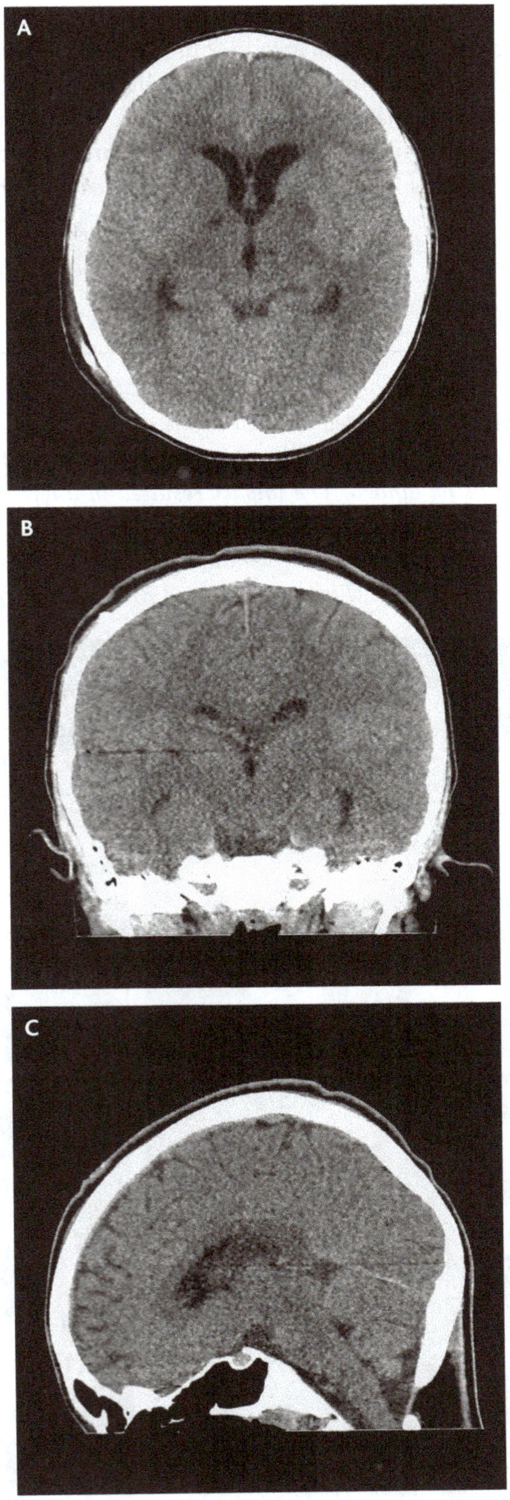

Figures 4-4A–C Examples of 3D multiplanar CT reformatting from the axial source image to coronal and sagittal planes.

imaging. Although the algorithms used in digital geometric processing are complex, the general process is one of taking a series of axial slices of brain tissue, stacking them on top of each other, and then using the reconstructed volume to produce images of varying orientation, usually orthogonal to the axial plane, such as coronal or sagittal. Because of the indirect process required to produce reconstructed images, resolution and clarity of the images are sometimes of poorer quality than that of the source axial images. With advances in technology and updated algorithms, the quality of the coronal and sagittal CT images is improving at a rapid pace and on some sequences matches that of scans obtained directly from the axial plane.

Recent advances in CT technology have also allowed for the reconstruction of tissue into a 3D matrix that can be presented and rotated on a computer screen. The most common methods employed to produce volume-rendered 3D images from single image planes are the maximum-intensity projection (MIP) and the minimum-intensity projection (mIP) techniques. Using predetermined threshold values corresponding to the density of certain types of tissue, such as bone, the image-processing algorithms can produce usable 3D models to be displayed on computer screens.

CLINICAL EXAMPLE

Jose: Skull Fracture with Traumatic Brain Injury

Jose and his friends were riding their skateboards when they became entangled and fell to the ground. Jose was not wearing a helmet and his head hit the corner of his friend's helmet as he landed. The impact resulted in a left parietal skull fracture and underlying injury to his parietal cortex. Jose's injury resulted in a fluent aphasia due to a bleed close to Wernicke's area (Figures 4-5D and E). His skull fracture can be easily visualized on the 3D CT reconstructed MIP images before repair (Figures 4-5A and B) and after repair (Figure 4-5C).

Three-dimensional volume rendering also allows for lateral rotation (Figures 4-6A–D) or vertical flipping (Figures 4-7A–D) of the images on a computer and provides the ability to see both the outside and the inside of cranial surfaces.

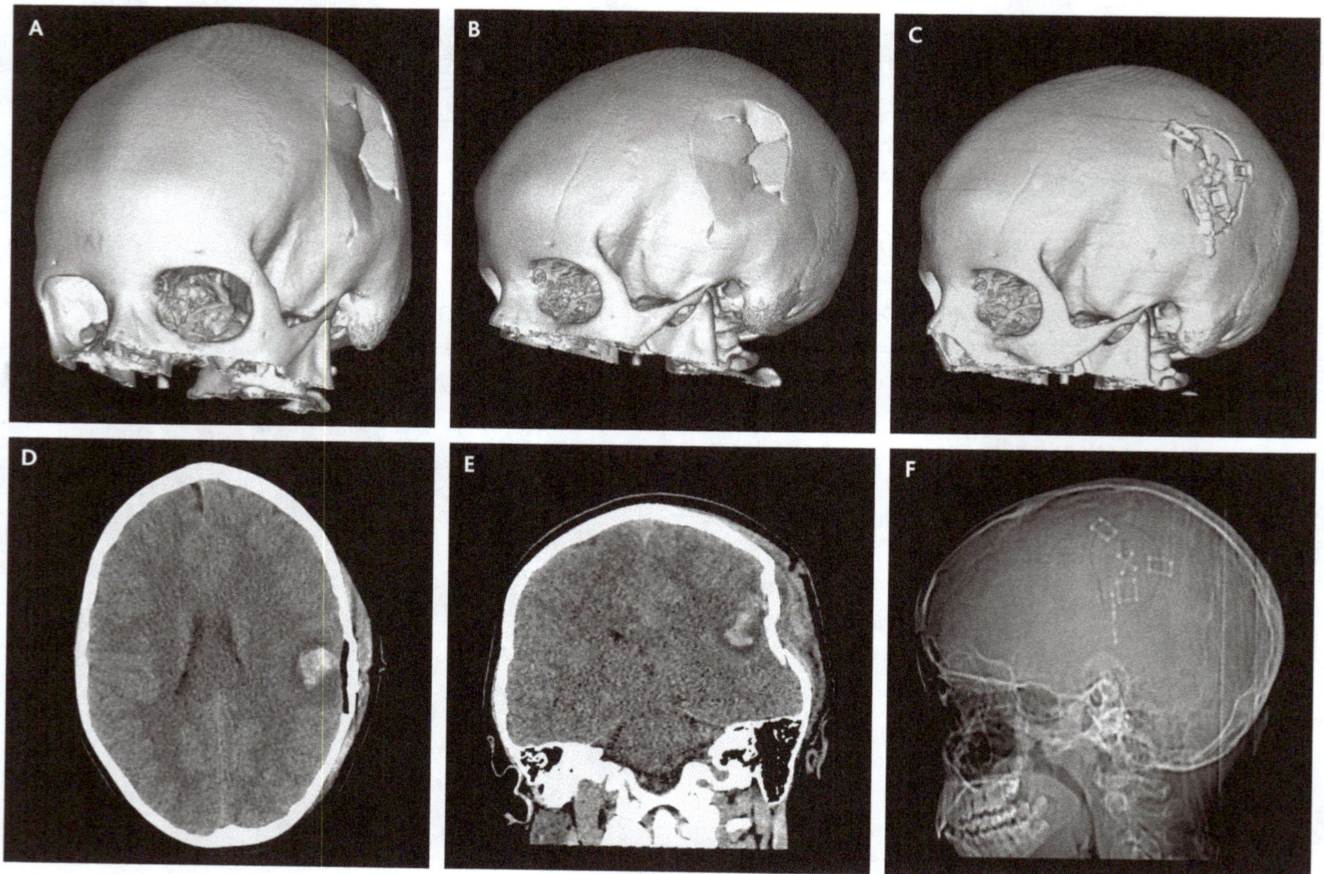

Figures 4-5A–F Clinical example Jose: skull fracture with traumatic brain injury. **A:** Prior to repair. **B:** Prior to repair. **C:** After repair. **D:** CT—axial slice with bleed. **E:** CT—coronal slice with bleed. **F:** CT x-ray after repair.

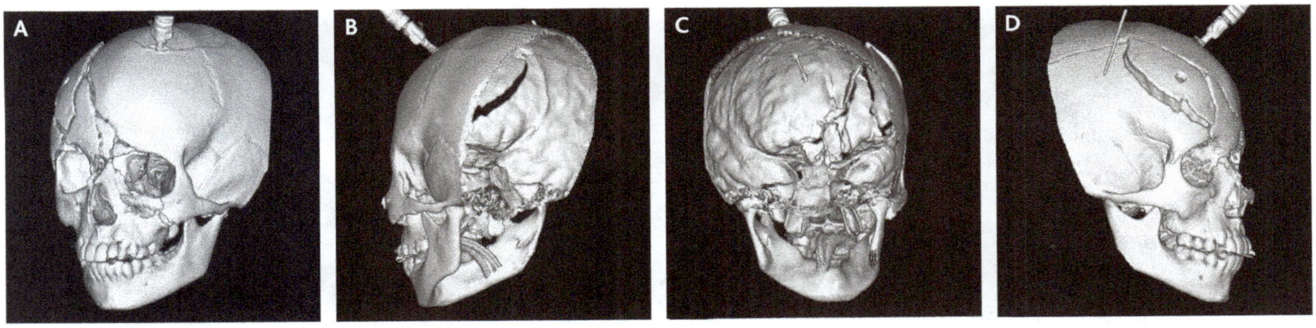

Figures 4-6A–D Three-dimensional volume rendering showing skull fracture: lateral rotation series.

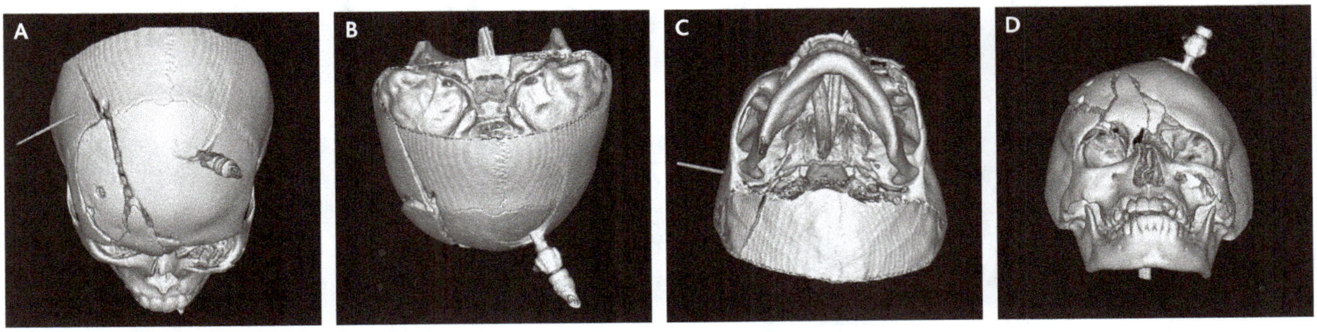

Figures 4-7A–D Three-dimensional volume rendering showing skull fracture: vertical flip series.

Absorption of X-rays

A simple x-ray uses ionizing radiation to produce images of tissue on the basis of absorption properties of the tissue. Dense tissue such as bone that readily absorbs x-rays will appear white or underexposed on a sheet of film. Tissue that is less dense and absorbs less radiation will appear dark or more exposed on a sheet of film. Because CT technology is based on the same concepts as that for simple x-rays, the image produced reflects the absorption profile of the tissue being scanned. The appearance of CT pixels on an image relates to the extent of x-ray absorption for the tissue at that location. The degree to which specific tissues block the transmission of x-rays is relatively constant and is represented by a value called an attenuation coefficient. CT attenuation coefficients are described using the Hounsfield scale, as described earlier.

Because of limitations in the dynamic range of CT scanners, or the range of Hounsfield units that can be captured with high resolution, radiologists can select a particular range of values to study. This allows for a higher degree of contrast variability for that specific tissue. The same difficulties are experienced when using a digital camera. Given the limitations in dynamic range, digital cameras are not able to capture all of the information from very bright to very dark, resulting in pictures that are blown-out on the bright end or clipped on the dark end. CT scanning has similar problems with dynamic range and is unable to fully capture all of the information at the most dense end for bone or the least dense end for water or air, without parts of the image becoming blown-out or clipped. Windowing enables assignment of the full range of grayscale values to a smaller range of tissue, thus allowing for expansion of the contrast spectrum to tissue of similar density. Selecting a range of contrast values for a CT is like choosing a camera's settings for a sunny day or for nighttime shooting: When set for a sunny day, the camera adjusts exposure levels to fit bright to very bright scenes; when set for nighttime, the camera sets exposure levels to capture dark to very dark scenes.

Windowing is often used to assess for fractures of the skull, with the entire grayscale spectrum being assigned to the limited range of density seen in bone. The trade-off with using a bone-window is that the soft tissues of the brain, being outside of the windowed range, will appear dark and have little contrast (Figures 4-8A–C).

On standard windowed CT scans, bone appears brightest, tissue has a medium grayscale level, liquid such as cerebrospinal fluid (CSF) looks dark, and air appears black. Within soft tissue, differences in density are apparent but can be minimal. The most obvious contrast differences in soft tissue involve the gray matter versus the white matter (Figures 4-9A–C). On CT imaging, gray matter appears

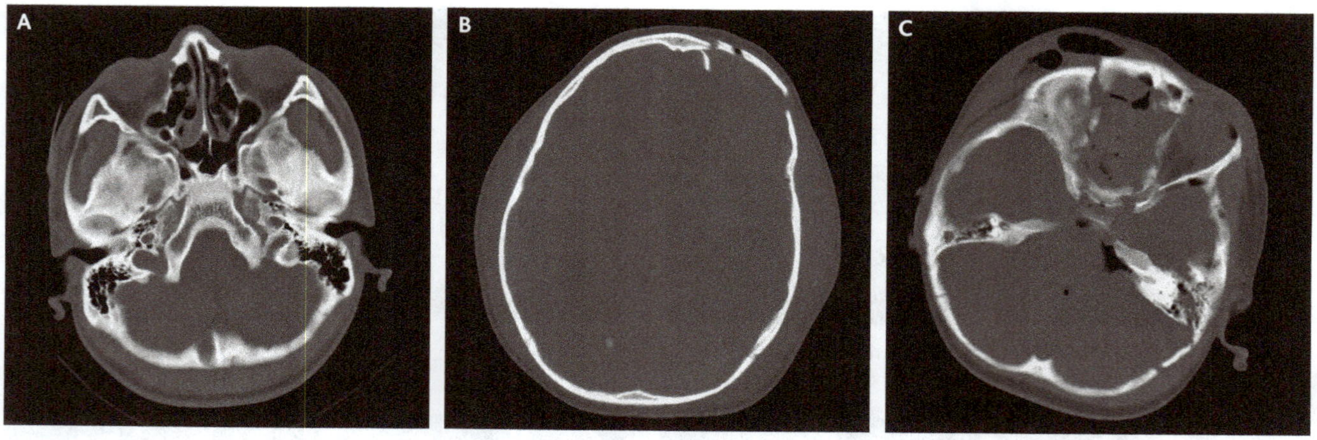

Figures 4-8A–C CT bone windowing. **A:** Normal. **B:** Left frontal fracture. **C:** Right orbital fracture.

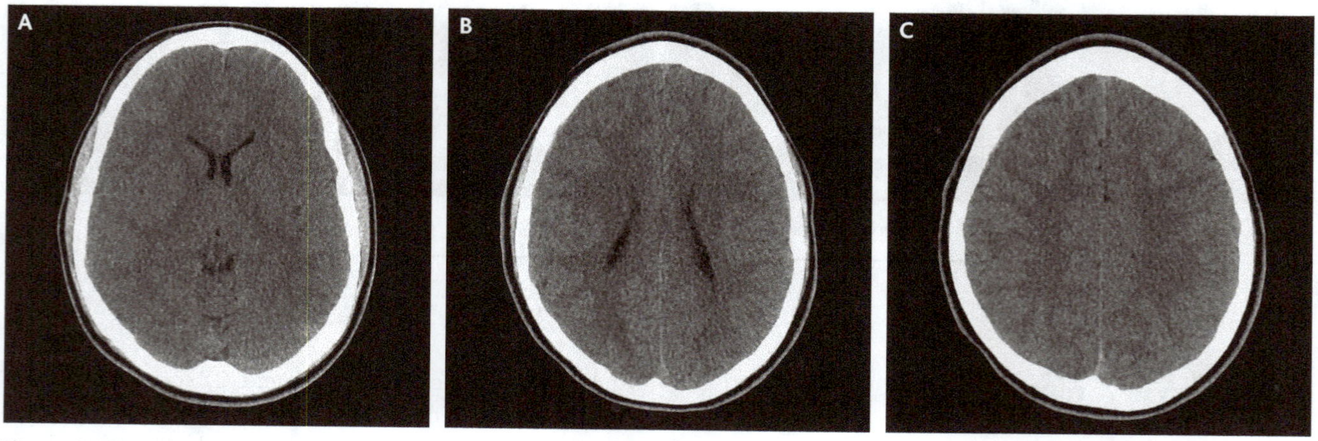

Figures 4-9A–C Standard CT images. Note soft-tissue distinction but little contrast resolution for bone.

slightly lighter than white matter because lipid has radiolucent properties, thus allowing more transmission of x-rays than other brain tissues.

> Radiologists use relative terms such as *hypodense*, *isodense*, or *hyperdense* to describe areas on a CT scan. Because the brightness on a CT image depends on absorption of x-rays and absorption increases with density, hypodense areas look darker, isodense areas have the same grayscale appearance as that of the reference tissue, and hyperdense areas look brighter. For example, swelling may appear hypodense or dark in comparison to normal tissue, as increased fluid reduces overall density. Conversely, areas of calcification may appear hyperdense, or bright, on a CT scan, in comparison to brain tissue. *Isodense* suggests an equivalent density to that of reference tissue—for example, a tumor may be described as isodense to brain parenchyma.

Safety Concerns with CT

Compared to single-plane film x-ray, CT scans use a relatively high amount of ionizing radiation. Repeat scanning, something that takes place quite often in patients with brain trauma, results in a cumulative increase in the patient's exposure to ionizing radiation. Children are at a greater risk for exposure side effects or complications. The risk is increased for children in part because of their smaller physical size, the greater number of cells that are actively dividing, and the greater life expectancy for future ionizing radiation exposure (Brenner et al., 2001; U.S. Food and Drug Administration [FDA], 2001).

The National Research Council's Committee on the Biological Effects of Ionizing Radiation estimates that the effect of radiation exposure on children less than 10 years of age is several times that of middle-aged adults. Even with this increased risk to children, one of the largest increases in CT use has been for diagnostics in pediatric patients (Beir, 1990). The primary reason for the increase in the number of CT scans performed in children relates to the

General Risks of CT

Risks associated with CT relate primarily to the increased lifetime exposure to radiation and the resulting increase in the risk of contracting cancer. Other risks include reddening of the skin, skin tissue damage, hair loss, or, potentially, birth defects to a fetus if high doses of radiation are used (FDA, 2001). The long-term health effects resulting from diagnostic CT imaging remain controversial, with most effects being indirectly related to CT scans. For reference purposes, the average individual is exposed to approximately 1 mSv of ionizing radiation over a period of 120 days, or approximately 3 mSv per year. The Sievert (Sv) is an internationally recognized unit of measurement relating to a dose-equivalency of radiation and is used to quantify the biological effects of ionizing radiation. An estimated average exposure from a single CT is approximately 1.8 to 3.8 mSv for adult protocols and 0.9 to 1.9 mSv for pediatric protocols adjusted for body weight (National Institutes of Health, National Cancer Institute [NIH-NCI], n.d.). In general, the individual cancer risks associated with CT scans remain very small and have been estimated at around 1 in 1000 or even lower (NIH-NCI, n.d.). Additional information regarding diagnostic imaging risks has been published by the health care accrediting agency The Joint Commission (2011).

speed at which the scans can be acquired. With current CT technology being able to produce clinically useful images in about a second, an anesthesiologist is not required to sedate a child for him or her to lie still long enough to allow for adequate image acquisition (Brenner & Hall, 2007).

The transition from film-based x-rays to computerized CT imaging has resulted in a greater chance of missing signs that a patient has been overexposed, especially a small child or adult. When using film to produce x-ray images, overexposure is readily evident as "overexposed," or dark, film. However, CT scans do not use film and the computer makes adjustments to the grayscale contrast following image acquisition. Without the cues to overexposure, it is more difficult to assess for unnecessary exposure to the patient.

To compensate for the smaller size of children in CT scanning, the U.S. Food and Drug Administartion (FDA) recommends adjusting the exposure settings on the basis of body weight in order to reduce exposure to the child. The FDA reports that the individual risk of exposure to ionizing radiation by having a CT scan is far outweighed by the diagnostic utility of such procedures. However, unnecessary exposure to CT-related ionizing radiation should be avoided, especially in children. Because the signal-to-noise ratio or quality of CT images increases with higher doses of ionizing radiation, decisions regarding the necessary image quality versus required exposure become important when using CT technology, especially with children or small adults.

REFERENCES

Beir, V., Committee on the Biological Effects of Ionizing Radiations, Board on Radiation Effects Research, Commission on Life Sciences, National Research Council. (1996). Health effects of exposure to low levels of ionizing radiation. *National Academy Press.*, Washington, DC.

Brenner, D. J., Elliston, C. D., Hall, E. J., & Berdon, W. E. (2001). Estimated risks of radiation-induced fatal cancer from pediatric CT. *American Journal of Roentgenology, 176*, 289–296.

Brenner, D. J., & Hall, E. J. (2007). Computed tomography—an increasing source of radiation exposure. *New England Journal of Medicine, 357*, 2277–2284.

Joint Commission (2011). Radiation risks of diagnostic imaging. The Joint Commission, Sentinel Event Alert Issue 47, August 24, 2011.

National Institutes of Health, National Cancer Institute (n.d.). Radiation Risks and Pediatric Computed Tomography (CT): A Guide for Health Care Providers. Web Page: http://www.cancer.gov/cancertopics/causes/radiation/radiation-risks-pediatric-CT

U.S. Food and Drug Administration (2001, November). Public health notification: Reducing radiation risk from computed tomography for pediatric and small adult patients. http://www.fda.gov/MedicalDevices/Safety/AlertsandNotices/PublicHealthNotifications/ucm062185.htm

Contrast CT Imaging

Contrast agents containing elements having a higher atomic number than that of normal brain tissue are often used during CT scanning in order to increase the contrast between certain substances within the brain. Substances with iodine or barium can be used for contrast CT imaging. Contrast-enhanced CT images are sometimes abbreviated CECT; regular CT images are sometimes abbreviated NECT, for nonenhanced computer tomography.

A primary reason for the use of contrast agents is to assess the integrity of the blood–brain barrier. By using contrast agents that do not normally cross the blood–brain barrier, any disruption to the barrier will be indicated by the appearance of contrast enhancement on a CT image. Some conditions that can disrupt blood–brain barrier integrity include rapidly growing neoplasms, infections or vascular damage. Blood vessels can also be made visible with contrast agents; contrast-enhanced angiography is discussed later in the chapter.

Measures to Minimize CT Radiation Exposure

1. Follow guidelines from the Imaging Gently Campaign and As Low As Reasonably Achievable (ALARA) Campaign.
2. Minimize unnecessary examinations through communication between the ordering physician and radiologist as to the appropriateness of the procedure for the specific condition or question.
3. When appropriate, use alternative diagnostic methods that do not use ionizing radiation, such as ultrasound or MRI.
4. Adjust exposure parameters on the basis of the patient's size, especially for small children or adults.
5. Limit the area of body scanned to the smallest possible region.
6. Determine the lowest resolution that will be clinically useful. Often, lower resolution scans are adequate, for example, when doing serial assessments of ventricular size.
7. Avoid multiple scans when not clinically necessary. Sometimes, patients receive multiple scans as they pass through a medical institution or from one medical center to another. Redundant scans may be ordered because previous scans taken at another institution are not available. With the current ability to readily transmitt CT scans via electronic means or store them on computer disks or external drives, the need for rescanning should be discouraged in lieu of obtaining the previous images.
8. Update CT scanning equipment to use systems with automatic exposure-control options, and more advanced technologies that requires less exposure to produce clinically useful images.

Contrast versus Non-Contrast CT Study

Indications for iodinated contrast-enhanced CT (CECT) examinations include the following:

- Neoplasms
- Inflammation
- Demyelination
- Infection
- Vascular conditions and malformations
- Used only when there is potential to increase diagnostic utility of an imaging examination

Indications for nonenhanced CT (NECT) examinations include the following:

- Anatomical abnormality or injury
- Bony abnormality or injury
- Refractory headache
- Suspected stroke or bleeding
- Seizures, especially partial
- Traumatic head injury (open- or closed-head injury)
- Unexplained mental status change

Computed tomography angiography/ venography (CTA/CTV)

Relying on an intact blood–brain barrier, the introduction of a contrast agent into the vascular system can allow for two and three-dimensional images of blood vessels. Contrast-enhanced CT images of the blood vessels are possible using computed tomography angiography (CTA). In CTA, rapid CT acquisition techniques are combined with the synchronized administration of a contrast agent into the blood vessels of the brain. Rapid scanning techniques are required, as the data acquisition often takes place during the first pass of the contrast bolus. CTA can produce both arteriograms and venograms, depending on when the image is acquired relative to the flow of the contrast agent. CTA is less invasive than traditional angiography and has notable diagnostic advantages. CTA is considered more sensitive for aneurysm detection than standard two-dimensional digital subtraction angiography (DSA) (Villablanca et al., 2002) and approximately equal to that of 3D-DSA, without the same degree of patient discomfort or risk of complications.

Even though DSA has higher contrast resolution than that of CTA, the three-dimensional nature of CTA has an advantage of providing views not possible with DSA. CTA is also considered superior to 3D time-of-flight (TOF) MRI sequences for the visualization of aneurysms, although the difference between the two modalities is small. Additional advantages of helical CTA include the speed at which it can be performed—less than a minute—and its relatively low cost, compared to that of traditional angiographic procedures. Disadvantages of CTA are that it is not yet able to reliably visualize very small vessels and the procedure subjects patients to ionizing radiation.

REFERENCE

Villablanca, J. P., Jahan, R., Hooshi, P., Lim, S., Duckwiler, G., Patel, A., Sayre, J., et al. (2002). Detection and characterization of very small cerebral aneurysms by using 2D and 3D helical CT angiography. *American Journal of Neuroradiology, 23,* 1187–1198.

NECT versus CECT of a Neoplasm

The CT scans in Figure 4-10 show a neoplasm within the left parietal lobe, without contrast (Figure 4-10A) and with contrast (Figure 4-10B) indicating slight enhancement within the mass. Other areas on the CECT enhance and include the choroid plexus within the lateral ventricles and some of the smaller vessels within the cortex. There are some small spots of hyperdensity shown on the NECT within the posterior horns of the lateral ventricles; this is from blood within the choroid plexus, which often appears bright on CT even without contrast enhancement. The edema surrounding the tumor is shown as a darker hypodense region on both the NECT and CECT images.

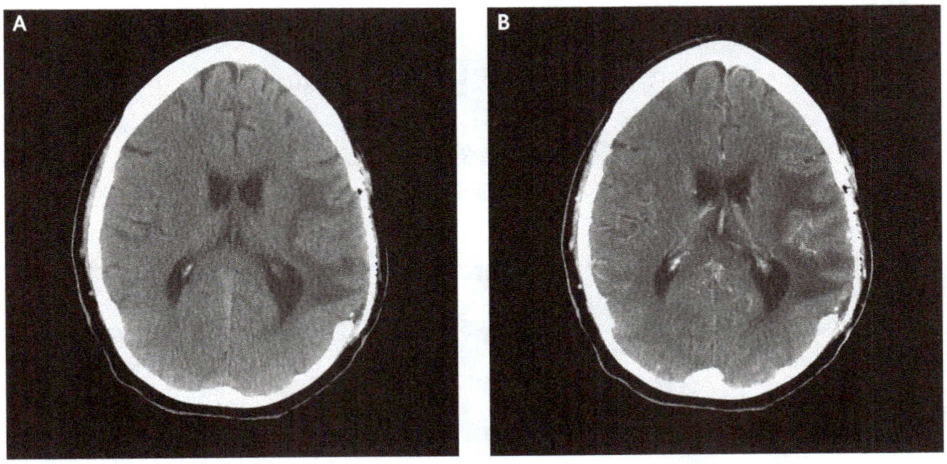

Figure 4-10 A: NECT of neoplasm within the left parietal lobe. **B:** CECT of neoplasm within the left parietal lobe.

CTA images can be presented in a standard two-dimensional axial plane (Figure 4-11A), reformatted to coronal or sagittal planes (Figures 4-11B and 4-11C), or presented as three-dimensional images via MIP/mIP volume rendering (Figures 4-12A–D).

Computed tomography ventriculography/cisternography

CT ventriculograms and cisternagrams are produced by injecting radio-opaque contrast agents into the ventricular system or arachnoid cisterns of the brain via a catheter. If an external ventricular drain is already in place, this can be used to introduce the contrast into the brain without having to place another catheter. Ventriculograms (Figures 4-13A and B) and cisternagrams are helpful in monitoring the flow of CSF through the ventricles or cisterns and can provide information regarding either blockage or a leak.

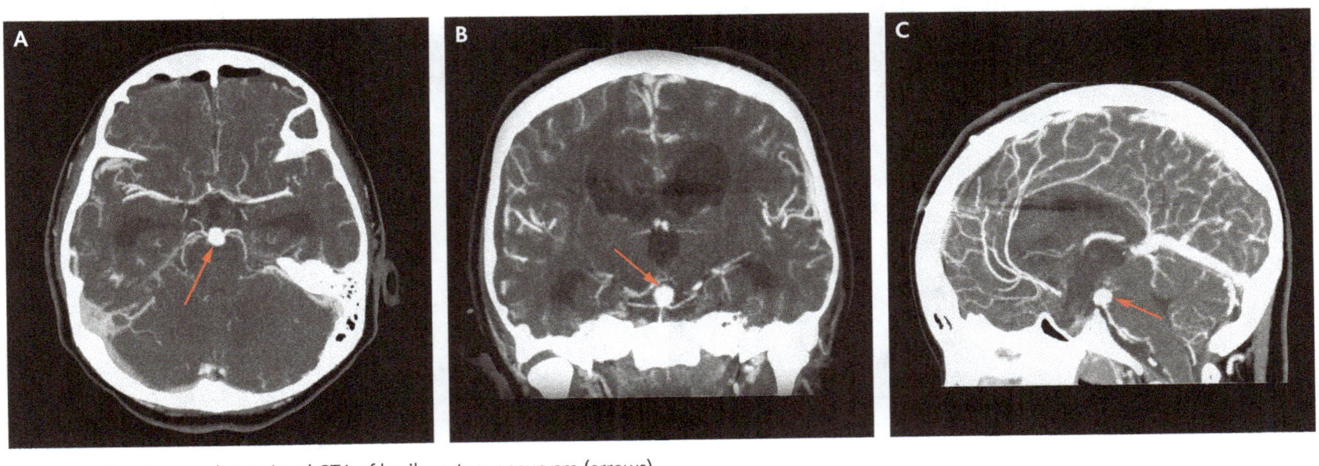

Figures 4-11A–C Two-dimensional CTA of basilar artery aneurysm (arrows).

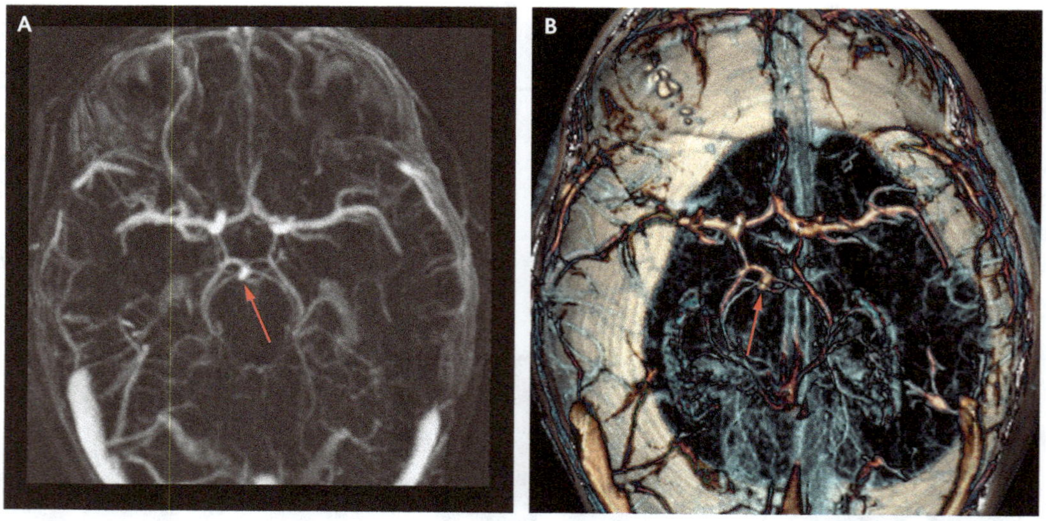

Figures 4-12A and B Three-dimensional CTA of basilar artery aneurysm in black and white and in color (arrows).

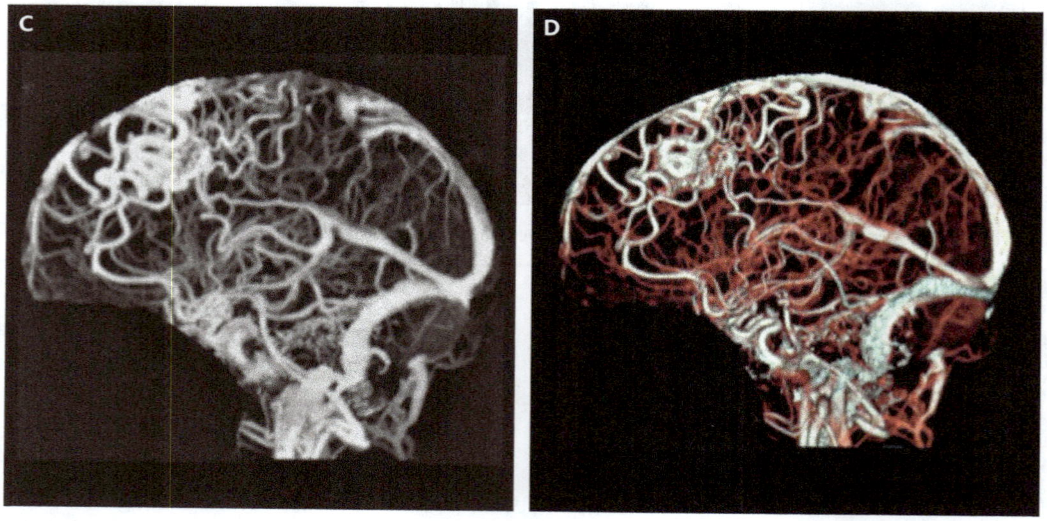

Figures 4-12C and D Three-dimensional CTA rendering of an arterial–venous malformation (AVM) in black and white and in color.

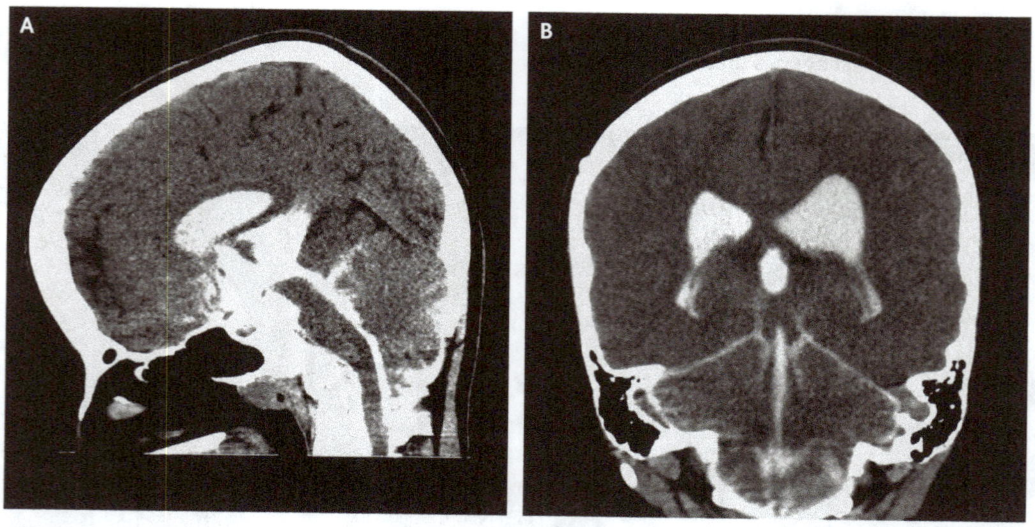

Figures 4-13A and B Ventriculograms showing normal flow of CSF through the lateral ventricles, third ventricle, cerebral aqueduct of Sylvius, and fourth ventricle. Note white contrast agent present within all of the ventricular cavities and cerebral aqueduct.

Andrea was diagnosed with fungal meningitis, resulting in significant inflammation of the arachnoid layer. During her illness, the viscosity of her CSF increased until it had the consistency of syrup. The combination of the viscous CSF and arachnoid inflammation resulted in a lack of CSF flow from the third ventricle down the cerebral aqueduct to the fourth ventricle (Figures 4-14A–D).

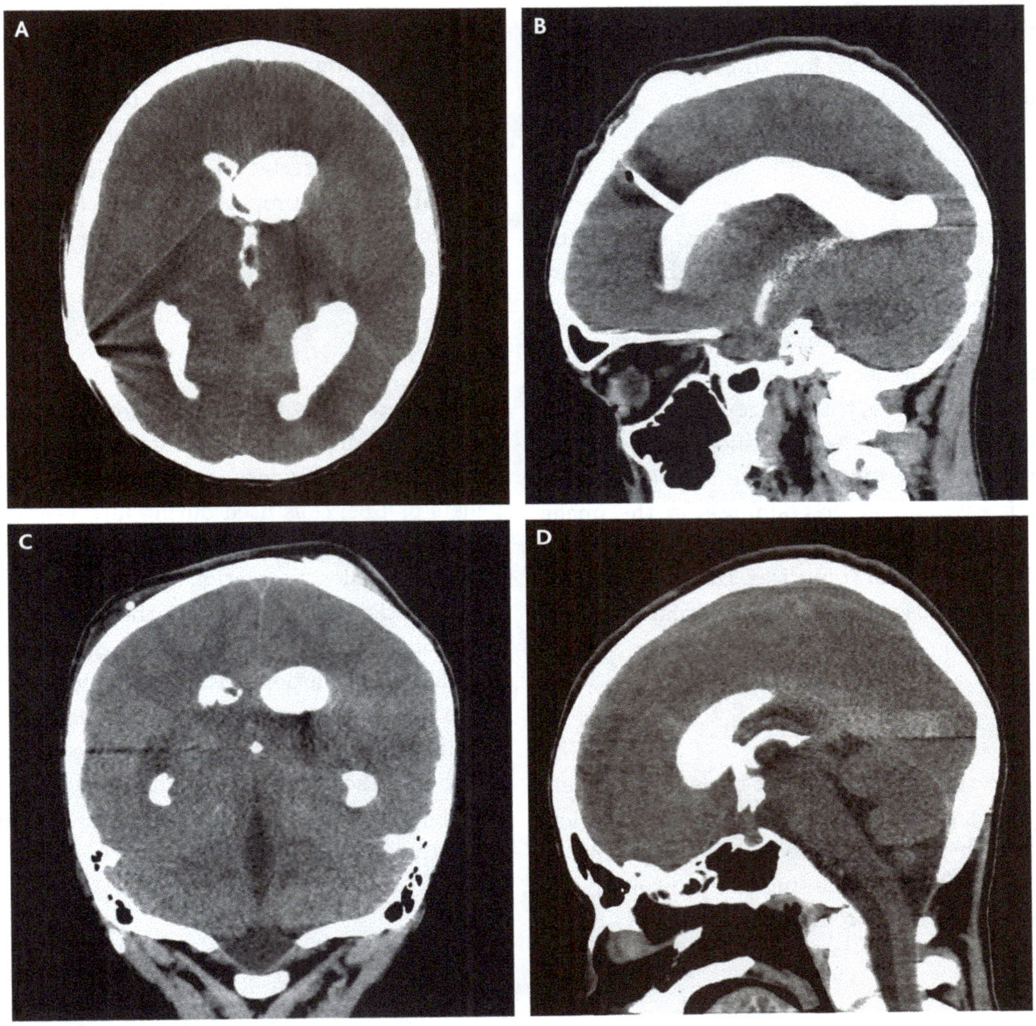

Figures 4-14A–D Clinical example Andrea: fungal meningitis. The dye can be seen in the right and left lateral ventricles, third ventricle, posterior (occipital) horns, and inferior (temporal) horns of the lateral ventricles (4-14a and 4-14b). However, no CSF is flowing through the cerebral aqueduct to the fourth ventricle or the subarachnoid cisterns (4-14c and 4-14d).

CT perfusion studies

CT perfusion sequences are used to assess a variety of hemodynamic properties of brain tissue. A contrast agent is injected at a rate of approximately 5–8 mL/sec, with an image set acquired approximately once per second for approximately 40 seconds. As the contrast agent passes through the vascular system, a variety of parameters are recorded on the basis of transient signal changes correlated with the flow of the contrast agent. For each voxel, in each brain slice (5–10 mm thick) the following data can be obtained:

- **Time to peak** (TTP), or the time it takes until maximum signal attenuation occurs
- **Mean transit time** (MTT), or the time it takes for the contrast bolus to pass from the arterial vessels to the venous vessels. MTT is measured from the first detection of the contrast to the time of maximum attenuation.

- **Relative cerebral blood volume** (rCBV), calculated on the basis of mathematical algorithms
- **Relative cerebral blood flow** (rCBF), calculated by dividing rCBV by MTT

CT Noise

CT imaging techniques are prone to noise, which reduces the spatial and contrast resolution of the generated image. CT-based noise can be classified into three primary groups, discussed below.

Quantum noise

Quantum noise results from too few photons reaching the detectors to allow a clear signal above the inherent noise. Any barrier between the source of ionizing radiation and the detectors can result in quantum noise. Barriers can be due to physical tissue, objects within the tissue, normal scatter of ionizing radiation, thin image-slice thickness, or even small voxel size. When the slice thickness is reduced, fewer photons are concentrated on the area of interest, resulting in increased noise or graininess in the image. Increasing the number of photons delivered to the tissue can counteract the effects of thin slices. However, this also increases the patient dose, which should be minimized if at all possible.

Electronic noise

Electronic noise results from variations in electrical current from the receptors, power fluctuations during acquisition, vibration in the physical structure of the equipment, or other factors that affect the recording and transmission of millions of data values to the computer.

Computational noise

Computational noise is derived from the statistical averaging, manipulation, and mathematical processing of the millions of data points and voxel values. The data must be rapidly processed and interpolated by reconstruction algorithms to form the final image sequences. As a general rule, the greater the required interpolation and mathematical manipulation of the data, the greater the chance of error (noise) being introduced into the system and resulting in image degradation.

CT Artifacts

An *artifact* is any graphical addition, omission, distortion, or error resulting from the scanning technique and unrelated to the tissue being imaged. Artifacts may be confused with pathology, obscure anatomical structures, or modify the appearance of tissue on an image. There are many reasons for artifacts being produced during the scanning process. The most common reasons for artifacts appearing on a CT scan are that metallic objects were scanned or the patient moved during image acquisition. Metallic objects are the most common cause of streak artifacts. Movement during image acquisition, while a relatively common cause of artifacts, is becoming less of an issue, with advances in technology and reduced time required for acquisition. Artifacts can also result from a close interface between tissues with different x-ray absorption properties or densities, causing linear streaks, blurring of the tissue margins, or distortion of the image.

Metallic artifacts

The most common CT artifacts are linear, radiating lines resulting from the presence of metallic objects, such as braces, filling, or bridges around teeth; bullet fragments or pellets or BBs; coils used during interventional radiology procedures; or external devices such as ventricular drains or shunts, halos or fixation devices that stabilize spinal cord or facial injuries. The appearance of metallic artifacts is one of radiating lines emanating from the metallic object, with loss of resolution close to the object. Metallic objects cause streaks because of their x-ray absorption properties attenuating the signal to a greater degree than the dynamic range of the scanner. The attenuation value is greater than the highest value assigned for the scanner, which is usually set to that of cortical bone.

CLINICAL EXAMPLE

Alejandro: Traumatic Brain Injury with Left Carotid Stroke

Alejandro was crushed under a large crate that fell from a warehouse rack. Not only did he suffer severe traumatic brain injury from the physical forces acting on his brain, but he also sustained numerous skull fractures (Figures 4-15A–C show fractures after repair). His injury was so severe that it resulted in damage to his left carotid artery, requiring it to be embolized with metallic coils. The coils produced notable linear artifacts evident on three-dimensional CT vessel reconstruction (Figures 4-16A and B), two-dimensional CT (Figures 4-17A–C) and three-dimensional CT bone reconstruction showing the internal structures of the skull (Figures 4-17D–F).

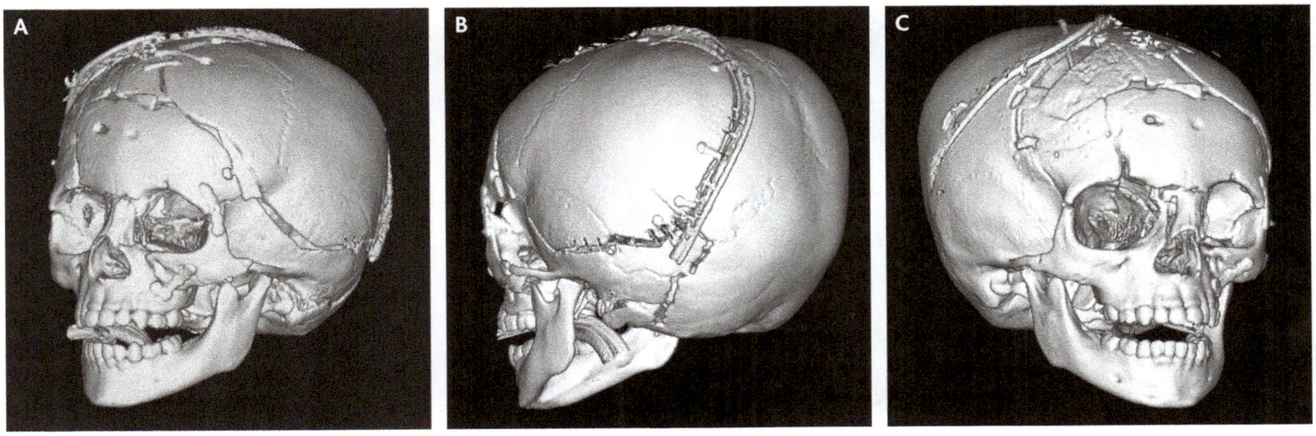

Figures 4-15A–C Alejandro's skull fractures after repair.

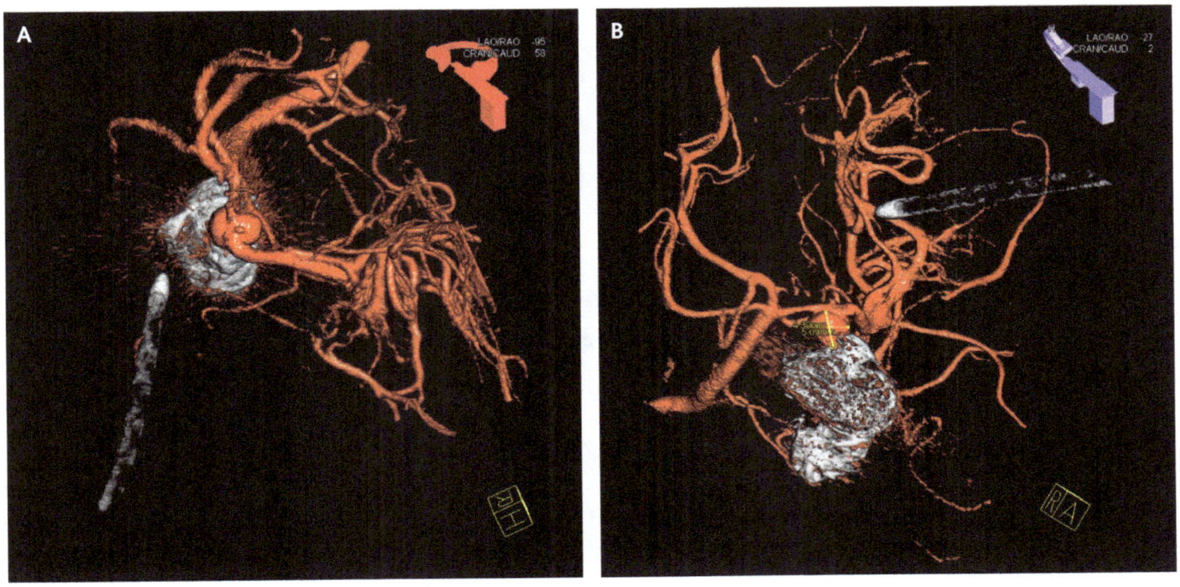

Figures 4-16A and B Vascular coiling, which resulted in the image artifacts (silver areas).

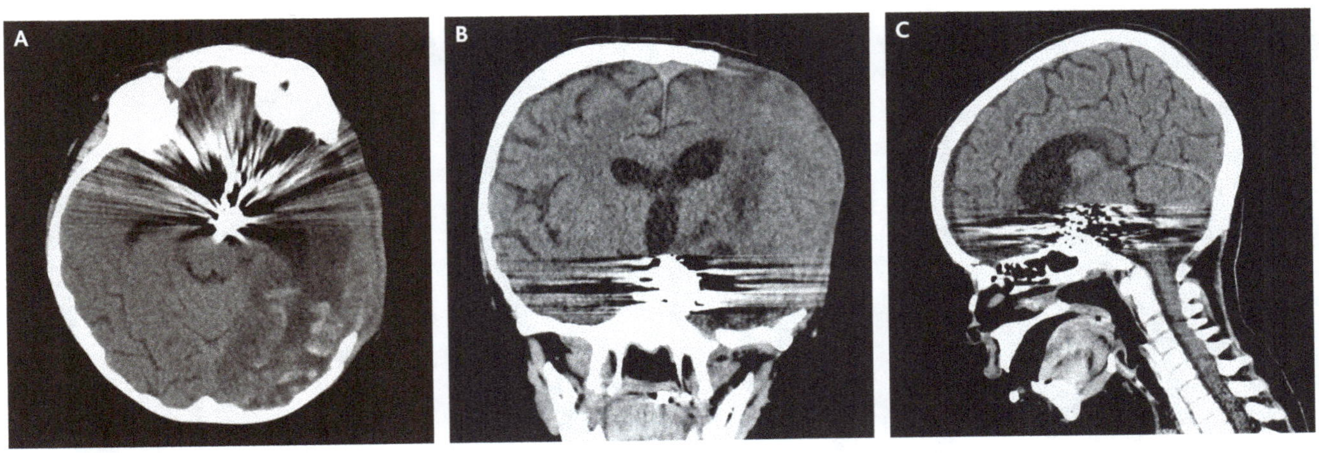

Figures 4-17A–C Two-dimensional CT images showing metallic artifacts from coiling.

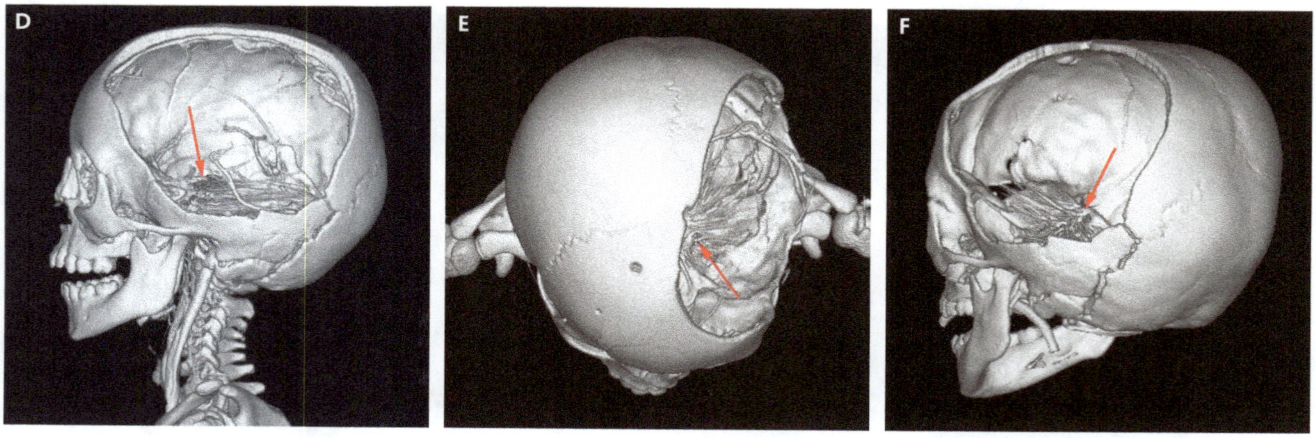

Figures 4-17D–F Three-dimensional MIP CT images with metallic artifacts (arrows).

Metallic objects outside of the brain and skull can also result in artifacts. This situation is common with devices such as external ventricular drains, intracranial pressure bolts, and shunts (Figures 4-18A–C).

Streak artifacts

Streak artifacts can be caused by motion, substances that fall outside the scanner's field, and borders between hard and soft tissues.

Motion of the patient or the machine during image acquisition results in the mathematical algorithms failing to reconcile inconsistencies in voxel value over location and time. When a grayscale value at a specific voxel location is not consistent over time, the computer is unable to allocate a specific value to the voxel and the reconstructed image will have linear or curved "movement" artifacts at that location. With more rapid acquisition times, motion artifacts are becoming less of a concern, although even small amounts of motion can cause streaks to occur on slices that transect both brain and bone tissue.

Streaks can also be produced by tissue that falls outside the scanner's field of view, with the extra tissue absorbing the x-ray energy before it reaches the tissue of interest. This is less of a concern for brain imaging as it is for full-body scans, as the head and brain rarely fall outside of the field of view.

Tissue borders can also cause streak artifacts when there is a large difference between the absorption properties of the tissues (Figures 4-19A–C). This is most evident when hard tissue is located between the x-ray beam and the soft tissue being scanned. The term *beam hardening* is used to describe the effects of dense tissue absorbing low-energy photons, thus leaving mostly high-energy photons to be recorded by the detectors. When a hardened beam travels across less-dense tissue such as brain parenchyma, a streak artifact can form across the image.

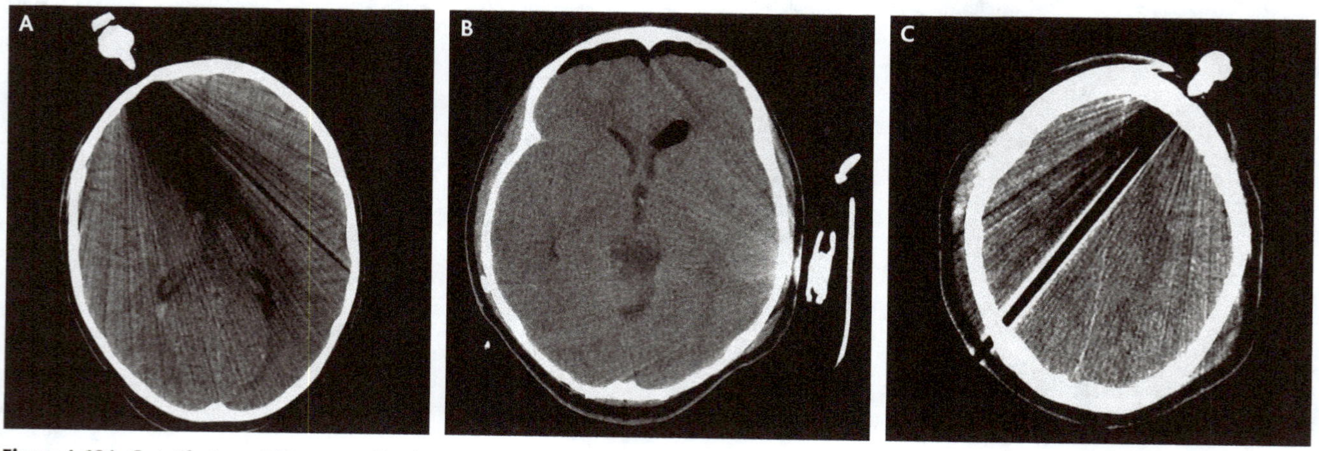

Figure 4-18A–C Artifacts on CT from metallic objects outside of the brain and skull.

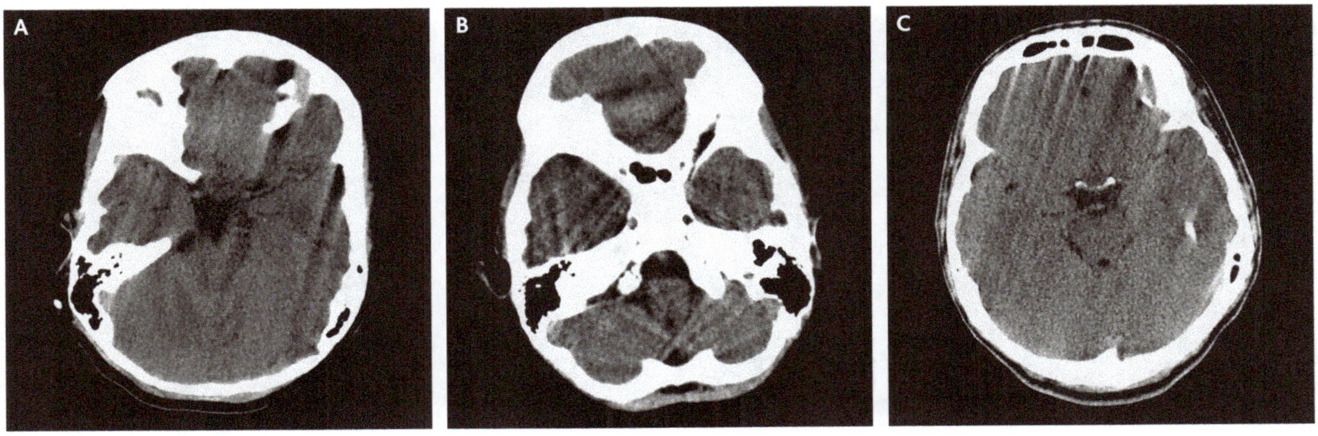

Figures 4-19A–C Examples of streak artifacts.

Angiography/Digital Subtraction Angiography (DSA)

Angiography falls partway between traditional film x-ray and CT scanning. Computers are used instead of film, and a series of images are captured over a short period of time (1–6 frames per second). Blood vessels are highlighted through the use of radio-opaque contrast agents injected via a transfemoral catheter. Traditional angiography produces images that contain the contrast-enhanced blood vessels in addition to other tissue and objects such as bone or EEG electrodes. DSA is a computer-adjusted angiographic sequence with only the blood vessels visible. In DSA, distracting visual images are removed on the screen by first making a mask image before contrast injection and then subtracting the mask from the final image of the vessels under contrast injection.

The grayscale contrast on the image is determined by the degree to which x-rays are absorbed. Traditional angiography produces a series of images in "AP" view, or looking through the head from anterior to posterior, or a lateral view, with the head facing the side. Oblique views that fall between AP and lateral are also useful for visualizing certain vessels.

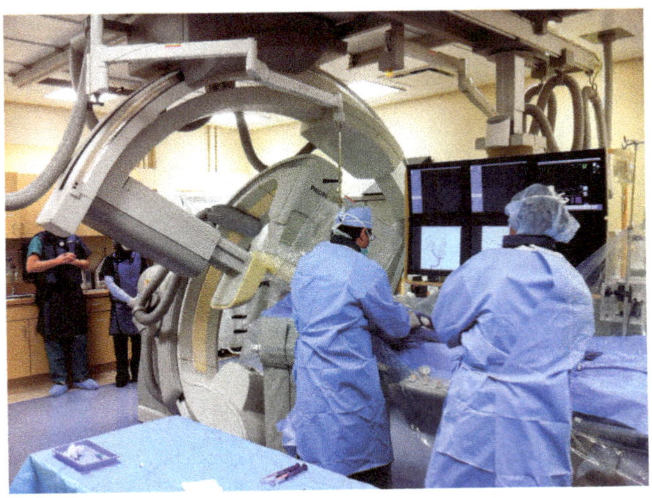

Figure 4-20 Biplane angiography system with two rotating frames.

With current biplane angiography systems, the x-ray source and sensors are located on two half-circle rotating frames, allowing for the acquisition of any image angle by the radiologist (Figure 4-20).

Phases of Angiography

Angiography has the advantage over many other imaging techniques of being able to visualize all stages of blood flow through the brain. Although blood flow is continuous, it is generally divided into seven distinct stages: the first three are arterial, the last three are venous, and the middle stage is capillary (Figures 4-21A–G and 4-22A–G).

Angiography can be performed via the internal carotid arteries (Figures 4-23A–C) or via the vertebral–basilar supply (Figures 4-24A and B).

Prior to the advances in CT and MRI angiography, standard angiography was the method of choice for visualizing vascular malformations in the brain (Figures 4-25A–D). Even with CT and MRI sequences that show blood vessels in two or three dimensions, vascular angiography remains highly useful to the clinician. An advantage of angiography over CT or MRI is that an interventional radiologist or vascular neurologist can treat many conditions via the catheter and without opening the cranial vault, as is necessary with standard neurosurgical procedures.

Three-Dimensional Angiography

Three-dimensional angiography is becoming more common and involves the acquisition of angiography images from around the head, combined with three-dimensional computer reconstruction (Figures 4-26A–E).

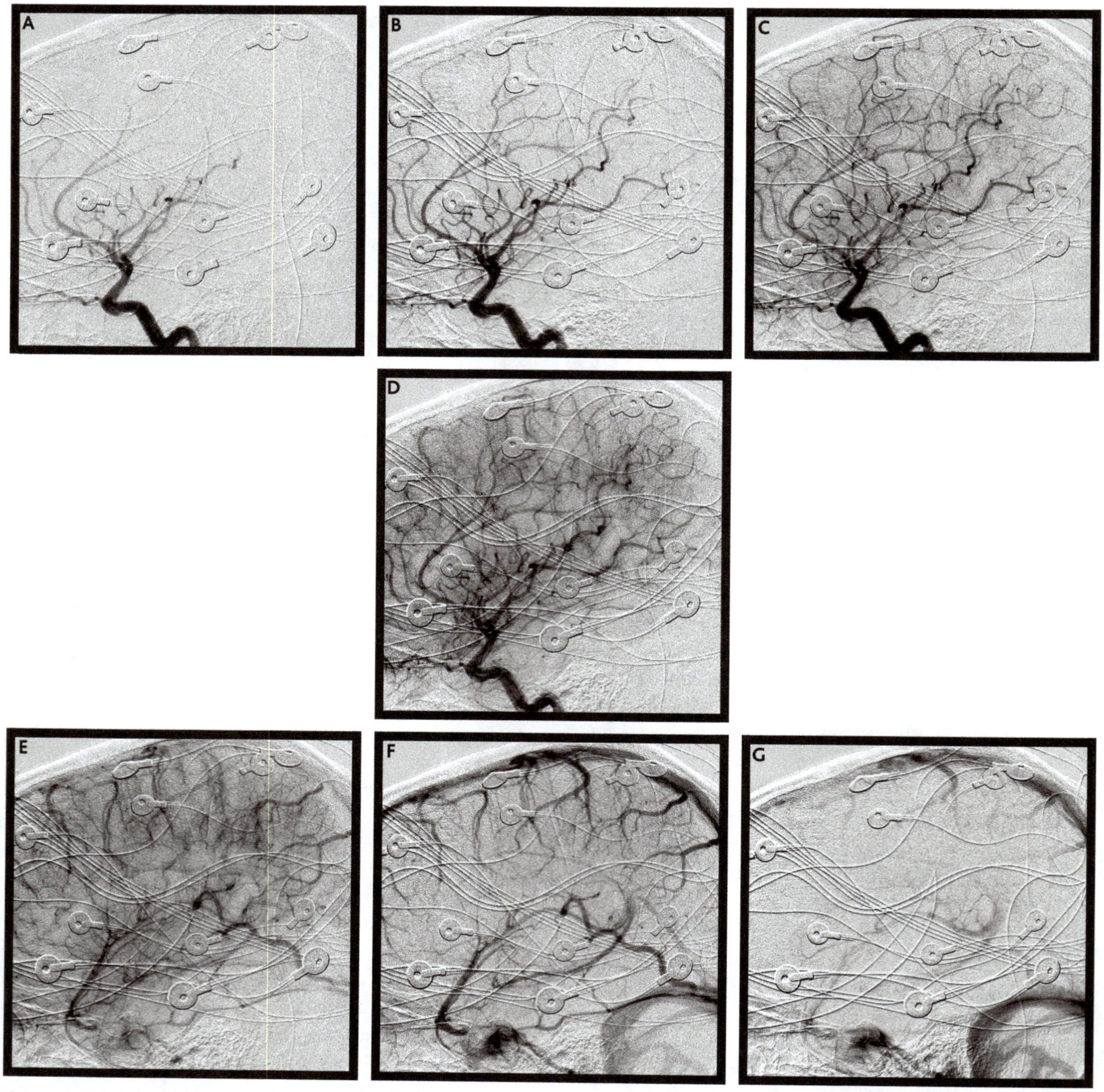

Figures 4-21A–G Phases of angiography: Lateral view. **A:** Early arterial. **B:** Mid-arterial. **C:** Late arterial. **D:** Capillary. **E:** Early venous. **F:** Mid-venous. **G:** Late venous.

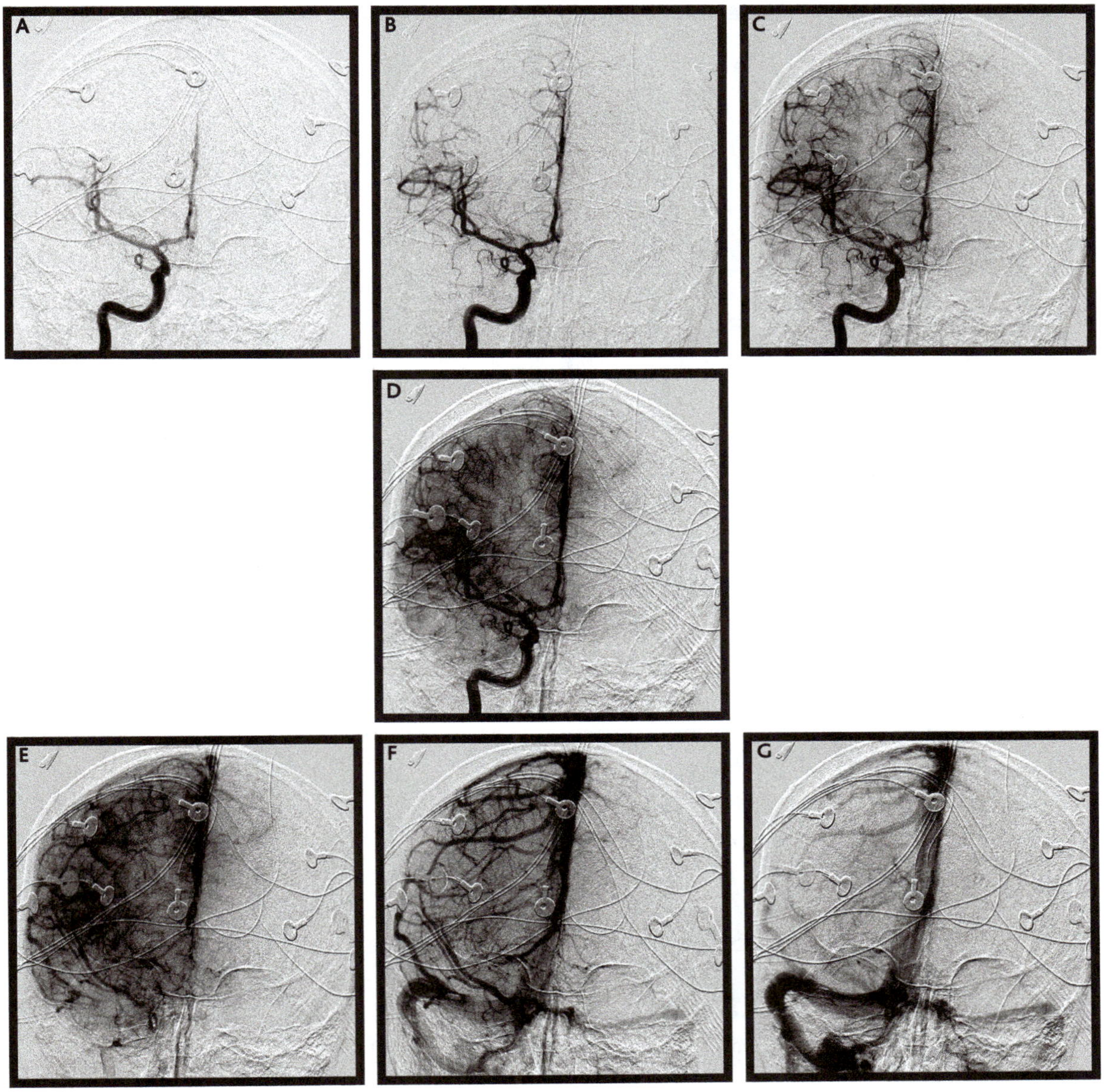

Figures 4-22A–G Phases of Angiography: Anterior–posterior (AP) view—right hemisphere injection. **A:** Early arterial. **B:** Mid-arterial. **C:** Late arterial. **D:** Capillary. **E:** Early venous. **F:** Mid-venous. **G:** Late venous.

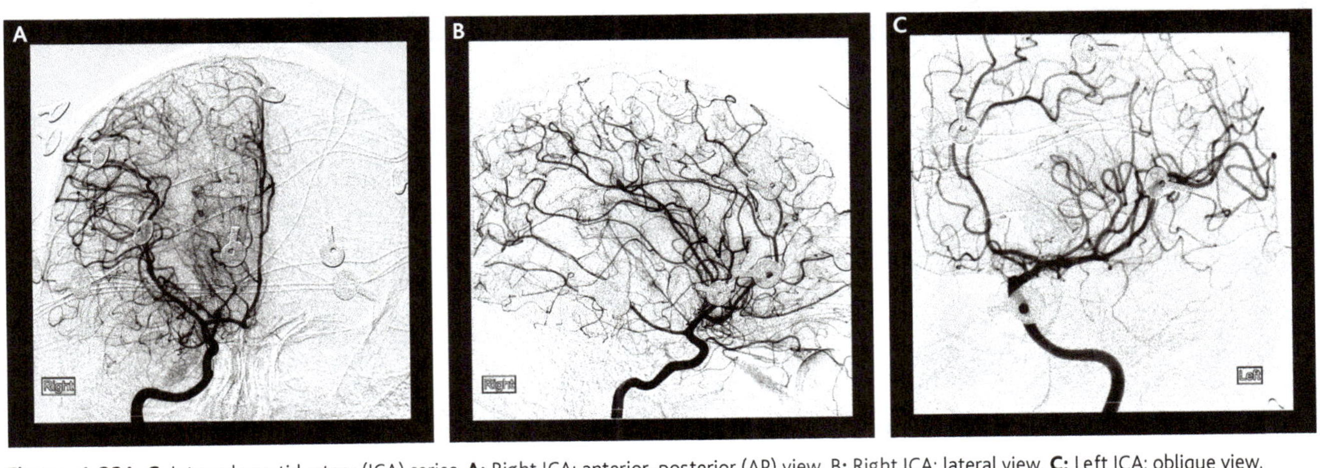

Figures 4-23A–C Internal carotid artery (ICA) series. **A:** Right ICA: anterior–posterior (AP) view. B: Right ICA: lateral view. **C:** Left ICA: oblique view.

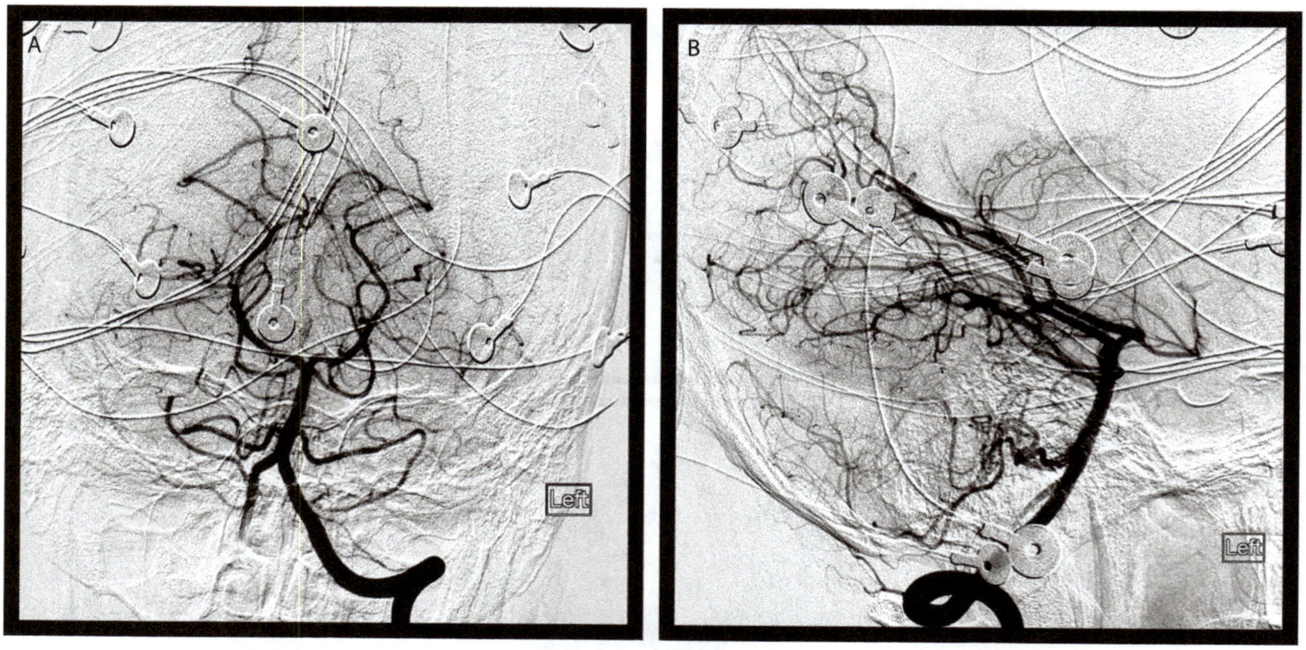

Figures 4-24A and B Vertebral series. **A:** Left vertebral: AP view. **B:** Left vertebral: lateral view.

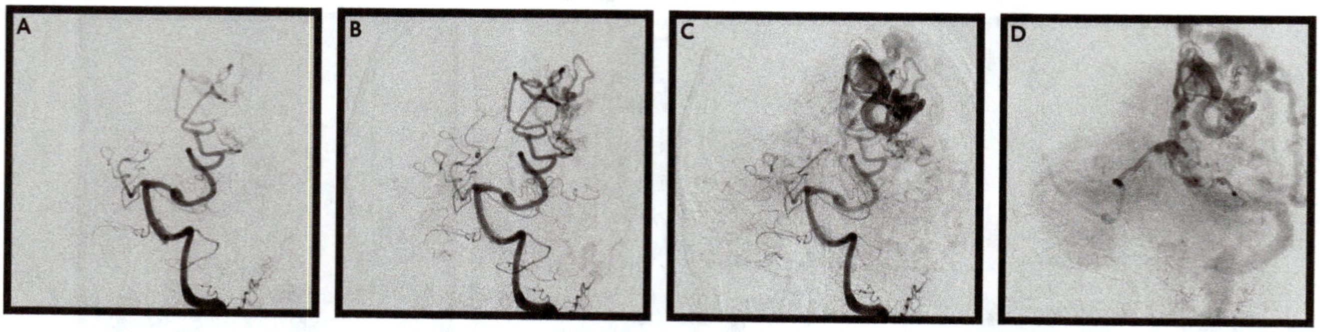

Figures 4-25A–D Vertebral angiograms of arterial venous malformation (AVM). **A:** Mid-arterial. **B:** Late arterial. **C:** Early venous. **D:** Mid-venous. *Courtesy of Lucian Maidan, M.D.*

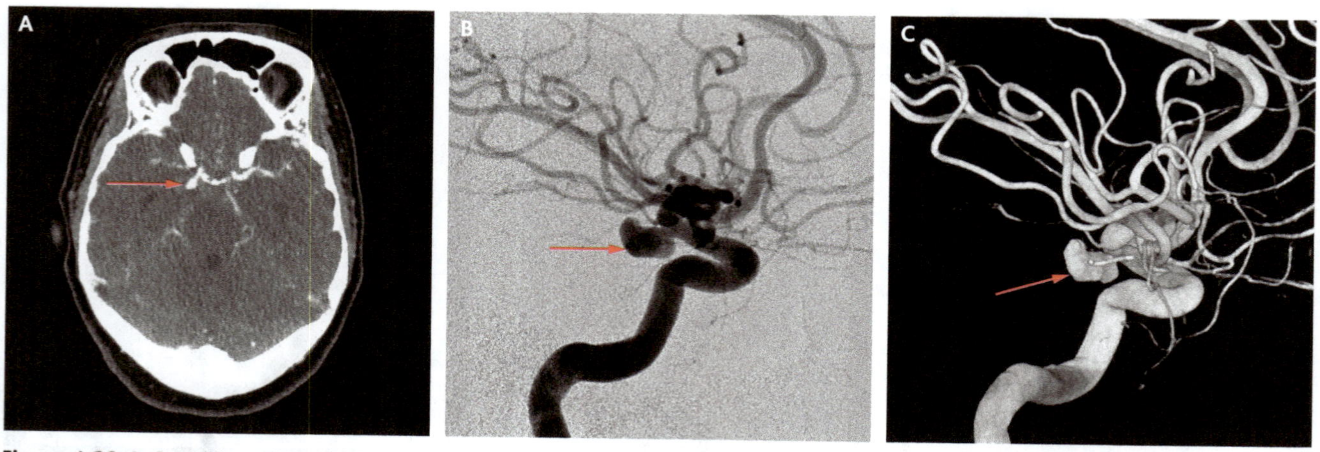

Figures 4-26aA–C Middle cerebral artery aneurysm (arrows) on CT and 2D and 3D DSA. **A:** CT scan. **B:** 2D angiogram. **C:** 3D angiogram. *Images courtesy of Lucian Maidan, M.D.*

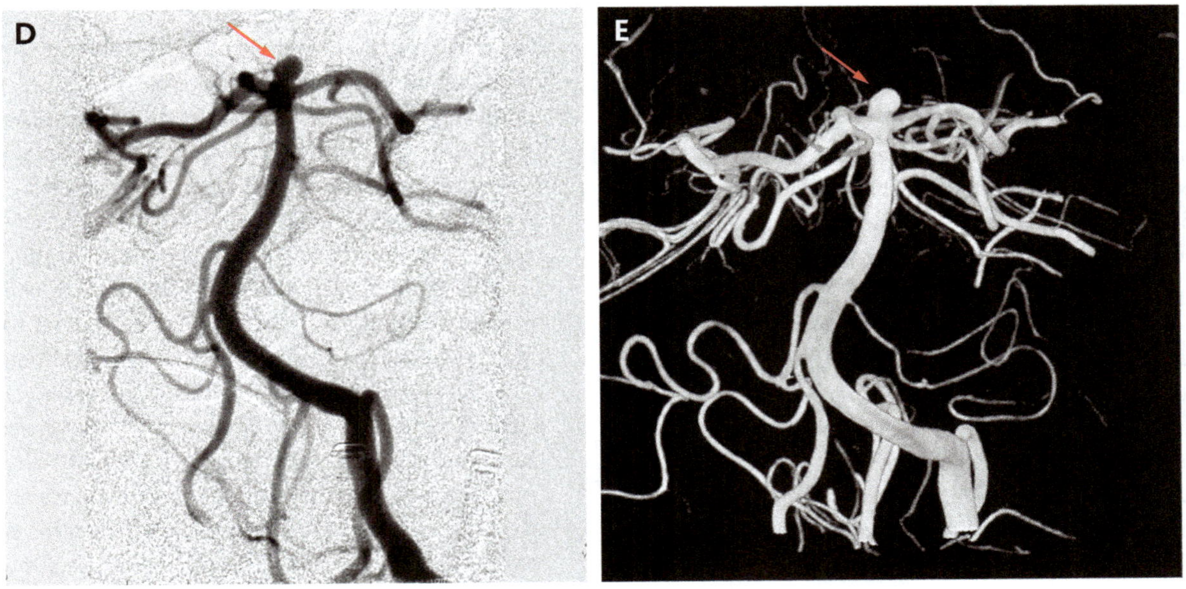

Figures 4-26D and E Basilar artery aneurysm (arrows) on 2D and 3D angiograms. **D:** 2D angiogram. **E:** 3D angiogram. *Images courtesy of Lucian Maidan, M.D.*

Magnetic Resonance Imaging (MRI)

The physics behind modern MRI imaging is extremely complex and is the fulltime purview of specially trained physicists or technicians. Even seasoned radiologists balk at most questions concerning how specific sequences are produced, why certain artifacts may be present, or why a particular pathological marker appears the way it does on a particular type of scan. This section will provide information on the basic concepts behind MRI imaging. Details of higher-level physics and computer image processing are beyond the scope of this text.

All MRI machines have the same basic components:

- A large magnet to produce a steady-state magnetic field. The magnet's strength usually ranges from 1 to 3 Teslas (T) for clinical use, although higher-strength magnets are available.
- Shim coils used to make the magnetic field uniform
- Radio frequency (RF) coils for transmitting the RF signal to the body
- Receiver coils used to record the RF emitted from the body
- Gradient coils to provide spatial localization of the emitted signal
- Computer algorithms to construct the image on the basis of received signals

At its most basic level, MRI takes advantage of the magnetic properties of protons, located within the nucleus of hydrogen atoms. Protons act like tiny magnets when exposed to a strong magnetic field, becoming uniformly aligned, similar to iron filings on a sheet of paper exposed to a magnet underneath.

Protons express magnetic properties to all magnetic fields, even those around us every day. What makes the MRI scan different is that the system produces a strong steady-state magnetic field that acts on all of the free protons within hydrogen in a uniform manner. Once the protons become aligned with the steady-state magnetic field, an RF pulse is used to perturb the orientation of the protons. After the RF signal is turned off, the protons return to their steady-state equilibrium, while emitting RF frequencies of a particular resonance. Measures relating to the relaxation back to equilibrium for the component parallel to the magnetic field result in T1-weighted images. Measures relating to the relaxation back to equilibrium for the component perpendicular to the magnetic field result in T2-weighted images. The RF signals are mapped onto voxels within a slice of brain, or a 3D matrix of the entire brain based on magnetic-field gradients.

Safety Concerns of MRI

The main magnetic field of a 1.5T magnet is approximately 30,000 times the strength of the earth's magnetic field and approximately the same as that used by the electromagnets used to pick up cars in junkyards; 3T magnets have twice this strength and pose an even greater risk to staff and patients. A primary concern of such high–magnet strength systems is the risk of pulling metallic objects into the scanner, in effect turning them into projectiles. At 3T, the magnetic strength is so high that even large metallic objects such as oxygen tanks or metal tables can become projectiles, posing significant risk of injury to patients and staff. When considering the effects of a magnet, it is important to consider how strong magnetic fields dissipate with distance. While the increase in "pull" from a magnet is somewhat gradual for lower-strength magnets, the higher-strength systems have a steep magnetic-strength gradient, and the pull on an object can go from weak to very strong in a very short distance (Figure 4-27). With staff, this means that objects that do not appear to be pulled to the magnet at one distance may experience rapid acceleration toward the bore of the scanner if taken just a short distance closer.

One particular safety concern for centers transitioning from 1.5T to 3T systems is that fewer medical devices have been tested on the 3T machines than on the older 1.5T machines. It is considered unsafe to scan a patient without confirmation of the effects of the 3T magnet on implanted medical devices. As the clinical use of 3T systems increases, more medical devices will be tested, and this will become less of an issue.

In addition to the dangers associated with the effects of increased magnet strength on metallic objects, the ambient noise level of a 3T system is approximately twice that of a 1.5T system, putting the patient at risk of hearing damage, without appropriate precautions. 3T systems can produce noise levels in excess of 130 dBA, greater than the upper limit of 99 dBA set by the FDA (1997). The use of hearing protection should thus be mandatory in such scanners, to protect patients' hearing.

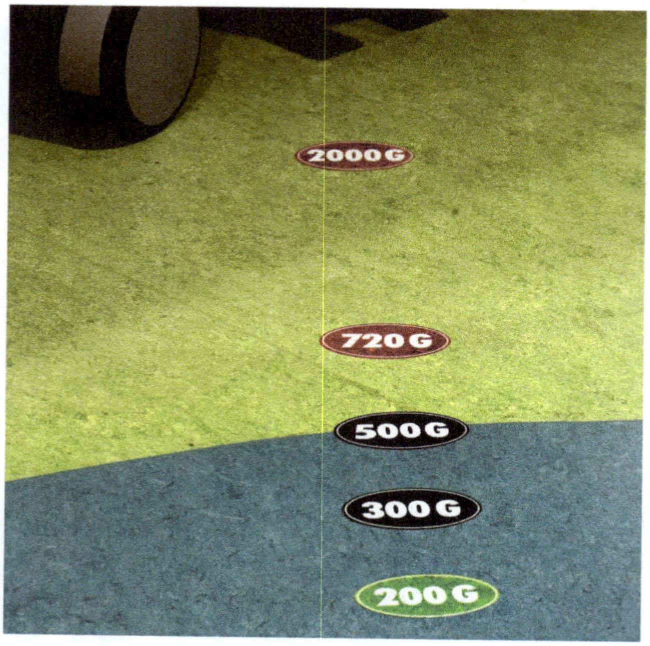

Figure 4-27 Graphical illustration of the nonlinear increase in magnetic field strength with diminishing distance from the core of an MRI scanner. The values are in Gauss (G) units, with 10,000 Gauss being equal to 1 Tesla. A 3-Tesla (3T) magnet will have a magnetic field strength of approximately 30,000 Gauss at the core or exact isocenter of the magnet. Note the nonlinear increase in Gauss values as distance to the scanner is decreased or moving from the bottom of the figure to the top. The distance between the 200 G and 300 G markers is approximately equal to the distance between the 300 G and 500 G markers, although there is a greater increase in magnetic strength for the latter.

The stronger the magnetic field, the clearer the radio frequency signal produced by the nuclei, the higher the signal-to-noise ratio, and the higher the spatial and contrast resolution of the image. Most current medical MRI scans use between 1- and 3-Tesla (T) magnets, although research centers are already using 7T magnets or higher for MRI imaging. Higher-strength magnets can provide more spatial and contrast resolution to an image. The signal-to-noise ratio increases linearly with the increase in the magnetic field strength, with 3T systems producing approximately twice the signal-to-noise ratio of a 1.5T magnet system. Image quality is also increased by the ability to use parallel acquisition techniques with stronger magnets. Higher magnetic field strengths allow for rapid image acquisition using echo planar or ultrafast gradient echo sequences, which are useful when assessing blood perfusion. There are some trade-offs when increasing magnet strength, such as increased sensitivity to susceptibility artifacts, image distortion, and signal loss. The increased susceptibility to paramagnetic artifacts has been used to produce sequences highly sensitive to blood products, such as susceptibility-weighted imaging (SWI), and for measures of brain functioning such as functional MRI (fMRI).

REFERENCE

U.S. Food and Drug Administration (1997). *A primer on medical device interactions with magnetic resonance imaging systems.* Retrieved from http://www.fda.gov/MedicalDevices/Device Regulationand Guidance/GuidanceDocuments/ucm107721.htm.

Problems with Higher-Strength Magnet Systems

Because magnet strength is an important determining factor in image quality, it is easy to believe that 3T systems are always better than 1.5T systems. However, not only do 3T systems increase potential risks related to use of the stronger magnets, but they are also more prone to producing many artifacts, especially those related to ferromagnetic susceptibility. A metallic object that resulted in weak magnetic interactions and artifact on a 1.5T MRI may cause substantial susceptibility artifact on a 3T system (Shellock, 2008). This is especially true for large metallic objects close to the brain, such as braces on teeth, and when using sequences susceptible to metallic artifacts, such as GRE or SWI (Figures 4-28A–C).

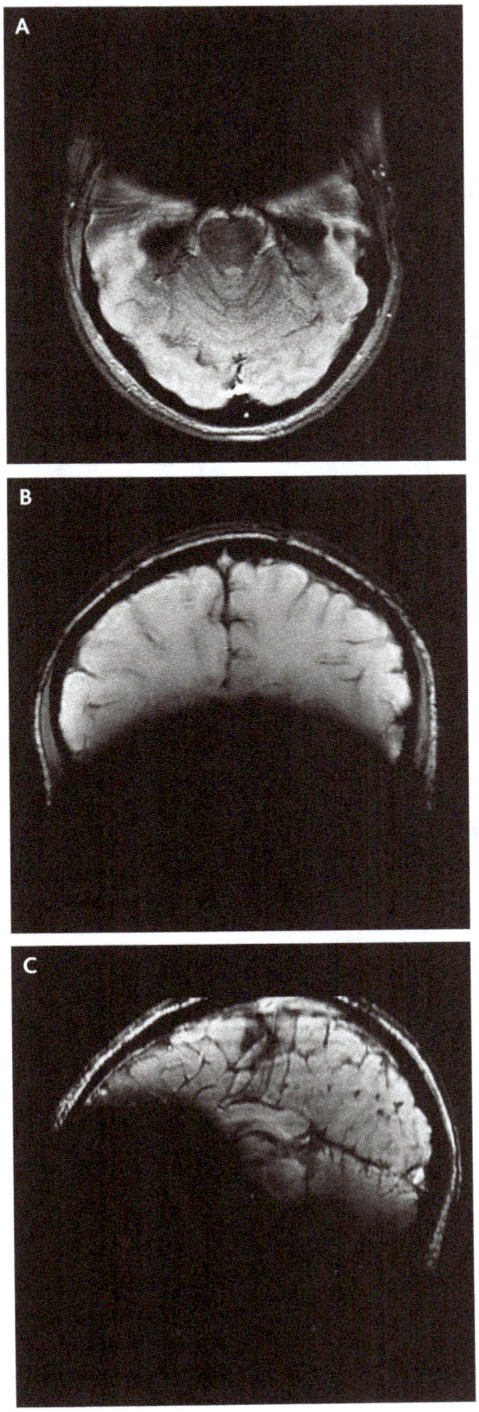

Figures 4-28A–C Susceptibility artifacts from braces on a high magnet-strength scanner. **A:** Axial GRE. **B:** Coronal SWI. **C:** Sagittal SWI.

REFERENCE

Shellock, F. G. (2008). *Reference manual for MR safety, implants, and devices*. Los Angeles: Biomedical Publishing Group.

Three-Dimensional Imaging

The ability to produce a full 3D matrix of data sets the MRI apart from CT. Because the data are recorded within a full 3D matrix of the brain, and voxels can be set to have sides of equal length, the data can be manipulated much easier on graphical workstations. From a clinical standpoint, this allows clearer images of brain lesions, which is especially helpful when consulting with patients and family members. In one instance, after two-dimensional images were shown to the parents of an infant patient, it became clear that they were having trouble understanding where the tumor was located in their baby's brain. Viewing of volume-rendered three-dimensional images, with a virtual window placed over the tumor was all it took for them to visualize their child's lesion (Figure 4-29).

Reformatting of MRI images

Although MRI images can be produced using multiplanar techniques, often only certain orientations are acquired. For example, during a particular patient session, T1 images may be acquired using sagittal or coronal planes, but not the axial plane. The determination of the specific plane used for a particular sequence is often dependent on the protocol requested by the radiologist. Some sequences are acquired in three dimensions using voxels with equal length sides, allowing for multiplanar reformatting through computer rendering software making it possible to visualize images from planes other than those acquired. Other MRI sequences are acquired as a series of slices, not unlike that of CT scanners (Figure 4-30A), making reformatting to orthogonal planes more problematic, with the final reformatted images being distorted with low spatial and contrast resolution (Figures 4-30B and C).

With advances in MRI technology, more sequences are being acquired using protocols that allow for 3D multiplanar reformatting. Acquiring MRI data in a 3D matrix using voxels with equal length sides allows for relatively simple reformatting to different planes and the production of higher-resolution volume-rendered images. In addition, the data matrix can be manipulated on a workstation to produce slices of varying thickness and at any angle.

There are many advantages to acquiring images in 3D format and reformatting them on a workstation post-acquisition. The most obvious advantage is that one can view scans in three orthogonal planes instead of only the

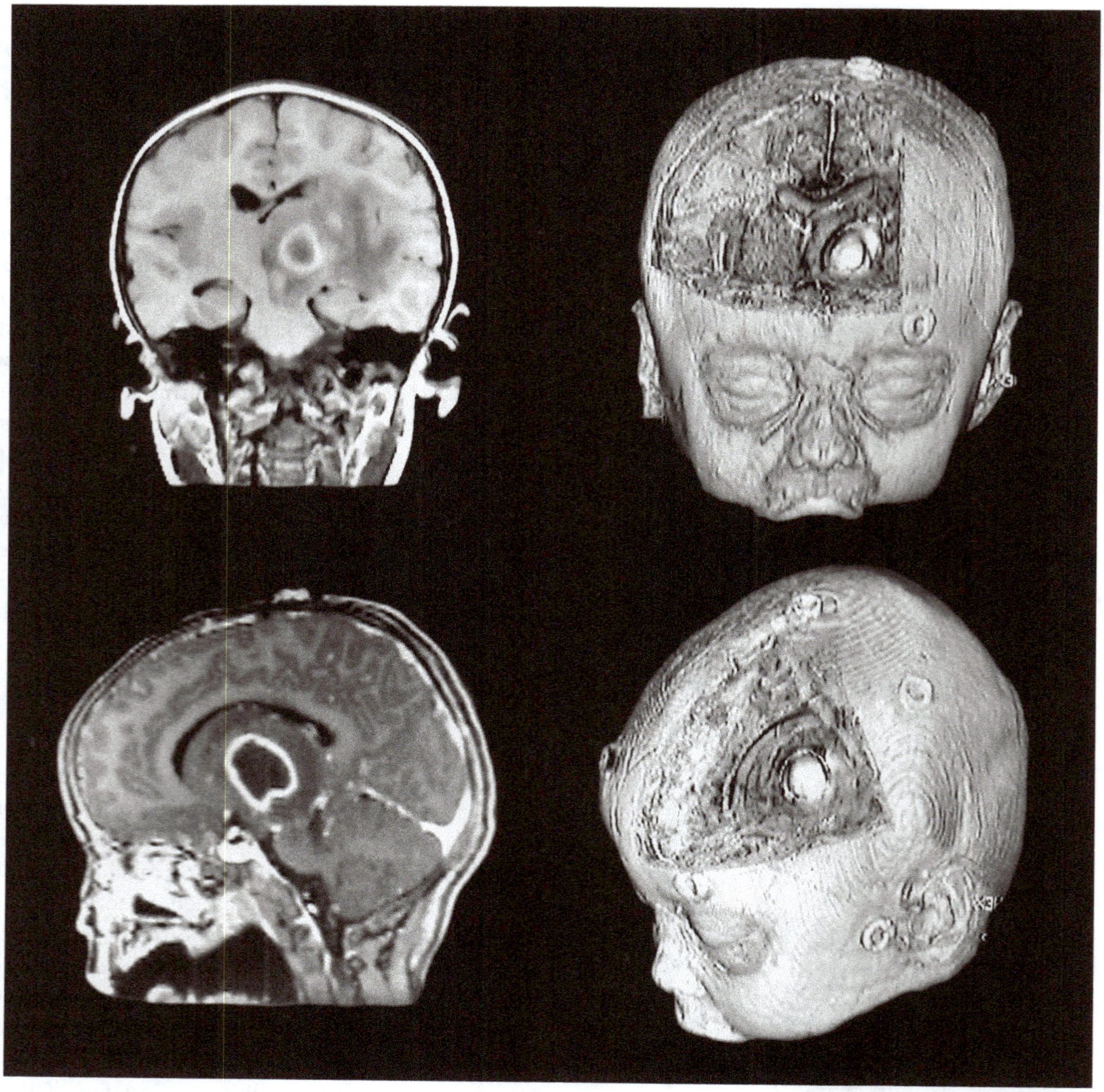

Figure 4-29 Two-dimensional MRI and three-dimensional volume rendering.

acquisition plane (Figures 4-31A–C). A less direct advantage is the ability to produce images in all three standard planes (axial, coronal, and sagittal) from a single acquisition session. In effect, condensing three scanning procedures into one means that the patient is in the scanner for less time.

An additional advantage of acquiring MRI data using a 3D protocol is the ability to manipulate the 3D matrix of data using a variety of proprietary software packages, after the patient has left the radiology department. Currently, some of the more sophisticated packages are only available on workstations produced by the scanner company; however, such programs are becoming increasingly available for use on hospital networks, desktop and laptop computers, and even portable devices such as smart phones and tablet computers. With increases in magnet strength and 3T scanners becoming more common, 3D multiplanar reformatting will likely become more available to the clinician, especially given the improved images produced by such systems. Many of the examples in the neuroanatomy, brain anatomy and brain atlas chapters (Chpaters 3, 5, 6 and 7) of this guide were reformatted from 3D FSPGR, BRAVO or MPRAGE spoiled gradient echo T1 sequences acquired in one plane and reformatted to other orientations using free, downloaded software on a notebook computer. For the brain atlas in Chapter 7, images were produced using segmentation and volume-rendering to provide a three-dimensional image of the head and brain. Multiplanar reformatting was used to produce two-dimensional slices of tissue in all three standard orientations. In addition, the brain images were resliced from a standard 5-mm thickness to 0.9 mm thick

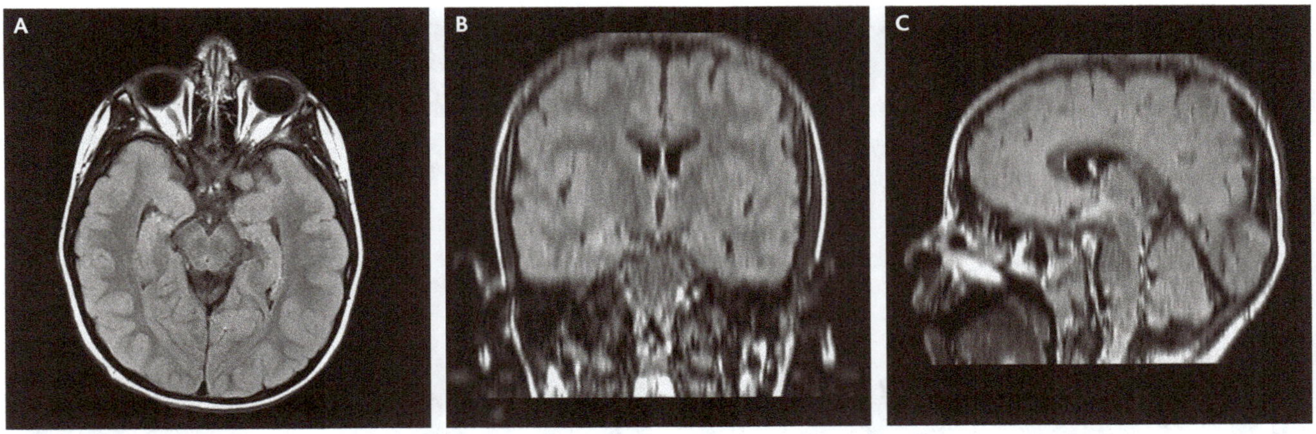

Figures 4-30A–C Reformatting of 2D-acquired images into other orientations. **A:** Original 2D source axial image. **B:** 2D axial reformatted to coronal image. **C:** 2D axial reformatted to sagittal image.

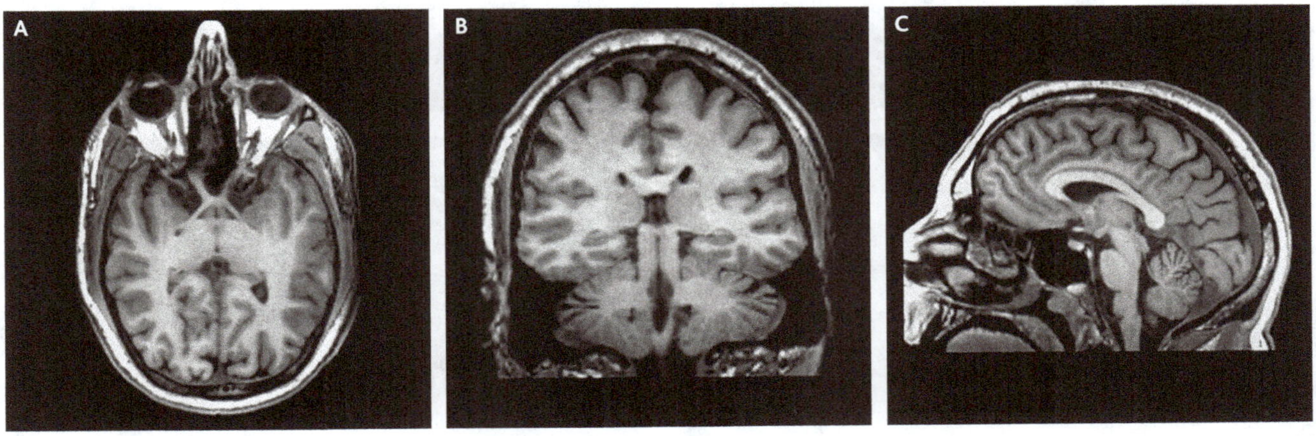

Figure 4-31A–C Reformatting of a 3D FSPGR image acquired in the axial plane. Note the greater resolution when compared to the reformatted images from 2D axial acquisition (Figures 4-30B and C). **A:** Original axial source image. **B:** Reformatted to coronal image. **C:** Reformatted to sagittal image.

in order to allow for better visualizion of the smaller structures and pathways.

Reslicing images using a thinner thickness and different slice angle

As stated above, images normally presented using 5-mm slices can be resliced using a thinner thickness and a different slice angle to more easily visualize small structures, for instance, the mammillary bodies. Figure 4-32 shows the slice angle used for a series of images through the mammillary bodies; the yellow reference line indicates the location of the new slices. All four axial images (Figures 4-33A–D) were acquired from within the yellow line. Note how the four 0.9 mm slices cut through approximately half the diameter of the mammillary bodies, structures no bigger than a small pea (arrow).

Three-dimensional volume rendering allows for real-time image slicing in all planes, individually or in combination (Figures 4-34A–F). There are a number of color-coding options available to highlight certain types of tissue or properties.

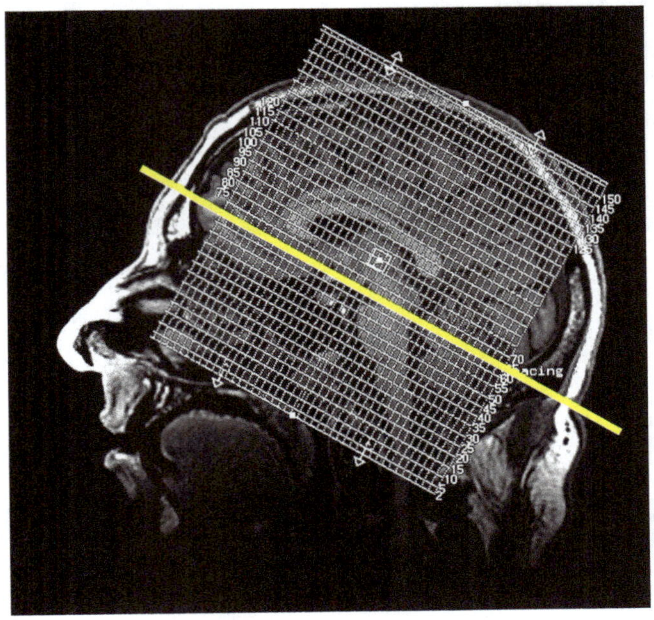

Figure 4-32 Sagittal reference image for Figures 3-33A–D. The four thinly sliced images shown in Figures 4-33A–D were acquired from within the yellow line on Figure 4-32.

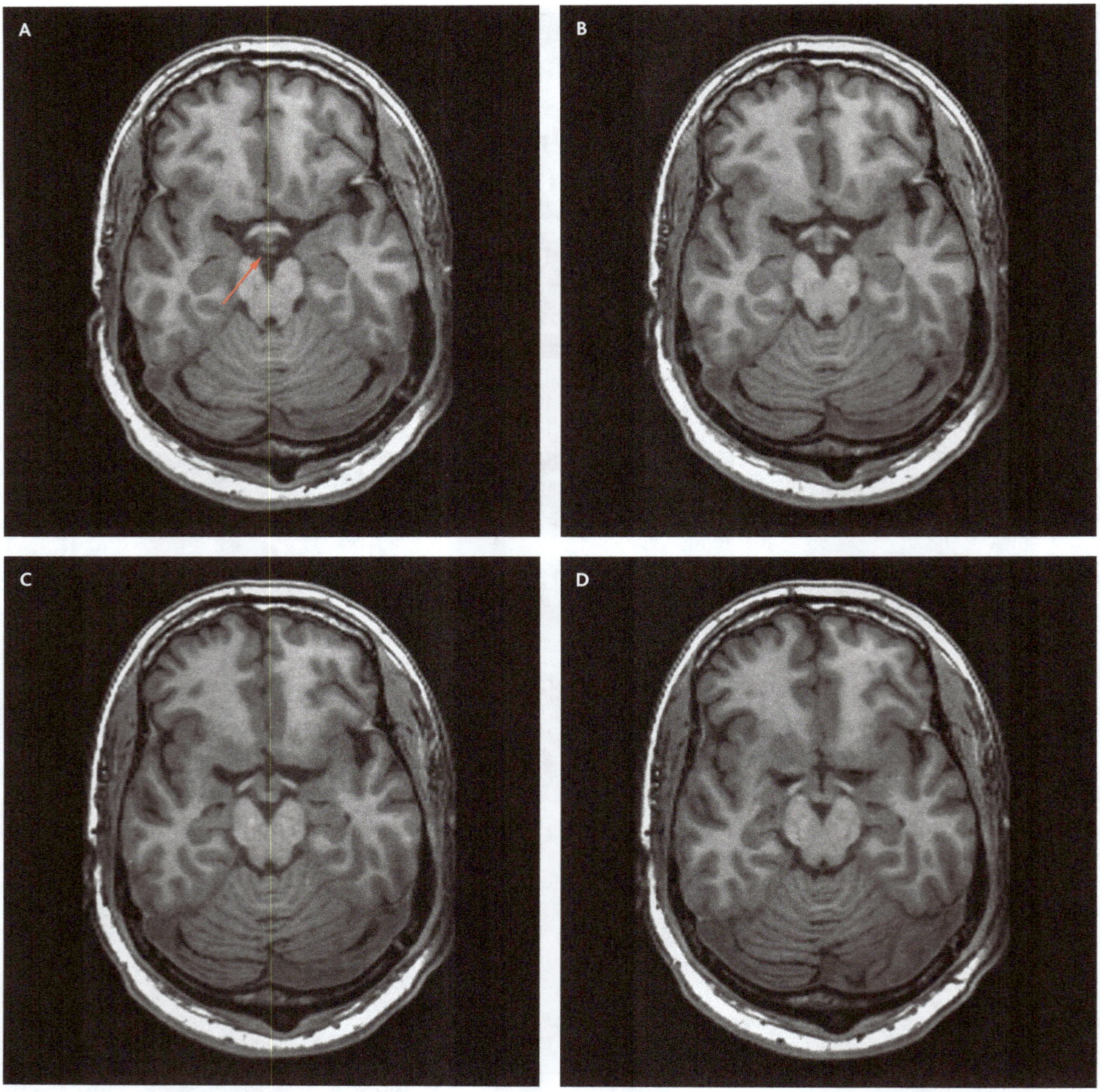

Figure 4-33A–D Thin sliced axial images showing the mammillary bodies (arrow). All four images were acquired from within the area indicated by the yellow line on Figure 4-32.

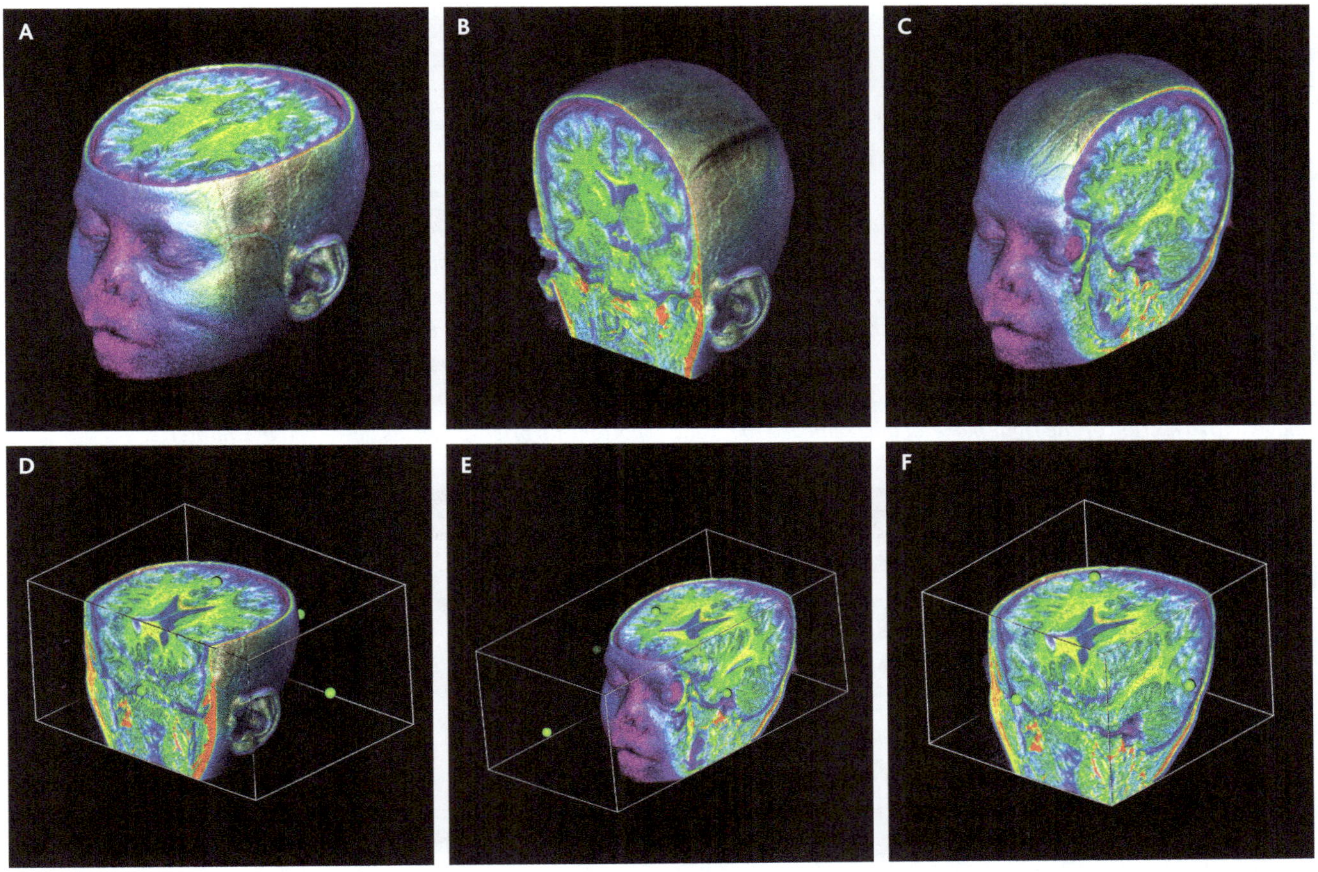

Figures 4-34A–F Examples of 3D volume-rendered and color-coded MRI images. **A:** Axial cut. **B:** Coronal cut. **C:** Sagittal cut. **D:** Axial and coronal cuts. **E:** Axial and sagittal cuts. **F:** Cuts through all three standard planes.

Cutting windows into an image

Through 3D volume rendering, combined with software-based graphics processors, images can be manipulated in a variety of ways to improve clinical utility. Sections of a person's skull and scalp can be removed to reveal the brain tissue beneath it (Figure 4-35A); windows can be "cut" into the side of a head to reveal specific structures (Figure 4-35B); or slices can be produced with reference to external features (Figure 4-35C).

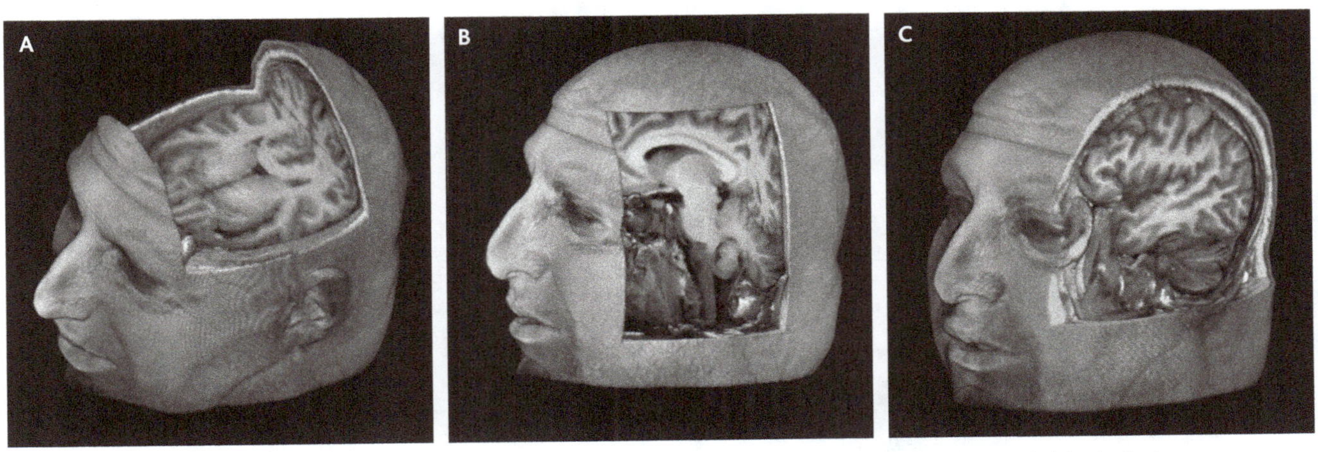

Figure 4-35A–C Three-dimensional volume-rendered MRI images with sections, windows or slices removed to show underlying brain tissue.

Mia: Motor Mapping Using 3D Images to Assist Interpretation

After fMRI motor mapping was completed for Mia's left hand, the information was presented to the surgeon in a standard two-dimensional (2D) axial format (Figure 4-36A). In addition, it was post-processed into coronal and sagittal planes (Figures 4-36B and C arrows). The activation maps (yellow) presented in Figures 4-36A–C are for Mia's left index finger, illustrating the degree to which small areas of motor activation can be localized within the brain using current fMRI technology.

The fMRI data were then presented in a 3D volume-rendered image with a section of the right parietal lobe removed to reveal the precise location of the activation map (Figure 4-36D). The area of greatest activation for Mia's left index finger is shown in Figure 4-36D in red and is located along the cortical edge of the right precentral gyrus or primary motor cortex (arrow). Note how much easier it is to visualize the activation area in the 3D volume-rendered image than in the standard 2D images. It may appear that the activation is on a different side of the brain on the 3D versus the 2D images; this is because the 3D image is viewed from the top, and 2D images are viewed from a bottom-up orientation, as described in Chapter 2.

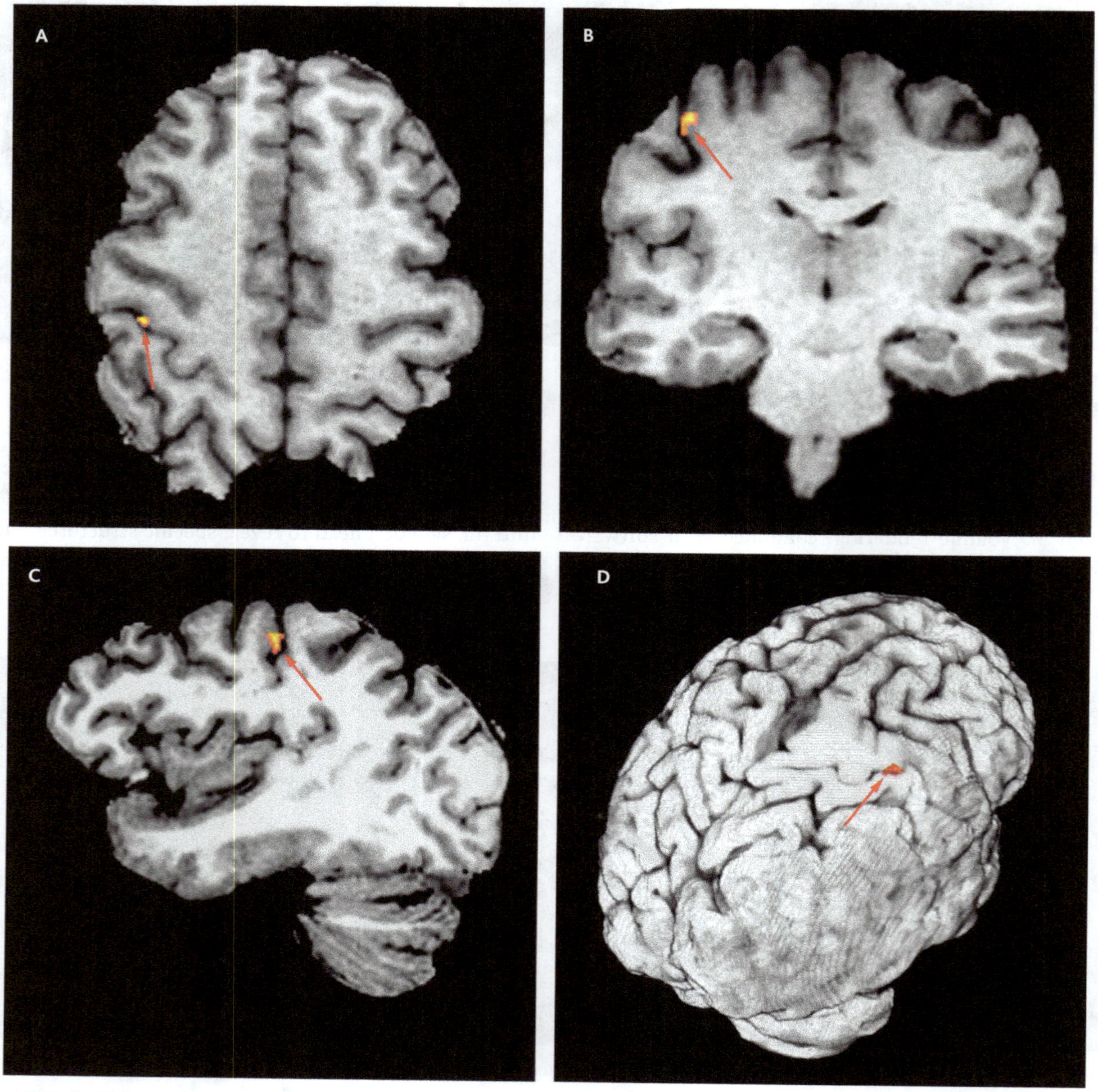

Figure 4-36A–D Clinical example Mia: motor mapping using 3D images to assist interpretation. The area of greatest activation for Mia's left index finger is shown in yellow (Figures 4-36A–C) and red (Figure 4-36D).

Signal Strength and Contrast on MRI

With a given strength of magnet, signal strength from tissue is dependent on a variety of physical features such as proton density, longitudinal relaxation time (T1), transverse or 90-degree relaxation time (T2), pulse sequence used, flow for fluids, and manipulation of a variety of imaging parameters. Signal intensity and the corresponding grayscale value on an MRI image are highly dependent on tissue characteristics, the sequence parameters, and flow. Flow can affect an MRI image because of the constant change in signal for a given location. Flow sequences such as a TOF sequence can be useful for imaging blood within the brain. Other forms of flow-sensitive sequences can be used to assess cerebral blood perfusion and oxygenation as it relates to brain metabolic activity.

MRI noise

Although electronic noise and computational noise apply to both CT and MRI scans, quantum noise is specific to imaging techniques using ionizing radiation. The primary source of MRI noise comes from the RF emissions from the patient's body that result from thermal motion. Few parameters can be adjusted to minimize noise, although a larger voxel size and selection of a surface coil over a whole-body coil can increase the signal-to-noise ratio. Surface coils are used when small anatomical structures such as the hippocampi need to be viewed in great detail. The smaller the coil, the less noise is picked up from adjacent tissue, leaving the tissue of interest cleaner, or with a higher signal-to-noise ratio. Another way to reduce noise is to average multiple excitations or measures of the same tissue. Because noise is random, each time the same tissue is scanned, the strength of the tissue signal increases in a linear fashion, as the random noise cancels itself out and decreases in strength. The same principle is applied in scientific research when multiple subjects are studied or multiple trials are performed by the same subject. Statistical averaging will result in a stronger signal and a reduction in error or noise.

MRI artifacts

Just as CT images may be marred by a variety of artifacts, so too are MRI images affected by artifacts. MR artifacts may decrease image quality or accuracy in a number of ways. As with CT scans, the two most common causes of artifacts on MRI involve movement of the patient during the image acquisition phase and metallic interference. Movement can increase noise or produce ripple or concentric lines on the image, and metallic objects can cause relatively large areas of signal loss due to the distortion of the magnetic field required for MRI acquisition. Turning a negative into a positive, magnetic susceptibility artifacts, like those seen with ferromagnetic metals, are now being used to image blood products because of the iron content (i.e. GRE, SWI).

Motion artifacts

Motion artifacts can be caused by random movement or by more periodic motion relating to a patient's respiratory or cardiac rhythm or to arterial or CSF pulses. Random movements result in images that may appear blurry or have increased noise or ripples (Figures 4-37A–C). Periodic motion tends to create ghosting of the image. Random-motion artifacts on an MRI are caused by tissue at a particular voxel having different spin properties between phase-encoding and recording of the signal. Consequently, the phase-encoding of values at that particular voxel will be corrupted, resulting in artifacts on the image. Rhythmic or periodic movements that produce ghosting result in an image with areas recorded with either increased or decreased signal intensity, unrelated to the tissue properties per se.

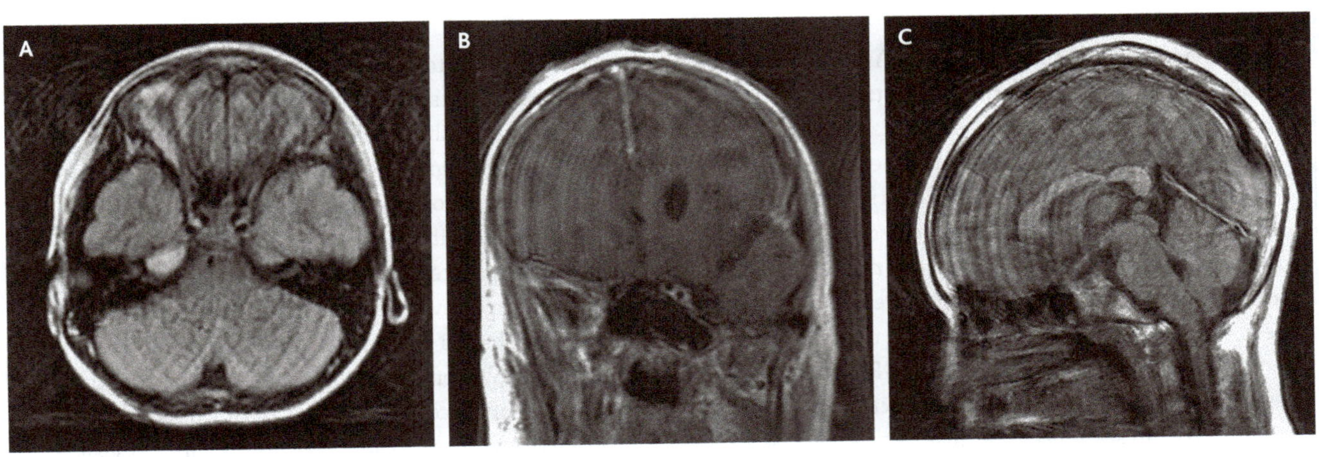

Figures 4-37A–C Examples of motion artifacts. **A:** Axial T1. **B:** Coronal T1. **C:** Sagittal T1.

Metallic objects

Metallic objects produce artifacts and distortion on MRI scans that radiate from the source, similar to that seen in CT scans (Figures 4-38A–F). The presence of a metallic object will disrupt the magnetic fields produced by the scanner. The disruption of the magnetic field will result in a change in the magnetic susceptibility of tissue or the internal magnetization of tissue as a function of its reaction to external magnetic fields. The degree to which the image contains artifacts or distortions depends on the specific metal type and pulse sequence used for the scan, as well as the strength of the magnetic field. Higher-strength magnets produce more disruption to magnetic susceptibility than lower-strength magnets.

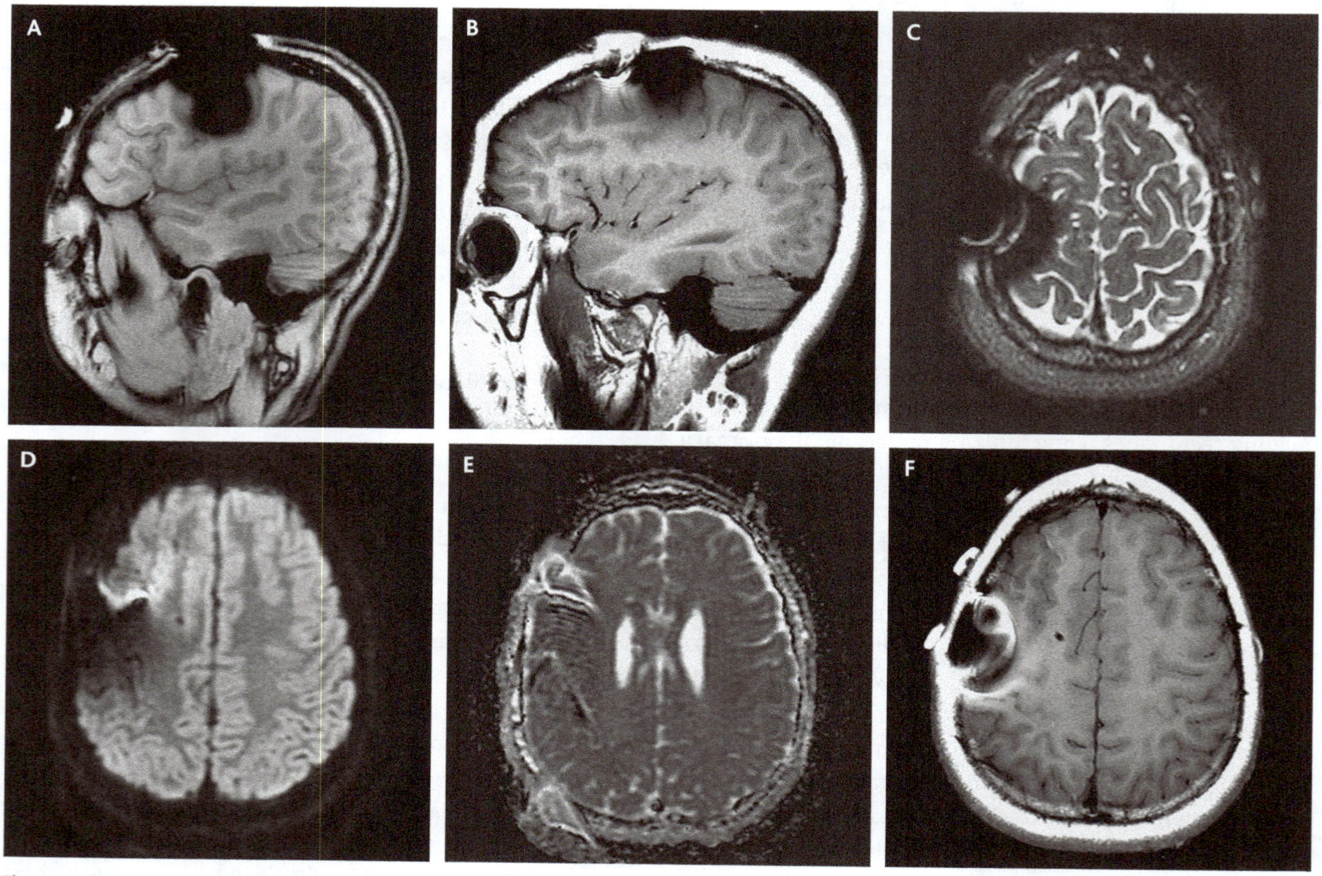

Figures 4-38A–F Examples of artifacts caused by metallic objects on the surface of the head, such as shunt systems, external ventricular drains, and staples. **A:** Sagittal SPGR. **B:** Sagittal T1. **C:** Axial T2 FSE. **D:** Axial DWI. **E:** Axial ADC. **F:** Axial T1.

Magnetic Susceptibility Artifacts Are Used to Produce Clinically Meaningful Sequences

Magnetic susceptibility can be summarized as the degree to which tissue becomes internally magnetized as a result of an external magnetic field. Bordering tissues with vastly different magnetic susceptibilities can cause distortions in the external magnetic field and can result in image artifact or distortion. Such artifacts are most commonly seen at the edges between air and soft tissue, or between bone and soft tissue. Gradient echo (GRE) sequences are more prone to susceptibility artifacts and distortion than spin echo sequences. Because of this increased sensitivity of GRE to susceptibility artifacts they can be used clinically to assess for blood. As blood breaks down, it causes susceptibility artifacts responsible for the loss in T2 signal on gradient echo images (GRE), which produces the visual marker for blood. Blood appears dark to black on GRE images owing to attenuation of the T2 signal. More recently, susceptibility-weighted images (SWI) have been shown to be even more sensitive to susceptibility artifacts and have a greater sensitivity for blood than GRE images. SWI produced on high–magnet strength systems can produce images showing tiny microbleeds resulting from diffuse axonal injuries that are not visible on T2 or GRE sequences. Susceptibility artifacts are also used to assess blood perfusion through the use of paramagnetic contrast agents. At its simplest level, the computer records the signal loss on T2-weighted images due to the contrast agent's susceptibility effect during the first pass of the contrast. The loss of signal (artifact) is then computed and provides a relative measure of perfusion in that area.

Magnetic Resonance Sequences

Only a couple of decades ago, MRIs produced either T1 spin-lattice or T2 spin-echo sequences. Radiologists and clinicians reviewed sheets of film with slices often depicted in a 4 × 4 or 4 × 5 matrix. When there were few sequences available, it was easy to determine whether a scan was acquired as a T1 or a T2. As additional sequences became available, it has become more difficult to determine the type of image just by appearance. This is especially true for sequences that combine parameters from other scans or use some parameters associated with T1 and some associated with T2, producing a hybrid that is neither. Adding to the complexity of MR imaging, sequences are now produced by manipulating parameters within a scanning session to highlight certain tissues or properties. When sequences are used that are not part of a specific protocol, the technologist must manually label them as a reminder of what was changed. This is why you may see sequence labels that do not make sense but instead indicate a specific protocol or parameter combination. For example, a radiology technologist labeled a series "EP GRE—SWI" to indicate that it was a sequence developed to mimic a standard SWI but by using an echo-planar gradient echo sequence. Interestingly, the sequence is neither a standard GRE nor a standard SWI; it is actually an image falling somewhere in between.

PEARL It is more important to develop a general idea of how common imaging sequences appear than to become confused by the many labels used in MRI. Not only are the labels different depending on the manufacturer of the scanner or workstation software (see Appendix 4-1), but sequence labels may also be unique to that particular scanning session.

PERIL Try to remain flexible when faced with many different MRI sequence labels; otherwise the complexity of the labeling nomenclature may prevent you from appreciating the clinical information provided by the images. Many sequences are labeled by the radiology technician immediately prior to acquisition, per the specific request of the radiologist. Sometimes, after post-processing data, the saved images may be given a unique label to reflect the general technique used. For example, after selecting or "seeding" a series of blood vessels, the technician may simply label them with the abbreviation *MRA* without reference as to how they were originally acquired. In addition, if the radiologist requests a nonstandard series of images using parameters that are not already stored as a protocol, the technician can name the series on the basis of parameters or a code that he or she can remember. For instance, when reslicing a series of images for this publication, the author renamed them "FSPGR BRAVO 0.9 ANG 45." This label referred to the source images being from an FSPGR BRAVO series, with a cut thickness set at 0.9 mm and the slice angle half-way between axial and coronal, or at a 45-degree plane. This label did not represent a sequence per se but was just a reminder of how the sequence was produced.

The complexity of available MRI sequences has increased substantially over the past decade and is now at a level that falls outside the scope of this introductory guide. Briefly, an MRI sequence consists of a few basic but essential components and a large number of available options. Sequences are formed from RF pulses and gradients. The RF pulses

As a general rule, if the CSF or the eyes are bright (have a high signal), the scan is a T2 sequence. If the CSF or eyes are dark (have a low signal), it is either a T1 sequence or a T2 FLAIR sequence. Looking at the gray or white matter can help to differentiate between a T1 and a T2 FLAIR image, with white matter appearing lighter on a T1 and darker on a T2.

Most brain pathologies produce the following appearance on MRI:

T1	Low signal (dark), except subacute blood (light) and fat (light)
T2	High signal (light)
GRE/SWI	Blood = dark

are used to produce the magnetic resonance characteristics for the tissue. The gradients are used for the spatial encoding of the resonance information in two-dimensional or three-dimensional space. The use of a variety of echo types (spin-echo, gradient-echo, etc.) and the evaluation of different relaxation times (e.g., T1 or T2) determine the appearance of tissue on a scan or the contrast of the image. The use of options such as inversion-recovery (IR) further allows for modification of how tissue is presented on the final image. Sequence parameters such as TR, TE, flip angle, field of view, etc. are user adjusted to find the best compromise between contrast, spatial resolution, scan time, and clinical requirements.

The primary determinant of how brain tissue is displayed is the specific pulse sequence parameters used or, more specifically, the repetition time between 90-degree RF pulses (TR) and the time between the first 90-degree RF pulse and the echo, or the echo time (TE). By manipulating TR and TE, various imaging sequences of the same tissue can appear quite different (e.g., T1 vs. T2).

One of the more complicated aspects of MRI involves the many abbreviations used to describe the sequences available to a radiologist. What makes it even more complex, especially for the non-radiologist, is the fact that there is no globally recognized abbreviation for a particular sequence. Each manufacturer uses unique proprietary labels for image sequences produced with their systems. For example, a steady-state gradient echo sequence (GE) is called a "GRE" or "MPGR" by General Electric, "FE" by Toshiba, "FFE" by Philips, "FISP" by Siemens, and "TRSG" by Hitachi (See Tables 4-1a and 4-1b provided at the end of this chapter for a list of current abbreviations). In medical centers that have multiple MRI machines made by different manufacturers, reviewing brain scans on the basis of specific sequence abbreviation becomes daunting at best and often time consuming. The same difficulty is experienced when reviewing brain scans from other institutions that use equipment made by a manufacturer different from the one you may be familiar with in your practice.

Adjusting TR (Repetition Time)
When using a long TR, the signal difference between gray and white matter is small. However, with a shorter TR, there is an increase in contrast between the soft tissues of the brain, such as between gray and white matter. Shorter TRs are thus good for visualizing soft-tissue anatomy and are used for T1 sequences.

Adjusting TE (Echo Time)
When using a short TE, the contrast between gray matter, white matter, and CSF is small. Longer TEs improve the contrast between these tissues and are used to produce T2-weighted images.

Manipulation of the angle of RF pulse can also change how a scan appears. As an example, gradient echo sequences differ from spin-echo sequences in that they use a flip angle often below 90 degrees and they lack a 180-degree rephasing pulse.

Because of the complexity of MRI physics, it is recommended that non-radiologists attend more to how the basic types of scans (T1, T2, FLAIR, GRE, SWI, etc.) appear, or how they can assist in clinical decision making, than to the specific parameters used to produce the sequences.

Another difficulty often encountered when first viewing MR images involves the combination of sequence type and image angles. Although it would seem logical to present a particular sequence in all three image planes, this is not the norm. With the exception of the sequences acquired using specific 3D protocols such as BRAVO or MPRAGE which can be reformatted easily in post processing, each image plane to be presented must be acquired separately. With individual sequences requiring, on average, several minutes to acquire, the acquisition of additional image planes can result in significantly longer imaging sessions for the patient. Fewer than six different sequences can mean more than 30 minutes in the scanner, and with three basic image planes, it would not require many different sequences to increase the scanning time beyond that which is comfortable for the patient or feasible in a busy radiology department. Generally, images are acquired using a combination of sequence types and image planes, dependending on the clinical question. For this reason, you may not be able to view all three image planes for a particular sequence (T1, T2, FLAIR, etc.), although the combination of image planes and sequences should be more than adequate to allow full visualization of the specific condition.

T1 spin-lattice sequences

Short TR (<1000 ms) and short TE (<30 ms)

T1 scans are produced using a short TR and short TE. They provide high resolution for soft tissue. T1 images are good at differentiating fat (light) from water (dark), thus they provide excellent anatomical clarity between the white matter with high fat concentration and gray matter. Because T1 images provide the best discrimination between different soft tissues, they are sometimes referred to as "anatomical scans." On T1 images, gray matter is gray, white matter is white, and CSF is black (Figures 4-39A and B).

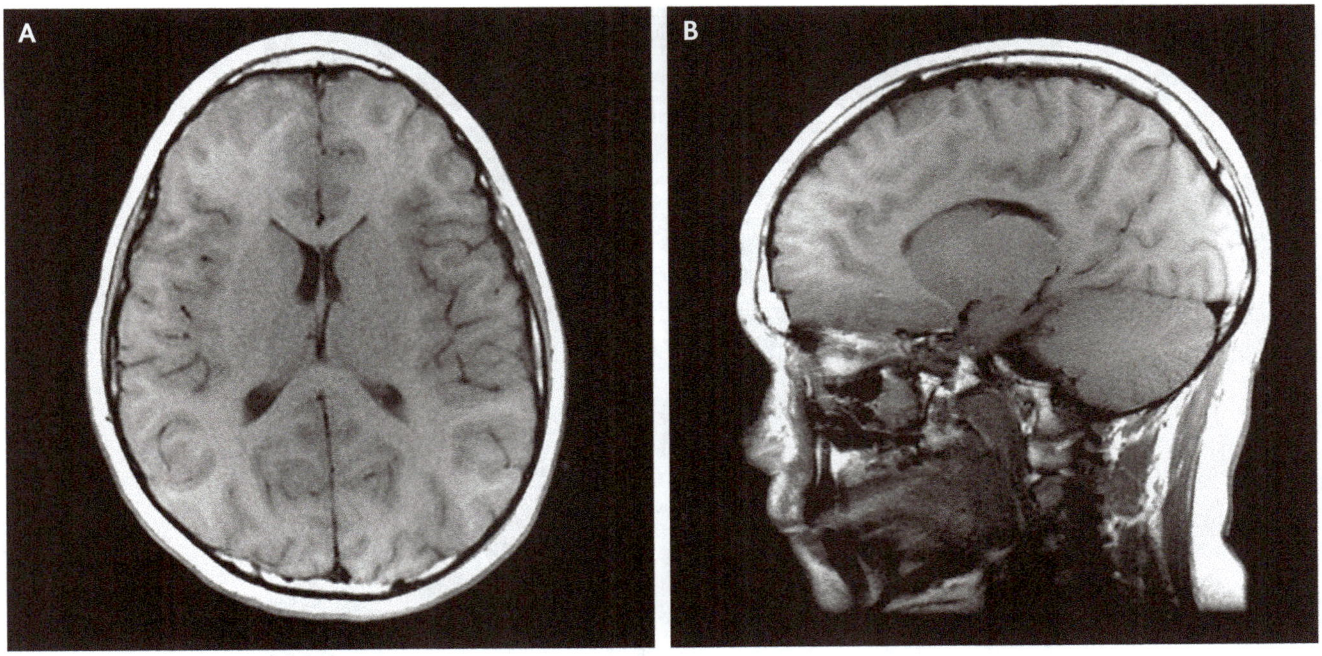

Figure 4-39A and B Image examples of T1 sequences.

3D spoiled gradient echo T1 images (i.e. FSPGR, BRAVO, MPRAGE)

T1 FSPGR, BRAVO, and MPRAGE type images are acquired using three dimensional protocols with voxels of equal length sides using thin-sliced T1 spoiled fast and ultrafast gradient-echo sequences. FSPGR, BRAVO, and MPRAGE sequences have excellent gray–white contrast differentiation, providing excellent images of anatomical structures. The thin acquisition slices enable visualization of the smaller structures of the brain, such as the pituitary, mammillary bodies, and hippocampi, in addition to thin white-matter tracts. The 3D acquisition protocols allow for multiplanar reformatting using a variety of image angles. Figures 4-40A–C provide examples of orthogonal axial, coronal, and sagittal images produced from a single axial acquisition source.

Because the images are acquired using a 3D protocol, they can be sliced and presented using any orientation or angle in post processing. Figure 4-40D shows a sagittal slice produced at an angle equal to that of the hippocampus, instead of the usual angle being equal to the longitudinal axis of the brain. By adjusting the slice angle to match the longitudinal axis of the hippocampus, the entire hippocampal structure can be viewed.

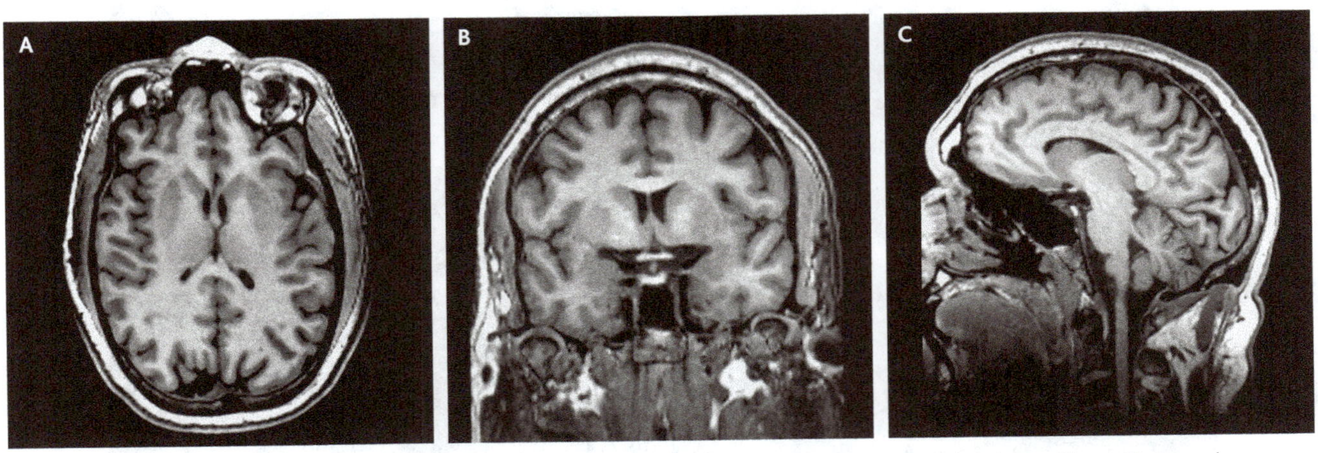

Figure 4-40A–C Reformatting of source axial BRAVO image into orthogonal coronal and sagittal slices. **A:** Axial–orthogonal image. **B:** Coronal–orthogonal image. **C:** Sagittal–orthogonal image.

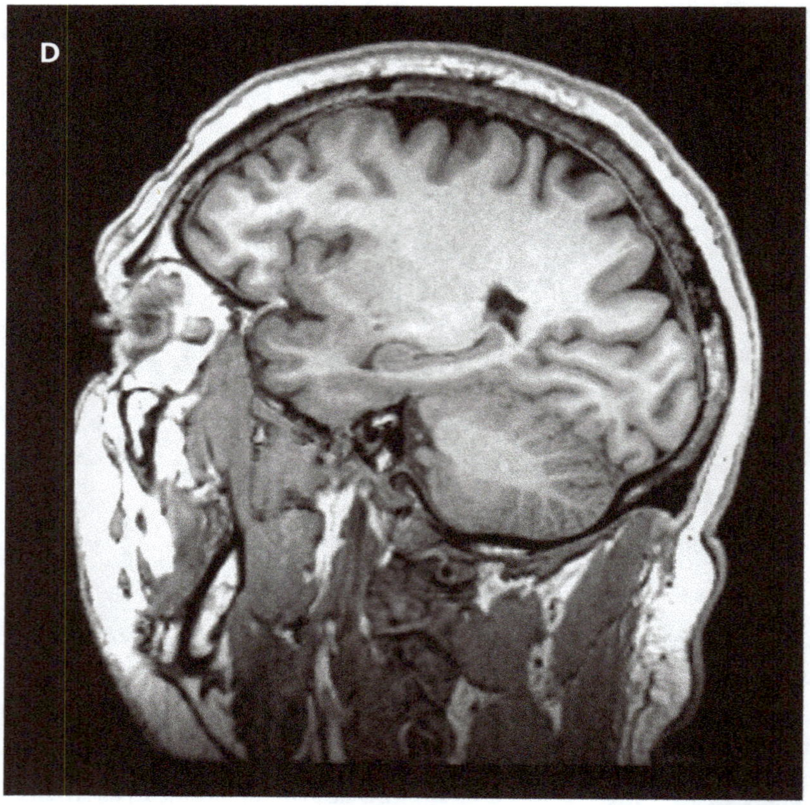

Figure 4-40D Sagittal slice using an angle to match that of the hippocampal structure to allow for fully visualization of the entire length of the hippocampus.

T2 spin-echo (spin-spin) sequences
Long TR (>2000 ms) and long TE (>80 ms)

T2 images also differentiate fat from water, although with opposite contrast to that of a T1 image; fat appears darker and water appears lighter. T2 images have lower resolution of soft tissue than T1 images but are better for visualizing most pathological processes involving the brain. Because T2 images provide relatively good resolution between normal and pathological tissue, they are sometimes referred to as "pathological scans" and have been the clinical workhorse of MRI for many decades. On T2 images, gray matter is light gray, white matter is darker gray, and CSF is white (Figures 4-41A and B).

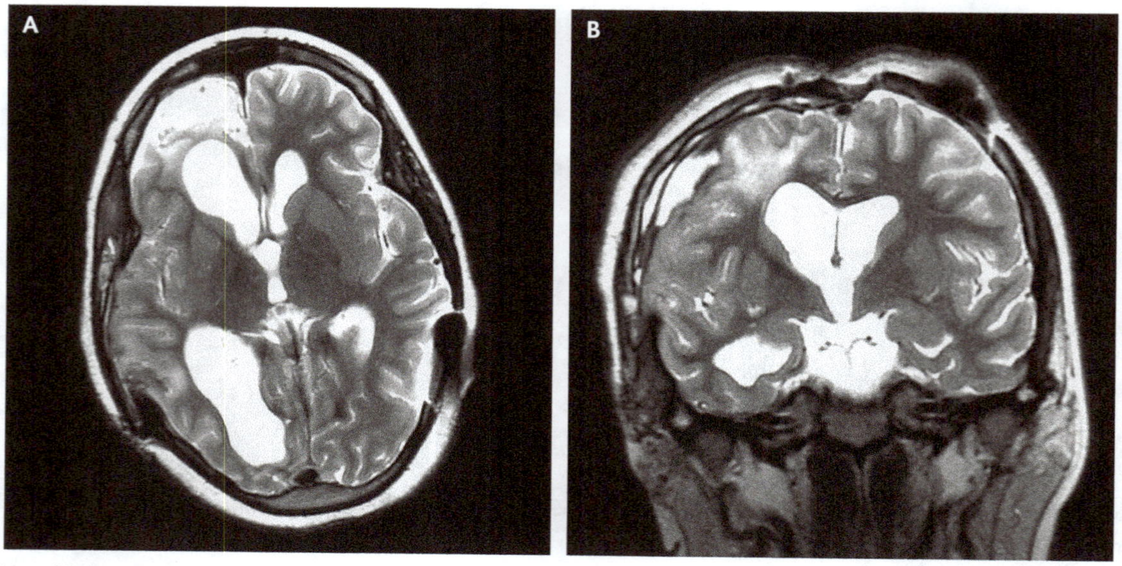

Figure 4-41A and B Image examples of T2 spin-echo sequences.

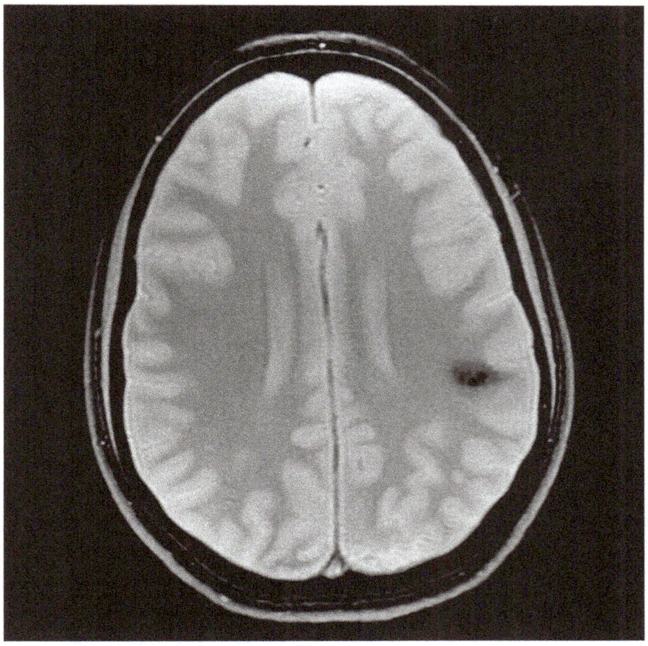

Figure 4-42 Image example of T2* "T2 star" spin-echo sequence.

T2 (T2-star) spin-echo (spin-spin) sequences*

T2*, pronounced "T2 star," images use a gradient echo (GRE) sequence with a long TR and a long TE. The GRE sequence used for T2* images is slightly different from a standard gradient echo sequence (described below) in that it does not have an extra refocusing pulse and so is not subject to additional attenuation above that of a T2 sequence. T2* sequences can be considered a standard T2 sequence that is more prone to magnetic susceptibility artifacts. The sensitivity to magnetic susceptibility artifacts makes the T2* useful for visualizing blood products, as is evident in Figure 4-42. The left parietal blood is evident as an area of hypointensity, referred to as "blooming."

T2 cube sequences

T2 cube sequences can be considered the T2 equivalent of a T1 sequence acquired using a 3D protocol, such as an FSPGR. T2 cube sequences are produced using a three-dimensional acquisition matrix and thin slices of approximately 1 mm in thickness. Similar to 3D FSPGR sequences, T2 cube images can be reformatted using a variety of image angles. Figures 4-43A–C illustrate T2 cube sequences of a patient with a cavernoma within the left parietal lobe just behind the central sulcus.

Proton-density (PD) or spin-density sequences

In spin-density images, also called proton-density images, the aim is to minimize any contrast caused by either T1

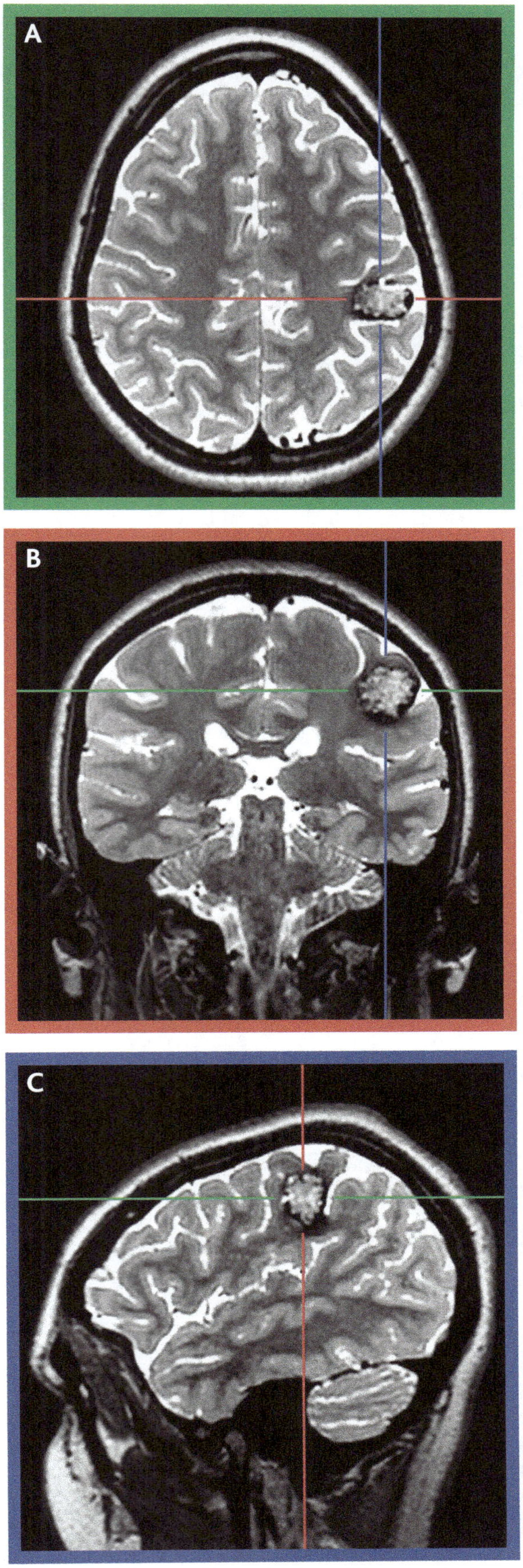

Figure 4-43A–C Image examples of T2 Cube sequences.

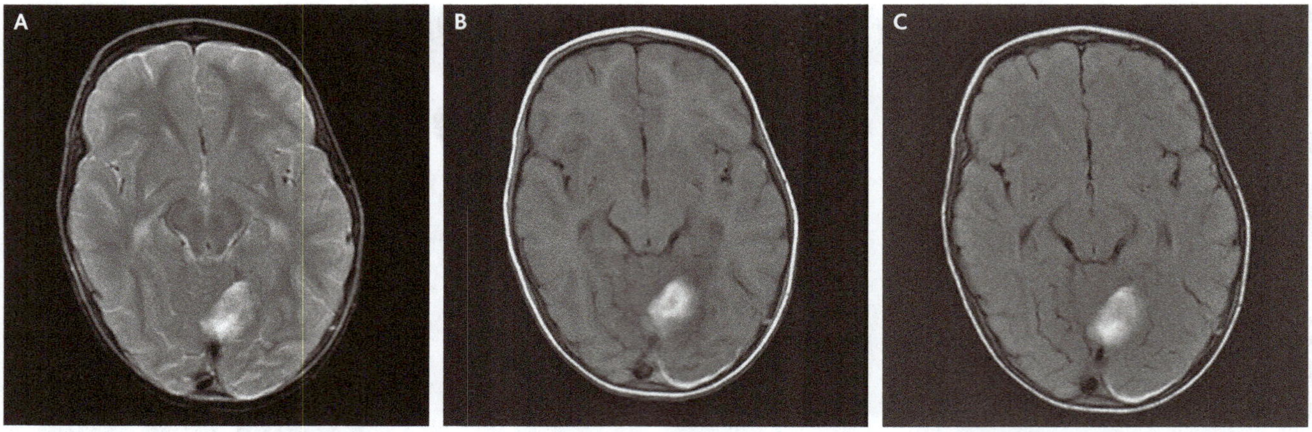

Figure 4-44A–C Example of a proton-density image, with additional image sequences provided for comparison. **a:** Proton density. **b:** T1. **c:** T2 FLAIR.

or T2 relaxation, with the signal being mostly dependent on the proton density of tissue (number of protons per volume of tissue relating to the amount of hydrogen). The sequences use either spin-echo (T2) or gradient echo (GRE) sequences with long TR and short TE. This lowers the signal from CSF, making assessment of periventricular white-matter pathology easier to appreciate. A proton density image is compared with standard T1 and T2 FLAIR images in Figures 4-44A–C.

Fluid-attenuated inversion recovery (FLAIR) sequences

For brain imaging, PD images have been replaced by **F**luid-**A**ttenuated **I**nversion **R**ecovery (FLAIR) sequences, which are sequences with the CSF signal suppressed. T1 FLAIR images are clinically helpful in that they have improved gray–white tissue distinction over that of standard T1 images and provide clearer information regarding anatomical structures. T2 FLAIR sequences are useful for assessing pathology without the markers of injury being clouded by bright CSF signal. By adjusting the time between the inversion and excitation pulses, the signal from any particular tissue can be suppressed; liquid such as CSF is the most common suppressed material. Contrast-enhanced FLAIR sequences can be helpful when assessing for infections of the brain or other conditions involving disruption to the blood–brain barrier. Figures 4-45A–C provides examples of T2 FLAIR and T1 FLAIR imaging of a right hemisphere low grade tumor).

Gradient echo (GRE) sequences

Gradient echo sequences differ from T2 spin-echo sequences in that they generally use a flip angle below 90 degees and do not use a 180-degree rephasing pulse. The low flip-angle allows for faster acquisition times. Although they are similar to T2 spin-echo sequences, they

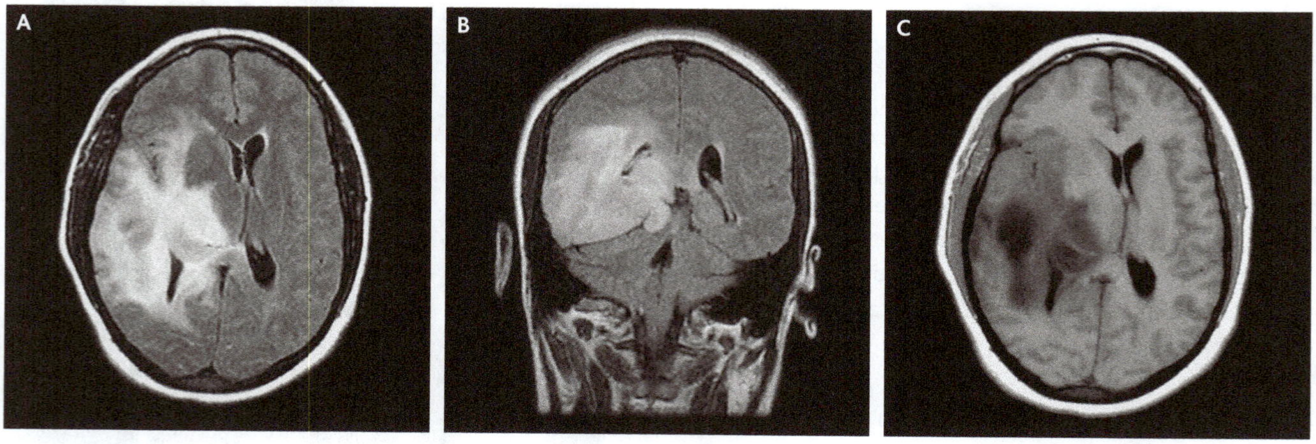

Figures 4-45A–C Image examples of FLAIR sequences showing low-grade astrocytoma. **a:** T2 FLAIR. **b:** T2 FLAIR. **c:** T1 FLAIR. *(Note: images labeled "Axial FLAIR," "Coronal FLAIR," or "Sagittal FLAIR" without other identifiers are generally produced using T2 weightings.)*

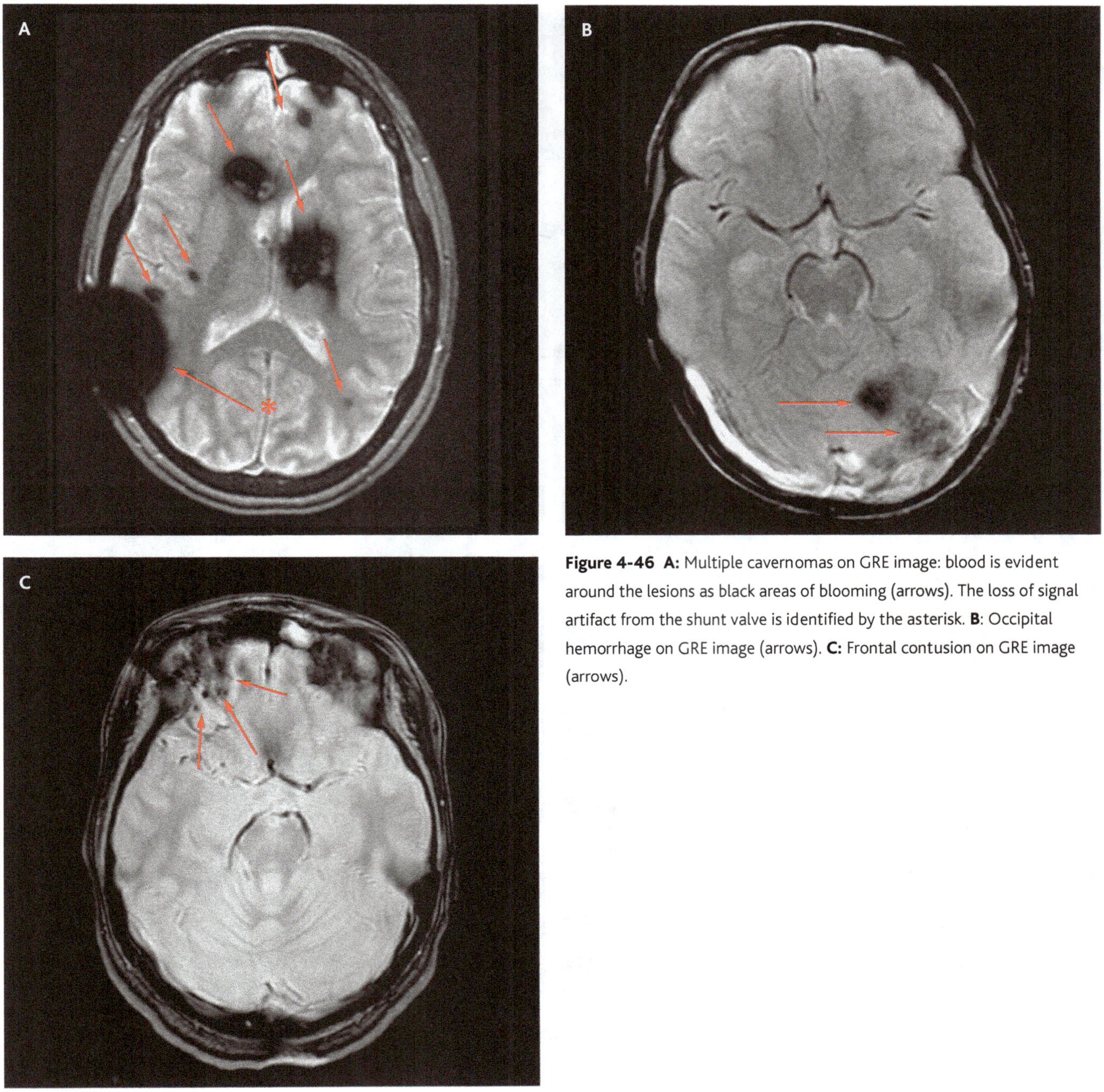

Figure 4-46 **A:** Multiple cavernomas on GRE image: blood is evident around the lesions as black areas of blooming (arrows). The loss of signal artifact from the shunt valve is identified by the asterisk. **B:** Occipital hemorrhage on GRE image (arrows). **C:** Frontal contusion on GRE image (arrows).

have both the advantage and disadvantage of being more sensitive to magnetic susceptibility artifacts. The disadvantage is that metal objects close to the brain, such as those found in shunt systems, cause marked loss of image signal (Figure 4-46A, arrow*). The advantage is that the scans are especially sensitive to acute or chronic hemorrhages. GRE sequences are most helpful for identifying blood within the brain, which shows as a black area of "blooming," due to the magnetic susceptibility of hemoglobin (Figures 4-46A–C, arrows).

Gradient echo–echo-planar sequences

Gradient echo–echo planar sequences (GRE-EPI) have increased sensitivity to susceptibility artifacts resulting from blood within the brain, and when produced with a 3T scanner, they provide images similar to those of susceptibility-weighted imaging on a 1.5T scanner (Figures 4-47A–C and 4-48A and B). GRE-EPI images can be difficult to interpret because of their susceptibility to artifacts resulting from tissue other than blood.

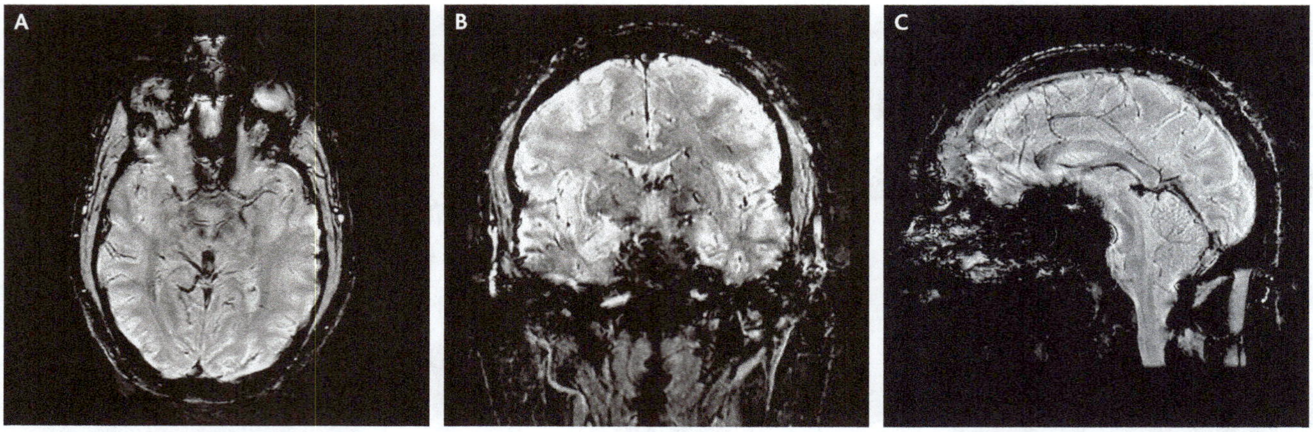

Figures 4-47A–C Normal GRE-EPI images acquired on the axial, coronal, and sagittal planes. *Note that some blood vessels are visible on these images as dark lines or dots if in cross section.*

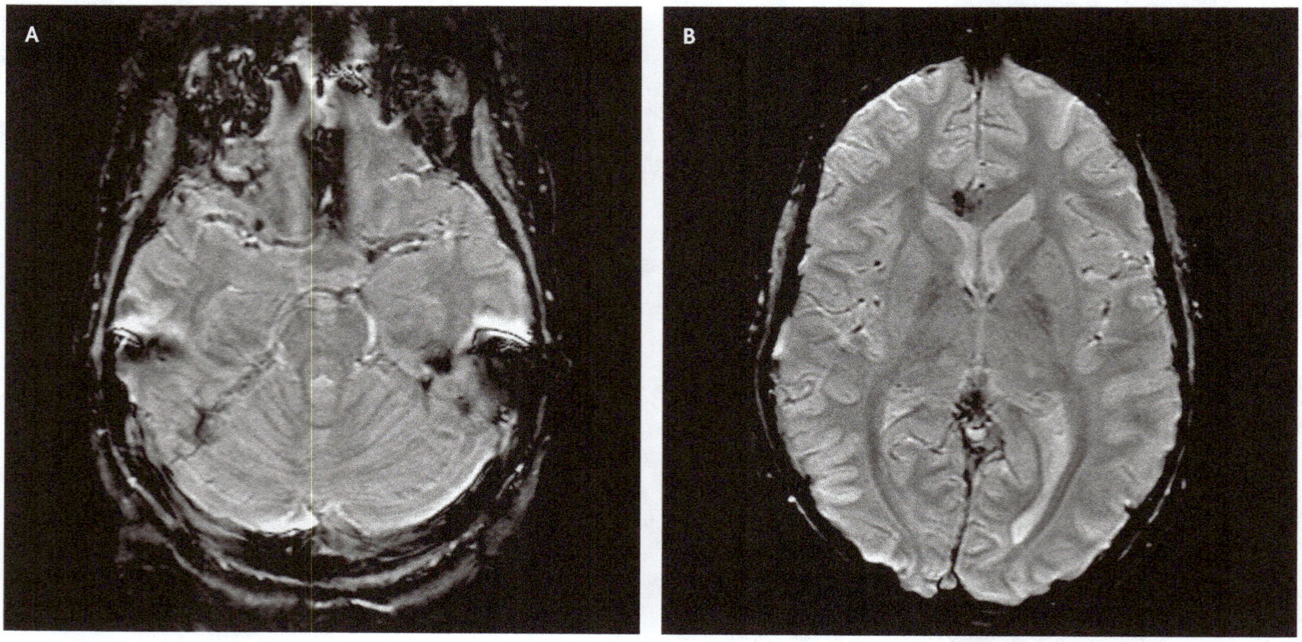

Figures 4-48A and B GRE-EPI patient studies. Note the right frontal hemorrhage just posterior to the orbit on 4-48a, and the corpus callosum bleed on 4-48b. **A:** Right frontal contusion. **B:** Corpus callosum hemorrhage.

Susceptibility-weighted MRI (SWI)

Susceptibility-weighted MRI takes advantage of the high sensitivity to magnetic susceptibility artifacts produced at higher magnet strengths. Although 1.5T scanners can produce SWI images, higher contrast and spatial resolution are evident with 3T or higher-strength magnets. Magnetic susceptibility relates to the degree to which a particular material will become magnetized when exposed to a magnetic field. Paramagnetic substances result in an increased magnetic field, while diamagnetic materials weaken a field. The change in the magnetic field shows up as an artifact on MR images. SWI capitalizes on the fact that some tissues produce much greater susceptibility artifacts on an MRI than others.

SWI images are created through a combination of several imaging techniques. High-resolution 3D T2* gradient echo images are produced with full flow compensation in all three planes. The 3D acquisition allows for the production of thin slices to reduce background interference or signal loss from background inhomogeneities. A phase mask is created and applied to the magnitude images in order to make images with both magnitude and phase contrast.

Minimum intensity projection (mIP) is performed over adjacent slices. Through the combination of these processes and manipulation of specific imaging parameters, images have improved contrast that is exquisitely sensitive to deoxyhemoglobin in venous blood, hemorrhages, and iron storage (Haacke, 2011).

SWI can be used to detect tiny petechial microhemorrhages caused by traumatic diffuse axonal-shear injuries that are often present at the gray–white matter borders but not visible on other imaging sequences (Figures 4-49A and B and 4-50A–C).

REFERENCE

Haacke, E. M. (Ed.) (2011). *Susceptibility weighted imaging in MRI: Basic concepts and clinical applications*. Hoboken, NJ: Wiley-Blackwell.

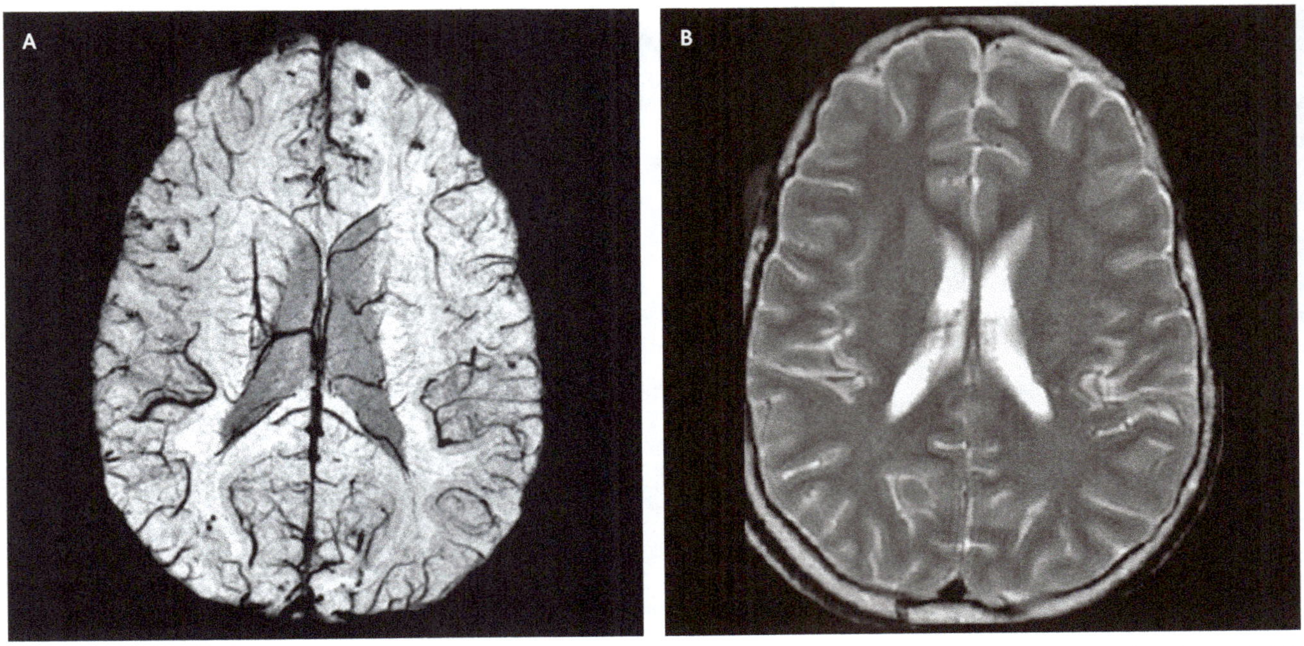

Figures 4-49A and B Traumatic brain injury with petechial hemorrhages shown as black spots on SWI but not visible on the T2-weighted image. **A:** SWI. **B:** T2 weighted image. *Courtesy of E. Mark Haacke, Ph.D.*

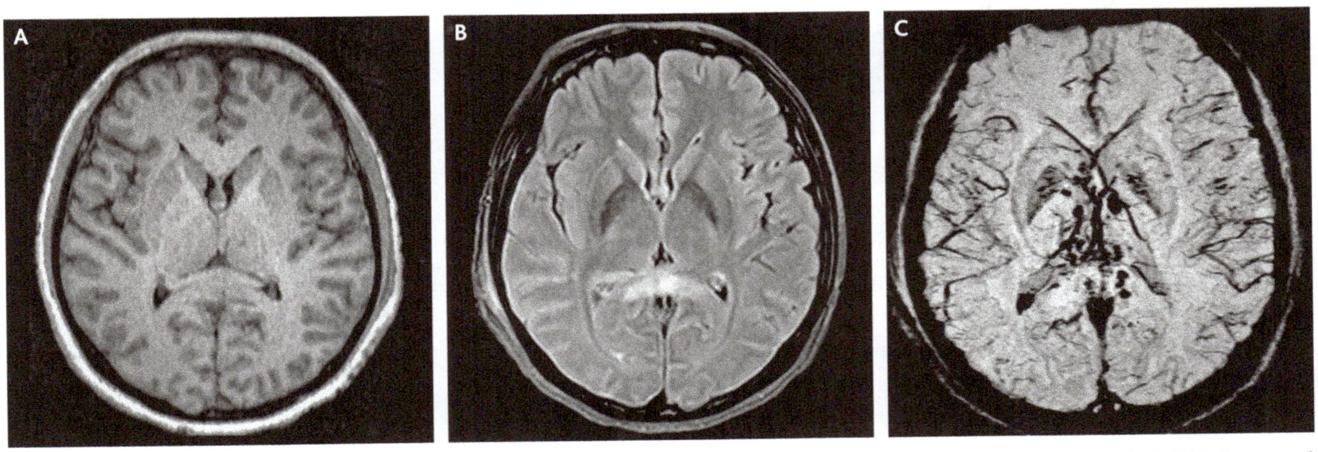

Figures 4-50A–C Traumatic brain injury with significant signs of subcortical microhemorrhage visible only on SWI. **A:** T1. **B:** T2 FLAIR. **C:** SWI. *Courtesy of E. Mark Haacke, Ph.D.*

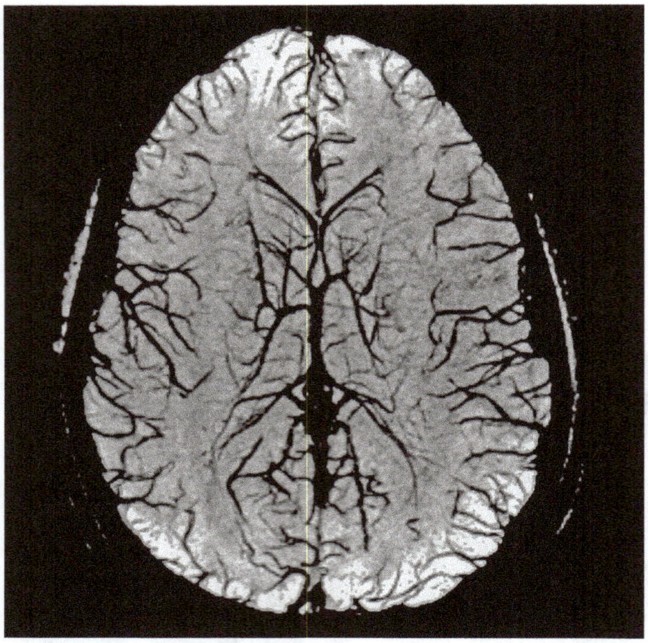

Figure 4-51 SWI showing high-resolution venography of the brain. Courtesy of E. Mark Haacke, Ph.D.

SWI is also helpful in the assessment of vascular anomalies or pathological processes such as stroke, hemorrhages, and vascular dementias. The high iron content present in multiple sclerosis means that SWI can be used to monitor disease severity and progression. Neoplasms with a high degree of vascularity, such as a glioblastoma multiforme (GBM), are dependent on angiogenesis or the rapid development of a vascular system to supply the new tumor cells. SWI can be used to monitor the angiogenic behavior of tumors, giving information on the most active growth regions or the effects of antiangiogenic medications. Because SWI is sensitive to venous blood, it can also be used to produce high-resolution venographies of the brain (Figure 4-51).

Propeller sequences

Propeller sequences are useful for minimizing motion artifact caused by head movement during the acquisition of an image series. Propeller sequences acquire data diagonally and in a concentric manner, much like a propeller blade turning over the brain. Algorithms are then used to realign the images using the edge of the skull to attenuate the effects of head movement within the scanner. Propeller sequences are much better at attenuating lateral movement than front-to-back movements and, as such, are more useful for axial and coronal images than for sagittal images.

When using susceptibility-based sequences such as a GRE, GRE-EPI, or SWI, it is important to remain aware of the limits to the technology. A primary limit concerns the spatial representation of substances that produce susceptibility artifacts. For example, the blooming appearance of blood on GRE images can give the impression that there is more blood present than in actuality. The appearance of a tiny spot of blood, barely visible on a T1 or T2 FLAIR image, may appear large on a GRE image because of the blooming caused by the susceptibility effects. This is not unlike taking a fountain pen and making a tiny mark on a regular sheet of paper and one on a sheet of tissue paper. The same amount of ink on each medium will appear differently: the spot will be very small on regular paper but will appear much larger or "blooming" on the tissue paper.

With the increasing sensitivity of MRI, such as the improvements in susceptibility-based imaging for blood, it is important to consider that some conditions may be detected even without clinical relevance. As technology improves and sensitivity increases for smaller areas of pathology, there will come a point when scanners may detect microscopic features thought to be pathological but which are in fact normal variants or questionably pathological and not clinically meaningful when considering a patient's overall functioning or condition.

Babies are particularly prone to movement during scanning, thus adding a propeller sequence can help ensure that sequences are produced without the detrimental effects of movement. The images in Figure 4-52 illustrate the difference in image clarity resulting from attenuating movement artifacts between the standard sequences (Figures 4-52A and C) and the corresponding propeller sequences (Figures 4-52B and 4-52D).

Fast imaging employing steady state acquisition (FIESTA) sequences

FIESTA sequences are useful when assessing the integrity of the ventricular system or cisterns within the brain, without the need to inject contrast agents into the CSF.

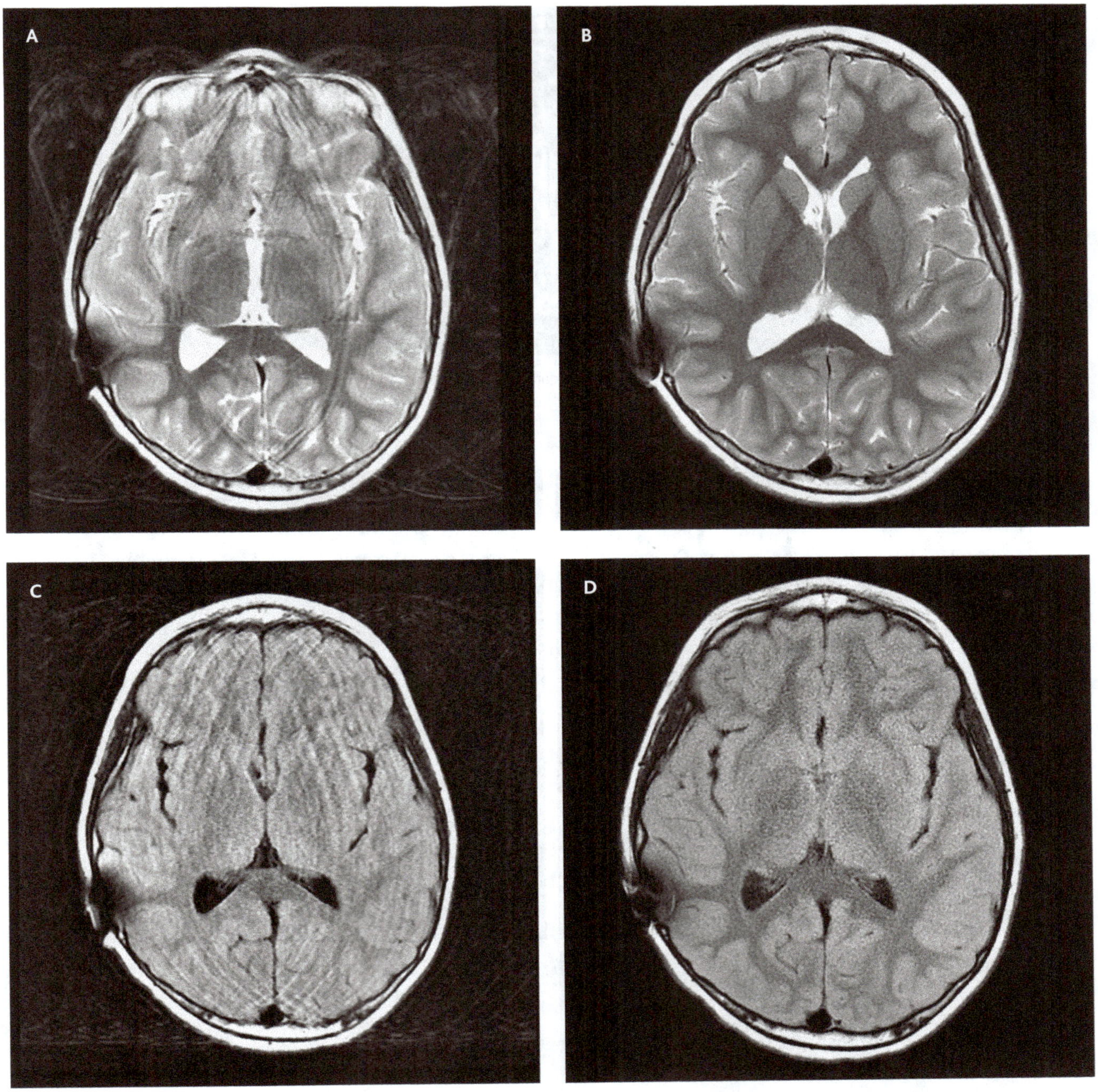

Figure 4-52A–D The ability of propeller sequences to attenuate head movement artifacts during image acquisition. **A:** Standard T2 sequence. **B:** T2 propeller sequence. **C:** Standard T2 FLAIR sequences. **D:** T2 FLAIR propeller sequence.

The images are produced with very short acquisition times using a T2 steady-state sequence. FIESTA sequences provide a strong signal from fluid while attenuating the signal from tissue, providing non-contrast images of the fluid cavities within the brain (Figures 4-53A–C). FIESTA sequences are acquired very rapidly and can be used to monitor flow of CSF through the ventricular system by using a stop-motion system similar to that of old cinema movies.

FIESTA sequences are also useful in assessing cranial nerves and structures of the internal auditory canal (IAC) or any structure surrounded by CSF. Figures 4-54A and B are axial and coronal FIESTA sequences of the IAC showing the VII and VIII cranial nerves (arrows). Figure 4-54C provides visualization of the right and left cochlear structures (arrows) and right and left V cranial nerves (arrows).

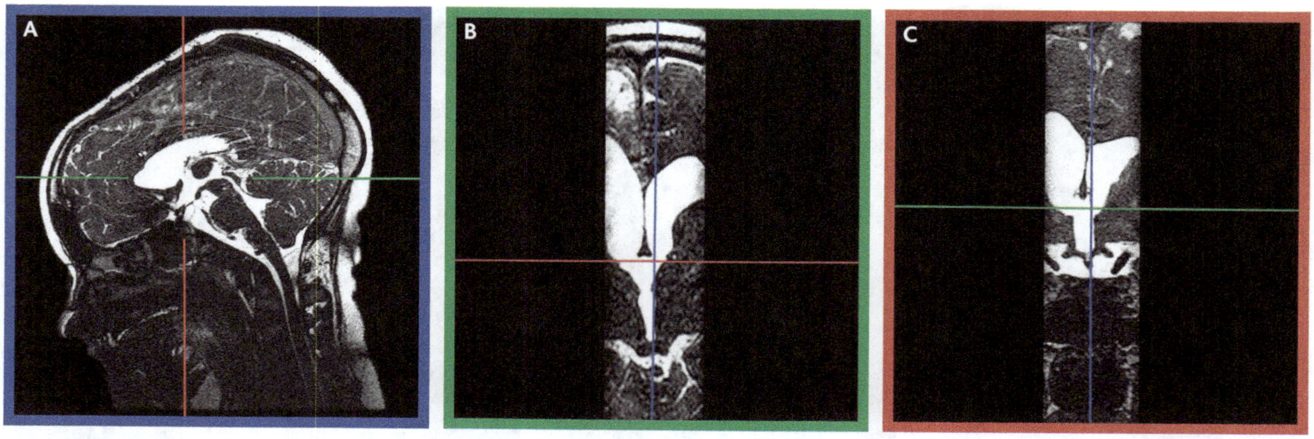

Figure 4-53A–C FIESTA sequences showing the ventricular system on standard width sagittal window (**A**) and narrow axial (**B**) and coronal (**C**) windows focused on the foramena of Monro.

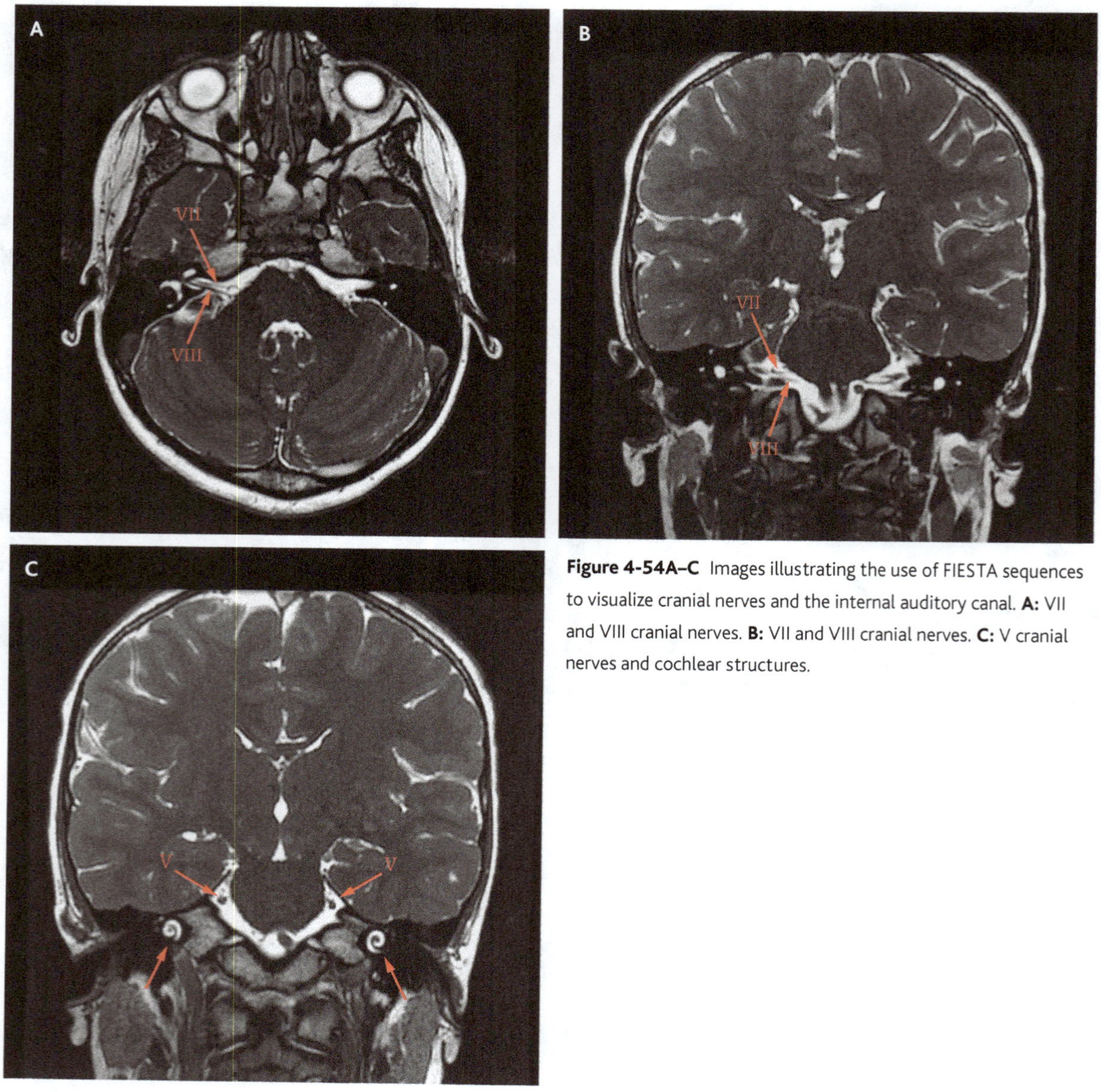

Figure 4-54A–C Images illustrating the use of FIESTA sequences to visualize cranial nerves and the internal auditory canal. **A:** VII and VIII cranial nerves. **B:** VII and VIII cranial nerves. **C:** V cranial nerves and cochlear structures.

MRI—Contrast-Enhanced Imaging

As with use of contrast agents in CT scanning, use of contrast in MRI is helpful for identifying disruption of the blood–brain barrier. Contrast imaging may be used to detect rapid neoplasm growth, infections, or vascular compromise. The most common contrast agents used with MRI are gadolinium based, as gadolinium is both paramagnetic and does not naturally cross the blood–brain barrier. Patient tolerance for gadolinium is excellent, without significant medical complications. Gadolinium shortens the T1 relaxation time of tissue, resulting in increased signal intensity (bright) on T1-weighted images.

Contrast-enhanced MRI is especially useful for identifying high-grade, isointense brain tumors such as a GBM. Often, because of the rapid growth of the tumor, there may be vascular compromise within and around the tumor. Figures 4-55A–C illustrate the appearance of post-surgery tumor regrowth on non-contrast and contrast imaging. The high-grade tumor appears edematous on non-contrast imaging (4-55a and b), but appears as a bright, enhancing ring around the resection cavity on contrast-enhanced imaging (4-55c) . Lack of tumor enhancement can suggest a lower-grade neoplasm, such as a grade II astrocytoma (Figures 4-56A–C).

Contrast enhancement is also useful for visualizing meningeal inflammation due to infection, as evident in the examples of severe meningoencephalitis shown in Figures 4-57A–D and mild viral encephalitis in Figures 4-58A–C.

Contrast enhancement is also useful when attempting to visualize vascular pathologies, such as cavernomas that have a tendency to seep or leak blood. The disruption to the blood-brain barrier around the vascular lesion results in localized enhancement on contrast imaging, as evident around a cavernoma in Figure 4-59A–F.

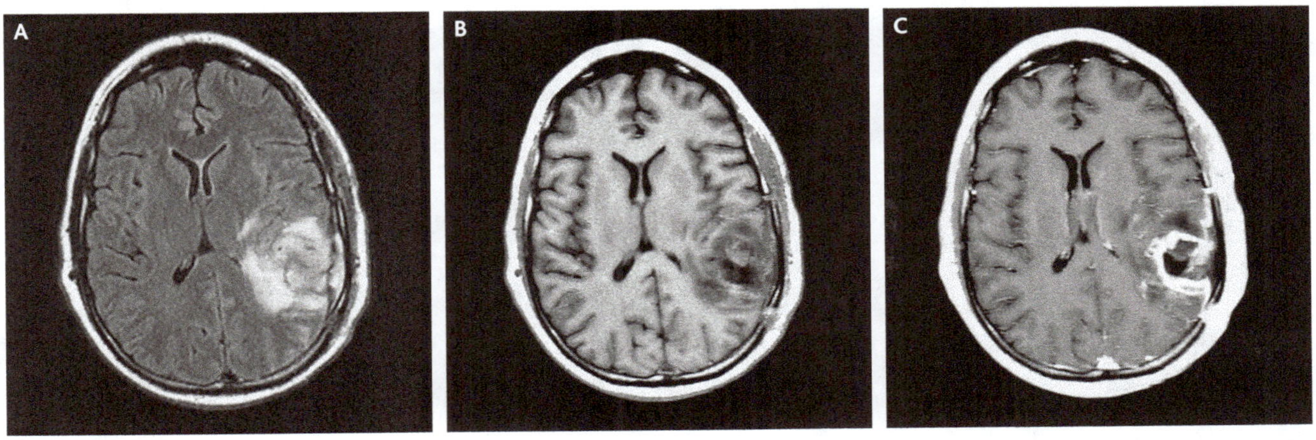

Figures 4-55A–C Non-contrast and contrast enhanced MRI images of an enhancing high-grade astrocytoma—gliobastoma multiforme (GBM). **A:** T2 FLAIR without contrast. **B:** T1 FLAIR without contrast. **C:** T1 FLAIR with contrast.

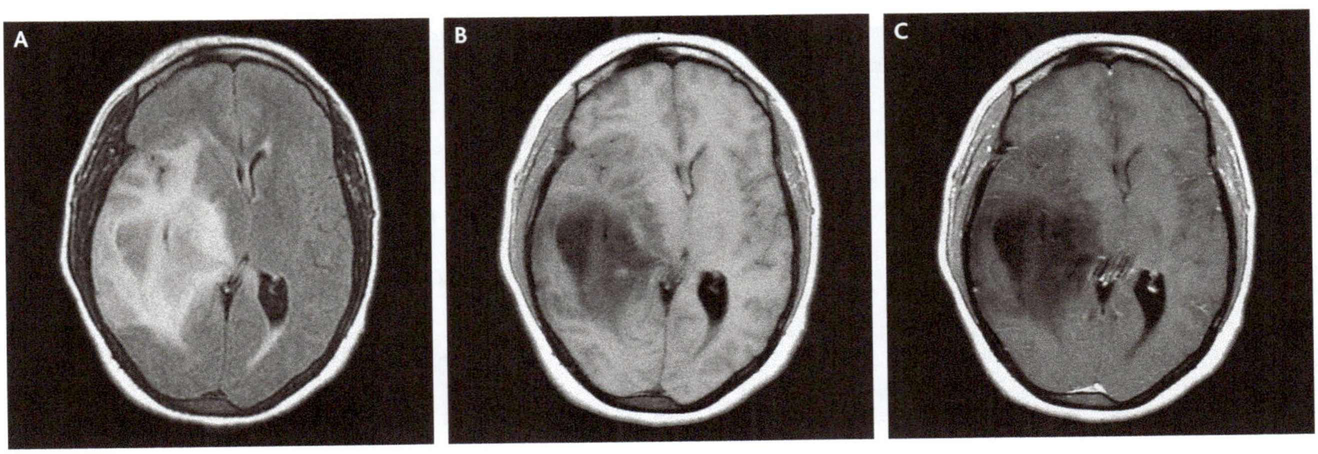

Figures 4-56A–C Non-contrast and contrast enhanced MRI images of a nonenhancing tumor—grade II astrocytoma. **A:** T2 FLAIR without contrast. **B:** T1 FLAIR without contrast. **C:** T1 FLAIR with contrast.

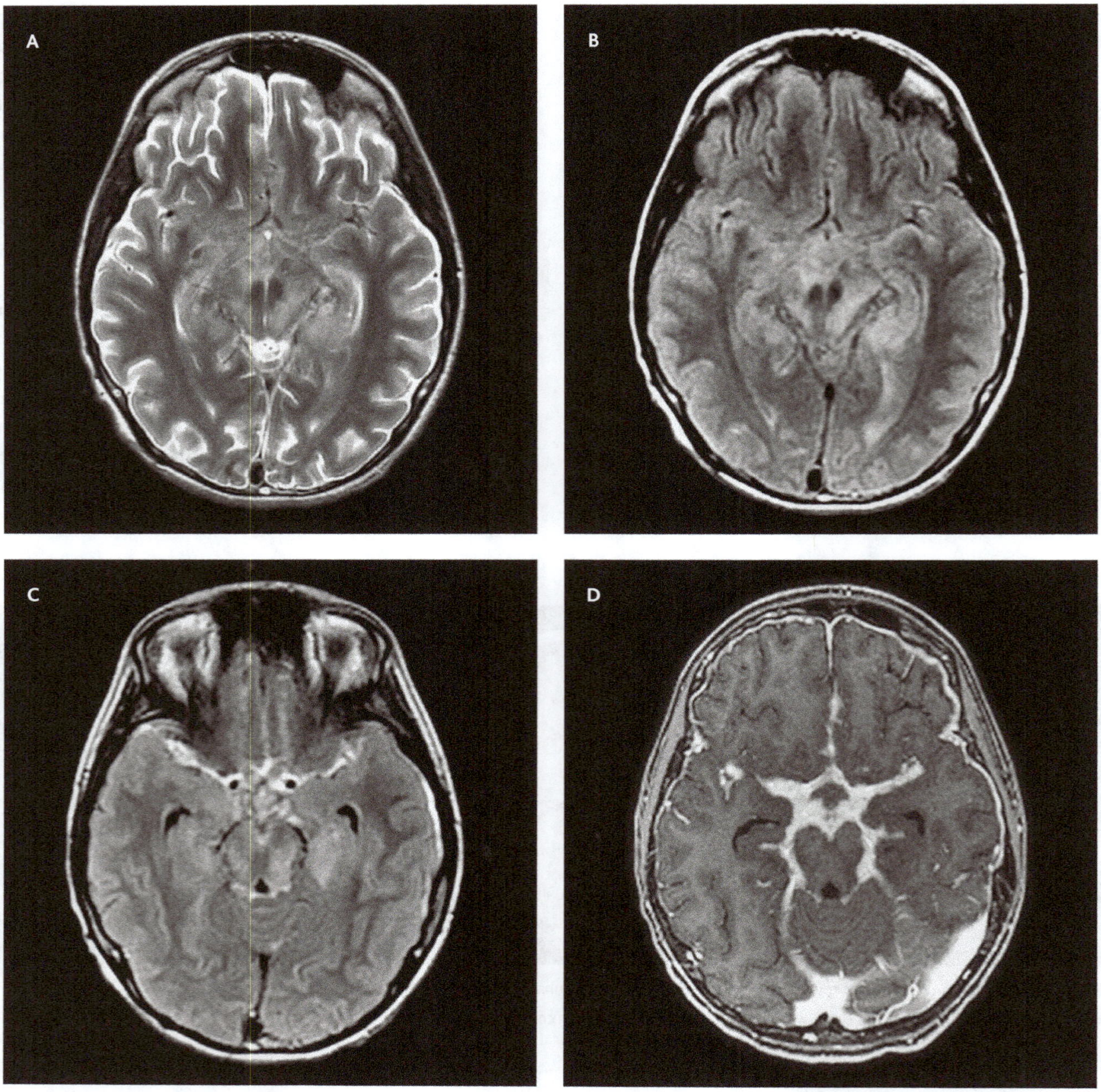

Figures 4-57A–D Non-contrast and contrast enhanced MRI images of severe meningoencephalitis, a combination of meningitis and encephalitis. **A:** T2 without contrast. **B:** T2 FLAIR without contrast **C:** T2 FLAIR with contrast **D:** T1 with contrast.

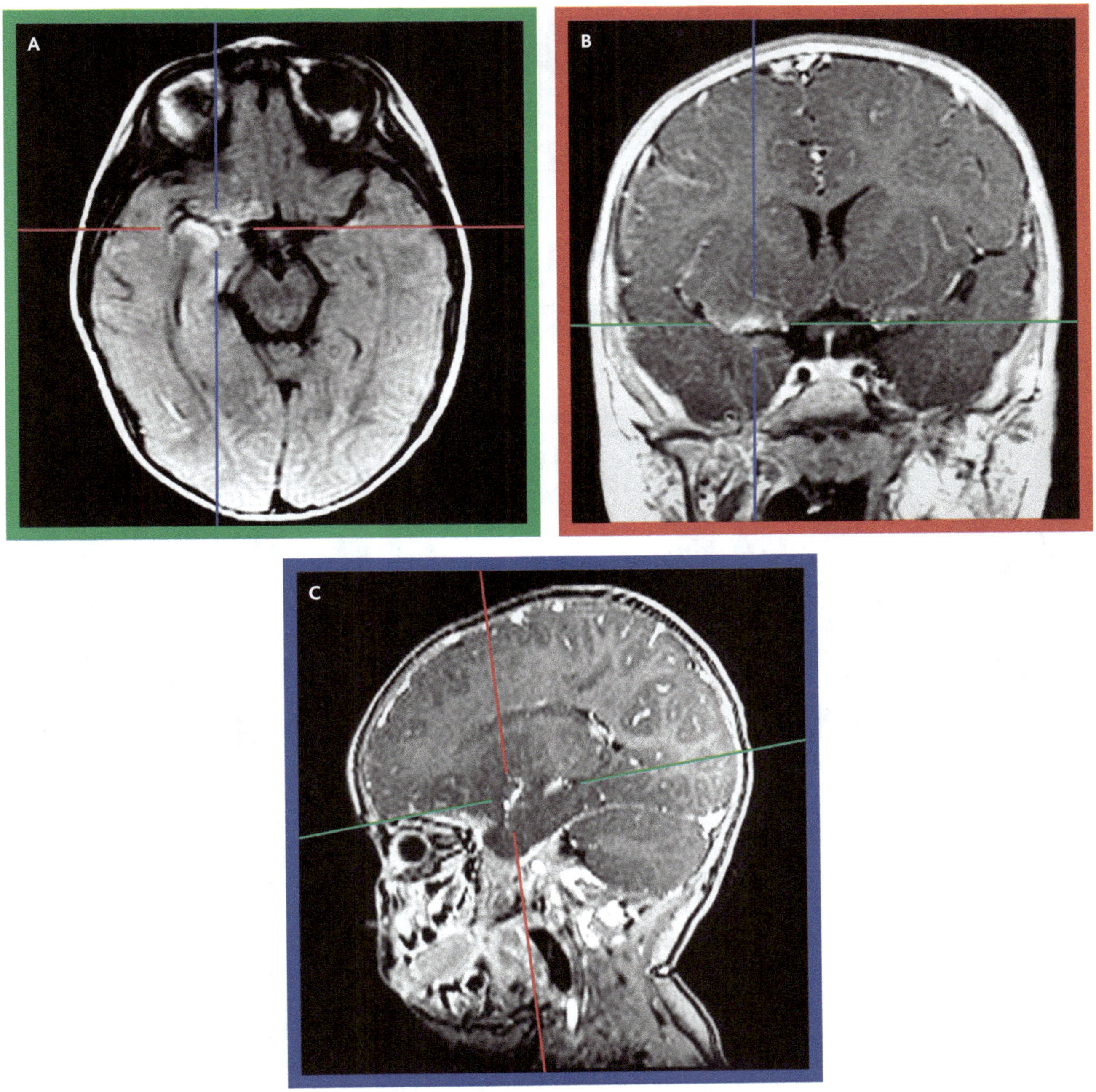

Figures 4-58A–C Contrast enhanced imaging of mild viral encephalitis. **A:** Contrast T2 FLAIR. **B:** Contrast T1. **C:** Contrast T1.

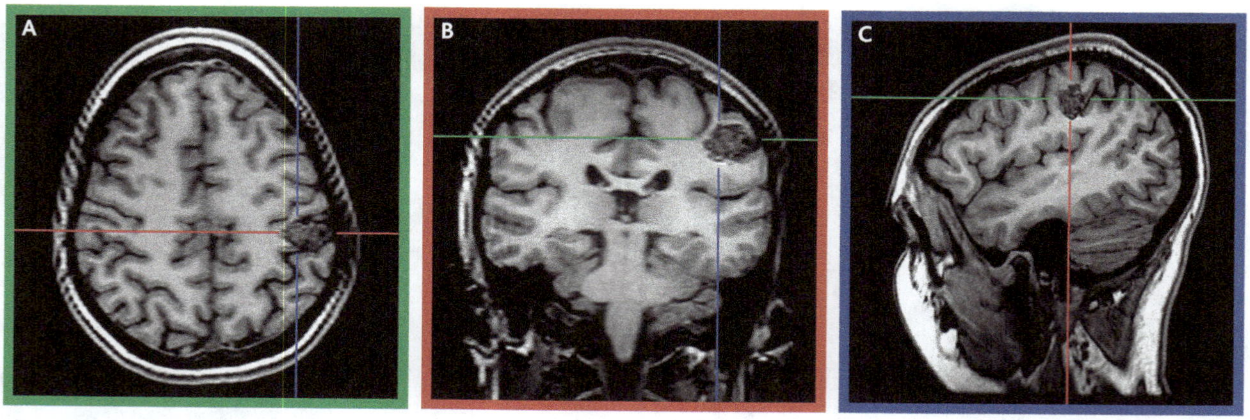

Figures 4-59A–C Left parietal cavernoma—non-contrast FSPGR series.

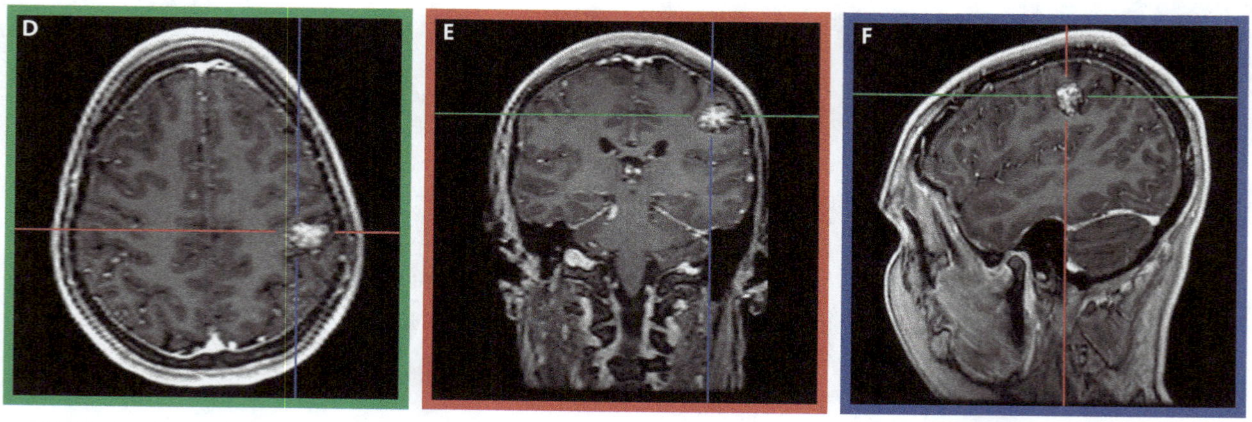

Figures 4-59D–F Left parietal cavernoma—contrast enhanced FSPGR series.

Contrast or Non-Contrast MRI Study

Indications for Gadolinium-Contrast MRI Examinations

- Neoplasms
- Inflammation
- Demyelination
- Infection
- Vascular conditions and malformations
- Only used when there is potential to increase diagnostic utility of an imaging examination

Indications for Non-Contrast MRI Examinations

- For a comparison with contrast images
- Anatomical abnormality or injury
- To assess for malformations involving cortex, nuclei, vessels, or other tissues
- To assess for ischemic tissue after injury, infection, or hypoxia
- Suspected stroke or bleeding
- Seizures, especially partial
- Traumatic head injury (open or closed-head injury)
- Unexplained mental status change

Magnetic Resonance Angiography (MRA)

Magnetic resonance angiography (MRA) is most commonly performed using non-contrast TOF sequences or contrast-enhanced magnetic resonance angiography (CE-MRA). Each method has its benefits and drawbacks, and the decision of which one to use often relates to the clinical question.

One confusing aspect of MRA is that TOF sequences can be used with or without contrast agents. When no contrast agent is used, the sequence is often labeled "TOF" but may also be labeled "MRA." To add to the confusion, contrast-enhanced MRA images may actually be labeled TOF+C, to indicate that a TOF sequence was acquired with the use of a contrast agent. Other times, contrast-enhanced images of the vessels will be labeled "CE-MRA." As noted previously, sequence labels are vendor specific and are often labeled by the technologist, resulting in labels from different centers varying to some degree. It is standard practice to call any MR images of the blood vessels an MRA, irrespective of the sequences or techniques used to acquire them. For the sake of simplicity, in this section we will use *TOF* to signify non-contrast images of the blood vessels and *CE-MRA* for contrast-enhanced images of the blood vessels.

Two- and Three-dimensional time-of-flight sequences (2D/3D-TOF)

Time-of-flight sequences are MR images that can capture the flow characteristics of rapidly moving blood. Usually, gradient echo sequences (GRE) with a short TR are used with acquisition slices perpendicular to the direction of blood flow. While the physics behind TOF sequences is highly complex and beyond the scope of this guide, the simple explanation is that TOF sequences are possible because they can detect the change in signal when blood flows from outside of the image slice and into the imaging plane. When entering the image plane, the blood produces a much higher signal on the GRE sequence, called the "entry slice phenomenon." For the greatest effect, fresh blood has to enter the imaging slice every repetition (TR), which makes the procedure sensitive to blood flow velocity. Direction of blood flow can also be mapped, producing both arteriograms and venograms. 3D-TOF images are acquired within all three planes, allowing for 3D reconstruction and rotation on a computer workstation.

Two-dimensional time-of-flight sequences (2D-TOF) can also be produced, although they have a much lower spatial and contrast resolution than that of 3D-TOF. 2D-TOF images are acquired as a series of very thin image slices that are stacked for reconstruction into pseudo-3D. Because 2D-TOF uses thin slices, it is more sensitive to slow-flowing blood through the slice but has poor resolution for flow along the slice axis.

Because TOF images are dependent on the relatively rapid flow of blood into the image plane, TOF sequences are better for imaging normal blood vessels (Figures 4-60A–C) than aneurysms, thrombi, or hematomas, where blood flow may be slow or even stagnant, turbulent, or in line with the acquisition plane.

TOF images are frequently interpreted using a standard axial image plane (Figure 4-61), with the vessels appearing brighter than surrounding tissue. The use of axial TOF

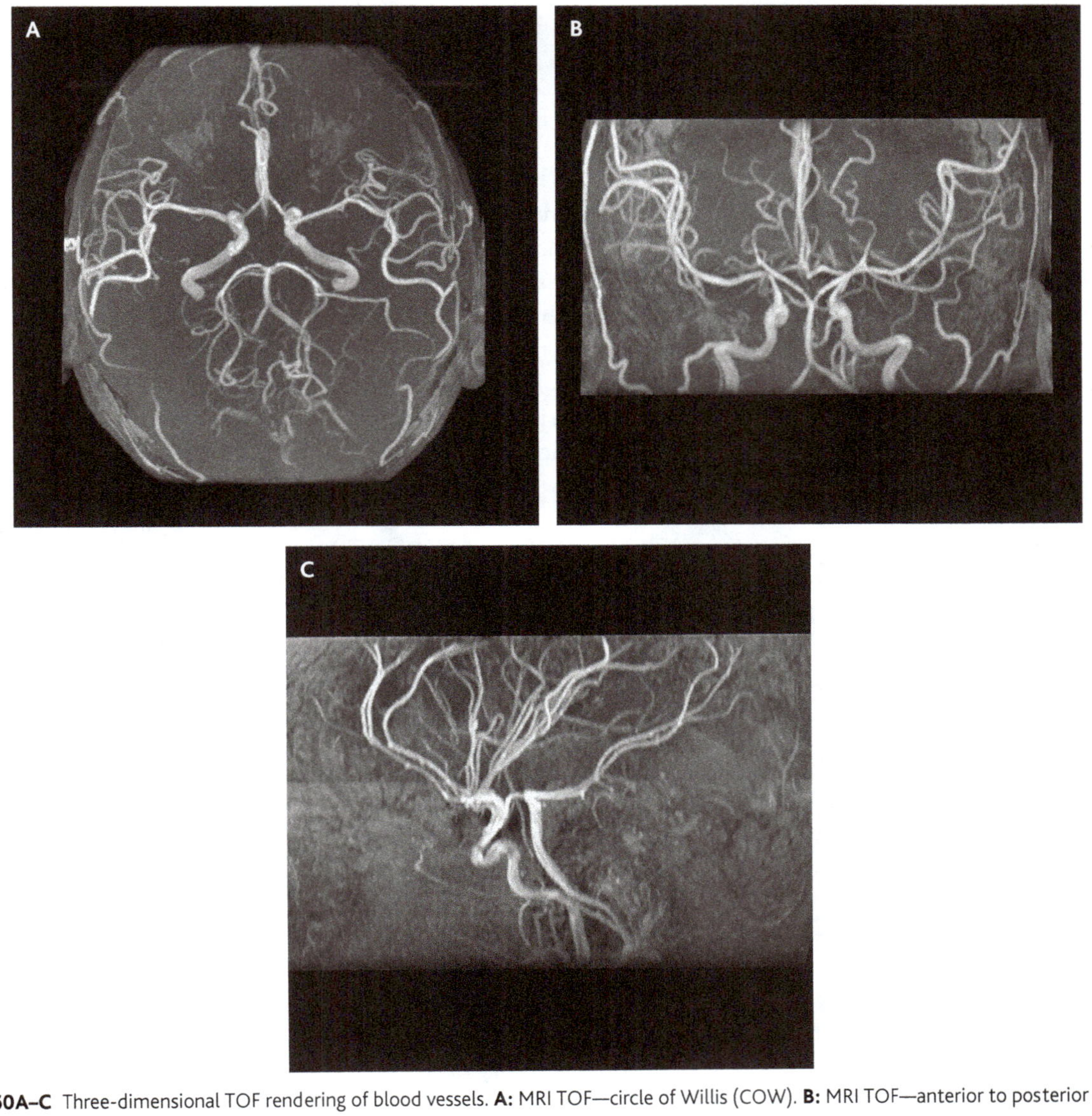

Figures 4-60A–C Three-dimensional TOF rendering of blood vessels. **A:** MRI TOF—circle of Willis (COW). **B:** MRI TOF—anterior to posterior (AP). **C:** MRI TOF—lateral.

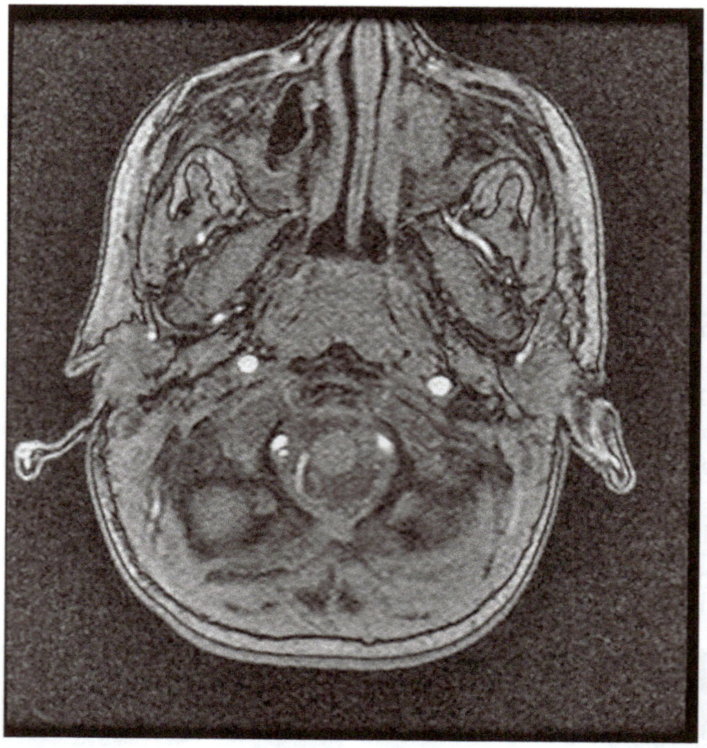

Figure 4-61 TOF displayed on 2D axial plane.

Most TOF images are produced using a 512 × 512 pixel per inch spatial resolution. While it is possible to acquire the same images with a 1024 × 1024 pixel resolution, the sequence requires almost 20 minutes to produce, a long time for a patient to be lying still without moving his or her head unless sedation is used. With TOF images, there appear to be diminishing returns with higher pixel resolution, at least with current 3T technology. Figure 4-62A was acquired using an 18-minute TOF sequence of the author's blood vessels. Not only is there little difference between the 1024 x 1024 image (Figure 4-62A) and another acquired at a 512 × 512 pixel resolution (Figure 4-62B), but the 512 × 512 image appears slightly more detailed and sharper. The long acquisition time increases the signal-to-noise ratio and resolution, but any gains in resolution are likely offset by tiny movements produced over the extended period required to acquire the image.

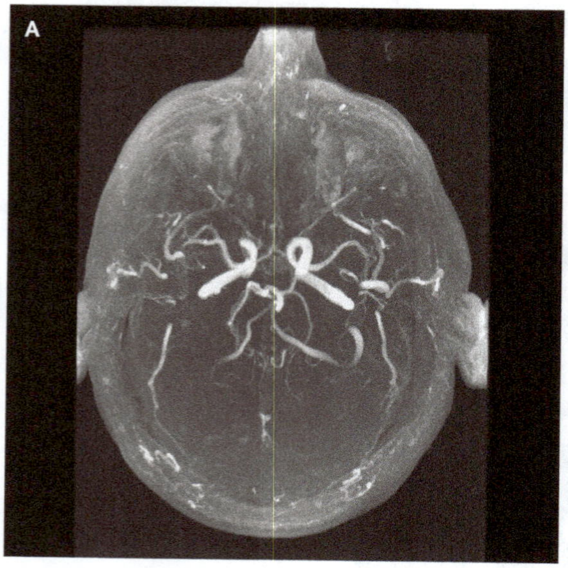

Figure 4-62A 1024 × 1024 ppi TOF image.

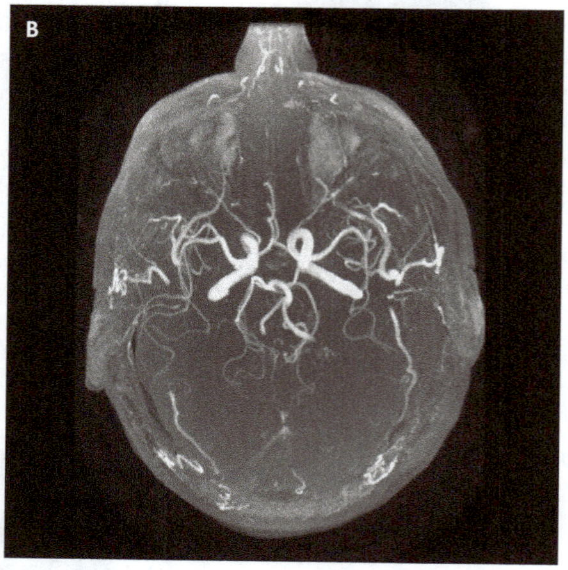

Figure 4-62B 512 × 512 ppi TOF image.

images requires interpretation of vessels on a thin slice, often acquired as a cross section of the vessel. The advantage of using axial TOF slices is that both blood vessels and soft tissues are displayed, providing the viewer with more information than that seen on TOF images presenting only the blood vessels.

Contrast-enhanced magnetic resonance angiograpy or venography (CE-MRA/ CE-MRV)

CE-MRA allows for full 3D visualization of blood vessels (Figures 4-63A–C). A bolus of gadolinium is injected while the scan records the flow of contrast through the vessels. CE-MRA requires a fast 3D gradient echo sequence, which provides four-dimensional recordings of blood flow (three graphic dimensions and one time dimension), or 4D-MRA. Timing the imaging to coincide with the flow of the contrast agent through the veins and sinuses enables the production of magnetic resonance venograms (CE-MRV). Use of the contrast agent improves the signal-to-noise ratio and the ability to differentiate vessels from background tissue.

CE-MRA and CE-MRV do not have the same flow concerns as in TOF imaging and are much better at differentiating pools of stagnant or turbulent blood, seen in aneurysms, large bleeds, or thrombotic conditions.

The combination of CE-MRA and CE-MRV can produce some remarkable images of the brain vasculature involving both the arterial and venous blood vessels (Figures 4-64A and B).

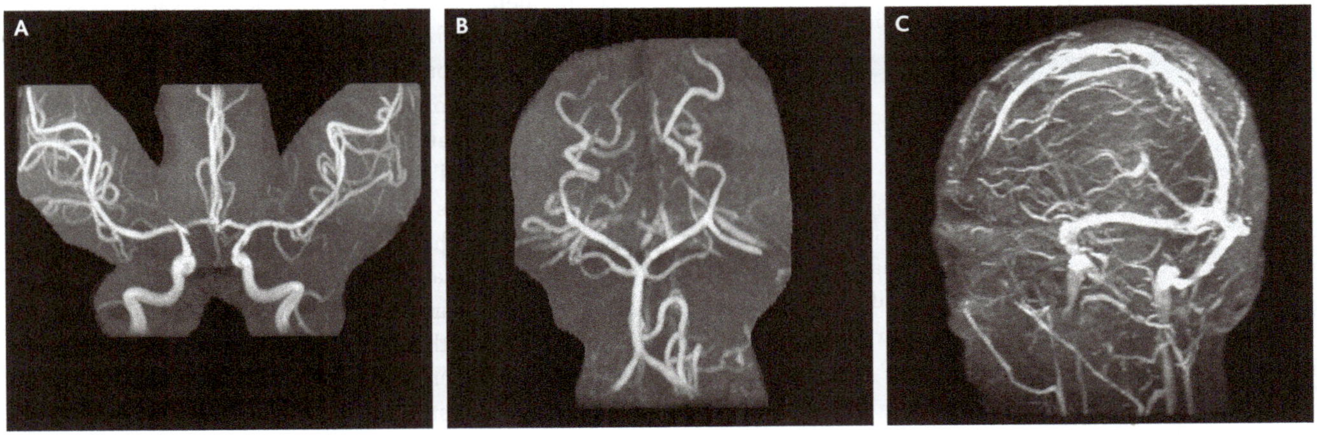

Figures 4-63A–C Contrast-enhanced MRA and MRV images. **A:** CE-MRA anterior vessels: internal carotid artery (ICA) and anterior (ACA) and middle cerebral (MCA) arteries. **B:** CE-MRA posterior vessels: vertebral, basilar, and posterior cerebral (PCA) arteries. **C:** CE-MRV: veins and sinuses.

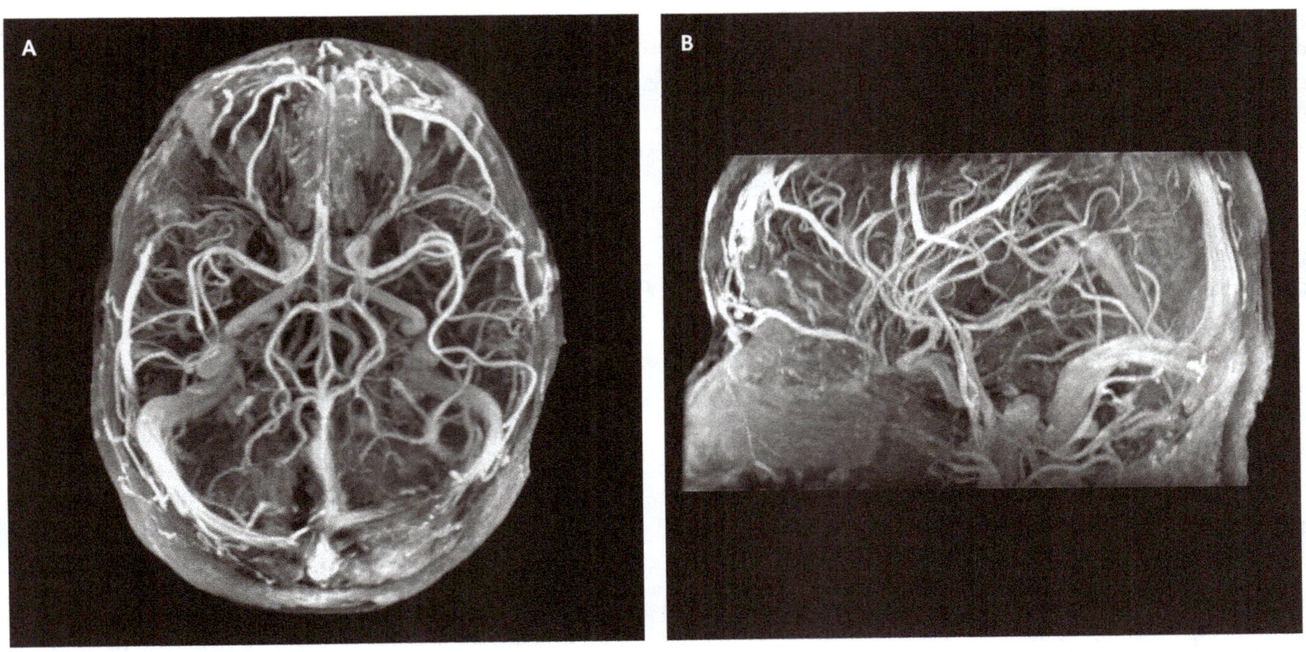

Figures 4-64A and B Contrast-enhanced combined MRA and MRV images. **A:** CE-MRA+MRV: arteries and veins, axial view. **B:** CE-MRA+MRV: arteries and veins, lateral view.

Aneurysms
TOF sequences may not show all aneurysms, and under some conditions, brain aneurysms may not be visible using TOF sequences. It becomes more difficult to visualize aneurysms with TOF sequences when they have slow or turbulent blood flow or are in-plane with the image axis. For aneurysms, contrast-enhanced CTA or MRA may be preferred, as flow is less of an issue and the lesion can be viewed in three dimensions, thus avoiding obscuration by other tissue and making full visualization possible. Traditional angiography or, more recently, digital subtraction angiography with transfemoral catheterization is also an option, but these modalities are more invasive and produce additional patient discomfort and risk of medical complications.

Hybrid Brain Imaging

Hybrid brain imaging techniques are sometimes considered static and at other times, functional. They enable the assessment of brain processes such as diffusion, perfusion, or metabolism, although they are not correlated with a specific activity, or "function."

Diffusion-Weighted MRI (DWI)

Until the last decade, CT scans were seen as the gold standard for assessing strokes, and for many situations, CT remains highly useful in this regard. However, diffusion imaging has enabled the visualization of effects of strokes and hypoxic injury at the molecular level, within the first hour following ischemia. Other applications of diffusion imaging include the assessment of neoplasms, cerebral lymphomas, cysts, infections, inflammatory and degenerative conditions, and traumatic injuries.

The basic determinants of how a diffusion image appears relate to the micromovement of water molecules at the cellular level. In large spaces, the diffusion, or movement, of water molecules follows the principle of random Brownian motion and can be described as isotropic (Greek, *iso* = equal, *tropos* = direction). Within the brain, water molecules can move either randomly in all directions, as when in the ventricles, or in a more restricted manner due to a barrier caused by cell membranes, proteins, fibers, macromolecules, etc. Diffusion imaging enables the assessment of water movement within the brain through the use of diffusion gradients to record differences in water mobility. In general, the faster the water molecules diffuse or move, the weaker (darker) the signal will be on the image; the more restricted the diffusion of water molecules, the stronger (brighter) the appearance on a diffusion-weighted image. Restricted diffusion or anisotropic diffusion can result from a variety of pathological process. For most pathologies, DWI imaging will appear hyperintense or brighter, although with severe damage and loss of the structural integrity of brain tissue and lacuna infarction, the area may appear hypointense or darker (see discussion that follows for more details regarding the appearance of pathology on diffusion imaging).

Apparent Diffusion Coefficient (ADC) Maps

Apparent diffusion coefficient maps are independent of the T2 component on a DWI image, allowing them to be used to clarify whether hyperintensity on a DWI image is due to reduced diffusion or T2 shine-through. Diffusion sequences are constructed on the basis of the relationship between the direction of water movement and a particular gradient designed to record this. Diffusion gradients are applied in multiple directions and multiple times to derive a full picture of diffusion that takes place in three dimensions. The ADC map is calculated using multiple diffusion sequences and provides a quantitative measure of water mobility. The advantage is that this quantitative measure is not affected by the T2 component and corresponds only to the degree of water mobility. Restricted diffusion appears hypointense or darker than normal tissue on an ADC map, which has the opposite appearance to that of a DWI sequence.

Exponential apparent diffusion coefficient (EADC) maps are also available and have the opposite contrast to that seen on ADC maps (restricted diffusion = bright, excessive diffusion = black). It may be helpful to attend only to the ADC map, not the EADC map, as a primary use of the ADC map is to rule out T2 shine-through, which is not as simple to do with EADC images.

Caution is warranted when assessing pathology through only diffusion-weighted images; you should always review DWI in combination with other sequences, especially an ADC sequence, if available.

Diffusion images are based on T2 sequences that are sensitized to the effects of diffusion through the use of special gradients. Therefore, the appearance of a diffusion-weighted image will depend on both the T2 component and a diffusion component. Put simply, anything that will cause T2 hyperintensity or a bright appearance on a T2 image may also make the same area appear bright on a DWI image. It is as if the brightness from the T2 component "shines through" the DWI sequences; this phenomena has been termed "T2 shine-through." When reviewing DWI sequences with a bright appearance, the area of interest may be from T2 prolongation resulting in hyperintensity, restricted diffusion, or both.

As a general guide, when the bright appearance on DWI is either caused by T2 prolongation or restricted diffusion alone, the tissue appears less bright than if both processes were present. If both T2 prolongation and restricted diffusion are present, there is a cumulative affect on the DWI, and the areas can look "light-bulb bright" or "blown-out," depending on your contrast settings for the image. Conversely, T2 shine-through and a low signal on the DWI (i.e., from an old stroke) may cancel each other out, resulting in the tissue appearing isodense or having the same density as surrounding tissue. Judging the "brightness" of a scan is not a reliable method of differentiating these two processes, especially when the image is viewed on a computer screen that allows adjustments to contrast and brightness.

As a rule, if you see hyperintensity or a bright appearance on a DWI image, you should also view the T2 or T2 FLAIR sequences and the ADC map. Review of T2 or T2 FLAIR sequences will determine whether shine-through may be a factor. If there is no hyperintensity on the T2 or T2 FLAIR images, then there is nothing to shine through to the DWI, and the bright appearance on DWI is likely the result of disrupted diffusion. If, however, the area is bright on T2 or T2 FLAIR sequences, then review of ADC sequences is required to determine whether the bright area on DWI is shine-through or disrupted diffusion; a darker appearance on ADC will confirm that the bright area on DWI is due to disrupted diffusion. It is a good idea to get into the habit of viewing the ADC map *every time* you review a DWI image, if it is available. Some centers do not have systems that can produce ADC maps, in which case, caution is warranted when interpreting DWI images. Where available, throughout this guide both DWI and ADC maps will be presented together to help you form the habit of viewing both images during your workflow.

Note: Diffusion-weighted images are prone to susceptibility artifacts from bone or metal, and so a bright appearance close to bone or metallic objects should be interpreted with caution.

Temporal Changes to Diffusion Images

When viewing diffusion images, it is important to take into account the changes in diffusion that can take place over time with injury to the brain, especially an ischemic event. Within minutes of an ischemic insult to the brain and up to a few days thereafter, there can be evidence of cytotoxic edema and reduced diffusion on DWI (appears bright) and ADC (appears dark). After a few days, the initial cytotoxic edema subsides, with a gradual increase in vasogenic edema, especially within the white matter, and eventually cell membrane breakdown. These conditions can result in a transient change in the appearance on DWI and ADC suggesting recovery of damage tissue. However, there may not be improvement in the extent and severity of pathology commensurate with the improved appearance of diffusion sequences. Any change from cytotoxic edema to encephalomalacia with loss of cell structure will result in a transition from restricted diffusion to unrestricted diffusion, with a period in between when diffusion may appear more normal on imaging. During this period, imaging may suggest recovery in the region, but this is an artifact of the changes in diffusion over time. During this intermediate period from restricted to unrestricted diffusion, the area of interest can appear bright on DWI images because of T2 shine-through, but the ADC images can appear neutral or isointense. With ongoing cell breakdown, encephalomalacia, and development of lacuni, the diffusion images may begin to suggest increased water mobility or increased isotropic diffusion in excess of that which is normal for brain tissue. During this stage, DWI images may appear hypointense, isointense, or hyperintense, depending on the relative effects of T2 shine-through and the state of diffusion. Eventually, the DWI images may appear hypointense or dark, reflecting isotropic or random water movement. Because ADC maps are not affected by T2 shine-through, the appearance of the lesion can progress from hypointense (dark) to isointense (neutral) during the intermediate stage, to hyperintense (bright) as the diffusion becomes isotropic and unrestrained by natural barriers such as cell walls. Monitoring the changes in the appearance of DWI and ADC images can be helpful when assessing the age of an ischemic insult or when determining long-term prognosis.

The interpretation of diffusion sequences can seem complex, but by following a few basic guidelines, it will become quickly apparent that diffusion-based images are very useful in diagnosing pathology to the brain. It is important to recognize that there are some exceptions to the rules presented below. For example, if there is hyperintensity on T2 and DWI, and the ADC map appears isointense, this may be explained by T2 shine-through or by the age of the lesion, with the lesion being too recent to result in changes to the ADC map.

How to Use DWI and ADC Maps to Assess Diffusion

A. With or without T2 hyperintensity: If the area of interest on the DWI sequence has increased signal (bright) and the ADC map has a reduced signal (dark), this suggests restricted or anisotropic diffusion.

Neal was diagnosed with encephalitis. His T2 and T2 FLAIR brain scans showed some hyperintensity within the right hemisphere just posterior to the splenium of the corpus callosum (Figures 4-65A and B). On the DWI image, the same area was bright, suggesting either restricted diffusion or T2 shine-through (Figure 4-65C). Because the area on the ADC map was darker than normal tissue, it was clear that this was not T2 shine-through and was restricted diffusion (Figure 4-65D).

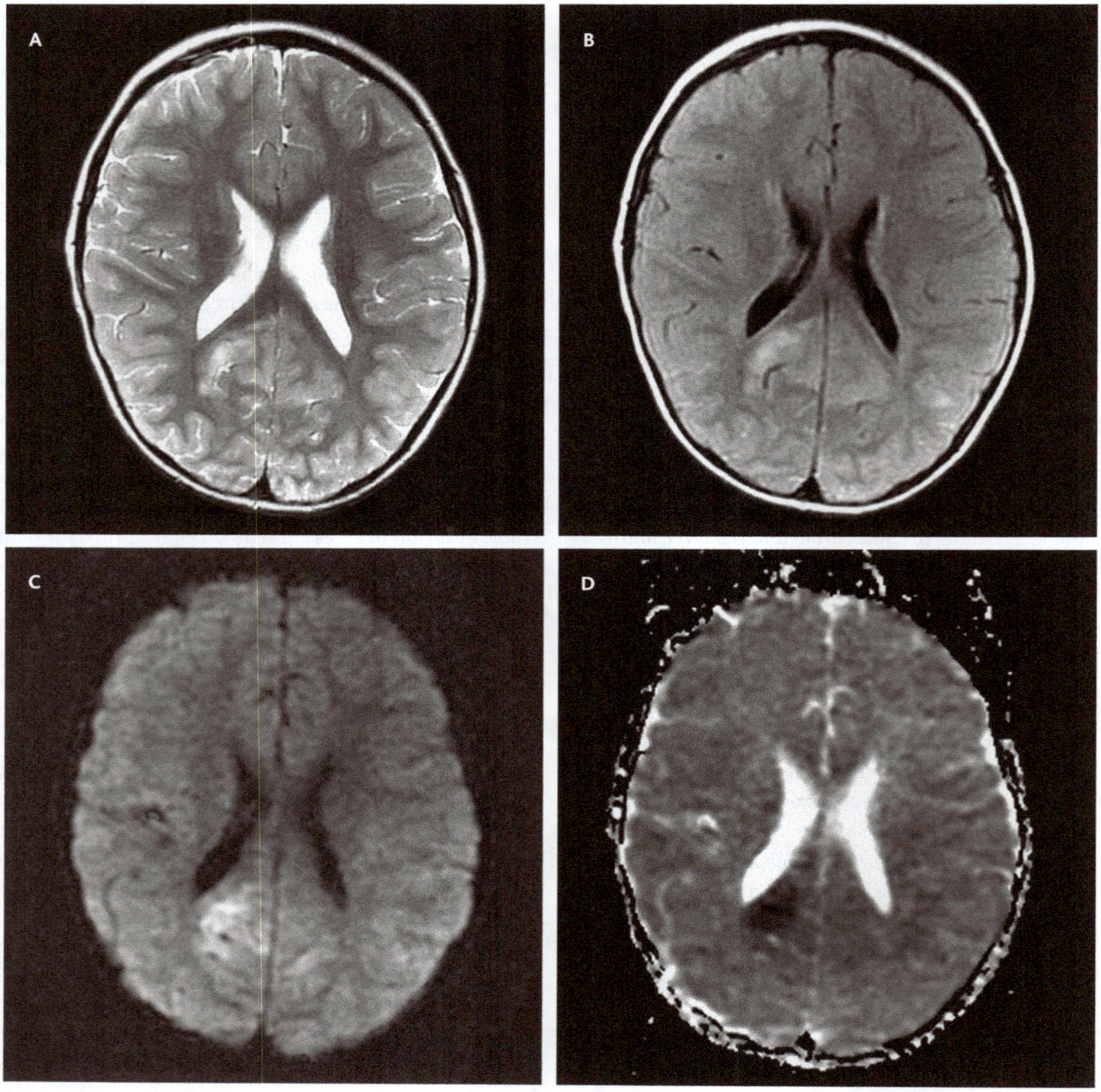

Figure 4-65A–D Brain imaging for Neal suggesting restricted or anisotropic diffusion in the right hemisphere just posterior to the corpus callosum. **A:** T2. **B:** T2 FLAIR. **C:** DWI. **D:** ADC.

B. With T2 hyperintensity: If the area of interest on the DWI sequence is also hyperintense (bright), but the same region does not appear hypointense (dark) on ADC, diffusion may not be restricted, and the bright appearance could be T2 shine-through. However, it is also possible that the appearance of the region on the ADC image will change over time, commensurate with subtle changes in diffusion. If the ADC remains isointense over time, the bright appearance on DWI is more likely shine-through than evidence of ischemia.

Mateo suffered bilateral thalamic and basal ganglia damage due to an embolic stroke. T2 hyperintensity on standard and FLAIR images was most notable within the left thalamic region (Figure 4-66A and B). The DWI image had a bright appearance in the left thalamic region, suggesting disrupted diffusion and hypoxic injury to the tissue (Figure 4-66C). However, this bright appearance on DWI may have been related to T2 shine-through and not to disrupted diffusion, as suggested by the isointense appearance (similar to normal tissue) of the left thalamus on ADC imaging (Figure 4-66D). To more accurately assess the integrity of the left thalamic region, follow-up diffusion imaging would have been helpful. Often, follow-up imaging is not always necessary, as a patient's clinical presentation can be helpful in confirming infarction, especially for

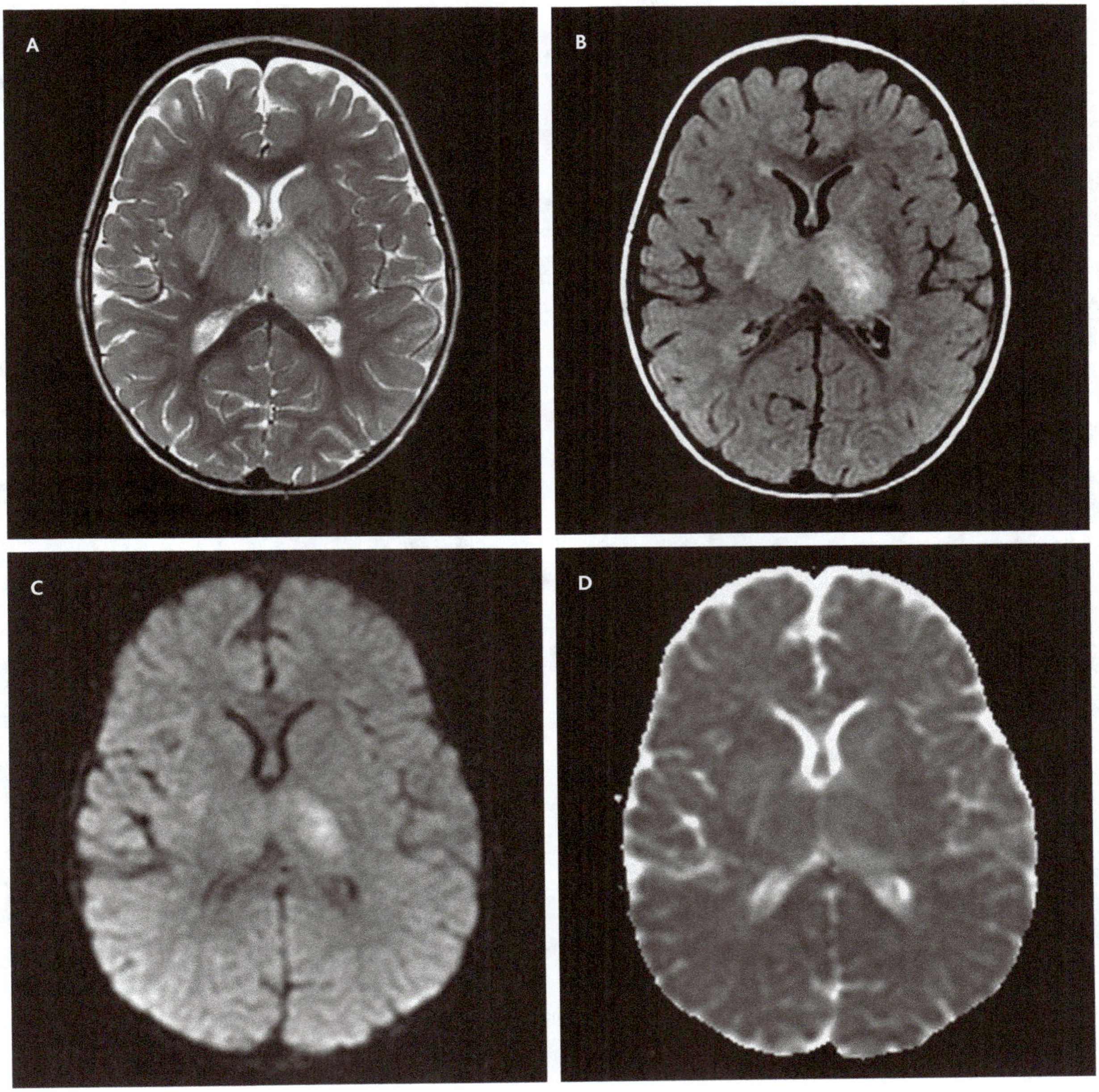

Figure 4-66A–D Brain imaging for Mateo suggesting possible T2 shine-through, most evident in the region of the left thalamus. **A:** T2. **B:** T2 FLAIR. **C:** DWI. **D:** ADC.

a focal region or specific anatomical structure such as the thalamus.

C. With T2 hyperintensity: If there is a bright appearance on both the DWI and the ADC map, this likely represents vasogenic edema, especially if the region of increased brightness or hyperintensity is within the white matter.

Several days following a severe traumatic brain injury, Conner's brain scans suggested vasogenic edema within the white matter of the right orbital and medial frontal lobe. Note the bright appearance or hyperintensity within the right medial frontal region on T2 and T2 FLAIR images (Figures 4-67A and B) in addition to corresponding hyperintensities on DWI and ADC (Figures 4-67C and D).

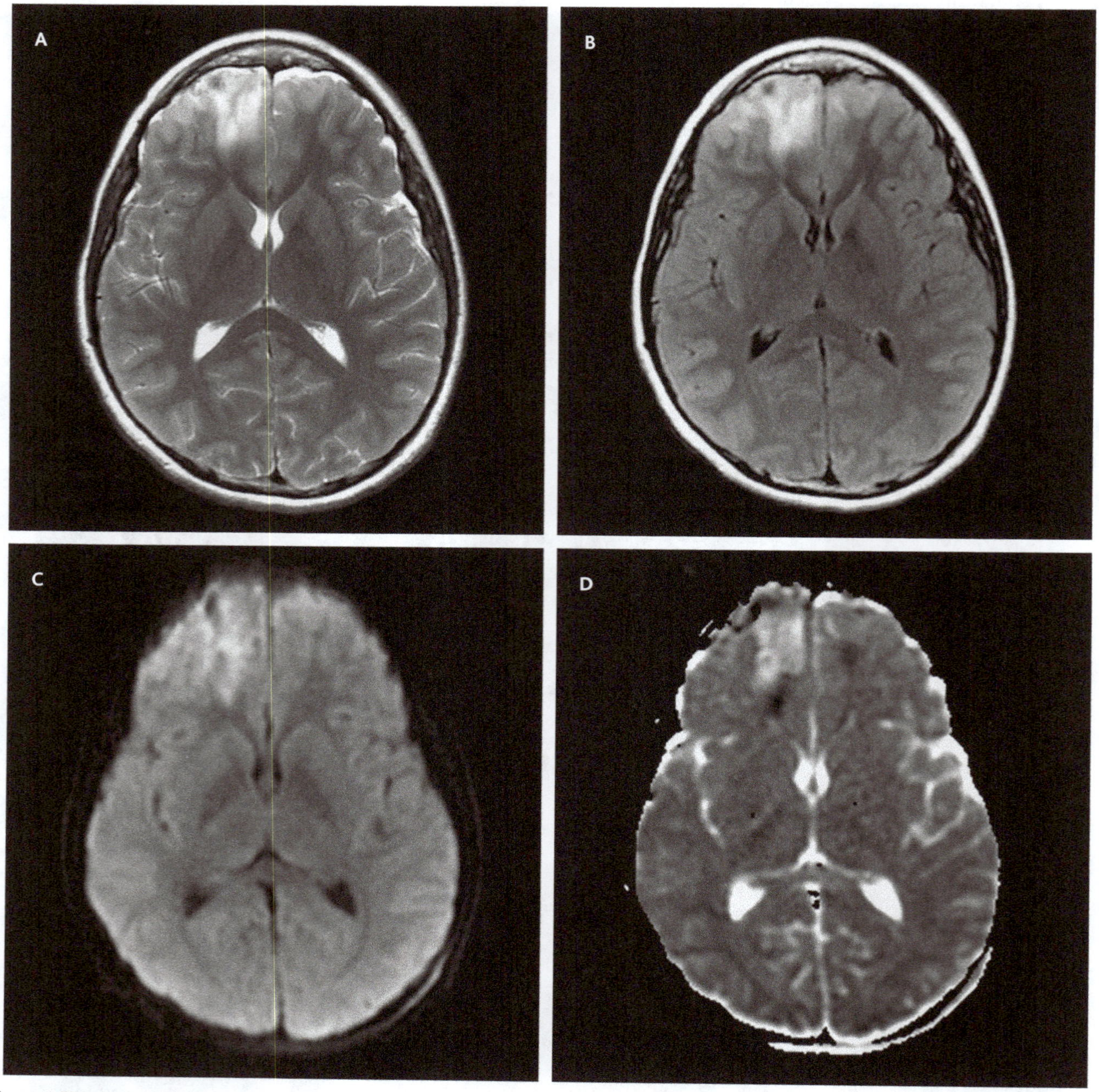

Figure 4-67A–D Conner's brain scans suggesting vasogenic edema, most evident in the right medial frontal region. **A:** T2. B: T2 FLAIR. **C:** DWI. **D:** ADC.

D. Areas of late-stage encephalomalacia with development of lacuna infarctions due to atrophy can appear dark on DWI and bright on ADC, a sign of increased or isotropic (unrestricted) diffusion.

Stephanie experienced progressive damage to her occipital lobes due to encephalitis. Two months following the onset of the encephalitis, Stephanie's diffusion scans suggested loss of tissue within the right hemisphere just posterior to the splenium of the corpus callosum. The region deteriorated into a lacuna infarction, or hole, in the tissue, filled with CSF. Similar to the water within the ventricles, the water within an area of atrophy due to infarction is best described as having isotropic or unrestricted diffusion. On MRI, this is suggested by the bright appearance on T2 and dark appearance on T2 FLAIR (Figures 4-68A and B), with a dark appearance on DWI (Figure 4-68C), and bright appearance on ADC (Figure 4-68D). Because lacunae in the brain parenchyma allow unrestricted and random water movement (isotropic diffusion), the appearance matches that of the ventricles: bright on T2, dark on T2 FLAIR, dark on DWI, and bright on ADC.

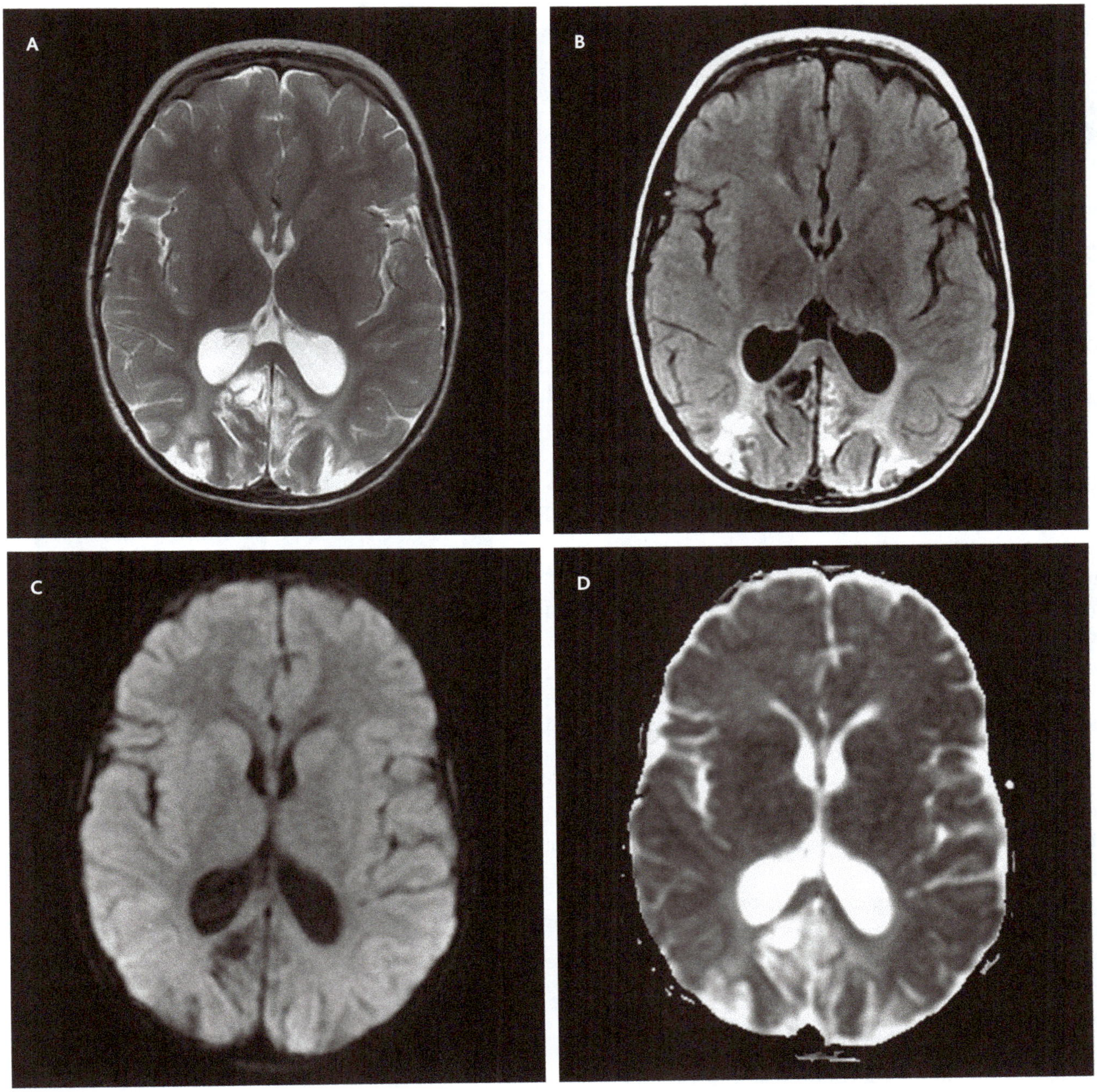

Figure 4-68A–D Stephanie's brain scans showing the appearance of a lacuna infarction on T2 weighted and diffusion imaging. **A:** T2. **B:** T2 FLAIR. **C:** DWI. **D:** ADC.

Summary of T2, DWI, and ADC Appearance for Different Types of Diffusion or Pathology

DIFFUSION/ PATHOLOGY	T2	T2 FLAIR	DWI	ADC
Restricted (anisotropic)	Bright or neutral	Bright or neutral	Bright	Dark
Unrestricted (isotropic)	Bright	Dark	Dark	Bright
Cytotoxic edema	Bright or neutral	Bright or neutral	Bright	Dark
Vasogenic edema	Bright	Bright	Bright	Bright
Possible T2 shine-through	Bright	Bright	Bright	Neutral

Diffusion Tensor Imaging—Fractional Anisotropy and Tractography

Diffusion tensor imaging (DTI) is based on the directional component of diffusion. When water molecules are unrestrained by barriers, the direction of movement is isotropic or random. However, if there is a barrier restricting movement, there will be an imbalance between the amount of movement against or across the barrier and the movement away from or along the barrier. In order to fully evaluate the various directional components of diffusion, many acquisition planes must be recorded, with the greater number of planes producing the clearest images. With multiple acquisition planes, computer algorithms can be used to determine the fractional anisotropy (FA) of water diffusion. *Fractional anisotropy* is a value that relates to the degree of random diffusion, with the values ranging from zero, for completely random or isotropic, to 1, for movement in only one direction or anisotropic. DTI can provide information regarding the direction, size, source, and destination of axon pathways, in addition to the integrity of the axonal wall.

When water diffusion is random or isotropic, the signal is attenuated and appears dark or black on the image. When water diffusion is restricted, it appears brighter on the image; the brightness is dependent on the FA value or degree of restriction. The FA values can also be presented on color-coded FA maps, with the colors representing the degree to which the area has diffusion that is isotropic (red) or anisotropic (blue) (Figures 3-69A–C).

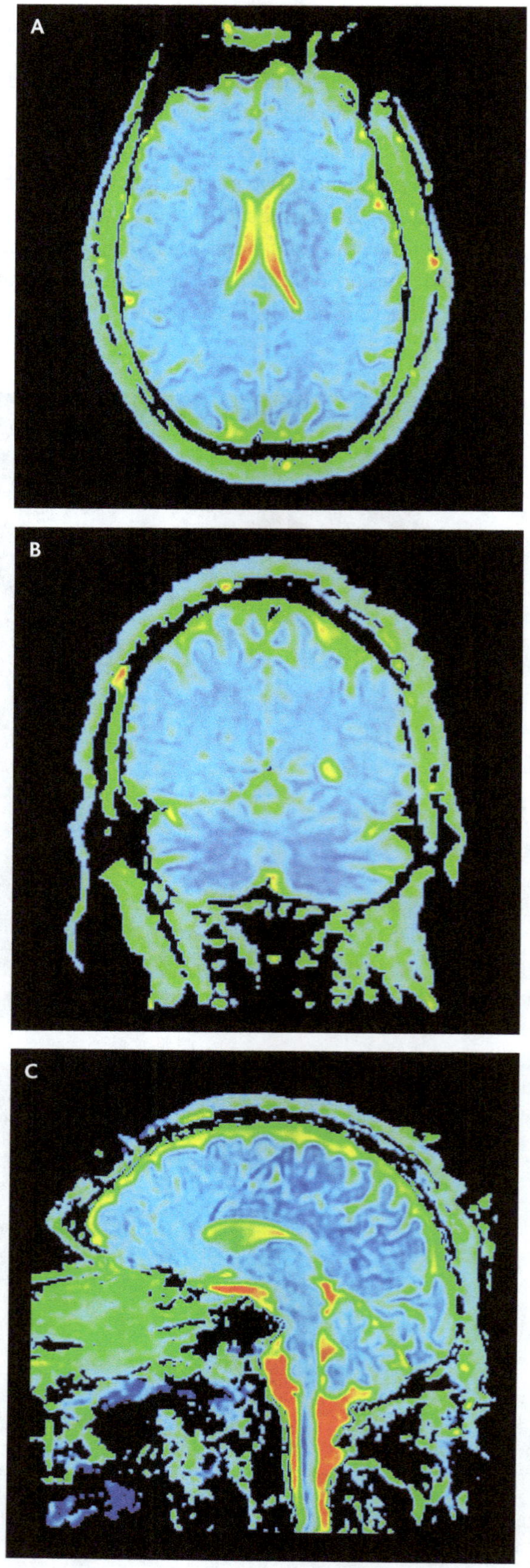

Figures 4-69A–C Color fractional anisotropy (FA) maps acquired in all three primary planes.

Structural FA Maps

FA maps provide information on the degree to which water diffusion is isotropic versus anisotropic. Structural FA maps take advantage of the directional component of diffusion to produce images showing the degree of FA in addition to the primary direction of diffusion. If water diffusion is restricted in one plane but not another, a directional component can be calculated. For example, imaging water in a glass would result in no unique directional component, as the water molecules can diffuse or move in any direction without restriction to flow (isotropic). However, if the water molecules are contained within a thin tube, diffusion would be more restricted across the diameter of the tube than along the length of the tube. In this case, the directional component would indicate more diffusion along the length of the tube than across the tube. Water in a tube is analogous to water within an axon, with diffusion being restricted or anisotropic. In an axon, there is greater restriction to water movement across the axon than along the length of the axon. Using computer algorithms, voxels are coded on the basis of the degree of FA or amount of restricted diffusion, in addition to the direction of greatest movement. When adjacent voxels have the same directional component, they are combined to form a line. For example, when voxels are isotropic with movement forming the shape of a round ball, they appear dark on the image. When voxels are anisotropic with movement forming the shape of a thin tube, they are placed end to end along the longest axis. By placing the anisotropic voxels end to end, tubes in the brain can be mapped. Put simply, this technology can be used to map axons within the brain through color coding based on their degree of FA and their directional component.

On grayscale images, the degree of FA is represented by the brightness of the area. The directional component is not fully represented, although it can be deduced from the position of the lines in relation to known anatomy. For example, although the image in Figure 4-70 does not provide directional information, the bright areas corresponding to the genu and splenium of the corpus callosum are clearly lateral fibers with a high degree of FA.

Color-Coded Structural FA Maps

Color FA maps show color coding of the directional component to diffusion, allowing for easier discrimination of white-matter tracts within the brain.

The standard color coding for DTI structural FA maps is as follows:

Red: Lateral fibers (across the brain)
Blue: Superior–inferior (top to the bottom)
Green: Anterior–posterior (front to back)

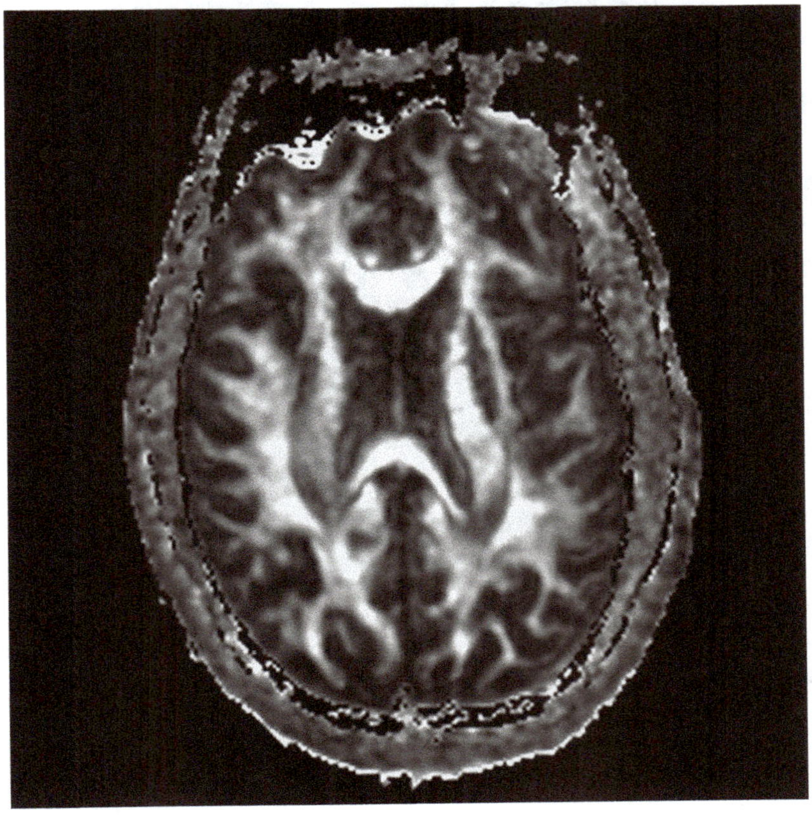

Figure 4-70 Black and white structural fractional anisotropy map.

Most protocols only call for sequences acquired within the axial plane (Figure 4-71A). However, some pathways are difficult to appreciate on axial structural maps but more easily appreciated on coronal (Figure 4-71B) or sagittal sequences (Figure 4-71C). Depending on the area of interest, the radiologist may acquire structural FA information in more than one plane, although each plane requires a separate acquisition run in the scanner.

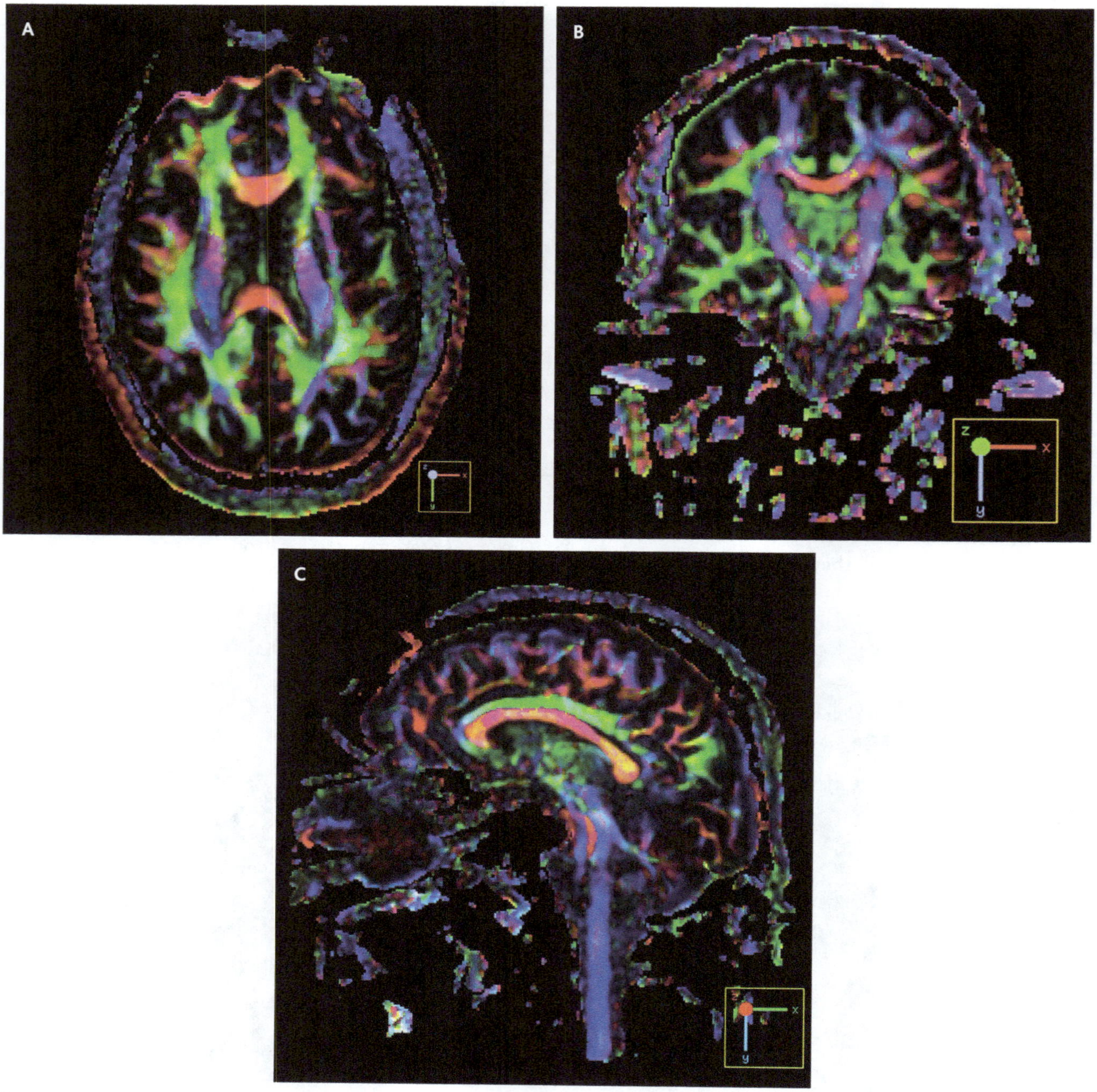

Figures 4-71A–C Color structural fractional anisotropy maps. Note that lateral corpus callosum fibers on all three images are red, the anterior–posterior aligned cingulate fibers are green, and the internal capsule and spinal cord fibers running superior–inferior are blue. Fibers that are aligned on a plane between axial, coronal, or sagittal may have a color other than red, green, or blue. For example, fibers aligned between lateral and vertical will be purple, a blending of red and blue.

DTI Tractography

Tractography can be used to connect voxels with a specific directional component and a high degree of FA.

DTI tractography is most useful in the mapping of white-matter axons within the brain. Water within the axons has greater diffusion along the longitudinal axis than across the membranes, resulting in a higher FA or unique directional component than that of water outside the axon. By graphically mapping the axons on the basis of their FA, images of white-matter pathways within the brain can be produced (Figures 4-72A–D).

The appearance of tracts on DTI is affected by axonal edema and the invasion of tissue by neoplasms, conditions that make tractography less precise.

Clinical Application of DTI

Traditionally, DTI has been restricted to research, and the anatomical mapping of brain structures. However, DTI can be a useful clinical tool, given the additional information provided by the sequences. Availability of DTI is increasing as medical and imaging centers replace older equipment with higher-Tesla systems capable of producing DTI. With

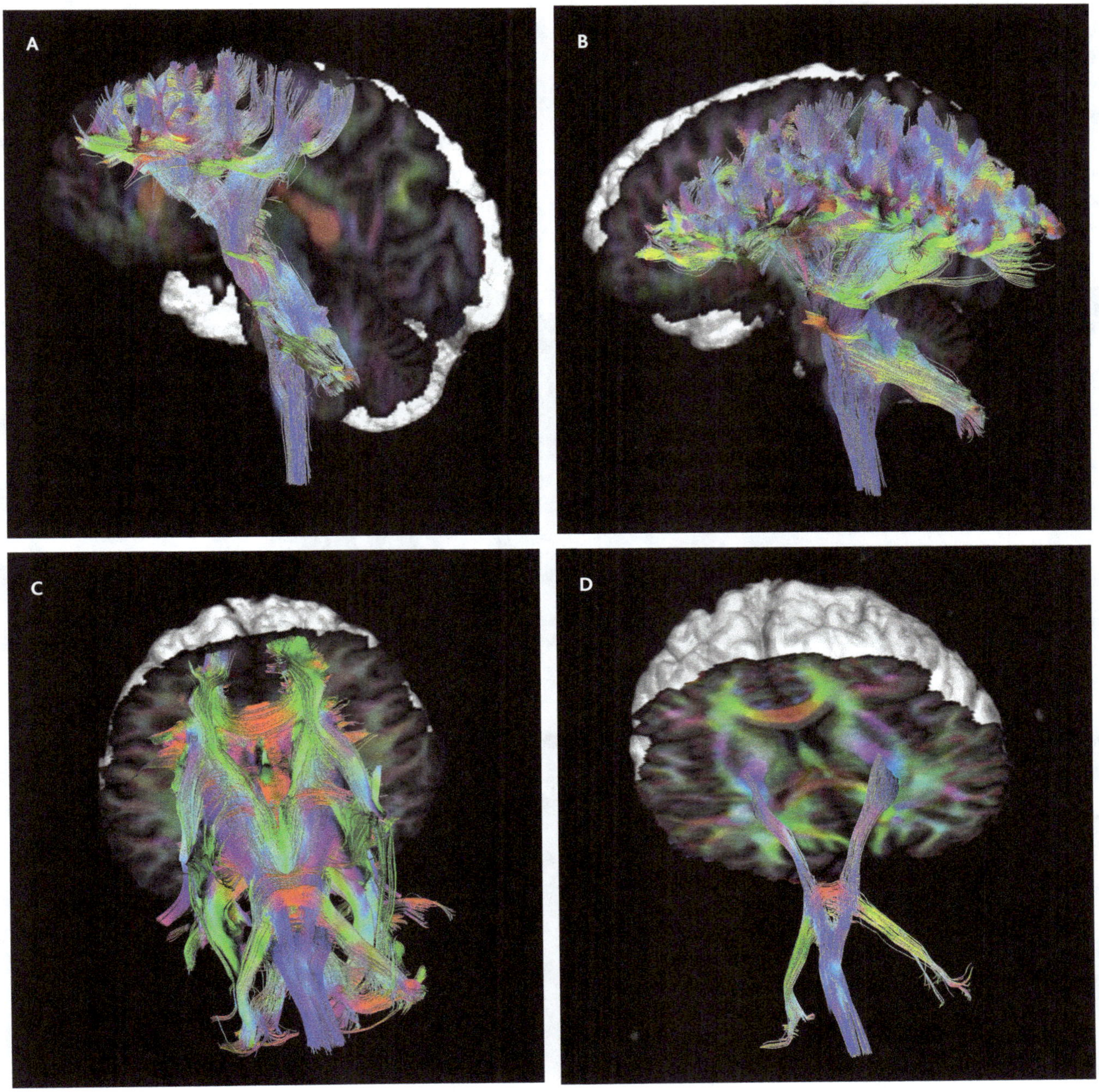

Figure 4-72A–D DTI tractography. **A:** Corona radiata and corticospinal tract. **B:** Corona radiata with intracortical connections and corticospinal tract. **C:** Anterior-inferior view of the primary pathways. **D:** Isolated ventral corticospinal pathways (motor).

Carson was scheduled to undergo resection of a large, recurrent right-hemisphere tumor. Standard CT imaging suggested a neoplasm centrally located within the right hemisphere. MRI with and without contrast was ordered to more accurately identify the location of the tumor, provide information on the tumor grade or type, and assist the surgeon in planning for resection. Imaging without contrast suggested a cystic tumor close to the midline subcortical structures of the thalamus and basal ganglia (Figures 4-73A–C). Post-contrast imaging revealed an enhancing ring around the tumor, often a sign of a higher-grade neoplasm (Figures 4-73D–F). Standard MR imaging was useful in identifying the precise location of the tumor, but the scans were less helpful in differentiating the white-matter tracts close to the tumor.

3T DTI was performed within the axial plane to better identify the white-matter tracts around the tumor. Review of the color-coded DTI structural FA maps indicated that the tumor was displacing a number of pathways (Figures 4-74A–C). It was clear from the FA maps that resection of the tumor would be complicated by the risk of damage to these pathways, especially the motor routes, and could result in the patient having a left hemiparesis post-surgery. On the color-coded FA map, the darker appearance within the right thalamic region represents an area of poor diffusion within and around the tumor, resulting in limited DTI resolution and contrast.

DTI tractography was performed to help isolate the white-matter tracts around the tumor, especially the motor pathways that form the corticospinal tract (Figures 4-75A–F). The location of the tumor is shown in Figures 4-75A and D as the lighter area within the medial right hemisphere. Note the splitting of the ventral motor pathways of the corticospinal tract within the right hemisphere, compared to the normal pathway in the left hemisphere (Figures 4-75E and F).

The tumor was resected without postoperative motor or sensory loss, something that may not have been possible before the use of 3T DTI, FA mapping, and tractography.

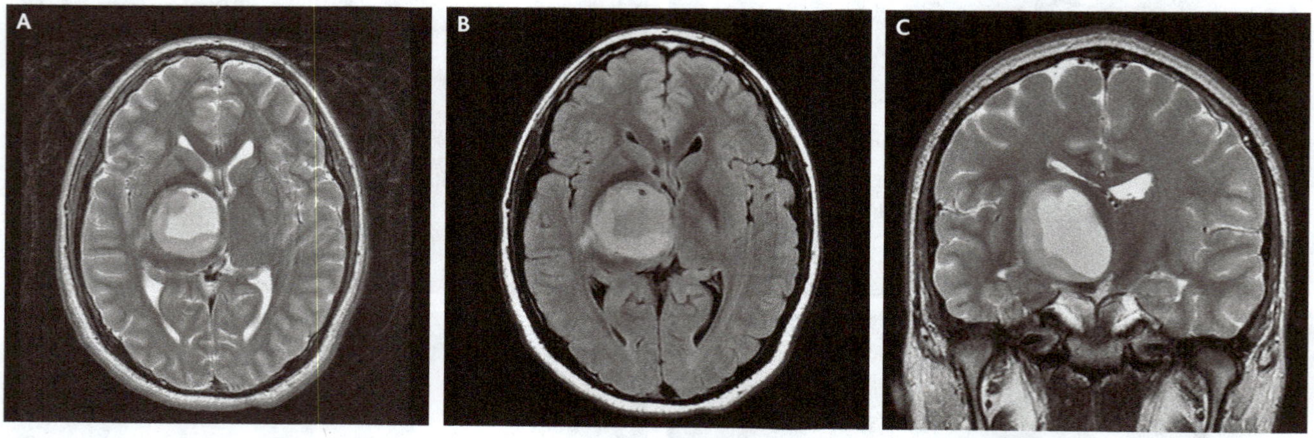

Figures 4-73A–C Clinical example Carson: non-contrast imaging of right thalamic neoplasm. **A:** T2 FSE. **B:** T2 FLAIR. **C:** T2 FRFSE.

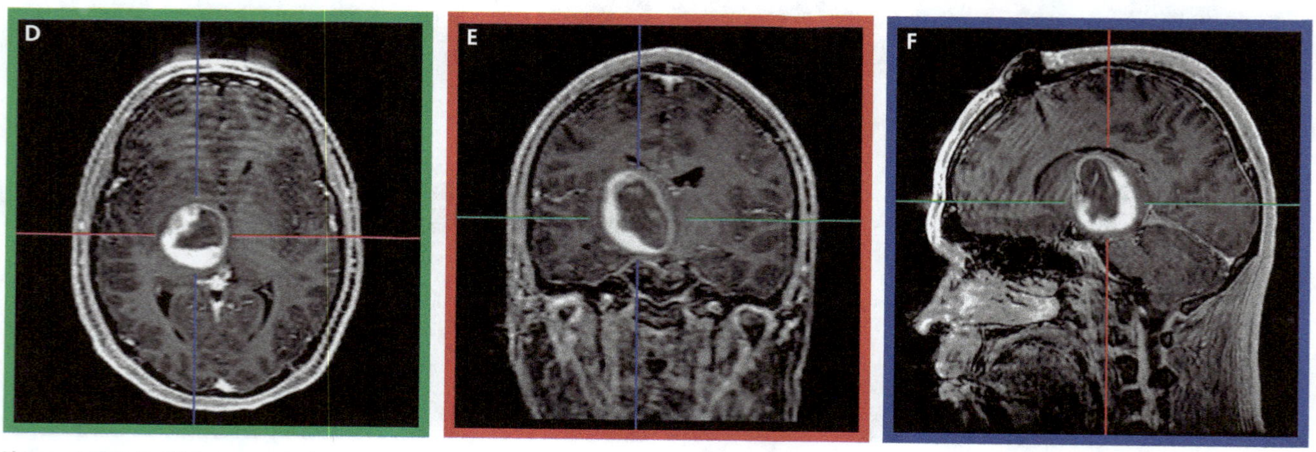

Figures 4-73D–F Clinical example Carson: contrast-enhanced imaging of right thalamic neoplasm. **D:** CE-3D T1 BRAVO. **E:** CE-3D T1 BRAVO. **F:** CE-3D T1 BRAVO.

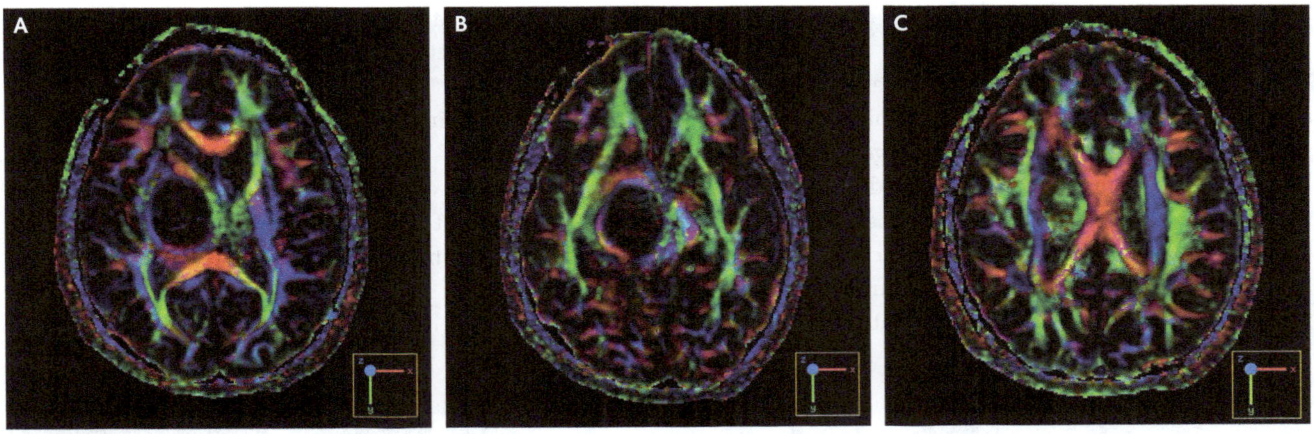

Figure 4-74A–C Clinical example Carson: color-coded DTI structural maps of white-matter tracts around the right thalamic tumor.

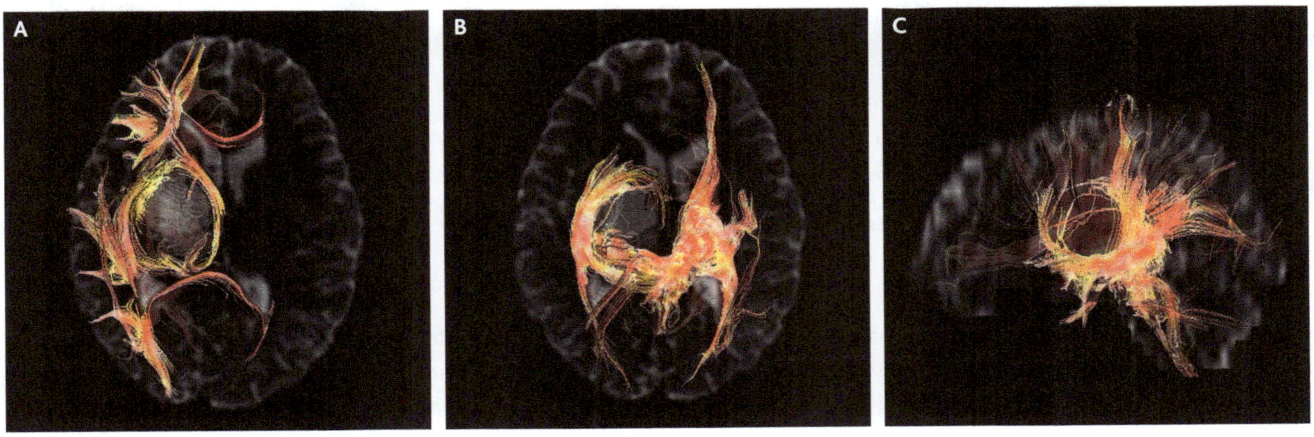

Figures 4-75A–C DTI tractography: primary pathways around the tumor.

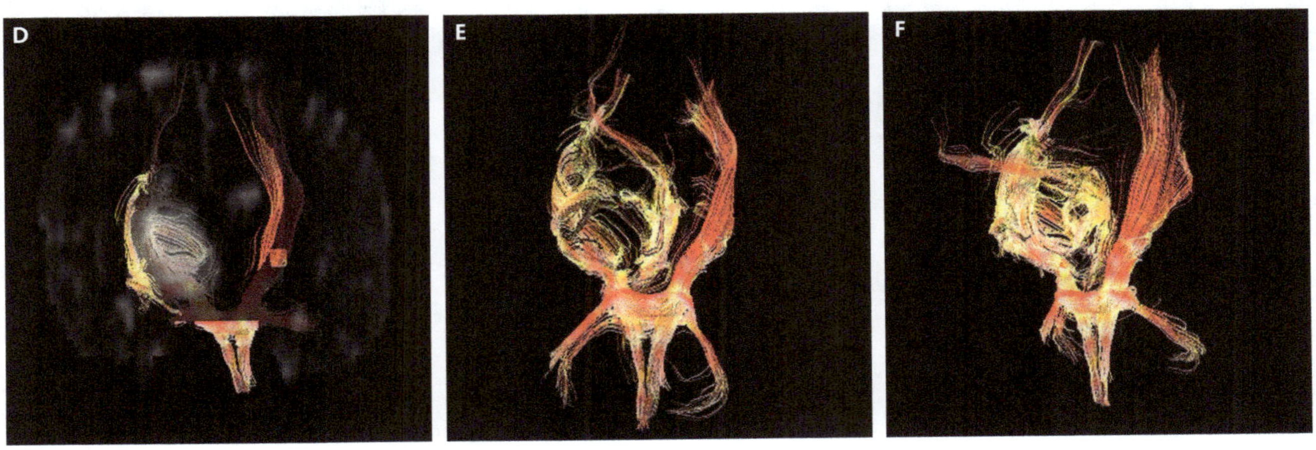

Figures 4-75D–F DTI tractography: ventral corticospinal fibers around the tumor.

more clinicians being exposed to DTI, it is expected that they will incorporate DTI into their clinical practice, especially if they have access to radiologists familiar with such sequences.

The clinical applications of color DTI tractography are numerous and include the assessment of normal and damaged pathways and presurgical evaluations. For example, resection of a tumor results in iatrogenic risk not only to nerve cells but also to the many pathways that run through the brain and close, to or even through a tumor. Color DTI can assist surgery teams in planning a surgical approach that avoids both eloquent cortex or nuclei and critical pathways close to the lesion, as was true for Carson, discussed in the clinical example presented above.

DTI as a Marker of Axonal Injury

With traumatic brain injuries, diffuse axonal injuries frequently result in significant compromise to a patient's functioning. Evidence is building to suggest that DTI-based FA values can confirm the presence of diffuse axonal injuries in patients suffering from traumatic brain injuries (Figures 4-76A–C and 4-77A–C), even in cases of mild injury.

Combining DTI tractography with functional MRI techniques is enabling study of how different parts of the brain are interconnected and how they communicate information during a variety of tasks, providing useful presurgical information.

One of the primary limitations of DTI involves the determination of FA values and the direction of diffusion when two or more axons cross within the same voxel. With greater measurements and smaller voxel sizes, this is becoming less of an issue; however, longer acquisition times and scanners with stronger magnets are required.

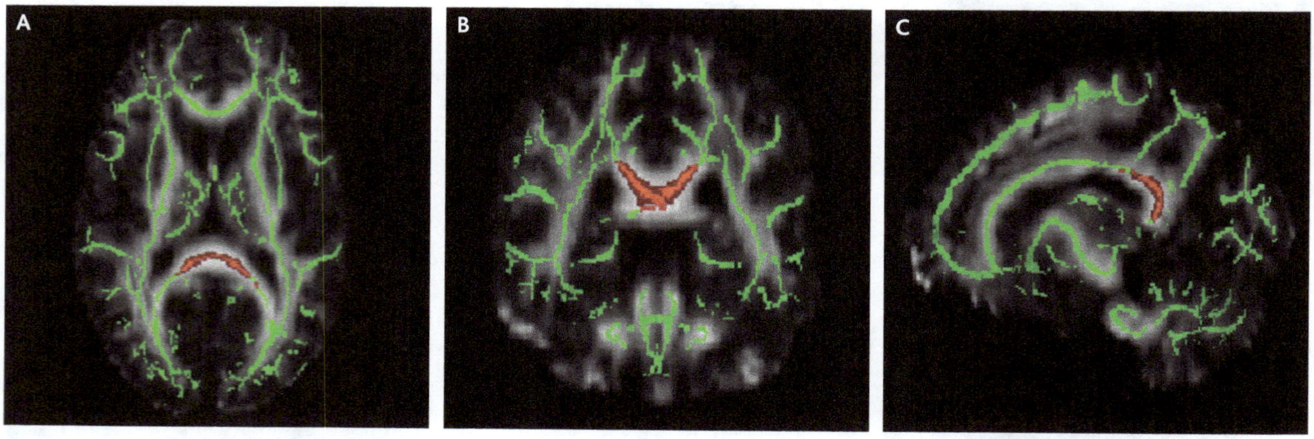

Figures 4-76A–C DTI of a patient with mild traumatic brain injury (TBI). The areas in green are skeletal paths of normal FA, while the areas in red have abnormally low FA values, representing a loss of directionality along fibers of the splenium of the corpus callosum. *Figures courtesy of E. Mark Haacke, Ph.D.*

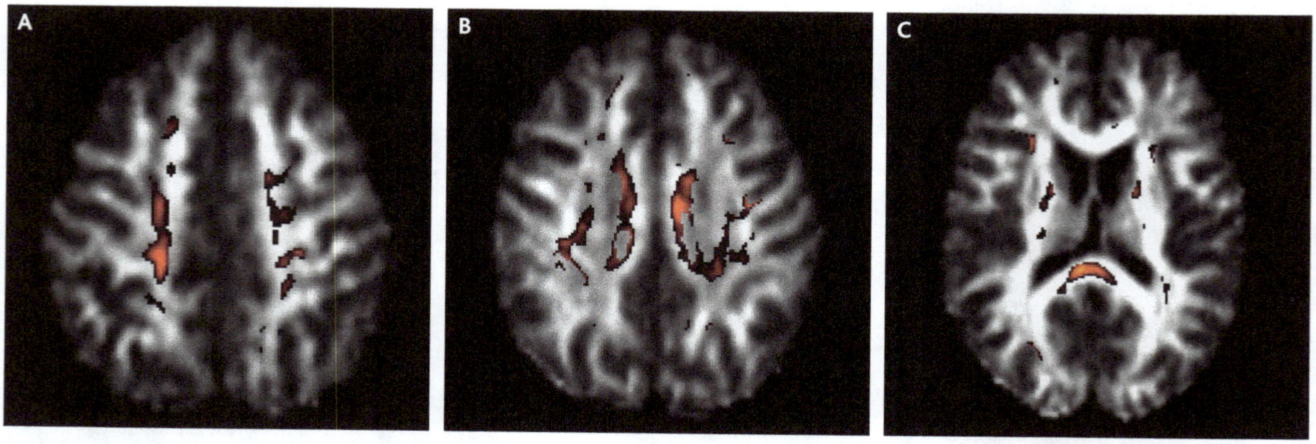

Figures 4-77A–C Regions of decreased FA (red) in traumatic brain injury, compared with healthy control subjects. **A:** Corona radiata. **B:** Superior longitudinal fasciculus, corona radiata, cingulum. **C:** Internal capsule, splenium, corpus callosum. *Figures courtesy of E. Mark Haacke, Ph.D.*

Cerebral Perfusion-Weighted MRI (PWI)

Cerebral perfusion-weighted images are produced through two primary processes. Dynamic susceptibility contrast-enhanced (DSC) perfusion studies use an exogenous paramagnetic contrast agent such as gadolinium. The susceptibility effects of gadolinium on either a T2-weighted or T2*-weighted image results in reduced signal due to magnetic field distortion caused by the gadolinium. The attenuation of T2 or T2* signal during contrast flow is dependent on the concentration of blood within the vessels and the number and diameter of vessels per volume of tissue. The change in the T2 or T2* signal is recorded during the first pass of the contrast agent through the capillary bed. Echo-planar sequences are used for rapid, sequential image acquisition, and baseline levels are calculated via computer, as well as data regarding the inflow and outflow of the contrast agent through the capillary bed. A drawback to gadolinium-enhanced perfusion sequences is that the study is dependent on the gadolinium remaining within the blood vessels. Gadolinium does not naturally pass through the blood–brain barrier and is thus appropriate for such studies. However, if there is damage to the blood–brain barrier, the leakage of gadolinium through the vessel walls will disrupt the study and may result in miscalculation of the perfusion variables.

In arterial spin-labeling perfusion studies, the saturated blood upstream of the slice of interest is used as an endogenous tracer. In this technique, comparison of the signals from within the area of interest and outside the area provides information regarding the hemodynamics of the tissue being studied. For both types of perfusion studies, post-processing is used to compute a variety of perfusion parameters.

The information obtained from perfusion studies relates to a variety of hemodynamic variables useful in determining the integrity of the vascular system or tissue of interest. The primary information provided is as follows:

- Time of arrival (T0) for the contrast agent
- Time to peak (TTP), or the time needed for maximum contrast variation between the area of interest and other tissue
- Mean transit time (MTT), or the time for the tracer to flow though the capillary bed of interest
- Regional cerebral blood volume (rCBV) within the area of interest relative to other reference tissue
- Regional cerebral blood flow (rCBF) based on the ratio of rCBV/MTT, for the area of interest relative to other reference tissue

Perfusion MRI is useful in the assessment of a number of clinical conditions, including vasospasm and vascular disease, ischemic stroke (changes are seen almost immediately), hemorrhagic conditions, multiple sclerosis (Figures 4-78A and B) and traumatic brain injury (Figures 4-79A and B), and in viewing the vascularity of neoplasms such as high-grade gliomas. Perfusion studies are also useful in the assessment of migraines and seizure-related disorders.

Autoregulation resulting in hypoperfusion following insult to the brain can result in secondary injury in the form of late-onset ischemic infarction, a reversible condition if treated soon enough. Quantification of this hypoperfusion may assist in prognosis and in the prediction of long-term outcome, and reducing the hypoperfusion may minimize the extent of secondary injury to the brain. The use of perfusion studies in assessing degenerative and psychiatric conditions is in its infancy, but it will likely increase in utility over time and with additional research.

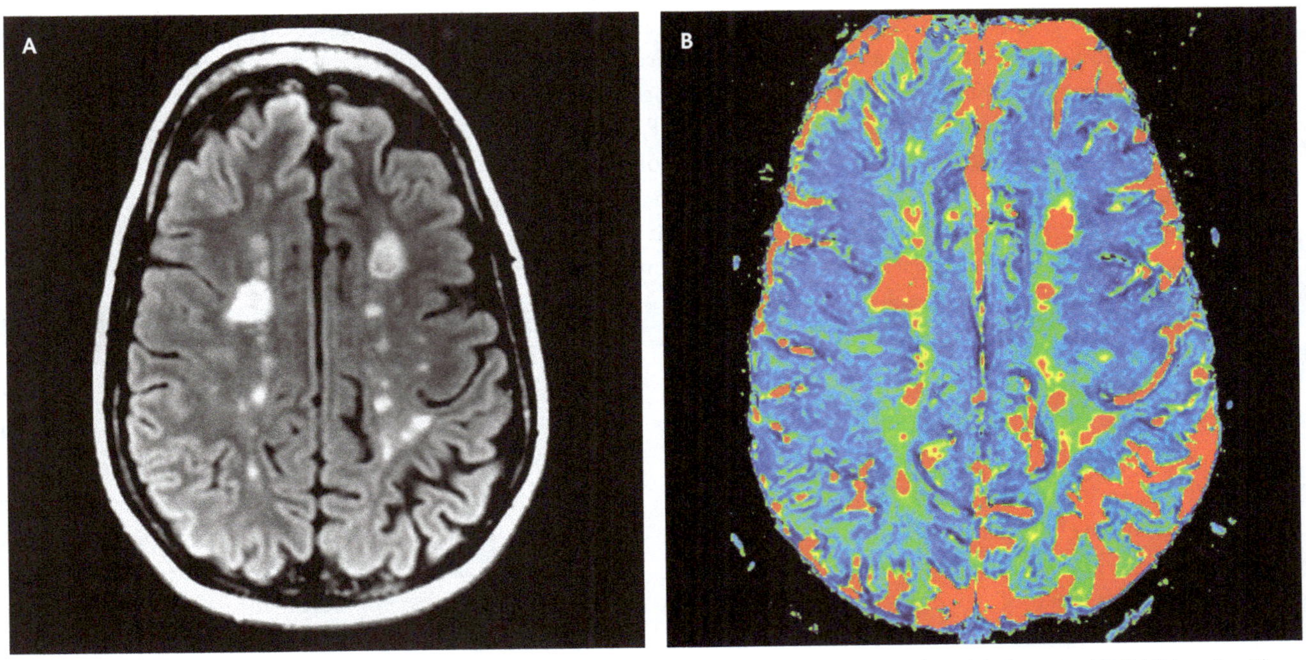

Figures 4-78A and B Clinical example: multiple sclerosis. Note disrupted perfusion (red) on PWI corresponding with plaques on T2 FLAIR imaging. Blue areas have good perfusion, red areas have disrupted perfusion or no perfusion due to the areas being outside of brain parenchyma, and green regions having an intermediate level of perfusion. **A:** T2 FLAIR. **B:** PWI. *Figures courtesy of E. Mark Haacke, Ph.D.*

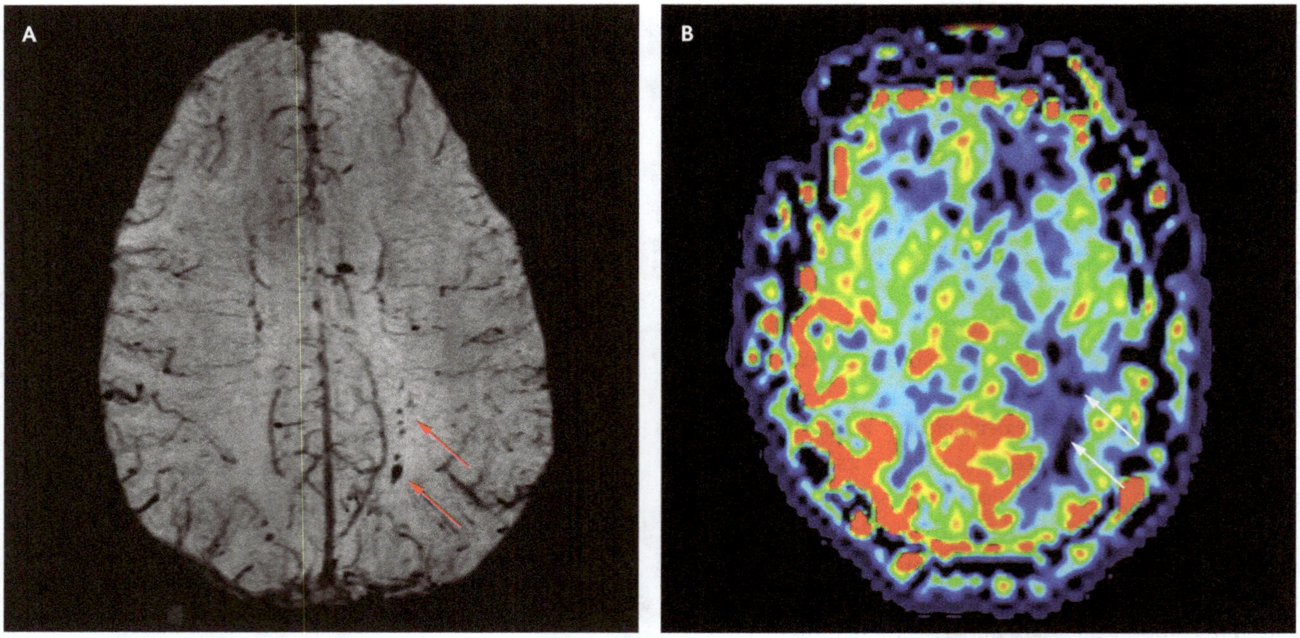

Figure 4-79A and B Clinical example: traumatic brain injury. Note evidence of diffuse axonal injury suggested by the microbleeds on SWI (arrows), which correspond to areas of reduced perfusion on PWI (arrows). On PWI, red areas have the greatest perfusion and black areas have the least perfusion. Green and blue areas have an intermediate level of perfusion, with green representing greater perfusion than blue. **A:** SWI. **B:** PWI. *Figures courtesy of E. Mark Haacke, Ph.D.*

Diffusion-Perfusion Ischemic Penumbra

In the field of light physics, a *penumbra* represents a partial or soft shadow where some light is obscured, but not all (Latin: *paene* = almost, nearly; *umbra* = shadow). The term is applied to a combination of perfusion and diffusion images. The areas of the brain that are only partially affected by an ischemic event, usually around an ischemic core, can be considered an ischemic penumbra or soft shadow. The inner core where the tissue is fully affected by ischemia is analogous to a full shadow. When diffusion images suggest significant disruption to diffusion and measures of rCBV (blood volume) suggest vascular-capillary compromise, the area is considered irreversibly damaged or infarcted. However, bordering the area there is often a zone that appears intact on diffusion sequences but has reduced blood perfusion. If a region has intact diffusion but reduced rCBF (blood flow) and MTT (speed of perfusion through the area), the region can represent an ischemic penumbra or soft shadow. Penumbra regions are not yet permanently damaged or infarcted but are at high risk of progressing to infarction if the blood supply (rCBF and MTT) is not resumed, to enable reperfusion of the area. Put simply, this region of tissue has the potential to be salvaged through reperfusion therapies, such as the use of thrombolytic agents or interventional radiology procedures.

Magnetic Resonance Spectroscopy (MRS)

Magnetic resonance spectroscopy (MRS) is a technique used to examine the chemical composition of tissue. MRS is based on NMR theory, which contends that different molecular arrangements of an excited isotope produce unique resonance frequencies. The spectrum of resonance frequencies produced by the excited isotope can be used to measure the level of certain metabolites in the body, each corresponding to a particular biological process. MRS involves the mapping of the metabolite levels onto an MR image. MRS requires a relatively strong and homogenous magnetic field to discriminate resonance peaks from the metabolites, thus 1.5T or higher magnets are preferred. A process called "shimming" is used to produce field homogeneity within the region of clinical interest. MRS has a relatively low signal-to-noise ratio, which results in low spatial resolution for the substance being assessed (approximately 15 mm × 15 mm × 15 mm), and each voxel contains data regarding a variety of metabolites.

TABLE 4-2 MRS Reference Guide

METABOLITE	GENERAL USE
Acetate (Ac)	Marker used to assess for an abscess, infections diseases
Choline (Cho)	Marker of cell membrane breakdown. Increased in demyelination, tumors, and cellular damage
Creatine (Cr)	Marker of cell metabolism. **Used as a reference for healthy tissue**
Free lipids (Lip)	Marker not found in healthy tissue. Suggests necrosis from conditions such as high-grade tumors
Glutamate/glutamine/ GABA complex (Glx)	Marker of neurotransmitter function
Lactate (Lac)	Marker of anaerobic respiration, not found in healthy tissue. Increased in anaerobic metabolism caused by ischemia, seizures, tumors, mitochondrial disorders
Myo-inositol (mI)	Marker found only in glial cells. Increased in gliomas and indicative of low-grade gliomas. Also a marker of gliosis and of demyelinating processes such as multiple sclerosis (MS) and metabolic and degenerative processes.
N-acetyl-aspartate (NAA)	Marker of healthy neurons. Used as a healthy marker; reduced levels show neuronal distress. Has the highest peak in normal brain tissue
Phosphocreatine (Pcr)	Marker of cell metabolism. **Used as a reference for healthy tissue**

There are two primary types of MRS: single-voxel spectroscopy (SVS), which analyzes the metabolic spectrum at a single voxel, and chemical shift imaging (CSI), which can be used to assess metabolites at a specific location on a slice of tissue (2D) and within a volume of tissue (3D).

MRS is used primarily to assess brain tumors, infectious or inflammatory processes, or pathologies with specific metabolic signatures (Table 4-2). MRS produces relative values, with the area of interest being compared to either choline or similar tissue outside of the region of pathological interest (often the analogous area in the other hemisphere).

Functional Brain Imaging

Functional brain imaging is different from the imaging presented earlier in this chapter in that its primary purpose is to measure the brain's reaction to a specific physical or mental activity. Functional brain imaging techniques involve a variety of technologies to accomplish their goal. Some use radioactive isotopes as tracers to track changes (PET, SPECT), some assess blood oxygen levels (fMRI), while others are designed to track tiny changes in magnetic field that result from neural firing (MEG-MSI). Each functional imaging technique carries both advantages and disadvantages and has a variety of spatial and temporal resolution levels. For example, SPECT has the lowest spatial resolution, followed by PET, MEG-MSI, and fMRI. To put the spatial resolution of the different techniques in perspective, SPECT and PET can be thought of as recording the activity of a stadium full of people. In this context, MEG-MSI would be used to record information from the bleachers, and the higher spatial resolution of fMRI would record a conversation among a group of fans.

Positron Emission Tomography (PET)

One of the earliest imaging techniques used to assess changes in brain functioning as a result of the subject completing a task was positron emission tomography (PET). PET is considered a branch of nuclear medicine, as it uses radioisotopes to measure brain functioning. Isotopes with short half-lives such as fluorine-18 (~110 minutes), carbon-11 (~20 minutes), nitrogen-13 (~10 minutes), and oxygen-15 (~2 minutes) are bound to other compounds in order to produce radiotracers. Radiotracers can be bound to any number of substances, such as water, glucose, ammonia, or even neurotransmitters. Because of the variety of substances that can be traced using radioisotopes, PET has many uses in the biological sciences. Currently, PET is used to measure such biological processes as glucose metabolism, regional cerebral blood flow, blood volume, oxygen uptake, tissue pH, drug activity, neurotransmitter function, enzyme function, and tumor growth and as a measure of cellular pathology.

The most common PET protocols involve the binding of fluorine-18 to glucose to produce fluorodeoxyglucose (FDG). The use of fluorine-18 has the advantage of a relative long half-life of 109.8 minutes, thus it can be transported from the source cyclotron to the PET facility. This feature is especially important for medical facilities without cyclotrons. Over time, more medical facilities are obtaining relatively compact on-site cyclotrons with integrated shielding and portable chemistry stations necessary to produce radioisotopes at the facility. Third-party vendors that supply multiple local medical and research facilities are also becoming more common.

The biggest advantage to PET is that the scanner can produce biologically based information not otherwise available through other brain imaging technologies.

CLINICAL EXAMPLE

Cameron: Glioblastoma Multiforme

As part of his neuro-oncology workup, Cameron underwent magnetic resonance spectroscopy. Four primary metabolites were reviewed using a 3 × 5 matrix over his glioblastoma multiforme a malignant brain tumor, and surrounding areas of normal brain tissue. For each of the 15 cells, MRS produced a spectrum with peaks and value data corresponding to each metabolite. A color map was produced for the composite metabolite activity and for individually selected metabolites (Figures 4-80A–G).

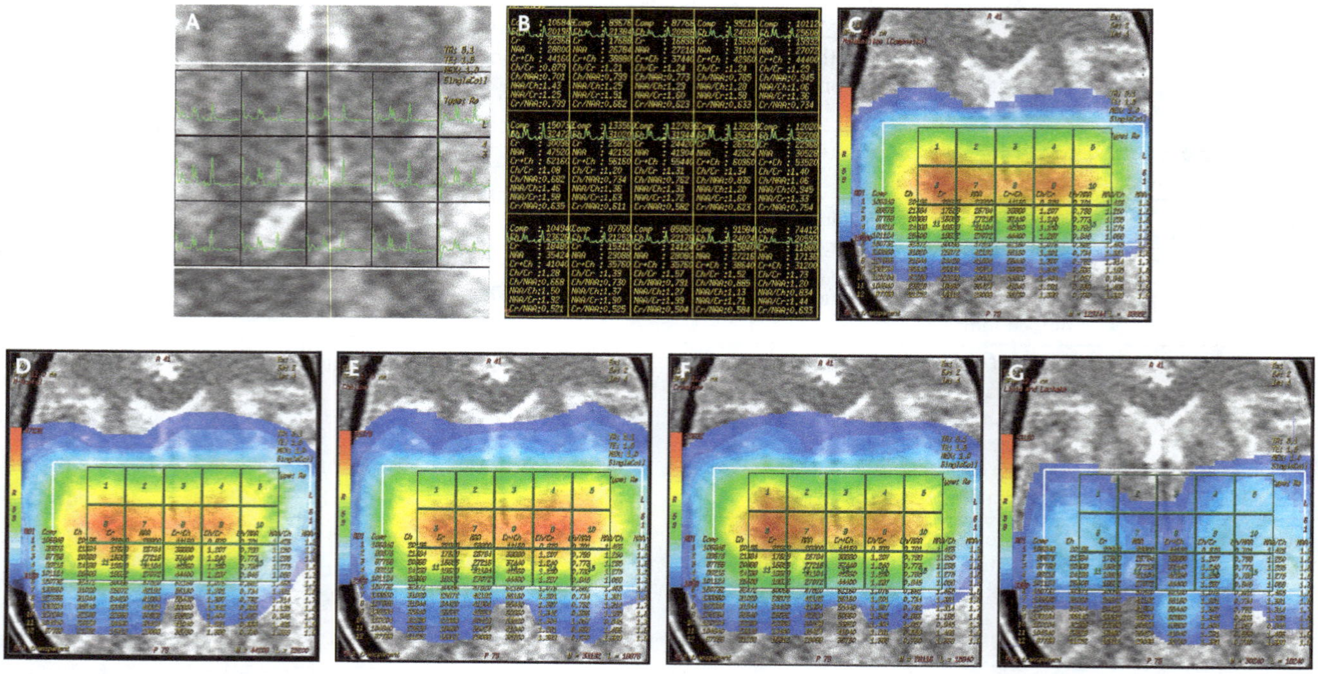

Figure 4-80A–G Clinical example Cameron: MRS of a high-grade astrocytoma (glioblastoma multiforme) and normal tissue around the tumor. **A:** Spectrum map. **B:** Spectrum with data. **C:** Composite map. **D:** N-acetyl map. **E:** Choline map. **F:** Creatine map. **G:** Lipid/lactate map.

Several factors limit the utility of PET studies. The exposure of the patient to radioisotopes is of concern, although as is true with CT scanning, the risks of ionizing radiation exposure need to be balanced against the probative value of the study. The total dose of ionizing radiation from a PET study is around 5 to 7 mSv; it is higher when using a combined PET-CT, as discussed below (Brix et al., 2005).

REFERENCE

Brix, G., Lechel, U., Glatting, G., Ziegler, S. I., Münzing, W., Müller, S. P., & Beyer, T. (2005). Radiation exposure of patients undergoing whole-body dual-modality 18F-FDG PET/CT examinations. *Journal of Nuclear Medicine, 46*(4), 608–613.

Another limiting factor of PET is that radioisotopes decay quickly and are only effective for a short period of time. This requires the patient to be on time for the appointment and that there be little to no time lag during the study. The isotopes must be available when required, something that is a concern when the PET facility does not have an in-house cyclotron. In addition, compared to other imaging techniques, PET has relatively poor temporal and spatial resolution.

Temporal resolution is poor as it takes approximately an hour for the radioisotope-labeled glucose (FDG) to become chemically incorporated and concentrated in the most active tissue. With FDG, the subject undergoes an activity period followed by a steady-state waiting period of usually approximately 1 hour. Because of this steady-state waiting period, PET scans are often described as producing "resting images," not real-time images.

Spatial resolution is variable depending on the radioisotope used for the study. However, because a PET scanner does not record the actual location of isotope uptake but instead the location of positron annihilation, spatial resolution is compromised; positron annihilation can be up to approximately 10 mm away from the site of uptake. An additional factor that disrupts spatial resolution is

How FDG PET Works

1. The radiotracer is introduced to the subject, usually via injection into the blood circulation.
2. The subject participates in a particular activity designed to activate a region or system of the brain.
3. A steady-state waiting period then follows for the relatively slow uptake period of the tracer.
4. After being taken up by brain cells, FDG becomes phosphorylated and cannot cross the cell membrane, causing accumulation within the cell.
5. The brain cells that were most active during the "activity stage" increase their metabolic demands and, ultimately, their uptake of the labeled glucose (FDG).
6. The concentration of the tracer is mapped within the brain as the isotopes undergo positron emission decay.
7. During positron emission decay, the radioisotope emits a positron that travels away from the source for approximately 1 to 10 millimeters.
8. The positron loses kinetic energy and eventually collides with an electron, becoming annihilated.
9. At the point of positron–electron collision, two gamma photons are released at approximately 180 degrees from each other.
10. The two gamma photons are detected by the PET scanner and are recorded based on the angle and timing of their contact with the detector. Only photons arriving almost simultaneously (within a few nanoseconds) and approximately 180 degrees from each other are recorded.
11. The location of the source (where the positron was annihilated) is calculated from the time difference between the photons arriving at the detectors, along a common path resulting from the 180-degree movement of the particles. The greater the time resolution of the scanner, the higher the spatial resolution of the final image.
12. The number of annihilations per area of space relates to the amount of isotope taken up by the tissue being studied.
13. The isotope concentrations are mapped via triangulation in two, three, or sometimes four dimensions (including time) by means of computer software.

CLINICAL EXAMPLE

Evelyn: New-Onset Anterograde Amnesia

Evelyn was a highly educated professional employed by a large university system. After recovering from meningitis, she returned to work only to discover that she was having difficulty remembering information presented during meetings. A CT scan was read as normal, suggesting that her difficulties were not organic or the result of brain damage. Some emotional difficulties experienced by Evelyn led her care team to believe that there may have been a psychological component to her memory difficulties. Neuropsychological assessment indicated that Evelyn had superior intellect, verbal and nonverbal reasoning, and executive functioning. However, memory for new learning (anterograde memory) was severely compromised, and she was unable to remember newly presented information after only a few minutes of distraction. The assessment also indicated that her memory difficulties were not related to poor attention, poor processing ability, poor understanding of the material, or an emotional condition. Her pattern of performance on various memory tests was inconsistent with the effects of an emotional condition and suggested an organic etiology. It was serendipitous that Evelyn's physician was involved in the development of PET scanning technology and had access to one of the early PET systems. FDG-PET revealed hypometabolism within both anterior medial temporal lobes (Figure 4-81A: arrows), clearly evident when her images were compared to that of a normal control subject (Figure 4-81B).

Even though the PET used in this case was a low-resolution PET conducted many years ago, the images provided the only clear radiological evidence of organic disruption that could explain the symptoms. The suggestion of bilateral temporal lobe compromise on PET was fully consistent with the information and conclusions obtained through the neuropsychological evaluation. The anterograde amnesia was related to hypometabolism of the bilateral hippocampi, and the emotional difficulties were likely related to the bilateral amygdala hypometabolism and general disruption of the medial temporal lobe limbic system. The PET information provided a picture of the pathology, something that was not otherwise available at that time.

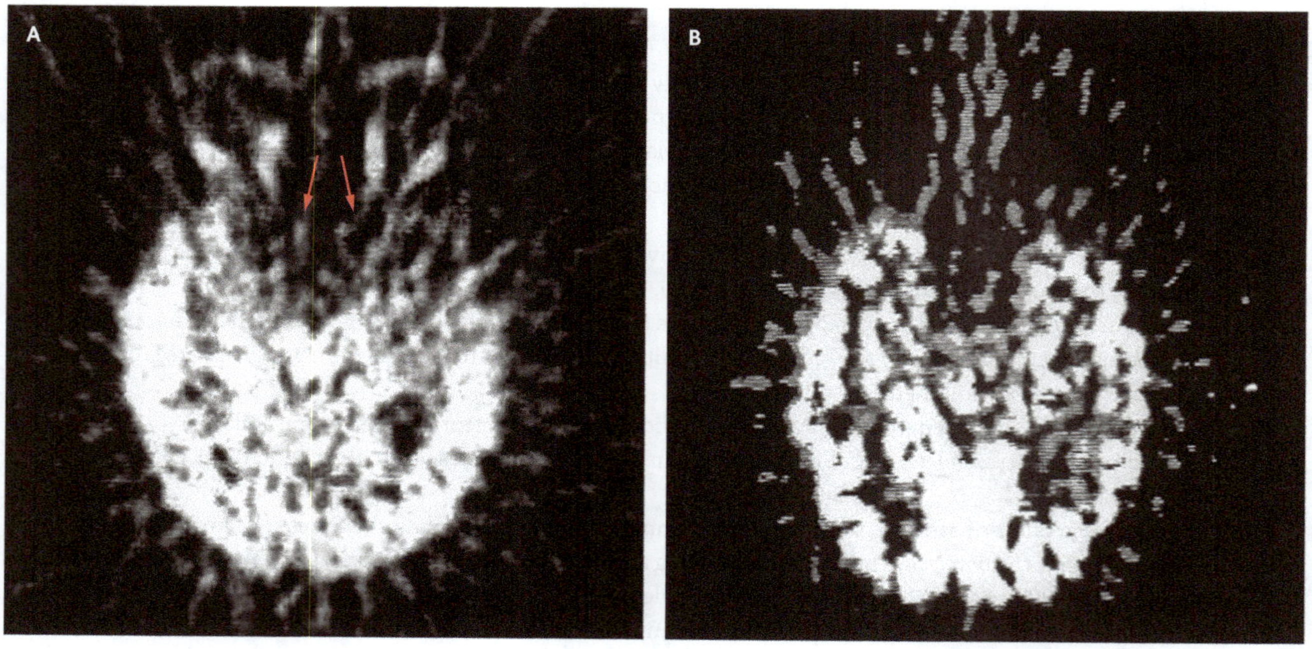

Figure 4-81 **A:** PET image of amnestic patient—Evelyn suggesting hypometabolism within the bilateral anterior and medial temporal lobes. **B:** PET image of a control subject showing normal levels of metabolism within the bilateral anterior and medial temporal lobes.

the variability in the path of the gamma photons, which are not always at exactly 180 degrees. Poor resolution as a result of data averaging is also a concern with PET, especially given the relatively small number of data points compared to the number used in other brain imaging techniques. Because the data averaging is conducted on less information, there is a greater effect of noise, random coincidences of non-paired photons (photons that hit the sensor at 180 degrees close in time but that were from different positrons), and detector dead-time (time required for the sensor to reset).

Spatial resolution is also dependent on the ability of the system to detect the timing difference between photon pairs as they contact the detector. Current systems have timing mechanisms that function at the 3- to 9-nanosecond level; greater accuracy is evident with shorter time windows. Some systems are being developed with time accuracy at the picosecond level, requiring fewer events to produce an image, and a higher signal-to-noise ratio and spatial resolution. As the timing accuracy of signal detection has improved, the images have become more precise and clinically useful. Even with the ongoing advances in PET technology, images produced more than two decades ago were helpful to clinicians, especially given that other brain imaging systems did not have the spatial resolution necessary to explain some clinical conditions (see clinical example Evelyn).

Combined Positron Emission Tomography and Computed Tomography (PET-CT) or Magnetic Resonance Imaging (PET-MRI)

Historically, PET scans were reviewed alongside CT images to provide an anatomical reference to the metabolic information exhibited on the PET image. Later, computer display systems were used to coregister separately obtained PET and CT or MR images, with the hybrid image providing anatomical and metabolic information. The logical evolution of PET technology has resulted in the development of PET-CT and PET-MRI systems having the capability of producing PET and CT or PET and MRI images simultaneously (Figures 4-82A–C). Because two scans are produced simultaneously, the position of the patient remains the same for the PET and CT or MRI, resulting in a higher level of precision when the images are coregistered.

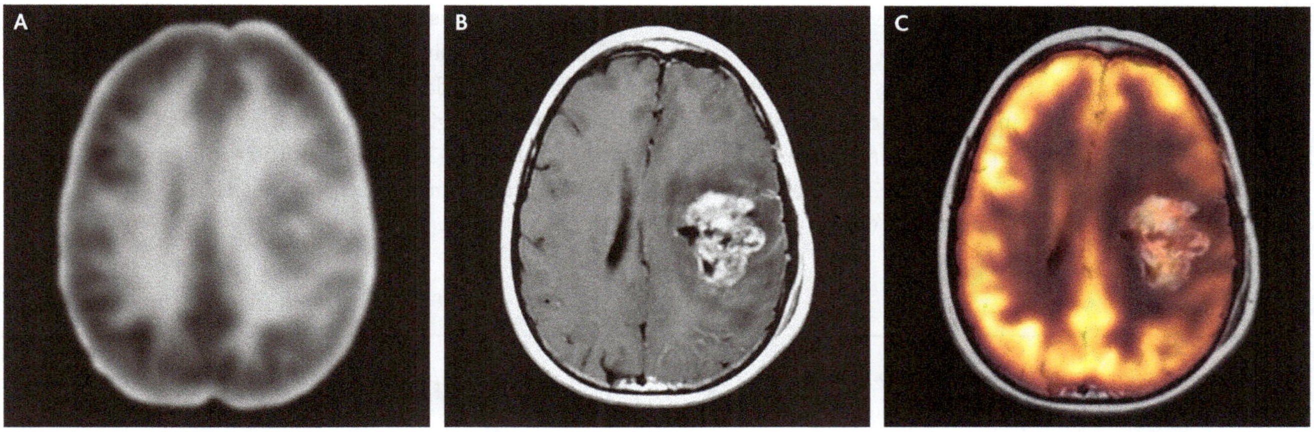

Figures 4-82A–C PET, MRI, and PET+MRI acquired from a patient with a left parietal tumor. **A:** PET. **B:** CE-T1 MRI. **C:** PET+MRI (brighter orange-yellow signifies greater metabolic activity).

Single-Photon Emission Computed Tomography (SPECT)

Single-photo emission computed tomography (SPECT) has many similarities with PET imaging, but with a few differences. Both SPECT and PET are considered nuclear medicine techniques, each using radioisotopes as tracers. One primary difference between the two techniques is in the isotopes used. SPECT uses isotopes that directly emit gamma particles; the isotopes used in PET emit positrons that eventually release gamma particles after collision with an electron. The gamma particles emitted by SPECT are recorded within two-dimensional space but are then often reconstructed into three-dimensional space. For brain SPECT, the most common isotope is technetium-99m (^{99}mTc), combined with hexamethylpropylene amine oxime to produce ^{99}mTc-HMPAO. This radiopharmaceutical compound is absorbed by brain tissue in a manner directly proportional to regional cerebral blood flow (rCBF). As rCBF is tightly coupled to the metabolic demands of a particular brain region, SPECT can provide graphical information correlated with brain metabolic activity. Most SPECT images are color coded, with blue representing low rCBF, orange a medium level of rCBF, red a high level, and white the highest level of rCBF and assumed metabolic activity.

On SPECT, a patchy appearance with "holes" on the image, especially those that are asymmetrical, can be suggestive of hypometabolism in that area. Focal areas of hypometabolism may correspond to damaged tissue as seen in medial temporal sclerosis, traumatic brain damage, infections of the brain, or neurodegenerative conditions. Genetic conditions that affect brain development may also show up on SPECT, especially if there is a specific focus of dysplasia. Hypermetabolism may be evident on SPECT for high-grade tumors or active seizure foci. Because SPECT is a type of perfusion study in that it measures rCBF, vascular integrity or pathologies such as moyamoya syndrome can also be studied using SPECT techniques.

A normal SPECT image appears relatively smooth and symmetrical, suggesting a consistent level of metabolic activity. Abnormal scans have a more heterogeneous appearance. Differentiating between a normal and abnormal SPECT scan for an individual patient is difficult given the many reasons for variations in normal rCBF. SPECT scans are easily degraded by movement of the subject. This is a concern, as a full series can take a relatively long time to produce, often 20 to 30 minutes. In addition, an uneven distribution of the radiotracer can produce artifacts on SPECT that appear to be regions of low rCBF and can be incorrectly interpreted as low metabolic activity. In addition, the attenuation of gamma particles by brain parenchyma can make deeper structures appear to have lower metabolism than that of surface areas, resulting in incorrect interpretation of neural damage or disruption. Attenuation by tissue is becoming less of an issue as newer systems are designed to compensate for these effects. SPECT scans are being combined with CT scans in much the same way as PET is with CT. Because the CT image is based on the density and absorption profile of brain tissue, it can provide a highly accurate map to compensate for the effects of gamma absorption by tissue. The CT image can also be precisely coregistered with SPECT images so that both functional–metabolic and anatomical information can be displayed on one image.

PET scans have a spatial-resolution advantage over SPECT scans. Both SPECT and PET images are constructed through the recording of gamma particles emitted by the radiotracer. However, PET scans record each source location based on the time-linked activation of two detectors 180 degrees apart for two separate gamma photons. With two "radiation events" for each data point for PET and only one for SPECT, PET can provide better spatial resolution.

SPECT is more available and less costly than PET. One of the primary reasons for SPECT being more widely available is that the radioisotope ^{99m}Tc has a longer half-life than that of FDG and can be produced relatively easily with a technetium-99m generator. Small, portable technetium-99m generators extract the isotope ^{99m}Tc from a source of decaying molybdenum-99 (^{99}Mo), which has a half-life of 66 hours. Once produced, the ^{99m}Tc has a half-life of 6 hours. The ability to have a fresh generator available and active for several days and to have an isotope for around 6 hours is a clear logistical advantage over FDG, which has a short half-life of ~110 minutes and requires an expensive cyclotron and chemical lab for production.

CLINICAL EXAMPLE
Mason: Moyamoya Syndrome

Mason was seen in the emergency room for rapid mental-status decline. Brain imaging suggested a demyelinating condition such as multiple sclerosis because of the dark spots within the white matter, evident on T1 imaging (Figure 4-83A), and corresponding bright spots on T2 imaging (Figure 4-83B). Further workup with MRI-TOF suggested a vascular etiology, possibly moyamoya syndrome, with evidence of bilateral middle cerebral artery vasospasm (Figure 4-83C).

Several SPECT studies were performed over time that showed changes to blood flow that were consistent with periods of vascular constriction followed by resolution. These studies also suggested moyamoya syndrome as the proximal cause of his white-matter damage (Figure 4-84).

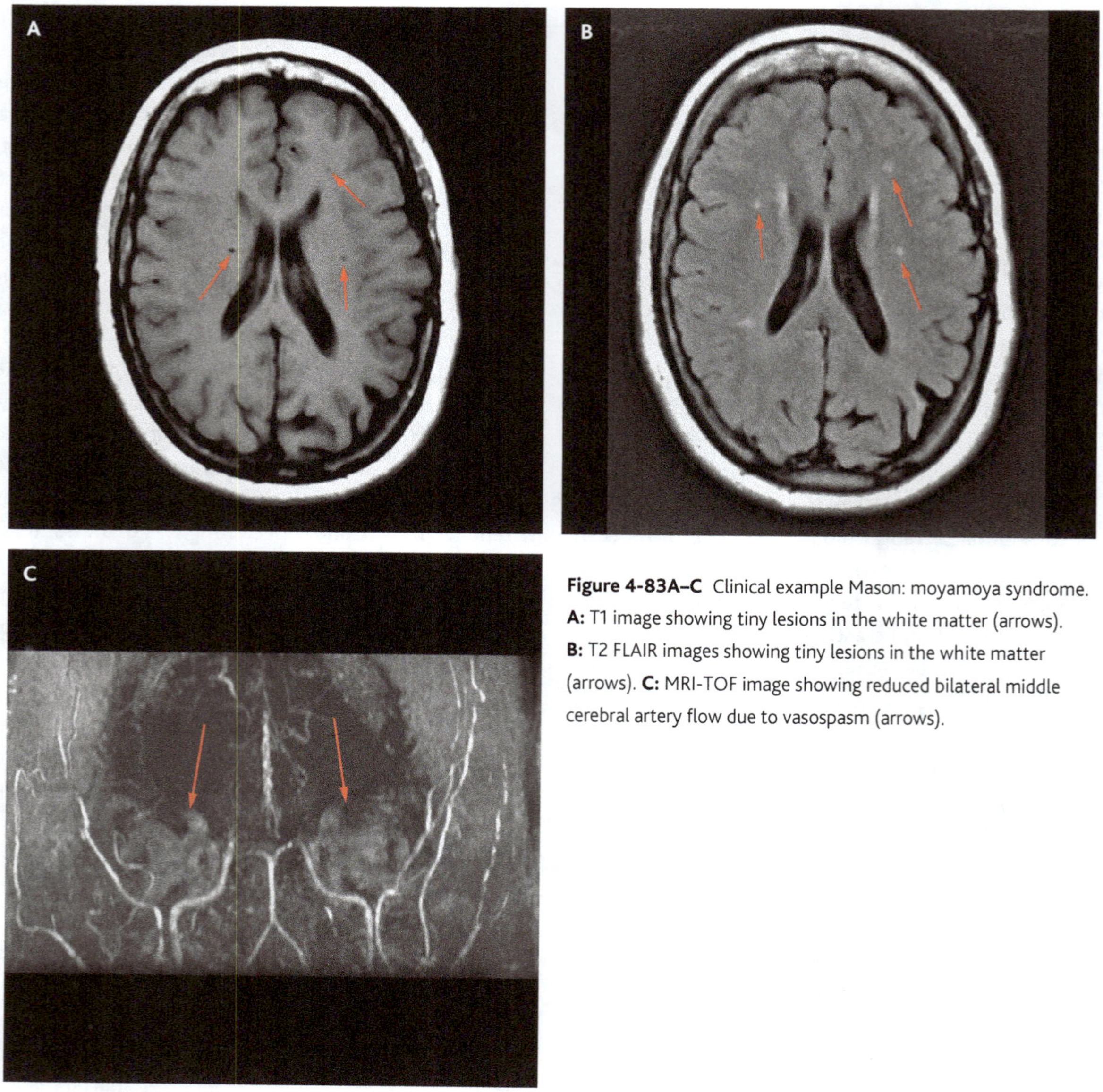

Figure 4-83A–C Clinical example Mason: moyamoya syndrome. **A:** T1 image showing tiny lesions in the white matter (arrows). **B:** T2 FLAIR images showing tiny lesions in the white matter (arrows). **C:** MRI-TOF image showing reduced bilateral middle cerebral artery flow due to vasospasm (arrows).

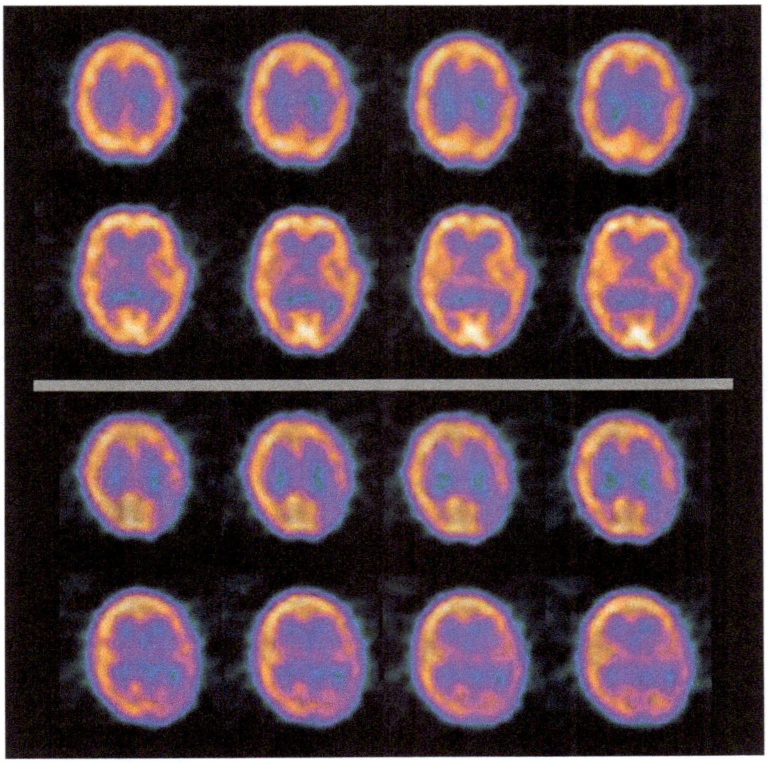

Top 8 images = normal without vasospasm

Bottom 8 images = vasospasm and constriction, most evident within the left middle cerebral artery distribution, posterior more than anterior. Subtle changes are also evident within the right middle cerebral artery distribution.

Figure 4-84 SPECT studies suggesting moyamoya syndrome (yellow areas have the greatest rCBF, and SPECT activation, with blue areas having the least rCBF and SPECT activation.

CLINICAL EXAMPLE

Preston: Right Internal Carotid Stroke

Preston was hospitalized after experiencing a right internal carotid artery stroke that resulted in loss of blood flow predominantly to the middle cerebral artery territory as well as partial loss of the anterior cerebral artery distribution. Hypodensity on CT imaging due to edema and onset of encephalomalacia suggested that the stroke involved much of the right middle cerebral artery distribution (4-85a). A SPECT scan suggested hypometabolism within the region supplied by the right internal carotid artery, including the basal ganglia and temporal lobe structures that receive blood from the middle cerebral artery. The slight diminution of luminance on SPECT corresponds to the area of vascular compromise. Comparison of the right and left hemispheres on axial (Figure 4-85B), coronal (Figures 4-85C and D), and sagittal (Figures 4-85E and F) SPECT images clearly suggests hypometabolism of the right middle cerebral distribution.

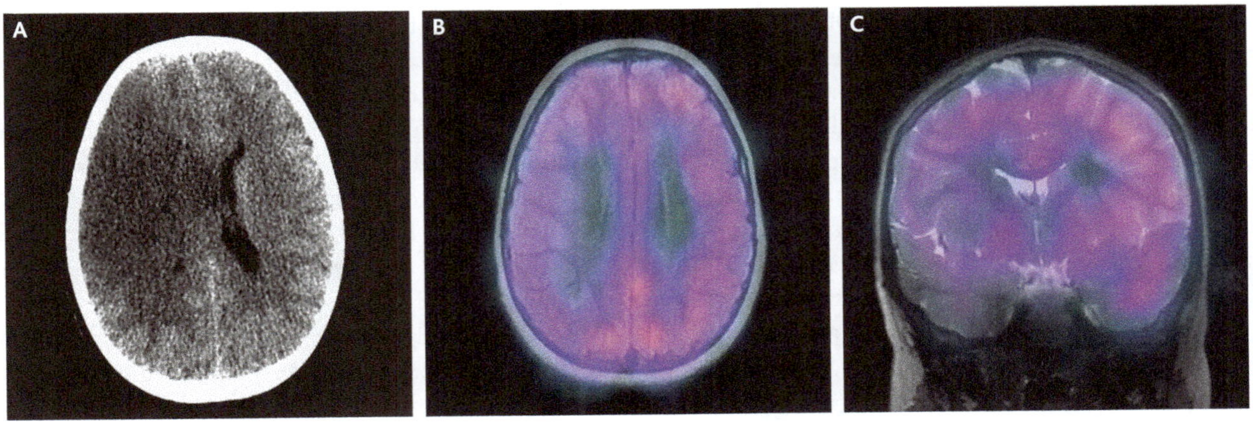

Figure 4-85A–C CT scan showing hypdensity of tissue within the right internal carotid and middle cerebral artery distributions. SPECT evidence of hypometabolism within the right internal carotid, middle cerebral and anterior cerebral distributions. For images 4-85b and c, the brightness or luminance of the purple corresponds to the extent of rCBF, with a brighter appearance corresponding to more flow. **B:** Axial SPECT+MRI. **C:** Coronal SPECT+MRI.

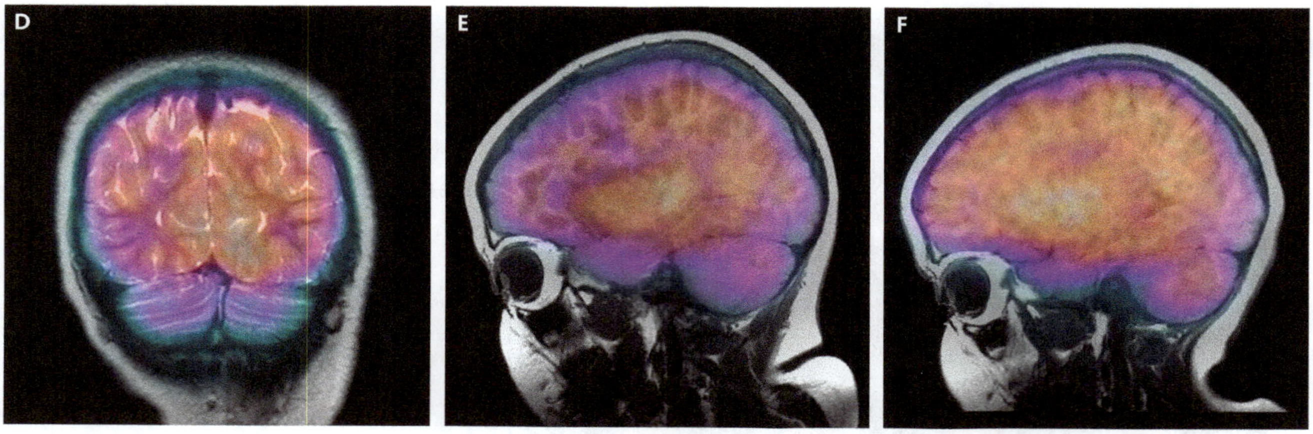

Figures 4-85D–F SPECT evidence of hypometabolism within the right internal carotid, middle cerebral and anterior cerebral distributions. For images 4-85d–f, the degree of rCBF is least for areas colored purple, greater for areas colored orange, and highest in areas that are yellow. **D:** Posterior coronal SPECT+MRI. **E:** Sagittal SPECT+MRI right hemisphere. **F:** Sagittal SPECT+MRI left hemisphere.

Functional Magnetic Resonance Imaging (fMRI)

Functional magnetic resonance imaging (fMRI) has become a relatively common research tool for measuring the effects of specific activities on brain functioning. fMRI can be considered the MRI equivalent of PET or SPECT in that it measures changes in regional demand for oxygenated blood commensurate with a specific task or activity. Brain areas with higher levels of metabolic activity produce a greater demand for regional cerebral blood flow and a disproportionate increase in the amount of oxygenated hemoglobin within that area. fMRI is able to detect small, rapid changes in blood oxygenation that correspond to a specific task or activity performed by the patient. The mechanism of fMRI involves the magnetic properties of hemoglobin, which differ according to the relative degree of oxygen saturation. Deoxygenated hemoglobin is paramagnetic and appears dark on a T2* sequence, whereas oxygenated hemoglobin is diamagnetic and appears brighter on a T2* image. The most common form of fMRI uses a blood oxygen level–dependent (BOLD) technique. An increase in neural activity results in oxygen demand greater than equilibrium in order to supply the increased metabolic load. When demand for oxygen rises, there is a vascular response in excess of need, producing an increase in oxyhemoglobin relative to deoxyhemoglobin. This results in a reduction of the T2 attenuation caused by the paramagnetic properties of deoxyhemoglobin, in addition to an increase in T2 signal (brighter) as a result of the increase in the diamagnetic oxyhemoglobin. BOLD techniques are based on the assumption that changes in blood oxygenation levels are positively correlated with increased metabolic demand by brain cells. The increased metabolic demand is thought to be correlated with increased activation of millions of neurons responding to the onset of a physical or mental task. While BOLD techniques are not the only form of fMRI, alternative methods are not yet common for clinical application and as such, will not be covered in this text.

During fMRI acquisition, patients are asked to perform a specific task paradigm, are presented with stimuli to one or more senses, or are asked to participate in active or passive (moved by someone else) physical movements. Activation of particular brain regions is recorded on the basis of degree of coincidence with the onset of patient activity or task paradigm. Multiple sets of images, often numbering in the thousands, are acquired from either response periods or resting periods. The image sets are then post-processed with sophisticated mathematical algorithms to assess for changes above a statistical threshold that would suggest a correlation between the change in BOLD signal and the activity of the task paradigm. The data are then graphically displayed according to brain location so that areas "most active" during the task can be identified.

fMRI has some notable advantages over functional imaging with PET or SPECT. fMRI is noninvasive, requiring no injection of tracer materials, and does not carry the same concerns regarding exposure of the patient to ionizing radiation via the radioisotope tracers. In addition, fMRI has greater spatial (1–2 mm) and temporal (1–2 seconds) resolution than that of PET or SPECT. Such resolution is considered high compared to alternate functional imaging techniques, but it is low when considered against the actual size of brain cells and neural microarchitecture or the millisecond timing of neural systems.

Because fMRI data need to be post-processed, the clinician can choose an appropriate statistical threshold to use for the specific case. Low statistical thresholds will identify larger areas of tissue with increased activation during a task, and higher thresholds can be used to show only the most active areas. For example, if a surgeon is primarily concerned with the functioning of larger regions of cortex, such as which hemisphere is used primarily for language processing, a low threshold can be used to show large areas of cortex activated by a language task, as in Figure 4-86. In this patient, only the left hemisphere was active during a varity of language-based tasks; the activation shown in Figure 4-86 is from a task involving fluent speech describing a favorite place to go to for vacation. Note the activation of both Wernicke's area and Broca's area, in addition to some activation over the arcuate fasciculus that joins these language areas.

Surgeons dealing with structures close to eloquent tissue may wish for a high degree of spatial resolution, thus a higher threshold can be used. For example, if the surgeon wishes to map the specific motor or sensory cortex associated with a particular finger or a hand, a higher threshold might be appropriate. Figures 4-87A–F were produced using a high statistical threshold, producing activation maps that show only the most active tissue corresponding to the specific task paradigm; right index finger movement in Figures 4-87A–C and left index finger movement in Figures 4-87D–F.

An advantage of using MR technology for functional applications such as fMRI relates to the use of three-dimensional protocols such as those used for BRAVO MRI sequences.

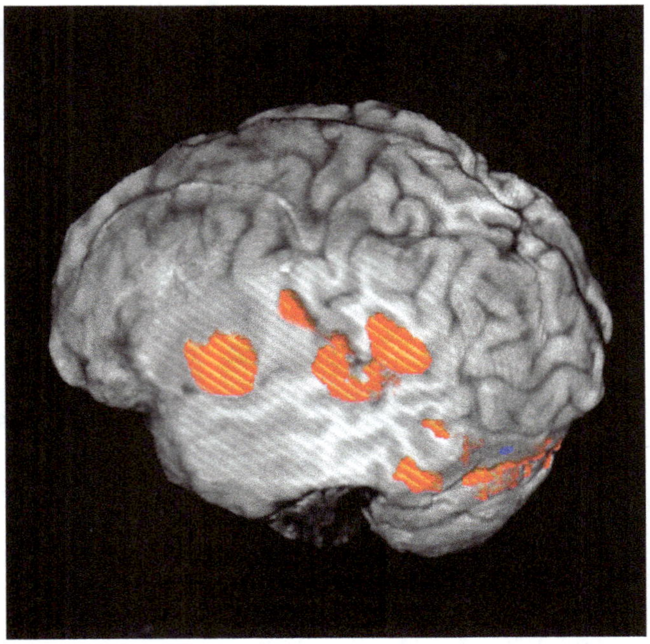

Figure 4-86 fMRI activation map for language processing using a relatively low statistical threshold.

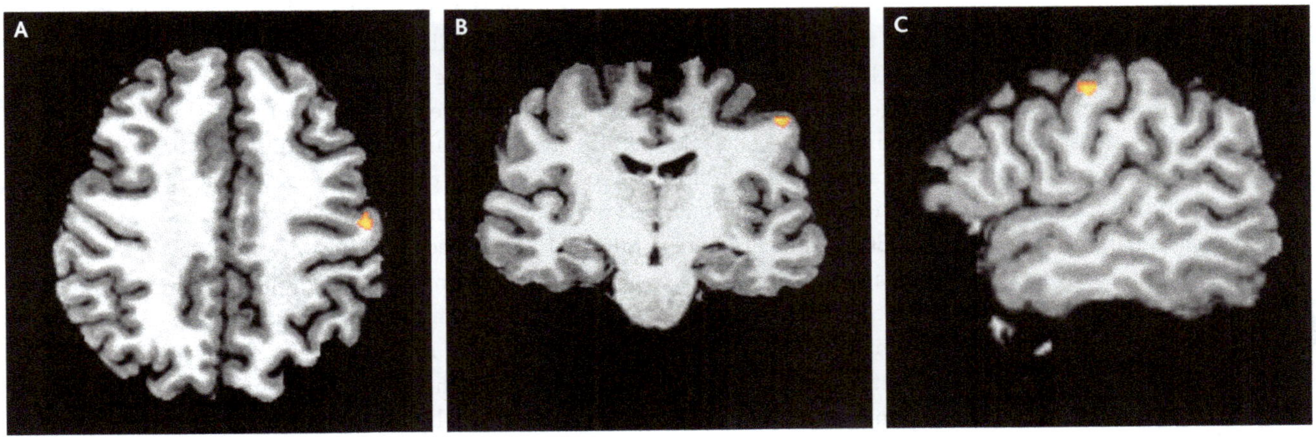

Figures 4-87A–C Right index finger BOLD activation maps (yellow-orange region).

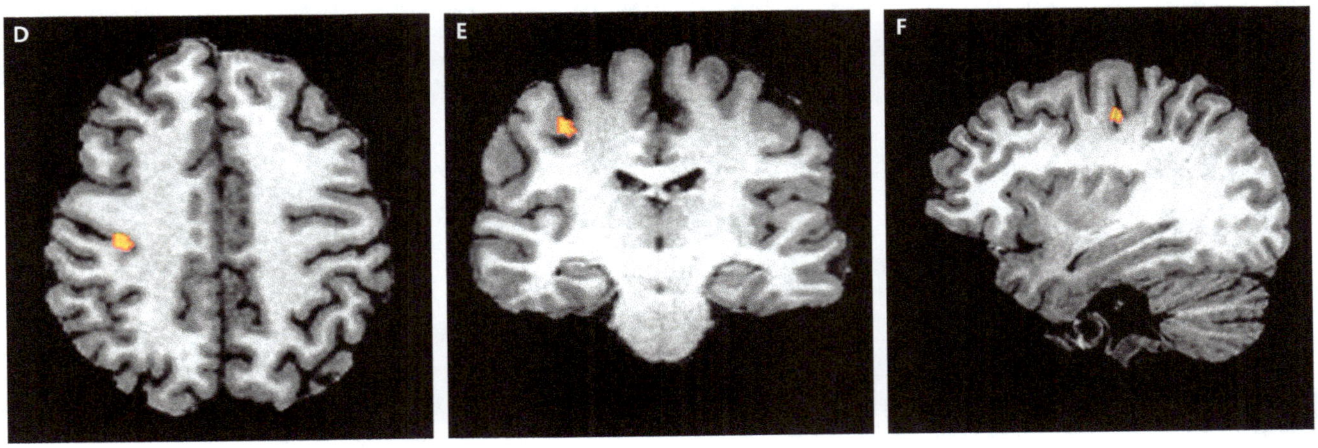

Figures 4-87D–F Left index finger BOLD activation maps (yellow-orange region).

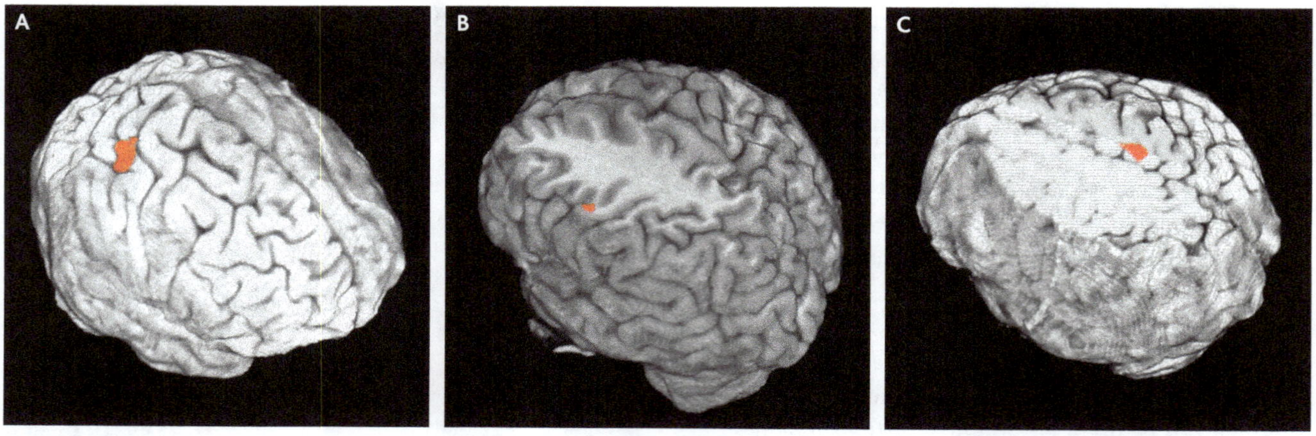

Figure 4-88A–C **A:** Left hand sensory BOLD activation map (red area). **B:** Right index finger motor BOLD activation map (red area). **C:** Left foot motor BOLD activation map (red area).

Using a base MR image acquired using a three dimensional protocol, such as BRAVO or FSPGR, the activation of brain areas can be displayed in two-dimensional axial, coronal, or sagittal slices in addition to three-dimensional graphical representations (Figures 4-88A–C).

Magnetic Encephalopathy (MEG-MSI)

While other functional brain scans detail the hemodynamics or metabolic activity of the brain, a MEG scanner measures fluctuations in the magnetic field that result from changes in the electrical potentials of active neurons. Magnetic field strength is related to the electrical potential of the source, thus fluctuations in the magnetic fields of neurons are extremely small. Because of this, MEG scanners require extremely sensitive sensors to convert magnetic fluctuations into electrical voltage changes, a task achieved by a superconducting quantum interference device (SQUID) magnetometer. Using a SQUID magnetometer, which requires cryogenic temperatures via liquid helium, the MEG scanner is capable of identifying tiny extracranial neuromagnetic fields at a femtotesla (10^{-15} T) level. The MEG scanner must be located within a shielded room to minimize ambient magnetic signals from electrical equipment such as computers, power cords, magnets found in many devices, and the earth's magnetic field. The task of isolating specific neuromagnetic fluctuations in the brain given all of the ambient magnetic fields within the environment is not unlike trying to record the sound of the footsteps of an ant during a rock concert. MEG scanners can detect neuromagnetic fluctuations at the millisecond (1/1000 second) temporal resolution but have relatively poor spatial resolution (from millimeters to around 2 centimeters).

As with fMRI, patients are presented stimuli or asked to perform a specific task during the acquisition stage. The information derived from MEG is correlated with the onset of stimulus presentation or the patient activity and presented on an MR image of the brain to produce what is called a magnetic source image (MSI). The MSI graphically codes the location of high activity in a manner similar to that used in other functional imaging techniques (Figures 4-89A–C).

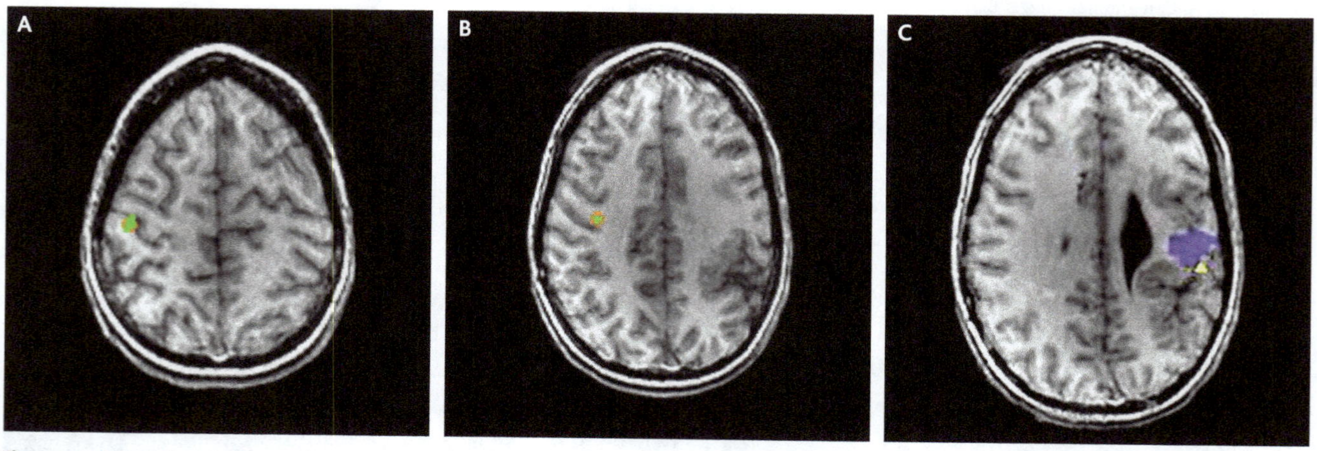

Figures 4-89A–C Functional mapping using MEG-MSI to localize areas of maximal activation during motor and sensory tasks (colored areas). **A:** Left index finger—sensory. **B:** Left lip—sensory. **C:** Right hand—motor. *Images courtesy of Joseph Sullivan, M.D.*

MEG-MSI can be used to measure evoked neural activity, such as that described above, or spontaneous neural activity when the patient remains passive during the acquisition stage.

Ictal MEG-MSI

Ictal MEG-MSI is used to localize abnormal electrical activity associated with seizures and is helpful in narrowing the location of seizure foci following initial EEG recording (Figures 4-90A–C). Ictal MEG-MSI can be combined with functional protocols to allow for the mapping of ictal spikes in addition to functional areas relating to specific activities performed by the patient. Figure 4-91 shows a MEG-MSI from a patient with spikes originating from his left periSylvian region, with language mapped to his right periSylvian region, consistent with the right hemisphere language laterality suggested by Wada examination.

An advantage of MEG-MSI is that it is a functional imaging technique that is noninvasive with no side effects. Also,

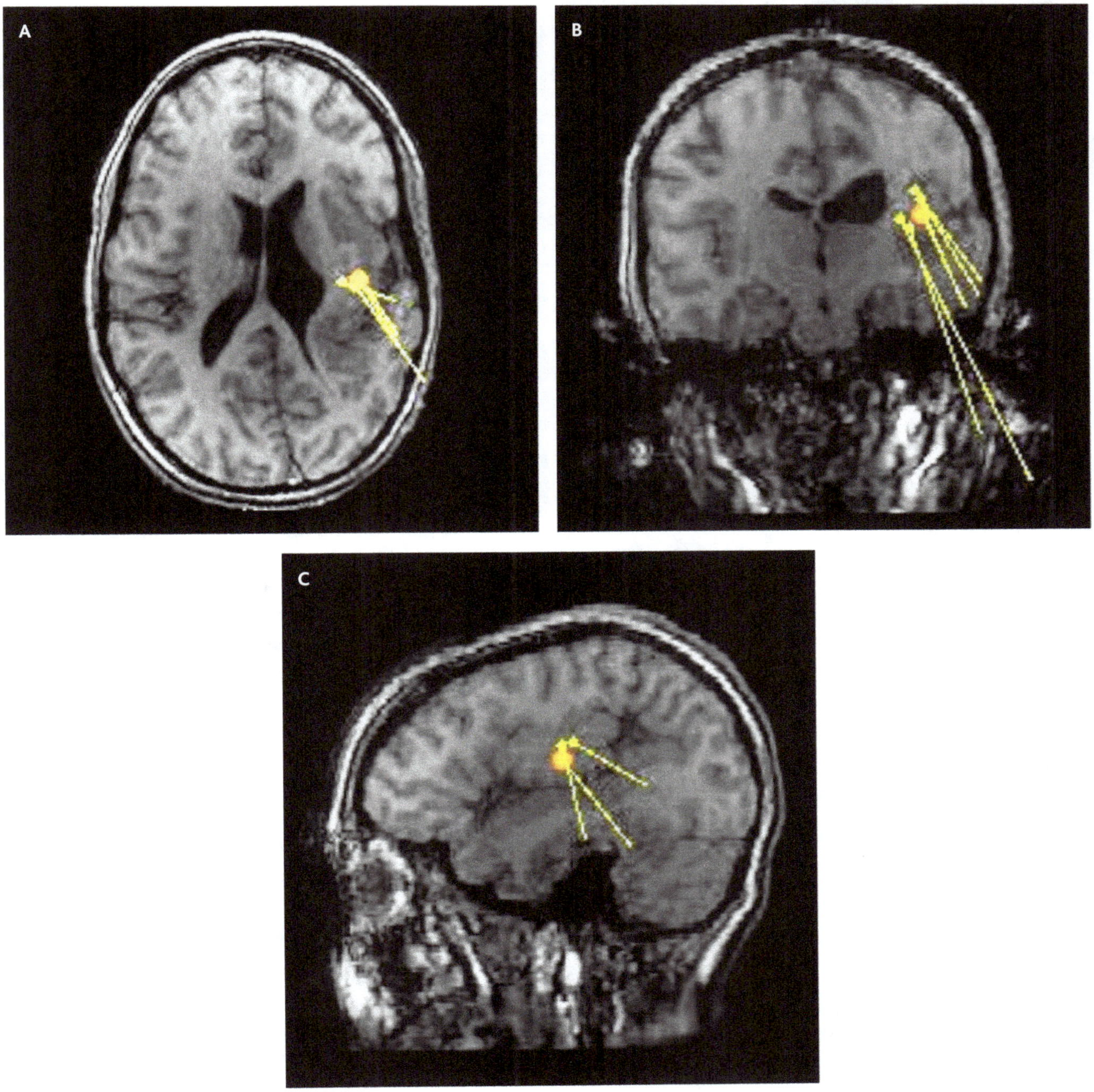

Figures 4-90A–C Ictal MEG-MSI used to localize seizure foci (yellow areas). *Images courtesy of Joseph Sullivan, M.D.*

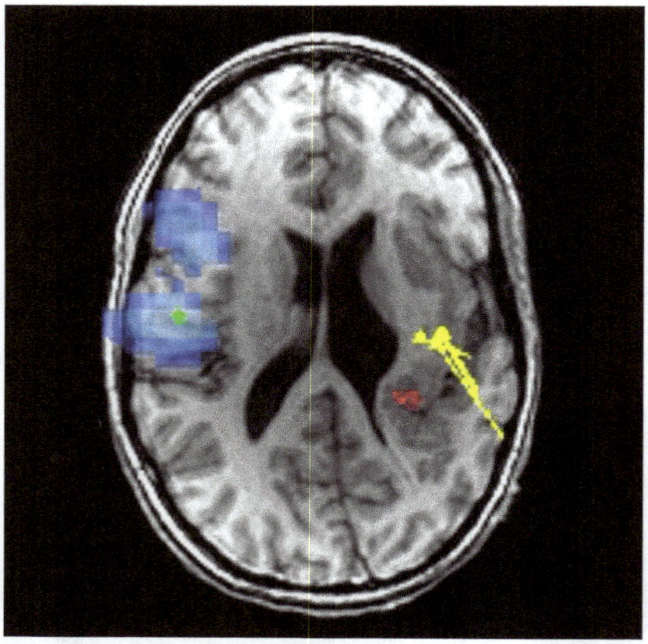

Figure 4-91 Speech and language mapping of a patient shown to have right hemisphere only langauge laterality on Wada examination. The yellow area indicates the location of ictal spikes, the blue areas represent tissue activated by language tasks, the green area represented the peak activation area of speech, and the red area represents the region activated during an auditory only task. *Image courtesy of Joseph Sullivan, M.D.*

it can produce real-time information to the clinician. Unlike fMRI, MEG scanning is silent, thus it is more appropriate for auditory paradigms.

Limitations of MEG-MSE

The primary limitation of MEG-MSE is the cost of the MEG scanner and special facilities required to shield the scanner from ambient magnetic field interference. Because of the requirement for a specific shielded facility, the cost is prohibitive for many institutions. Currently, MEG scanners are located primarily at large medical research facilities.

MEG scanners have relatively poor spatial resolution, but when combined with fMRI, this limitation can be minimized. Similarly, although MEG lacks structural and anatomical data, by combining MEG with MRI, information about a magnetic source and anatomical locations can be provided within the 3D MRI data matrix.

MEG–fMRI Combination

Just as PET and CT or PET and MRI are being combined to take advantage of the strengths of each systems, advances in technology have led to the introduction of MEG-fMRI systems. The combination of MEG-MSI and fMRI has the higher spatial resolution of fMRI, along with the higher temporal resolution of MEG-MSI. Thus combined MEG-fMRI systems can produce images with increased spatial and temporal resolution.

General Concerns About the Clinical Use of Functional Brain Imaging

A person is not a normalized population

For many years, functional imaging has been used for neuroscience research with great success. Functional brain imaging has only recently been applied to the clinical setting. Although the transition from research laboratory to clinic is a logical evolution for brain imaging, this change in application requires careful thought because there are many differences between these domains. A primary concern about the use of research-validated brain imaging techniques to assess patients relates to the application of normalized population data to an individual subject. Research studies using PET, SPECT, fMRI, and MEG rely on large population means and statistical procedures in order to carry out empirical norming and comparison between measures of central tendency (means, medians, and modes). Research methods and statistical procedures are designed to minimize noise (intra- and intersubject variability) so that the most accurate analysis of the data can be performed. However, clinical diagnostics and treatment planning are most beneficial when based on a patient's unique profile on imaging studies, something that may or may not match the standards and expectation derived from research protocols. If a patient's imaging does not match that expected from population data, the discrepancy may be seen as a clinically relevant issue or an inadequacy of the imaging technique, not one of normal variation. Such discrepancies may be relatively benign, having little effect on the patient's ultimate outcome. However, with the trend toward use of functional imaging for diagnoses and presurgical planning, small differences between a patient's functional brain imaging and that expected on the basis of research may make the difference between an appropriate and inappropriate diagnosis, or between a successful surgical outcome and one with profound functional deficits.

Is the "active" area a region of processing or a transmission hub?

Another concern regarding the small "active" areas suggested by functional imaging techniques relates to the understanding that the brain functions with a combination of discrete processing units and a highly complex, integrated network of neural systems. As such, an "active area" on a brain scan may not be the central processing unit for the activity being assessed but may instead be a transmission hub or nodal point within the distributed networks. This issue becomes especially important when attempting to map cortical regions before resection surgery. Avoiding an active hot spot may preserve part of the network, but it may put the patient at risk for resection of other areas that did not appear on the scan yet are still critical for functioning.

Local Activation versus Global or Distributed Activation

Caution is warranted when interpreting massive amounts of data and statistical outcomes that are ultimately represented as small, colored patches on a brain image. Such data can suggest that a stimulus or activity activates only a small area of tissue, but it may in fact be associated with a larger area. Adjustment to statistical threshold values on an fMRI can reduce the activation map from a relatively diffuse area to a small region where maximum activation was detected. Surgery around the small area of maximum activation may still be within critical eloquent cortex not visible on the image because the statistical threshold was set too high during post processing. One of the more difficult aspects of conducting functional imaging for clinical decision-making is determining where to set the threshold to highlight areas of highest activation, without missing other areas also involved in the task. Thresholds that are too low may result in images with activation evident in multiple regions of the brain. Thresholds that are too high may fail to show any area of activation or miss areas that are important but do not reach the threshold level and are not evident on the image.

Simple task paradigms are not the same as complex real-life activities

The use of a simple task paradigm for clinical assessment fails to take into consideration the complexity of normal functioning. For instance, when assessing "language functioning," a paradigm may consist of a simple linguistic task involving verbal fluency, word generation, rhyming, or naming. The functional study is predicated on the assumption that the task activates language-processing systems of the brain. However, cognitive tasks required for real-life activities are rarely simple and structured like those used during functional studies. Real-life cognitive activities rely on many other cognitive processes, such as arousal, attention, sensory processing, and executive functioning. Mapping cortex on the basis of a narrow task may fail to indicate the extent of tissue required for real-life activities within the same functional domain. Diagnostic and treatment planning based on a simple paradigm may not be adequate for all patients, especially given the complex nature of functioning in the real world.

Neuropathology can change metabolic functioning

Several functional imaging techniques are dependent on changes to metabolic activity or hemodynamics of brain tissue (PET, SPECT, fMRI). When using such data, it is important to consider the effects of a particular neuropathogical process on metabolic activity and hemodynamics. Conditions such as traumatic brain injury, hypoxic encephalopathy, encephalitis and meningitis, and neoplasms change the metabolic and hemodynamic status of involved tissue, a change that may affect interpretation of a functional brain image.

Functional imaging techniques are indirect measures of neural activity.

Functional imaging techniques do not directly measure neural activity. SPECT and fMRI rely on changes in blood flow and oxygenation that are assumed to correlate with neural activity. PET is considered by some to be the most direct measure of neural activity, given that it relies on metabolic demands at the cellular level. However, the actual measures are based on the gamma rays produced by the annihilation of a positron when it connects with an electron, often several millimeters from the source of the tracer or "active tissue." MEG-MSI is also considered a direct measure of neural activity. However, MEG-MSI is actually an indirect measure of neural activity, as the images are based on the recording of magnetic field fluctuations, correlated with neural firing.

Because functional brain imaging techniques are really indirect measures of neural functioning, interpretation is based on the assumption that the measures are highly correlated with neural activity. As taught in freshman statistics, correlation does not imply causation, a lesson to heed when using functional data to determine critical patient care needs. Because functional imaging techniques have a degree of inherent noise (technical and biological), with enough statistical comparisons, over time it is not only possible but actually expected that noise in the system will appear as a "signal." The somewhat unpredictable nature of thought processes, cell metabolism, blood flow, and neuron firing will at times result in an area of the brain becoming active at the same time that a stimulus is presented or a task is completed, purely by chance. Thus it is critical that findings from functional neuroimaging studies be replicated using multiple paradigms (stimuli or task activities), or confirmed by other methods before such findings are used in clinical decision-making.

When findings are clear and unambiguous across measures, clinical decisions can comfortably be made with indirect measures of neural activity. However, the more equivocal the findings, the more critical the assumptions of causation become and the lower the reliance on the data should be for the clinical team. Combining results from a variety of measures is recommended, when possible, to ensure that the data are valid and not a statistical anomaly.

Neural Activation Functions at the Submillisecond Level

MEG-MSI is the only functional neuroimaging technique that functions at the millisecond level of temporal resolution. PET, SPECT, and fMRI all function at a temporal resolution greater than 1 second, or 1000 milliseconds. As such, the activity at the cellular or nerve level of analysis is taking place at more than 1/1000th the rate of the measures commonly being employed to assess such activity. A further concern regarding the temporal resolution of functional imaging techniques relates to the lag time between activation of nerve cells and the change in physiological markers used to measure the activation. This is most pronounced in PET, in which long lag times are required to ensure that the radiotracer accumulates in the "active" tissue. SPECT relies on vascular changes, which are also relatively slow in comparison to the millisecond speed of neural firing. Even with the relatively rapid acquisition sequences of fMRI there can be a lag of several seconds between nerve cell activation and measurement of oxygenation levels for the hemoglobin. MEG-MSI has the highest temporal resolution, and combining this technique with other techniques such as fMRI has shown some promise in alleviating the concerns about temporal lag time.

The Problem of Type I (False Positive) Errors

Once a patient has been scanned by functional imaging techniques, massive amounts of data must be analyzed by means of complex computer algorithms or statistical packages. The greater the amount of data and number of comparisons to be analyzed, the more important it is to control for error, especially type I error, or a false-positive result. Put another way, conducting multiple comparisons on large datasets will increase the probability that a "significant finding" will be discovered purely by chance. fMRI paradigms are especially prone to this type of error in that there are a lot of data comparisons, often around 130,000, resulting in a high probability that some will be significant by chance. Recently, fMRI packages have incorporated statistical controls for multiple comparisons, thus minimizing false discovery rates and family-wise error. The use of high statistical thresholds can also minimize type I error, although it will increase occurrence of type II errors or the failure to detect a signal when one is present.

The Problem of Nonindependence

With fMRI, an additional concern relates to the technique of first evaluating which parts of the brain are most responsive to a stimulus or task activity and then re-evaluating the paradigm with focus only on that region. Statistically, this is akin to conducting post hoc analyses without adjusting for the increased error rate, or the statistical problem of nonindependence. When there is nonindepedence, a hypothesis is not independent of manipulation by the experimenters and can be affected in a manner to maximize not only findings but also type I error (false alarms). In nonstatistical terms, this is akin to trawling for fish in a large ocean, finding an area populated by fish, studying that area in depth, and then applying the results to the entire ocean. By statistically double-dipping, both type I and type II error are increased. The study is more likely to find "activation" in the area of interest by chance (type I error) but also miss activation in other areas that are not the focus of interest (type II error).

Time Required to Complete a Study

With functional neuroimaging, problems can arise because of the extended time period required for many of the studies. Even the most cooperative patients can have difficulty maintaining the same head position for many minutes at a time. Any head movement during a study can result in artifacts that obscure actual signals and result in increased noise. Such head movements decrease the signal-to-noise ratio and can produce type II errors, or the failure to detect a signal when one is present.

Interpretation of Functional Imaging Data

The use of brain imaging to evaluate functioning has revolutionized the field of clinical neuroscience, and the benefits of such techniques have been immeasurable. Functional imaging techniques have improved scientific understanding of the brain and allowed for new clinical procedures to be developed that minimize patient discomfort, morbidity, and mortality. For example, invasive Wada procedures are being replaced by data provided by a combination of functional imaging techniques, thus reducing the risk of iatrogenic stroke caused by the catheterization of the patient. However, when interpreting functional imaging findings, many assumptions are required, and many caveats are necessary in order to control for the concerns described earlier. Such clinical rigor will only benefit the field. These concerns are not advanced as criticism of the methods but as a way to encourage advancements in technique and appropriate caution when formulating clinical decisions based on research findings.

Benefits of Using Multiple Functional Imaging Techniques for Each Patient

Many large medical centers now use diagnostic and treatment planning protocols that employ multiple redundant functional brain imaging measures. For example, a presurgical workup for a patient with partial seizures may include neurological and neuropsychological assessments to highlight the patient's functional profile, fMRI and MEG-MSI to assess for language laterality or location of eloquent sensory, motor, or language cortex, and sometimes PET or SPECT studies to assess for areas of hypo- or hypermetabolism. A comparison of data from all functional assessment methods allows a higher level of clinical decision-making. Data that are consistent between methods may be seen as clinically valid and reliable enough to allow the patient to progress to surgery or to a particular treatment regimen. When data are less consistent between measures, other more invasive procedures may be employed, such as transfemoral sodium amytal Wada testing or awake surgical procedures with electrocorticography and electrical stimulation-based brain mapping. Combining a variety of functional brain imaging methods for an individual patient provides clinical information based on the strengths of each method while minimizing the limitations inherent in each procedure.

CLOSING REMARKS

Chapter 4 provided a guide to the various imaging technologies available to the clinician. Although not all of these modalities may be available to you, it is important to know the basics of how they work and what information they can provide. Even though you may not have access to some imaging modalities, with the ease of storing multiple scanning series on a CD or DVD, it is likely that you will receive scans from other institutions that use modalities different from those available to you. Thus you should be prepared to review data from a variety of scanning technologies, not just standard CT or MRI. Once you develop a foundation of knowledge of the various types of scanning technologies, it is important to apply that information to a variety of clinical situations.

The next two chapters provide clinical examples of common conditions encountered in a clinical setting. Various brain imaging techniques were selected for visualizing the clinical examples in order to give you practice at interpreting a variety of scans. For most of the clinical examples, standard imaging sequences are used, such as CT, MRI-T1 and T2, and DWI/ADC, as these will be the ones you will most likely encounter in your clinic. Where necessary, the examples are of scans from more advanced systems, as well as 3D reconstruction for CT and MRI, to assist you in identifying the primary areas of pathology.

Chapter 5 covers injuries resulting primarily from physical trauma to the brain, such as contusion, diffuse axonal injuries, hemorrhages, and swelling. Chapter 6 covers conditions mostly unrelated to physical trauma, such as infections, neoplasms, hypoxemia, and neurodevelopmental syndromes. It is important to consider the overlap between conditions presented in Chapters 5 and 6 and to understand that many conditions from one chapter may include pathologies from the other, and vice versa. For example, edema is a complication of both physical trauma and infection or hypoxia, and hemorrhages or strokes can be caused by trauma or nontraumatic conditions. The division of conditions according to primary etiology as trauma or non-trauma is intended to simplify the presentation of conditions and should not be interpreted as evidence of mutual exclusivity between the various disorders.

Because this is a guide to brain imaging, most clinical examples were chosen for their ease of interpretation. Many cases that you encounter in the clinic may be less obvious, more subtle, or even ambiguous compared to those in this guide. However, the primary features will likely be similar to those presented here, with the severity and extent of injury differing from case to case. When in doubt, consult a radiologist or clinician more familiar with the type and severity of pathology being assessed.

The clinical examples presented in Chapters 5 and 6 were selected on the basis of a variety of criteria. The primary focus was to use exemplar cases that were neither too subtle nor too obvious. Cases that are very subtle are difficult to visualize using only a few static images and may be missed by many readers. Cases that are obvious do not require close inspection or analysis on the part of the viewer and can result in a passive approach to learning. To facilitate your skill acquisition, many of the examples chosen represent pathologies that are readily evident but not always obvious without close attention to the image. Furthermore, to increase the use of active learning, arrows are not used on all cases to identify areas of pathology. The anatomical descriptions provided, as well as the specific slice choices and use of crosshairs, should make it relatively simple for you to visualize the regions of interest, without the use of arrows. Where appropriate, arrows are used to assist you in identifying specific image features relevant to the case or useful in your clinical interpretation and learning.

TABLE 4-1a Common Abbreviations for Sequences, Based on Vendor Sources

SEQUENCE LABEL	SIEMENS	GE	PHILIPS	HITACHI	TOSHIBA
Spin echo	SE	SE	SE	SE	SE
Gradient echo	GRE	GRE	Fast field echo (FFE)	GE	Field echo (FE)
Spoiled gradient echo	FLASH	SPGR, MPSPGR	T1-FFE	RF-spoiled SARGE, RSSG	Fast FE, RF-spoiled FE
Steady-state gradient echo	FISP	MPGR, GRE	FFE	TRSG	FE
Coherent gradient echo	FISP	GRASS	FFE	Rephased SARGE	SSFP
Steady-state free precession/ gradient echo	PSIF	SSFP	T2-FFE	Time-reversed SARGE	
Balanced gradient echo—true FISP	TrueFISP	FIESTA	Balanced FFE	Balanced SARGE, BASG	True SSFP
True FISP/duel excitation	CISS	FIESTA-C		Phase-balanced SARGE, PBSG	
Double echo steady state	DESS				
Multi-echo data image combination	MEDIC	MERGE	M-FFE		
Ultrafast gradient echo	TurboFLASH	FAST GRE, FAST SPGR	TFE	RGE	Fast FE
Ultrafast gradient echo 3D	MPRAGE	3D FGRE, 3D Fast SPGR, MPRAGE, FSPGR BRAVO (half K-space)	3D TFE	MPRAGE	3D fast FE
Ultrafast gradient echo with magnetization preparation	T_1/T_2-TurboFLASH	IR-FSPGR, DE-FSPGR	IR-TFE		Fast FE
Volume-interpolated GRE	VIBE	LAVA-XV	THRIVE	TIGRE	
Susceptibility-weighted imaging	SWI	SWAN	Venous BOLD		
Dynamic MRA with K-space manipulation	TWIST	TRICKS-XV	Keyhole 4D-TRAK		
Non-contrast TSE-based MRA	NATIVE-SPACE		TRANCE	VASC FSE	FBI, CIA
Non-contrast true FISP-based MRA	NATIVE-TrueFISP	Inhance inflow IR	B-TRANCE	VASC ASL	Time-SLIP
Inversion recovery	IR, Turbo IR (TIR)	IR, MPIR, FastIR	IR-TSE	IR	IR
Short tau inversion recovery	STIR	STIR	STIR	STIR	FastSTIR
Long tau inversion recovery	Turbo dark fluid	FLAIR	FLAIR	FLAIR	FastFLAIR
True inversion recovery	True IR		Real IR		FastIR

(Continued)

Table 4-1a (Continued)

Sequence Label	Siemens	GE	Philips	Hitachi	Toshiba
Fast spin echo, turbo spin echo	Turbo spin echo (TSE)	Fast spin echo (FSE)	Turbo spin echo (TSE)	Fast spin echo (FSE)	Fast spin echo (FSE)
Ultra-fast spin echo	SSTSE, HASTE	SS-FSE	SSH-TSE, UFSE	FSE-ADA	(Super) FASE, DIET
Single-shot fast spin echo/turbo spin echo	HASTE	Single-shot FSE	Single-shot TSE	Single-shot FSE	FASE
Multi-echo spin echo	Multi echo	SE	Multi SE	SE	Multi écho
FSE/TSE with 90° flip-back pulse	RESTORE	Fast recovery FSE (FRFSE)	DRIVE	Drive equilibrium FSE	T2 pulse FSE
Hyper echoes	Hyperecho				
3D TSE with variable flip angle	SPACE	CUBE	VISTA		
Turbo gradient spin echo (GRASE)	TurboGSE, TGSE		GRASE		Hybrid EPI
Hybrid echo planar	TurboGSE, TGSE		GRASE		Hybrid EPI
Motion correction with radial blades	BLADE	PROPELLER	MultiVane	RADAR	JET
Echo planar imaging (EPI)	EPI	EPI	EPI	EPI	EPI
Spin echo-echo planar	EPI SE	SE EPI	SE EPI	SE EPI	SE EPI
GE-echo planar	EPI Perf, EPIFI	GRE EPI	FFE-EPI, TFE-EPI	SG-EPI	FE-EPI
Hybrid echo planar	TurboGSE, TGSE		GRASE		Hybrid EPI
Diffusion-weighted imaging (DWI)	DWI	DWI	DWI	DWI	DWI
Apparent diffusion coefficient map	ADC	ADC	ADC	ADC Map	ADC

Table 4-1b Abbreviations for Parameters Based on Vendor Source

Parameter	Siemens	GE	Philips	Hitachi	Toshiba
Echo time	TE	TE	TE	TE	TE
Repetition time	TR	TR	TR	TR	TR
Inversion time	TI	TI	TI	TI	TI
Averages	Averages	NEX	NSA	NSA	NSA
Simultaneous extinction	Simultaneous extinction	Phase offset multiplanar (POMP)	Multi-slice	Dual slice	QuadScan
RF pulse in gradient echo	Flip angle	Flip angle	Flip angle	Flip angle	Flip angle
Scan measurement time	Acquisition time, TA	Acquisition time	Acquisition time	Scan time	Acquisition time
Distance between slices	Distance factor (% of slice thicknes)	Gap	Gap	Slice interval	Gap
Shifting slice off center	Off-center shift	Off-center FoV	Off-center FoV	Off-center FoV	Phase & frequency shift
Field of view (FoV)	FoV (mm)	FoV (cm)	FoV (mm)	FoV	FoV
Rectangular FoV	FoV phase rectangular FoV	Partial FoV (PFoV)	Rectangular FoV	Rectangular FoV	Rectangular FoV
Bandwidth	Bandwidth (Hz/Px)	Receive bandwidth (kHz)	Fat/water shift (pixel)	Bandwidth	Bandwidth
Variable bandwidth	Optimized bandwidth	Variable bandwidth	Optimized bandwidth	Variable bandwidth	Matched bandwidth
Frequency oversampling	Oversampling	Anti-aliasing	Frequency oversampling	Frequency oversampling	Frequency wrap suppression
Phase oversampling	Phase oversampling	No phase wrap	Fold-over suppression	Anti-wrap	Phase wrap suppression
Segmented K-space	Lines/segments	Views per segment	Views/segment		Segments
Time delay/block k-space	Time delay	Intersegment delay	TD		TD
Half Fourier imaging	Half Fourier	1/2 NEX fractional NEX	Half scan	Half scan	AFI
Partial echo	Asymmetric echo	Partial Echo	Partial echo	Half echo	Matched bandwidth
Gradient moment nulling	GMR/flow comp	Flow comp	Flow comp; flag	GR	FC
Ramped RF pulse	TONE	Ramped pulse	TONE	SSP	ISCE
Magnetization transfer contrast	MTC, MTS	MTC	MTC	MTC	SORS-STC
Prep pulse—chemically	Fat sat	Fat sat/chem sat	SPIR	Fat Sat	MSOFT
Water excitation	Water excitation		Proset	Water excitation	PASTA
Fat–water separation	DIXON	IDEAL		FatSep	
Prep pulse—spatially	Presat	SAT	REST	Pre sat	Pre sat
Moving sat pulse	Travel sat, Tracking sat	Walking sat	Travel REST	Sequential pre sat	BFAST
Multichannel RF coil sensitivity normalization	Prescan normalize	PURE	CLEAR	NATURAL	
Central k-space filling arterial visualization	Elliptical scanning	Elliptical centric	CENTRA	PEAKS	DRKS

5 NEUROIMAGING OF TRAUMATIC BRAIN INJURIES

Traumatic brain injuries comprise a very heterogeneous group of conditions. Thus it is not unusual for a patient to receive more than one series of images acquired with a variety of modalities. Emergency or critical-care imaging with CT may be used to provide information regarding imminent herniation or bleeds, or other conditions requiring immediate neurosurgical intervention. Follow-up MRI may become necessary if the initial CT does not fully explain a patient's clinical presentation. Until recently, MRI was considered elective, not emergent, as scans required long acquisition times. However, with increased magnet strength and more advanced sequences, MRI can now be acquired rapidly enough for some utility in the emergency department. Even with advances in MRI, within the emergency department, CT remains the primary imaging resource for traumatic brain injuries. Although MRI may result in a small increase in one's ability to visualize injury not visible on CT, this does not outweigh the risks of placing an acutely ill patient into a device where monitoring is difficult and all ferro-magnetic materials must be removed from the patient and treatment team.

Patients who have sustained concussions or mild closed-head injuries may have "normal"-appearing CT scans, especially if done acutely and prior to significant development of edema. CT scans and most MRI sequences are poor measures of subtle brain injury because of their limited spatial and contrast resolution. Neuroimaging may fail to show smaller microbleeds at the cellular level or areas of axonal shearing, although newer sequences such as susceptibility-weighted imaging (SWI) have made advances in this area and show some promise. CT imaging is the technique of choice for fractures of the calvarium, especially with a dedicated bone-window or with three-dimensional reconstruction and volume rendering.

CT imaging is less useful than MRI in determining the extent and severity of traumatic damage to brain parenchyma because of the poor contrast resolution for soft tissues or those of similar density. Over time, damaged areas of parenchyma may be more easily identified on CT as tissue density decreases and the area starts to atrophy. Severe diffuse injury to the brain, such as that sustained in an unrestrained high-speed motor vehicle accident or in cases of nonaccidental trauma (NAT) to a baby or infant, can result in changes to the brain that are easily identified on CT. Hemorrhages are frequently evident on CT after traumatic brain injury, especially larger bleeds within the meningeal layers. For fractures of the cranium, CT imaging remains the modality of choice, with high spatial and contrast resolution for bone. In addition, 3D reconstruction and volume rendering of the calvarium can provide excellent visualization of fractures.

MRI is the method of choice for post-acute assessment of traumatic brain injuries, especially when the patient's symptom constellation is not explained by CT. With the higher spatial and contrast resolution, injuries not evident on CT may be readily apparent on MRI. Diffusion and perfusion sequences enable assessment of ischemia or infarction, which are frequent consequences of physical trauma to the brain. Diffusion tensor imaging (DTI) is showing promise in assessing pathway damage due to diffuse axonal injuries and the effects of trauma or compression and shock waves acting on the soft brain tissue.

With increasing severity of traumatic brain injury, damage becomes more readily appreciated on all forms of brain imaging.

FOCAL INJURY, DIFFUSE INJURY, OR A COMBINATION?

When first learning about traumatic brain injuries, many students are instructed that there are two types of injury, focal and diffuse. In general, *focal injuries* affect small areas of tissue and result in symptoms specific to only that area. In contrast, *diffuse injuries* affect large areas of tissue, without focal damage to any one region. The reality of most traumatic brain injuries is that both focal and diffuse damage to the brain often coexist, resulting in some focal deficits and some general compromise to brain systems. Closed-head injuries almost without exception result in a combination of focal and diffuse injury to the brain. Focal injuries are most often the result of contusions, hemorrhages, or both, while diffuse injuries are often the result of twisting forces or shearing of thin axons or blood vessels. Shock waves that travel through the soft brain tissue owing to the compression wave from high-speed impacts can result in diffuse damage to tissue some distance from the contact point. Shock waves from explosions can damage the brain diffusely, although focal injuries may be caused by damage to specific blood vessels. Penetrating injuries, sometimes called "missile injuries," may or may not result in both focal

CLINICAL EXAMPLE

Joshua: Focal Injury Suggested by Imaging but with Focal and Diffuse Pathology

Joshua was injured by a piece of lumber that fell from a scaffold at a construction site. He was not wearing a construction safety helmet, and the heavy piece of wood caused a skull fracture and a relatively focal hemorrhagic contusion of the right frontal lobe. There was no loss of consciousness at the scene and he was responsive following the injury. Shortly after the injury, Joshua experienced a rapid deterioration of mental status; his Glasgow coma score (GCS) dropped from 15 to 8 during transport to the emergency department. He was intubated and an intracranial pressure monitor was placed. Head CT showed a right frontal depressed skull fracture with subarachnoid and subdural hemorrhages localized primarily to the right frontal region (Figures 5-1A–D).

Follow-up MRI also suggested a relatively focal injury to the right orbital frontal region, without evidence of diffuse damage to the brain (Figures 5-2A–D).

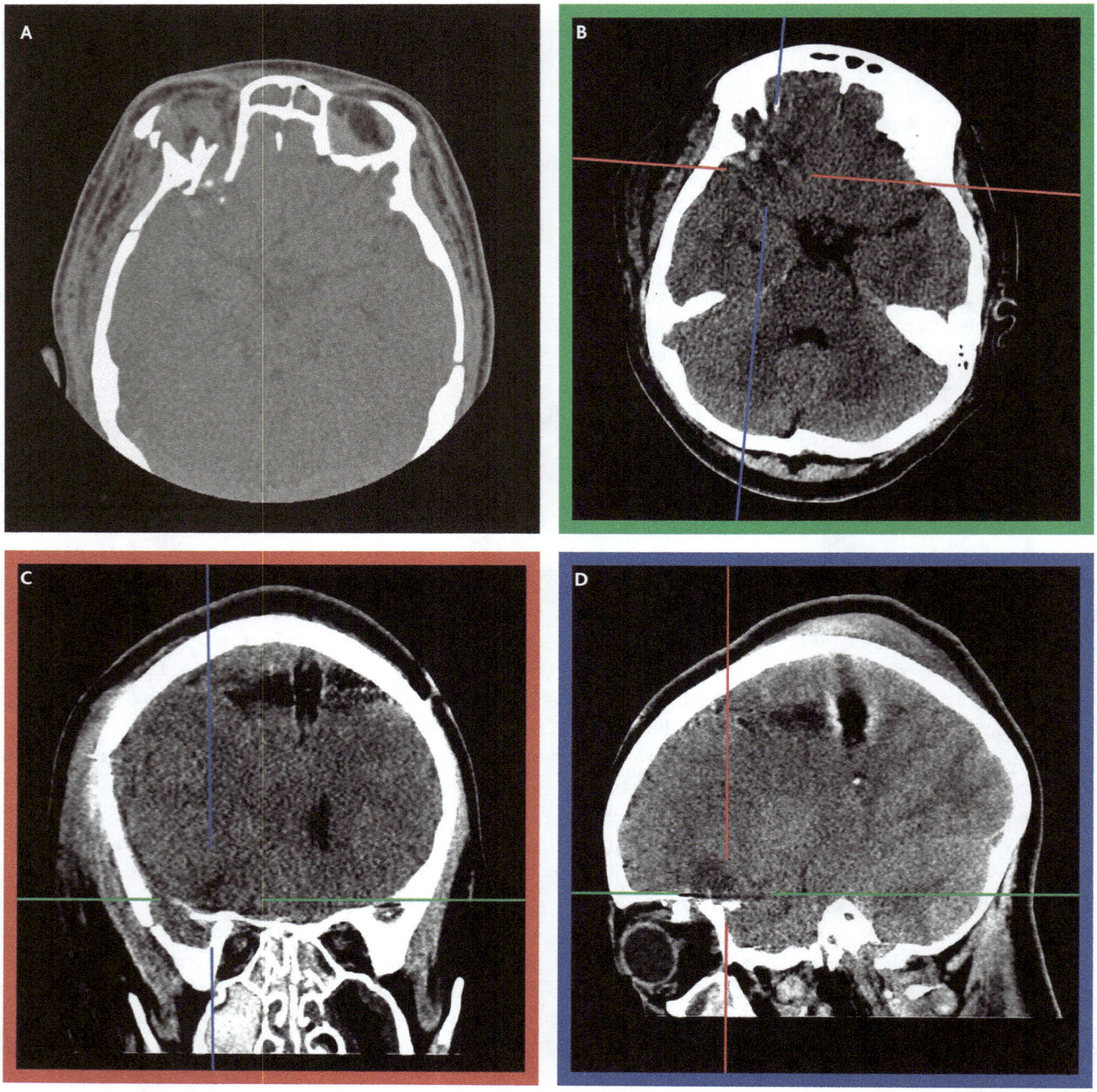

Figures 5-1A–D Clinical example Joshua: CT series showing right orbital skull fracture and focal injury to the right frontal lobe.

Review of the CT and MRI scans suggested that Joshua's brain injury was focal, and there was no reason to believe that the impact was of the severity to cause significant shock waves that could damage the brain diffusely or cause axonal shear injury. However, clinical assessment was remarkable for Joshua presenting with significant global cognitive and functional compromise, which are more consistent with a diffuse injury than a focal injury to the right frontal lobe. Review of his medical chart indicated that his intracranial pressures were extremely high (above 40 mmHg) during his intensive-care stay. Normal intracranial pressure ranges from a little below 10 to approximately 15 mmHg for an adult lying down. Pressures above 20 mmHg are considered abnormal, and pressures above 40 mmHg almost universally result in brain damage. Although Joshua's injury was of the type to cause mostly focal damage and his acute brain scans suggested focal damage, his excessive intracranial pressure resulted in significant diffuse secondary injury to his brain. Six months after his injury, Joshua continued to present with evidence of diffuse neurological compromise, consistent with deficient executive functioning, attentional abilities, memory, and higher-order reasoning skills.

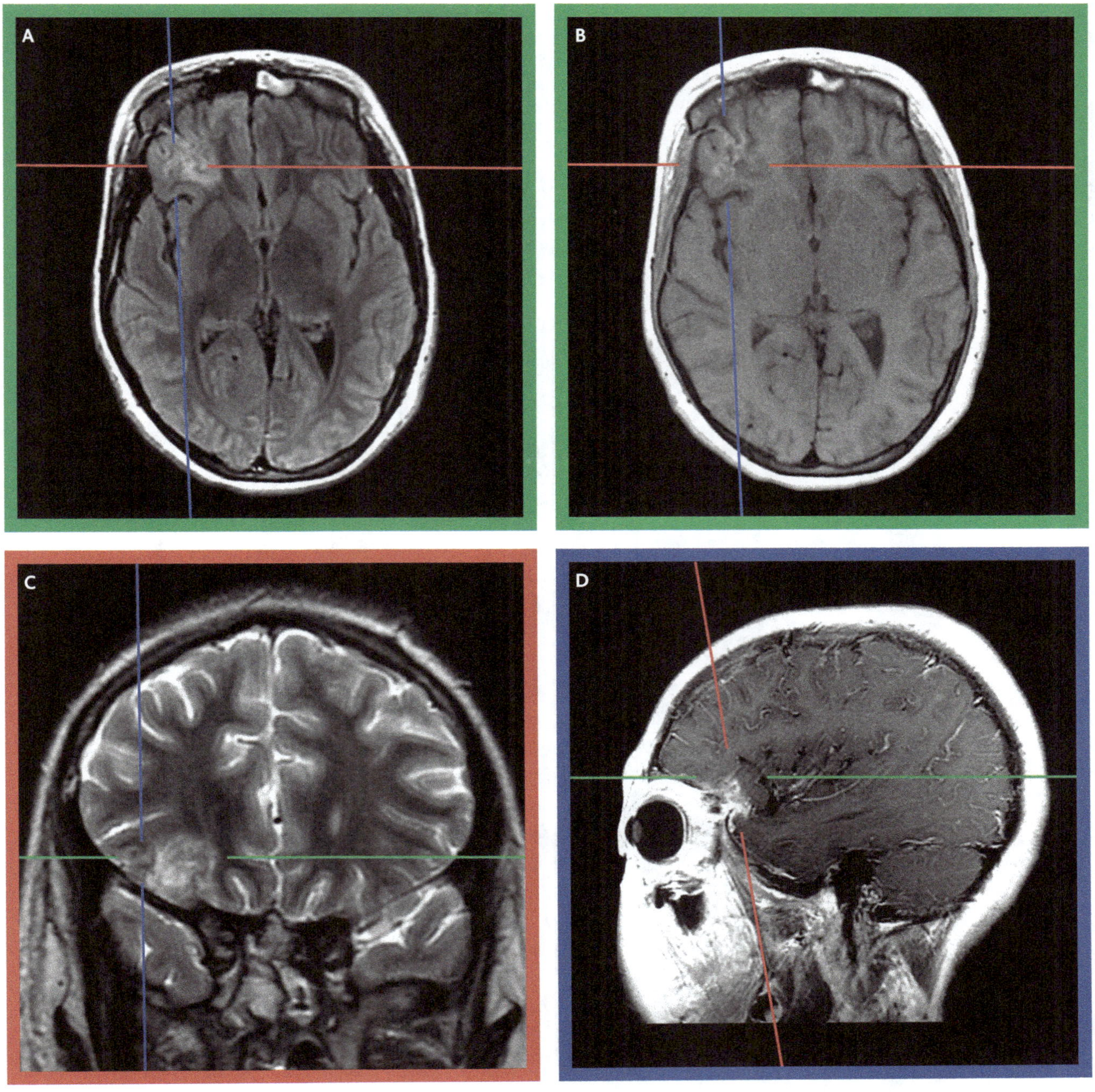

Figures 5-2A–D Clinical example Joshua: follow-up MRI series showing focal right frontal injury. **A:** T2 FLAIR. **B:** T1. **C:** T2. **D:** CE-T1.

and diffuse injury, the most critical factor being the velocity of the penetrating object. High-velocity projectiles not only result in a focal wound track but also diffuse injury radiating from the projectile path caused by the pressure wave and heat relating to the dispersing energy of the object. Even in cases where imaging suggests focal trauma, secondary mechanisms such as increased intracranial pressure, release of excitatory amino acids, compromised autoregulation, and other processes can result in diffuse damage in excess of that expected given the focal injury evident on imaging.

POST-TRAUMATIC HEMORRHAGES

One of the primary neuroimaging indicators of physical trauma to the brain is blood within the meningeal layers, brain parenchyma, or ventricular system. CT is sensitive to hemorrhages that result from tearing of bridging vessels within meningeal layers; this tearing produces epidural (outside the dura), subdural (under the dura), or subarachnoid (within the arachnoid layer) hemorrhages. Intraparenchymal and intraventricular hemorrhages are also evident on CT, making it the technique of choice for post-traumatic bleeds, especially in the emergency department. MR imaging is often used for follow-up assessments to more accurately visualize the severity and extent of hemorrhage and soft-tissue damage to the brain.

Epidural Hematoma/ Hemorrhage (EDH)

Epidural hematomas (EDH) result from blood pooling between the cranium and the dural layer. Epidural bleeds are often associated with fractures of the skull and the severing of vessels lying between the dura and the skull. As the area between the dura and skull fills with blood, the dura dissects away from the skull, producing a lenticular (lens-shaped) mass on the scan (Figures 5-3A–C). The mass can deform the underlying brain tissue and result in midline shift, asymmetrical compression of the ventricles, and, ultimately, herniation of the brain.

Herniation of the brain involves the pushing or extruding of soft tissue across a dural membrane. Two common areas for herniation are the uncus, which is located on the

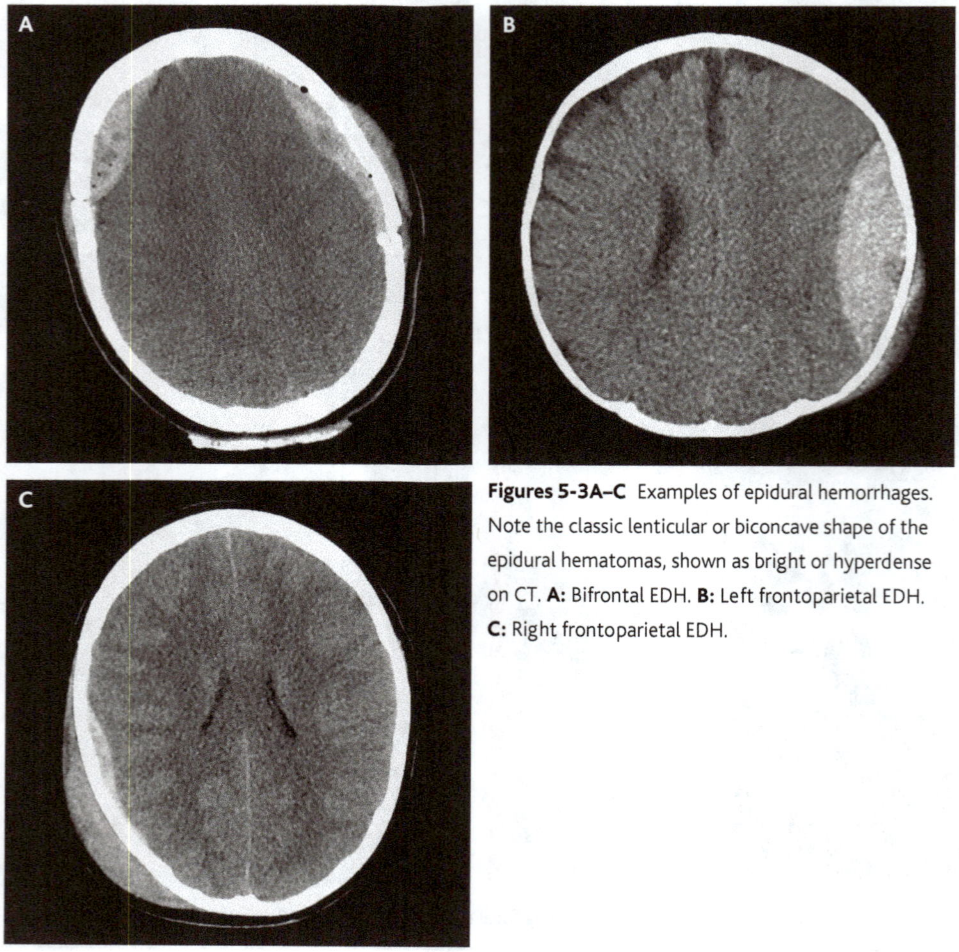

Figures 5-3A–C Examples of epidural hemorrhages. Note the classic lenticular or biconcave shape of the epidural hematomas, shown as bright or hyperdense on CT. **A:** Bifrontal EDH. **B:** Left frontoparietal EDH. **C:** Right frontoparietal EDH.

medial aspect of the temporal lobe, and the medulla, which can be pushed inferiorally through the foramen magnum (Latin: large hole), at the base of the skull. Herniation of the brain stem structures is life threatening and requires rapid, emergent surgical treatment, often involving evacuation of the hematoma, in addition to decompressive craniotomy, to release pressure inside the cranium if swelling is a concern.

In addition to the risk of herniation, if the pressure on brain tissue exceeds cerebral perfusion pressure or the pressure required to push the blood through the capillary beds, hypoxic ischemic injuries can result and cause damage to brain tissues. Other than the mass effect and the resulting pressure exerted on the brain, there may be little damage to brain tissue from an epidural hemorrhage, especially if evacuated acutely and prior to herniation (Hutchison & Lebby, 2009). Epidural hematomas can form rapidly if major vessels such as the main branches of the middle meningeal artery are severed. Conversely, if smaller vessels are breached, it may take several hours before an epidural hemorrhage causes enough neural disruption to warrant medical attention. Epidural bleeds from arterial sources have a greater risk of pressure effects and herniation than venous epidural bleeds because of the reduced pressure of the venous system. Skull fractures are a frequent cause of epidural bleeds, and the review of images should include an assessment of cranial fractures.

It is important to note that the appearance of blood on imaging changes over time (see Table 2-4); this should be taken into account when viewing epidural hematomas. For example, on CT, hyperacute bleeds of less than a few hours may appear isodense to brain or heterogeneous, with the hemorrhage increasing in density for a few hours to days and eventually becoming hyperdense (bright) (Figures 5-3A–C). After a few days, the hemorrhage may again decrease in density and appear isodense or even hypodense.

REFERENCE

Hutchison, T., & Lebby, P. C. (2009). Traumatic encephalopathies In R. B. David (Ed)., *Clinical pediatric neurology* (3rd ed.). New York: Demos Medical Publishing.

At times, epidural hematomas may appear to have a heterogeneous appearance, something that is referred to as a "swirl sign." A *swirl sign* is suggestive of active bleeding, with fresh blood that is less dense mixing with older blood that has clotted and has become more dense. There are times when a heterogeneous or swirl appearance is not caused by active bleeding, thus caution is warranted when interpreting this appearance. For example, chronic epidural hematomas can take on a hypodense or mixed-density appearance on CT imaging, which can be mistaken for ongoing bleeding or the swirl sign (Figures 5-4A–F).

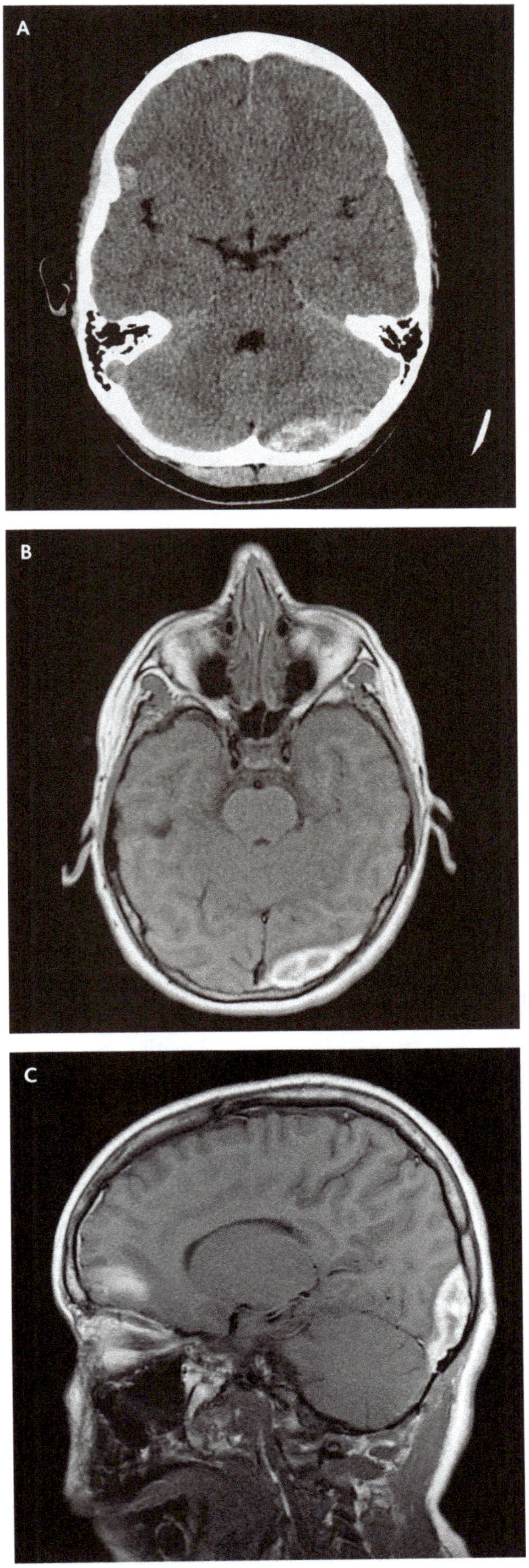

Figures 5-4A–C Non-contrast imaging of a venous occipital epidural hematoma with swirl sign. **A:** CT. **B:** T2 FLAIR. **C:** T1.

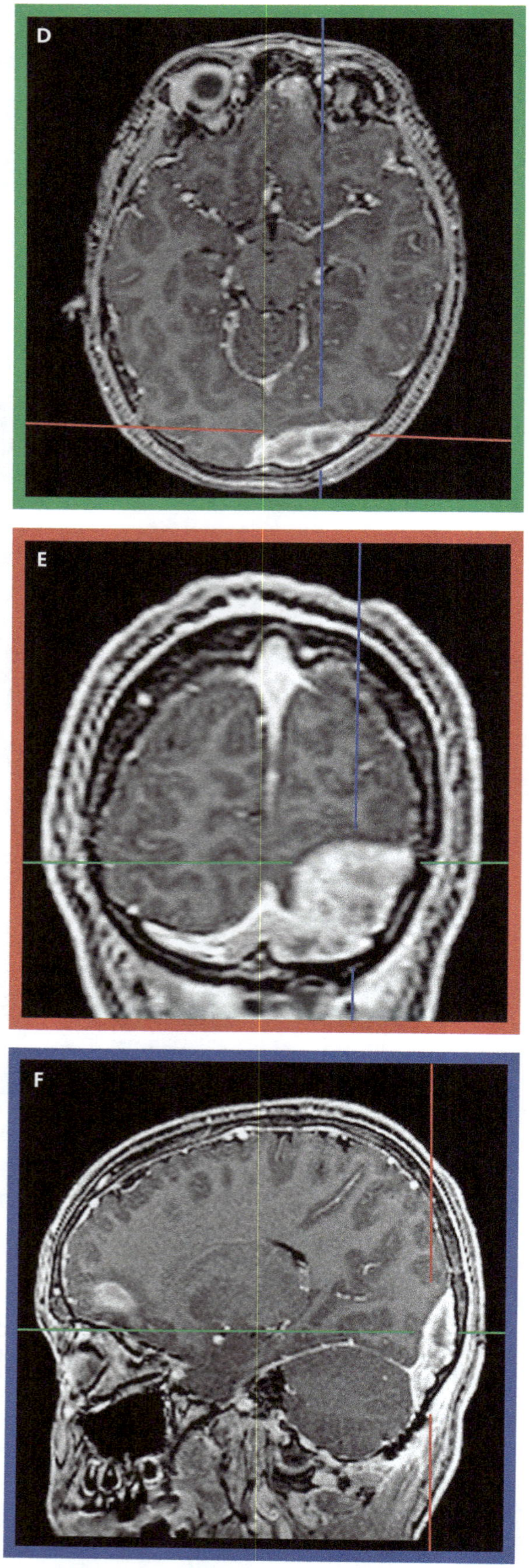

Figures 5-4D–F Contrast-enhanced (3D CE FSPGR T1) series showing a venous occipital epidural hematoma with swirl sign.

Epidural Hematomas/Hemorrhages

- For trauma-based EDH, CT imaging is the study of choice.
- Follow-up MRI may be useful in some cases.
- The epidural hematoma takes on a lenticular or biconvex appearance.
- A heterogeneous appearance or a "swirl sign" can suggest ongoing bleeding.
- Most epidural hematomas are caused by trauma to arteries, not venous structures.
- Brain injury is primarily caused by the mass effect exerted on the brain, with secondary compression and displacement of brain tissue resulting in herniation.
- Skull fractures are common in patients with EDH.
- Most injuries are located supratentorially, although they can be infratentorial (posterior fossa), a condition that is more emergent because of the sensitive nature of brain stem structures.
- CT density/MRI intensity varies with the age of the bleed and the effects of ongoing bleeding.
- CT density changes from hypodense or isodense (minutes to hours) to hyperdense (hours to weeks) and back to hypodense (chronic).
- MRI intensity changes from hypointense to hyperintense over time for T1 and T2 sequences.
- Classic symptoms include a lucid interval prior to deterioration of mental status.
- Outcome can be good if the EDH is promptly treated and before excessive intracranial pressure or herniation occurs.

Subdural Hematoma/ Hemorrhage (SDH)

Subdural hematomas (SDH) are caused by blood pooling between the dura and the arachnoid layer and are generally associated with underlying brain injury. Subdural bleeds often result from tearing of bridging veins within the subdural space resulting from shearing forces. When shearing forces are strong enough to cause tearing of subdural veins, they are also strong enough to cause damage to cortical nerve fibers; microscopic evidence of axonal shear injury frequently is present under a subdural bleed (Hoskote et al., 2002; Tomita et al., 1997). Accordingly, subdural bleeds are often associated with underlying injury to the brain and long-term functional compromise for the patient. The tissue underlying a subdural hemorrhage can become quite edematous or appear dark on a CT scan, contrasting the brighter appearance of blood. Because the hemorrhage is venous, subdural bleeds often form at a slower rate than that of epidural hematomas and exert less pressure on the underlying brain parenchyma. Nonenhanced CT imaging is the method of choice in the emergency department, although follow-up MRI is helpful in fully appreciating the extent of damage to the soft tissue of the brain. MRI is also indicated when the patient's symptoms appear in excess of that expected given the size of the hemorrhage and extent of any pressure effect.

REFERENCES

Hoskote, A., Richards. P., Anslow, P., & McShane, T. (2002). Subdural haematoma and non-accidental head injury in children. *Childs Nervous System, 18,* 311–317.

Tomita, H., Tonem O., & Ito. U. (1997). Hemispheric cerebral atrophy after traumatic extra-axial hematoma in adults. *Neurological and Medical Chirurgie 37,* 819–824.

On CT imaging, hyperacute bleeds less than a few hours may appear hypodense (dark) or heterogeneous. The hemorrhage becomes increasingly dense over the next few hours to days, with acute bleeds appearing hyperdense (bright) on a CT. After a few days, the hemorrhage may again appear isodense or even hypodense on CT imaging. When the hematoma becomes isodense and takes on the same appearance of brain tissue, displacement of the cortical mantle becomes an excellent marker of the extent of the bleed. Effacement of the sulci along the hemorrhage can also be evident on imaging, with the outer surface of the sulci failing to reach the inner surface of the skull. Over time, an EDH may appear to spread diffusely over the extra-axial space between the dura and arachnoid layer. Contrast-enhanced CT imaging may highlight the dura and membranes; the cortical blood vessels will be displaced medially.

The appearance on MRI will depend on the sequence used and the age of the bleed. In general, T1 and T2 imaging will show the subdural bleed as hypointense during the early stages (hours to a few days), with increasing intensity becoming evident over the next few days to weeks. Gradient echo (GRE) imaging and SWI are useful for assessing subdural bleeds; the blood appears dark to black and with a blooming appearance.

Unlike epidural bleeds, which have a lenticular appearance, SDH are often crescent shaped and follow the contours of the brain. In addition, SDH may be less clearly defined than epidural bleeds. Like epidural bleeds, a heterogeneous appearance or swirl sign with both hyperdense and hypodense regions may suggest ongoing bleeding. Tearing of the subarchnoid layer is more evident in SDH than EDH, resulting in cerebrospinal fluid (CSF) leaking into the hemorrhage. The mixing of blood and CSF can easily be mistaken for a swirl sign, given the heterogeneous appearance. Larger bleeds can produce compression and displacement of brain parenchyma and increased intracranial pressure with risk of herniation. However, pressure effect and risk of herniation are much less for SDH than for EDH, because the blood source for SDH is venous instead of mostly arterial for EDH. Subdural hemorrhages can be found anywhere within the brain where there is dura, although SDH do not cross the dural reflections or folds that form the falx cerebri and tentorium cerebelli.

Examples of Subdural Hematomas/ Hemorrhages

Examples of subdural hematomas are shown in Figures 5-5A–C, along the edge of the left tentorium and transverse sinus, and in Figures 5-5D–F, along the left superior lateral convexity.

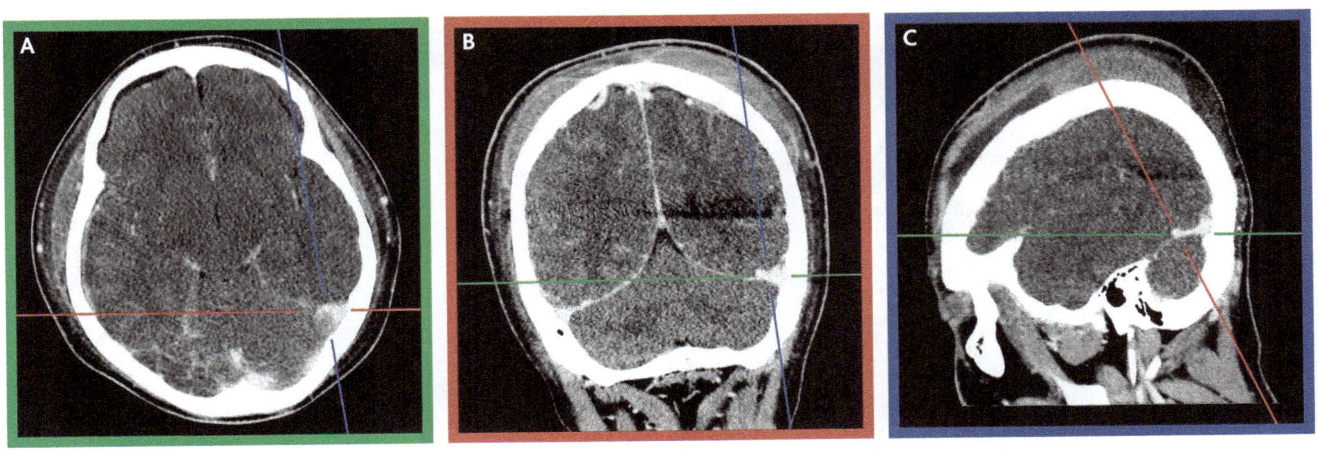

Figures 5-5A–C CT series—subdural hematoma along the edge of the left tentorium and transverse sinus.

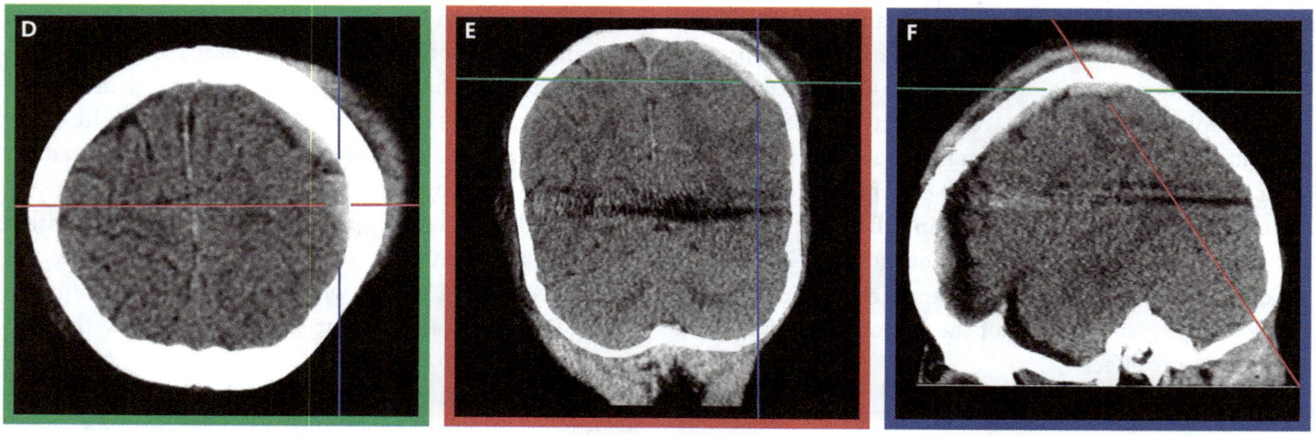

Figures 5-5D–F CT series—subdural hematoma along the left superior lateral convexity.

Although large subdural hemorrhages suggest significant physical trauma to the brain, sometimes extensive bleeding can result from a minor physical injury. This was the case with Lucius, an infant who fell while trying to stand. His subdural hemorrhage was excessive for the severity of his fall.

CLINICAL EXAMPLE

Lucius: Mild Head Injury with a Large Subdural Hematoma

Lucius was an infant who fell onto carpeted floor while pulling to stand. Brain imaging revealed extensive subdural hemorrhaging over the left hemisphere (Figures 5-6A–C). Additional studies indicated that his fall likely damaged a bridging vessel attached to the superior sagittal sinus, resulting in the subdural hemorrhage being in excess of that expected for the mild physical trauma to the head and brain.

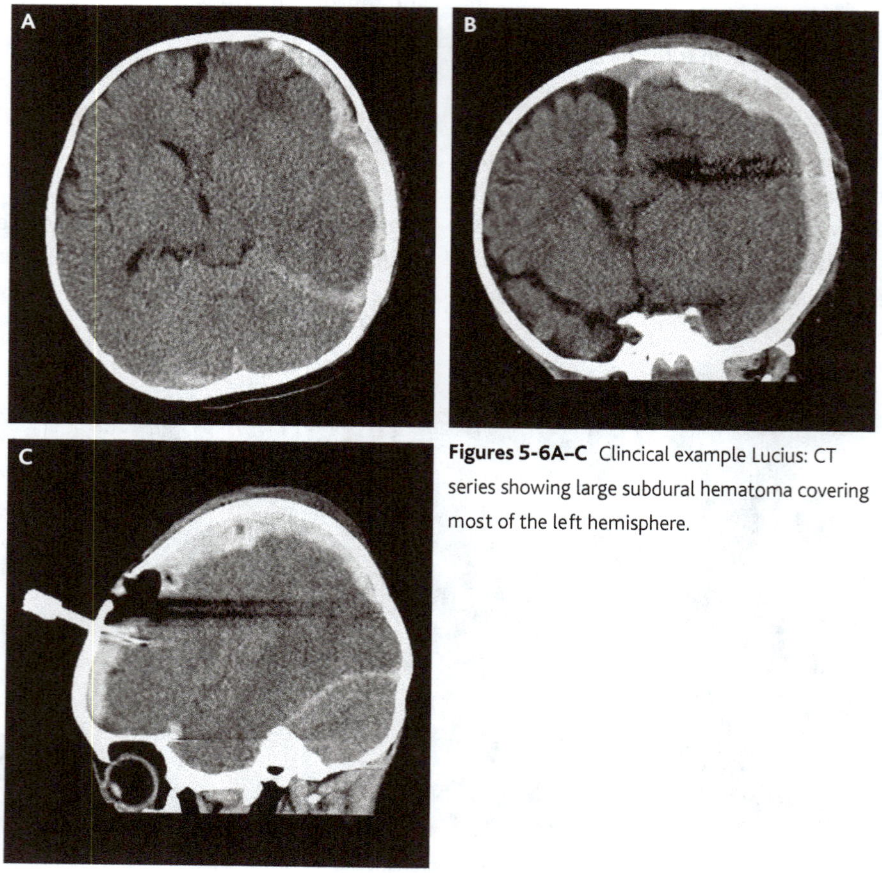

Figures 5-6A–C Clincical example Lucius: CT series showing large subdural hematoma covering most of the left hemisphere.

Subdural Hematoma/Hemorrhages

- SDH are collections of blood between the dural layer and the brain.
- SDH are often crescent shaped and follow the contours of the dural membrane around the cortex, along the falx cerebri, and along the tentorium. A unique feature of SDH is that they do not cross the dural reflections (folds), making them easier to recognize.
- SDH are most often supratentorial (above the tentorium) and around the lateral cortical convexity of the cortex.
- Non-contrast-enhanced CT is the method of choice for initial examination. The use of MRI may help if the patient's symptoms are out of proportion to the extent of hemorrhage.
- CT density/MRI intensity varies with the age of the bleed, the effects of ongoing bleeding, and the dilution of blood with CSF due to tearing of the arachnoid layer.
- CT density changes from hypodense or isodense (minutes to hours) to hyperdense (hours to weeks) and back to hypodense (chronic).
- MRI intensity changes from hypointense to hyperintense over time for T1 and T2 sequences.
- SDH may appear black due to susceptibility effects on GRE or SWI sequences.
- When the blood is isodense on CT or isointense on MRI and difficult to appreciate, the extent of the hematoma may be evident by observing any displacement of the cortical mantle with effacement of the sulci. Displacement of the cortical veins, evident with contrast enhancement, may also be helpful.
- A mixed density of blood may indicate nonaccidental trauma, owing to the presence of blood at different ages.

Subarachnoid Hematoma/ Hemorrhage (SAH)

A bleed between the arachnoid layer and the brain is called a *subarachnoid hemorrhage*. Subarachnoid hemorrhages (SAH) follow the contours of the cortical mantle and arachnoid layer.

Unlike other hemorrhages such as subdural or intraparenchymal bleeds, subarachnoid hemorrhages do not show the same pattern of hemoglobin changes over time. Subarachnoid bleeds have a slower progression of degradation, which is most likely due to the high ambient oxygen saturation of the CSF within the subarachnoid space.

Subarachnoid hemorrhages are often located adjacent to subdural or intraparenchymal bleeds and soft-tissue contusions. Areas around the cisterns and Sylvian fissure, above the corpus callosum, and around the inferior frontal subarachnoid spaces and the convexity of the cortical sulci are common locations for subarachnoid hemorrhages. Subtle subarachnoid bleeds within the basal or interpeduncular cistern may be the only evidence of post-traumatic subarachnoid hemorrhaging. Subarachnoid hemorrhages are often associated with additional injury to the brain, such as diffuse axonal injury, and are frequently seen in combination with subdural and intraparenchymal hematomas (see section below for more information on intraparenchymal hematomas).

On CT imaging, subarachnoid bleeds are relatively simple to visualize as thin strips of hyperdensity relative to CSF or brain parenchyma. The appearance on MRI will depend on the sequence used. T2 FLAIR can be the most useful sequence to assess for post-traumatic hemorrhages; subarachnoid bleeds appear as areas of hyperintensity around the sulci, cisterns, and cortical mantle. GRE and SW imaging may also show subarachnoid bleeds as areas of hypointensity or dark regions of blooming.

Examples of Subarachnoid Hematomas/ Hemorrhages

Examples of subarachnoid hematomas presented here involve a variety of anatomical locations, with many images showing SAH in more than one location. The figure crosshairs identify the location of subarachnoid hemorrhages close to the corpus callosum (Figures 5-7A–C), in the basal or interpeduncular cistern (Figures 5-8A–C), along the tenorium (Figures 5-9A–C), and along the Sylvian fissure (Figures 5-10A–C).

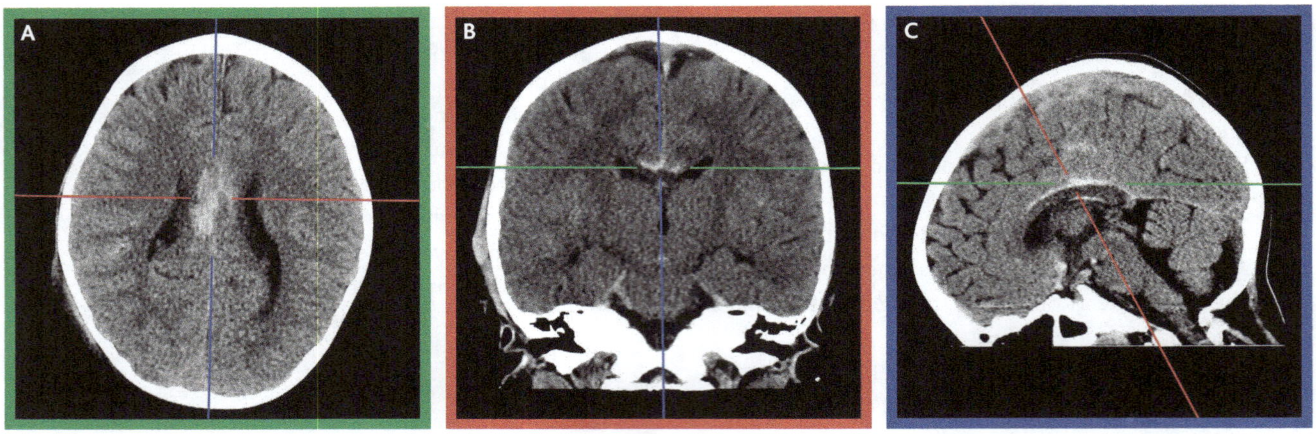

Figures 5-7A–C CT series showing a subarachnoid bleed above the corpus callosum.

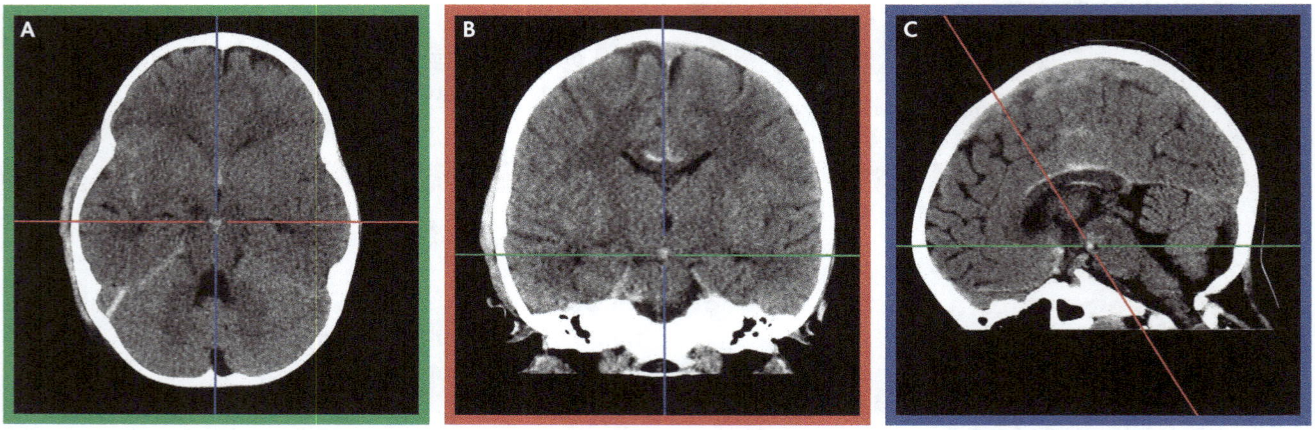

Figures 5-8A–C CT series showing a subarachnoid bleed within the basal or interpeduncular cistern, often the only sign of a diffuse injury to the brain.

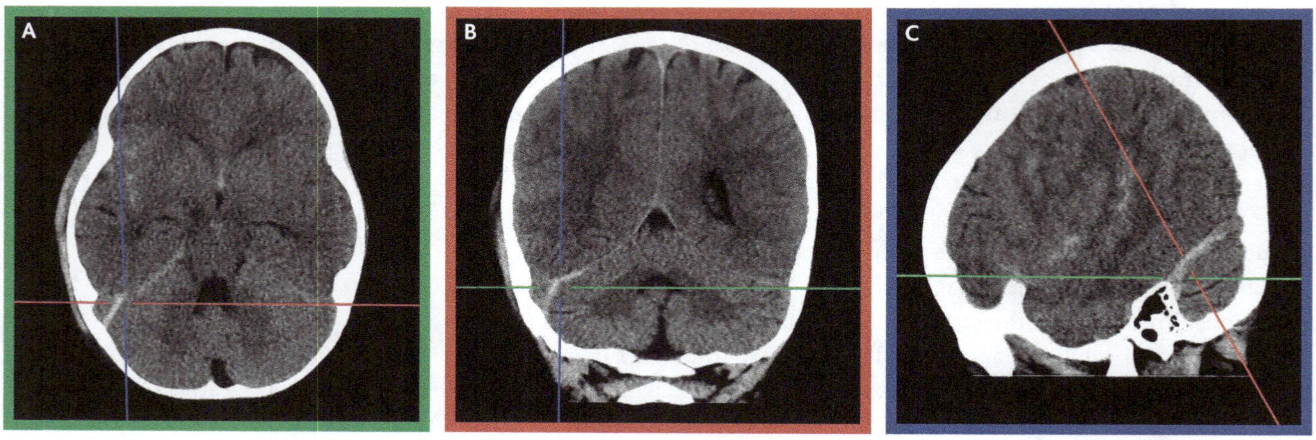

Figures 5-9A–C CT series showing a subarachnoid bleed under the tentorium, a relatively common place for SAH. Note also the subarachnoid blood around the right Sylvian fissure evident on axial and sagittal slices.

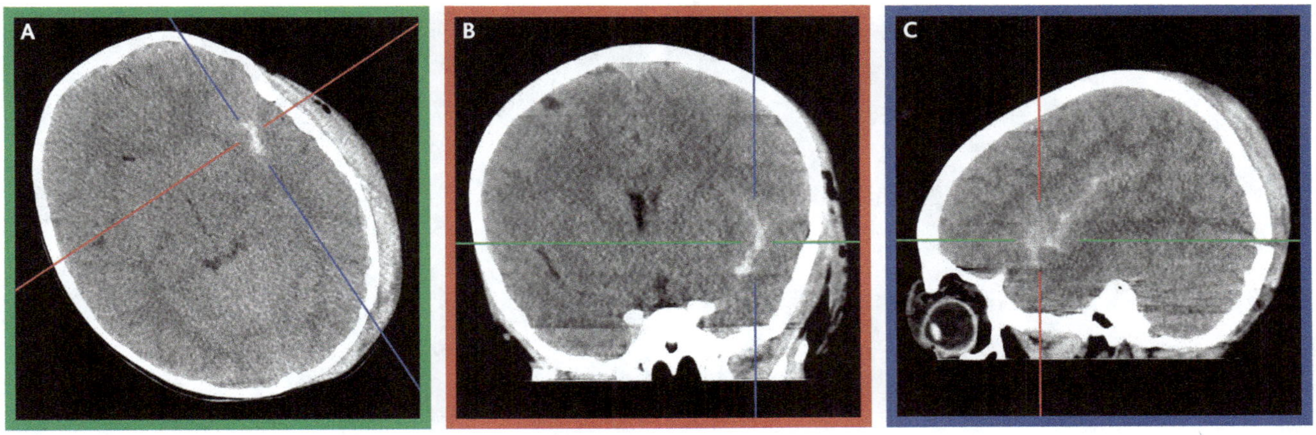

Figures 5-10A–C CT series showing a subarachnoid bleed within the Sylvian fissure, a frequent location for SAH.

Intraparenchymal Hemorrhages

Traumatic intraparenchymal hemorrhages are often associated with contusions or lacerations of the parenchyma. They are often accompanied by focal edema and diffuse axonal injury. Intraparenchymal hemorrhages can range from microbleeds not evident on brain imaging to bleeds that involve large areas of tissue. With increasing magnet strength, specialized sequences, and higher-resolution scanning, some microbleeds not evident on brain images a few years ago are now appreciable on sequences such as SWI. Larger petechial hemorrhages are often readily evident on CT imaging and some MRI sequences, especially T2 FLAIR, GRE, and SWI, with the latter method being highly sensitive to such bleeds.

Petechial Hemorrhages

Petechial hemorrhages, especially within the white matter or at the gray–white junction, corpus callosum, or brain stem, suggest diffuse axonal injury (Hutchison & Lebby, 2009). Because petechial hemorrhages are associated with diffuse axonal injuries, their prognostic value is greater than that expected for the degree of bleeding evident within the brain.

REFERENCE

Hutchison, T., & Lebby, P. C. (2009). Traumatic encephalopathies. In R. B. David (Ed.), *Clinical pediatric neurology* (3rd ed.). New York: Demos Medical Publishing.

Diffuse Axonal Injury

CT is sensitive to small petechial hemorrhages resulting from tearing of tiny blood vessels within the brain parenchyma. From a basic physical standpoint, forces excessive enough to cause tearing of blood vessels throughout the brain are also of the magnitude to cause diffuse injury to tiny nerve fibers, a condition called *diffuse axonal injury* (DAI). When injury to blood vessels and nerve fibers is caused by shearing or twisting forces, they are most often evident at the frontal gray–white junction. Injury at the gray–white junction is generally a result of the physical forces affecting tissues of varying densities to a different degree.

Diffuse axonal injuries can be widespread and cause profound loss of brain functioning, even without notable evidence of tissue damage on neuroimaging. Brain imaging is quite limited when it comes to visualizing diffuse microscopic damage, although DTI is showing some promise for the assessment of damage to larger white-matter tracts. Even though brain scans do not have the spatial resolution to enable visualization of axonal shearing at the microscopic level, markers of such damage are often readily evident on a variety of brain images, even CT. A primary marker of DAI results from the tearing of tiny blood vessels within the brain parenchyma. Even though axonal shearing may not be visible on a scan, the appearance of petechial hemorrhages or tiny spots of blood throughout the parenchyma is highly suggestive of DAI (Figures 5-11A and B) .

When physical forces act on the brain secondary to rapid acceleration and deceleration of the structure, the tissue is affected by both compression and shock waves that pass through the tissue. For example, in a motor vehicle accident, when the skull hits the windshield of a car, a compression wave will be transmitted from the part of the brain contacting the inner surface of the brain to the rest of the tissue. In addition, the overall deceleration of the remaining tissue will result in a number of shock waves traveling around the soft brain tissue. If rotational forces are involved, there will be a combination of a shock/compression wave and

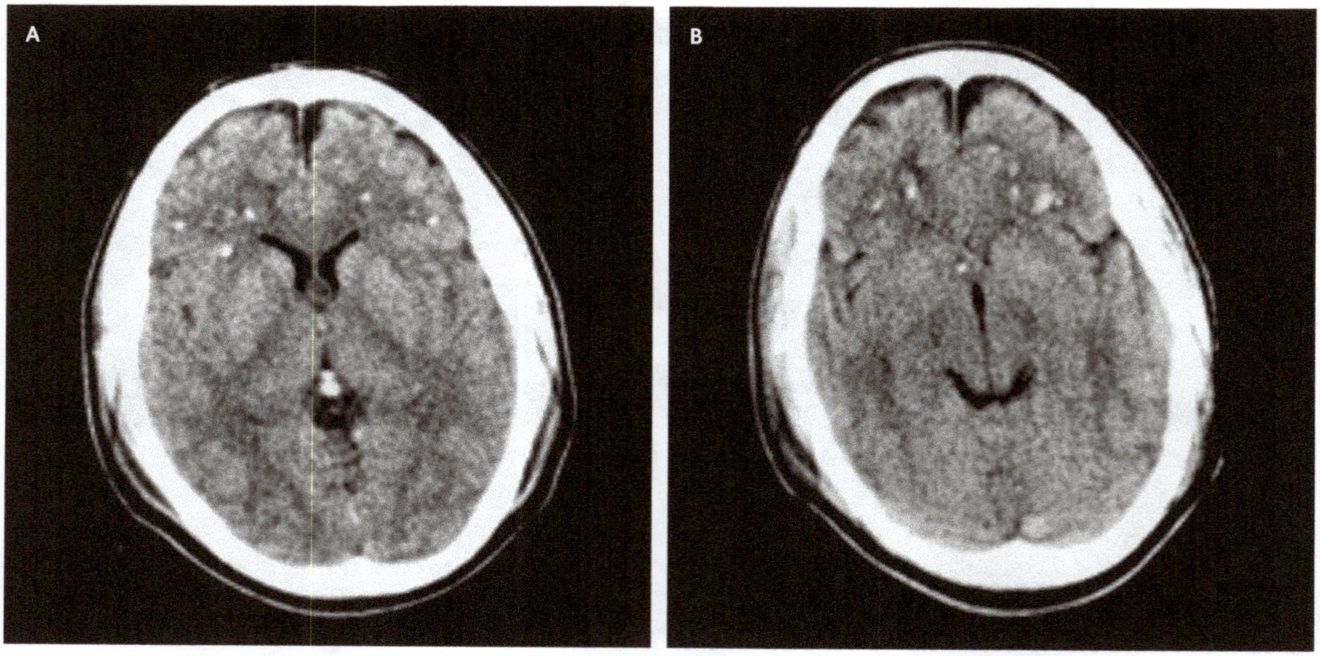

Figures 5-11A and B CT examples of petechial hemorrhages, predominantly at the frontal gray–white borders.

twisting torque applied to the tissue, resulting in more severe damage to the white matter. As shock waves and rotational forces travel through brain parenchyma, the effects of the forces will differ depending on the specific density of the tissue. Because tissues of different density are not affected equally by forces acting on the brain, they tend to move against each other, resulting in tearing or shearing of connections. Following a brain injury, axonal shear injuries are most commen in areas where different densities of tissue meet, such as at the gray–white junction. Shearing of axons at the gray–white junction is more common in infants and children than in adults, although older children and adults are more prone to shearing at both the gray–white junction and the corpus callosum (Hutchison & Lebby, 2009).

REFERENCE

Hutchison, T., & Lebby, P. C. (2009). Traumatic encephalopathies. In R. B. David (Ed.), *Clinical pediatric neurology* (3rd ed.). New York: Demos Medical Publishing.

Following traumatic brain injury, petechial hemorrhages are also frequently found within the corpus callosum and subcortical white matter or centrum semiovale (Figures 5-12A–E). Persistent evidence of hemorrhagic contusions and DAI on brain imaging suggests a worse prognosis for the patient.

Axonal injuries involving the corpus callosum are common following trauma to the brain but may not be evident on brain imaging. While severe tearing of corpus callosum fibers is often evident on imaging, it may not be obvious; any review of brain scans following a traumatic brain injury should include this structure. Figures 5-13A–C provide examples of damage to the posterior corpus callosum just anterior to the splenium. Mid-sagittal T1 images may provide the clearest picture of damage, although coronal views can also be quite revealing, especially on T2 or T2 FLAIR sequences. Axial sequences are often the least clear for corpus callosum injuries, as the structure is arched and the slice only cuts through a small section at a time. Figures 5-14A–C provide examples of damage to almost the entire corpus callosum structure, with Figures 4-14A–C being aligned with the anterior part of the structure, and Figures 4-14D–F being aligned with a more posterior section of the corpus callosum.

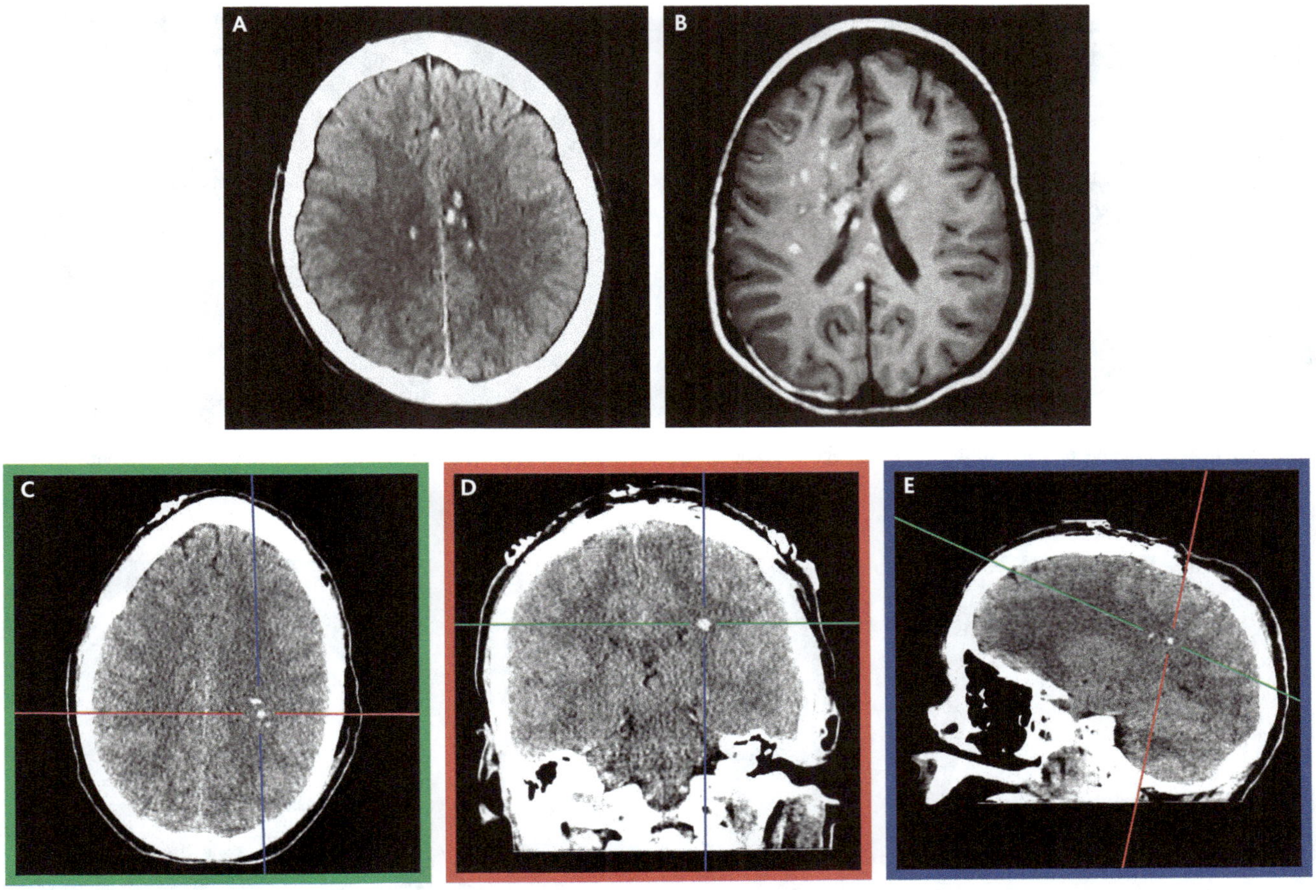

Figures 5-12A–E Examples of petechial hemorrhages around the corpus callosum and within the subcortical white matter of the centrum semiovale. **A:** CT. **B:** MRI T1. **C:** CT **D:** CT **E:** CT

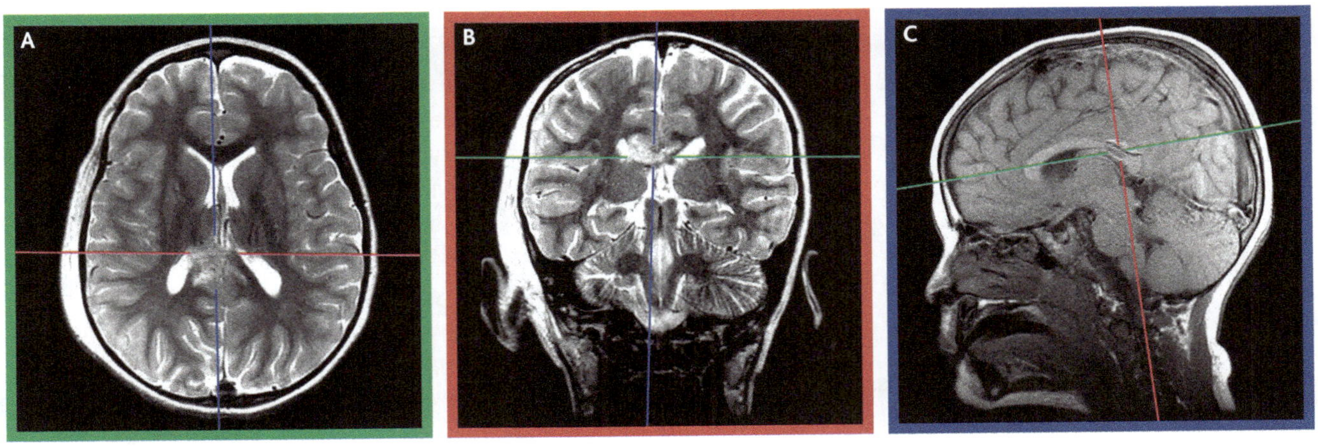

Figures 5-13A–C Example of posterior corpus callosum injury due to physical trauma. **A:** T2. **B:** T2. **C:** T1.

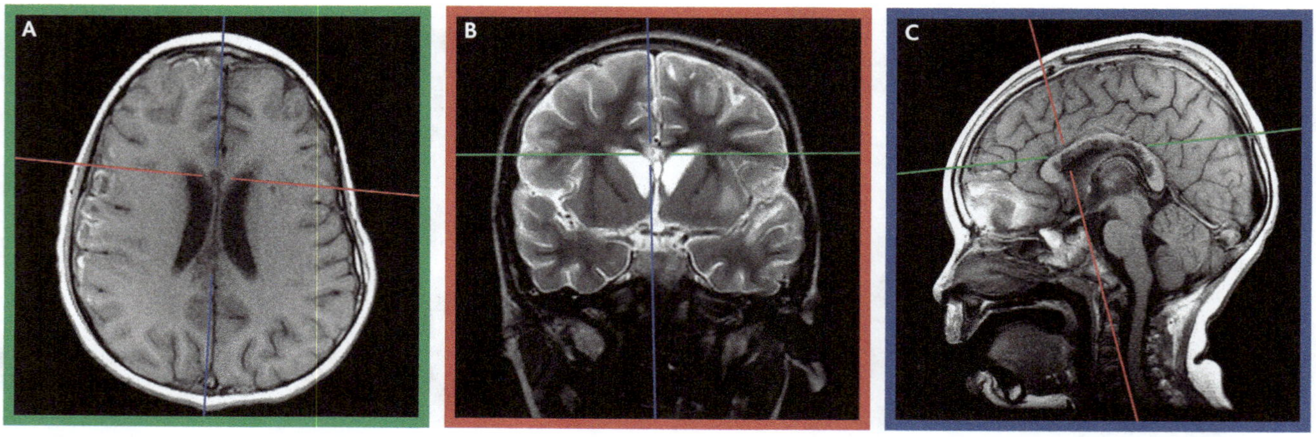

Figures 5-14A–C Example of severe white matter damage involving almost the entire corpus callosum. Images are aligned to best show the anterior corpus callosum injury. **A:** T1. **B:** T2. **C:** T1.

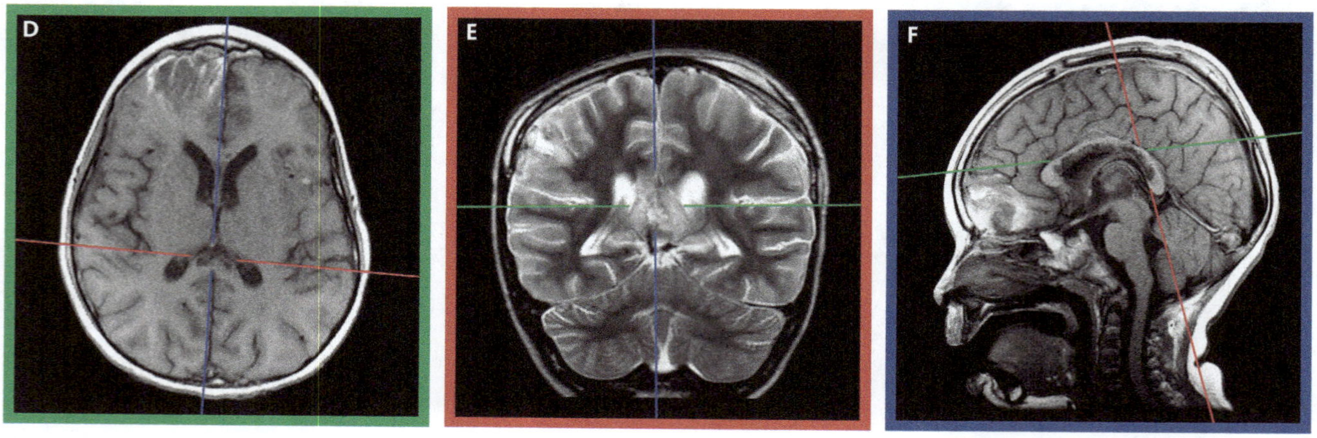

Figures 5-14D–F Examples of severe white matter damage involving almost the entire corpus callosum. Images are aligned to best show the posterior corpus callosum injury. **D:** T1. **E:** T2. **F:** T1.

PEARL Microbleeds may not be evident on CT imaging, especially close to the bony structures at the front of the brain. If the CT appears normal and the patient's symptoms suggest diffuse axonal injury, an MRI study may help to identify microbleeds or smaller petechial hemorrhages not visible on CT imaging. The best sequences to review include T2 FLAIR, GRE/GRE-EPI, and SWI.

PERIL A normal CT scan with abnormal patient functioning can be interpreted many ways. For example, the patient may be viewed as having a psychiatric condition or as malingering. This is especially true for those cases with secondary-gain issues, such as legal involvement. Even with a normal CT, many patients experience significant functional deficits involving cognition, emotion, behavior, social skills, and motor or sensory functioning, because of undetected diffuse axonal injuries. Medication management may also disrupt the patient's functioning, irrespective of any brain injury, or in addition to the injury. Mild cognitive compromise from DAI may be exacerbated by medications used to control pain, resulting in a level of deficit in excess of that suggested by the normal CT scan. Similarly, cognitive difficulties may be exaggerated by the effects of acute emotional disturbances such as depression or anxiety, which frequently follow a traumatic event.

Do not rely so heavily on brain imaging that you minimize the importance of your clinical examination.

Absence of evidence is not evidence of absence, especially with brain imaging.

Hemorrhagic Contusions

Immediately following an injury, hemorrhagic contusions may be difficult to appreciate on brain scans, especially CT. With blood first appearing hypodense on CT then, after a few hours, transitioning to hyperdense, there is a period of time, a few hours after a hemorrhagic

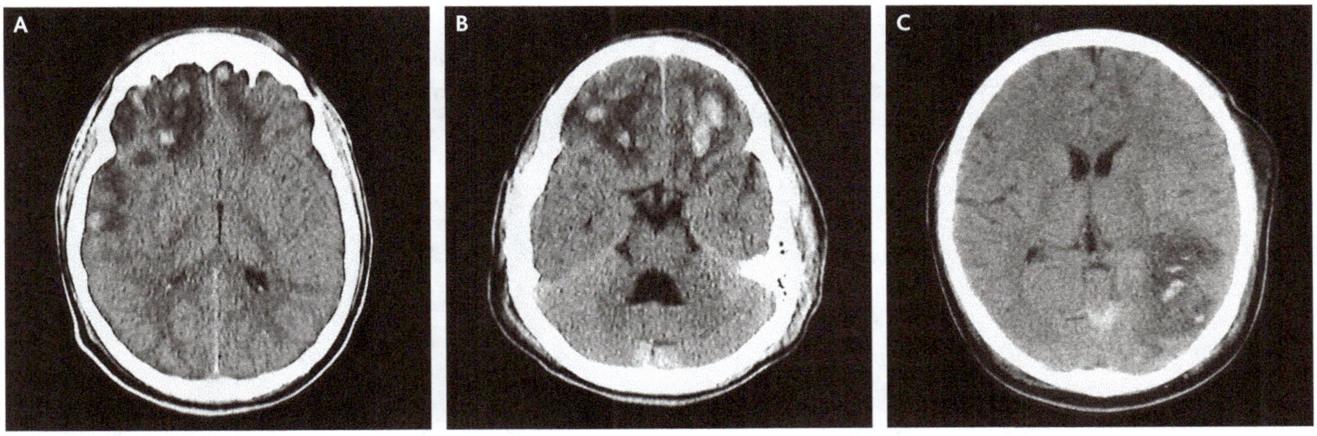

Figures 5-15A–C Examples of hemorrhagic contusions. **A:** Bifrontal-temporal. **B:** Bifrontal-temporal. **C:** Left parietal-occipital.

contusion, when the blood may not be readily evident on CT imaging. Similarly, edema that usually surrounds a contusion takes time to form and may not be apparent shortly after an injury. After the first few hours, hemorrhagic contusions become readily evident on CT as well as other types of brain imaging (Figures 5-15A–C). On CT, the most common examination in the emergency department, blood will become hyperdense, or bright, on the scan within a few hours and contrast with the darker, or hypodense, appearance of emerging surrounding edema. Hemorrhagic contusions are often identified as a small area of blood surrounded by a region of soft-tissue swelling. Depending on the MRI sequence, this may appear as a bright area of blood surrounded by darker swelling (T1) or a larger area of hyperintensity from the blood and edema (T2/T2FLAIR). On GRE and SWI images, the blood may appear black surrounded by slightly hyperintense edema.

CLINICAL EXAMPLE
Caydon: Right Parietal Hemorrhagic Contusion

Caydon was injured during a fall from his bicycle. He was not wearing a helmet and his head hit the ground, causing a hemorrhagic contusion within the right parietal lobe (Figure 5-16). Caydon experienced focal deficits relating to the area of injury, with other functions remaining mostly intact. While in the hospital, Caydon's neuropsychological examination indicated a verbal intelligence quotient (IQ) of 127, within the superior range, but with a performance IQ for visual spatial reasoning being 47, or severely impaired. Even though he was 23 years old, he was unable to do simple visual spatial tasks expected of 6-year-old children. He had a severe visual agnosia and was unable to identify objects around his room or pictures presented to him. He was also unable to recognize friends and family because of prosopagnosia. Visual neglect was evident for information on the left side of space, which was most evident on complex tasks, and with divided attention or simultaneous stimulation.

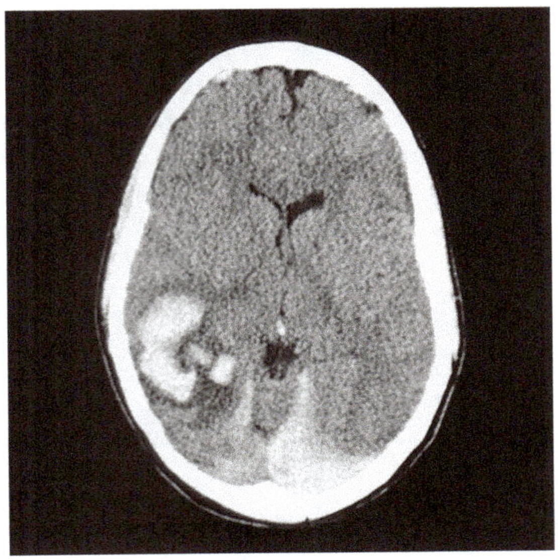

Figure 5-16 Clinical example Caydon: right parietal hemorrhagic contusion.

CLINICAL EXAMPLE

Michael: Left Parietal Hemorrhagic Contusion

Following an accident while riding his skateboard without a helmet, Michael was unable to understand what others said or to express himself with spoken or written language. His speech was intact, although the words he said did not make sense. When describing a picture of a boy fishing by a bridge, Michael said, "You can siddlerock, with volantic." Michael had Wernicke's type aphasia, also called fluent or receptive aphasia, due to a hemorrhagic contusion within the left temporal-parietal region (Figure 5-17). During Michael's rehabilitation, his ability to understand and communicate with spoken and written language improved, although several months later he still produced errors in his speech (paraphasias and neologisms) and had difficulty following multipart compound directions containing more than two details.

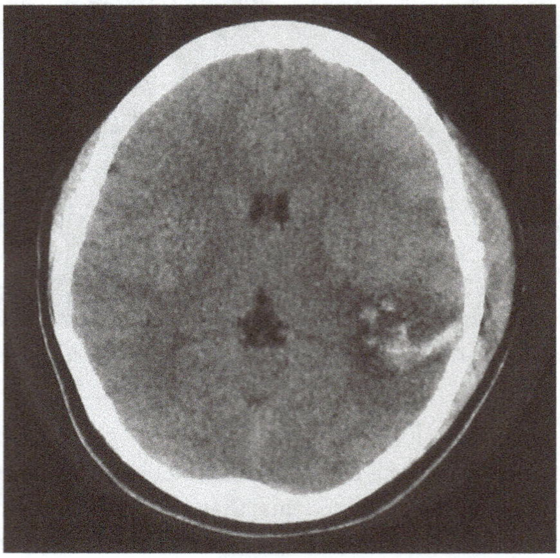

Figure 5-17 Clinical example Michael: left parietal hemorrhagic contusion.

CLINICAL EXAMPLE

Katie: Left Frontal Hemorrhagic Contusion

Katie was injured in a motor vehicle accident, the damage being mostly restricted to her left frontal region (Figure 5-18). Along with a right-sided hemiparesis, Katie had difficulty expressing herself verbally. She was dysnomic, having difficulty with word finding, especially for nouns. She could say a few words, but verbal formulation was effortful and speech was highly dysfluent. Speech was telegraphic in that she used mostly content words to express herself, with long pauses between utterances. Many paraphasic errors (inappropriate words) were evident in her speech. When asked to describe a picture, she said, "Um ... errr ... table ... cookie ... errr ... hmmm ... falling ... errr ... errr ... bed ... no ... errr ... boy."

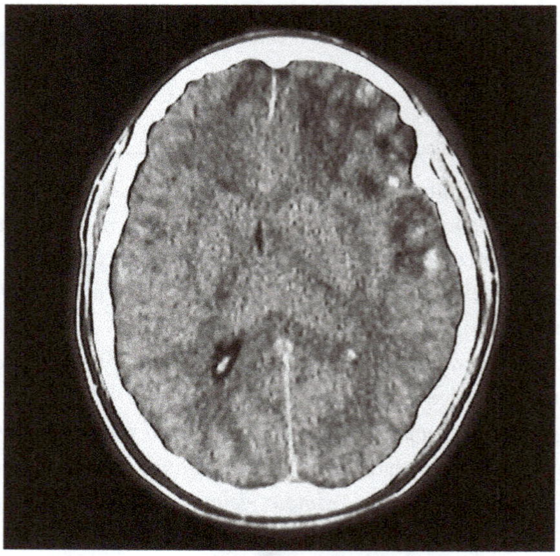

Figure 5-18 Clinical example Katie: left frontal hemorrhagic contusion.

With post-traumatic intraparenchymal hemorrhages, it is important to remain cautious when interpreting the extent and severity of a bleed from images acquired shortly after an injury. The use of serial scans over several days or weeks is optimal for determining the extent and severity of post-traumatic intraparenchymal hemorrhages, as acute scans may underrepresent the amount of bleeding or damaged tissue. MRI is preferred over CT, as there is no cumulative exposure to ionizing radiation, and many sequences are highly sensitive to the presence of blood products.

Change in Appearance of a Hemorrhagic Contusion over Time

Figures 5-19 thorugh 5-21 show the changes in appearance on brain scans of a hemorrhagic constusion over time. CT imaging acquired on the day of the injury (Figures 5-19A–C) revealed a skull fracture and underlying hemorrhagic contusion identified by the small bright area of hyperdensity indicating blood, surrounded by the darker area of hypodensity caused by the edema. CT imaging taken one day following the injury (Figures 5-20A–C) revealed a clear change in the appearance of blood from the day of the injury. A few hours after the injury, the blood appeared isodense to slightly hyperdense (Figures 5-19A–C). One day following the injury, the hemorrhage has a much brighter appearance and is more extensive (Figures 5-20A–C). Also note the darker appearance of the surrounding edema. The difference in the CT images over a period of 1 day is quite marked, with the scans acquired 1 day post-injury suggesting a more severe injury than that on the scans from the day of injury. Four days following the injury, the lesion appeared as a hyperintense area on T1 MRI (Figure 5-21A), and the edema was more evident as a bright border of hyperintensity on T2 FLAIR MRI (Figure 5-21B). Blood was easily appreciated on GRE imaging as the areas of black at the core of the lesion (Figure 5-21C). Follow-up CT and MRI suggested a larger area of injury than that suggested by the original CT scans taken only a few hours after the injury.

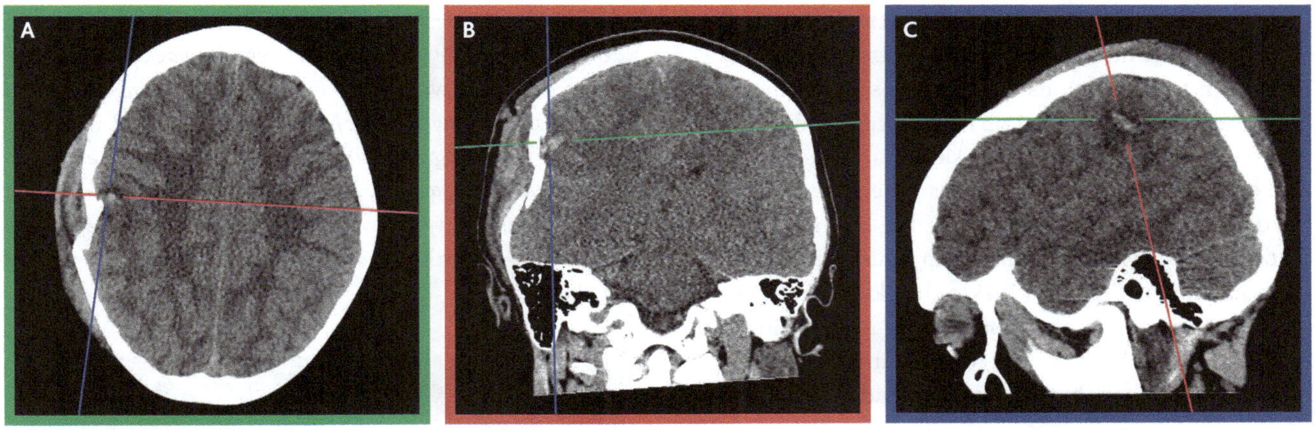

Figures 5-19A–C CT scans taken on the day of the injury.

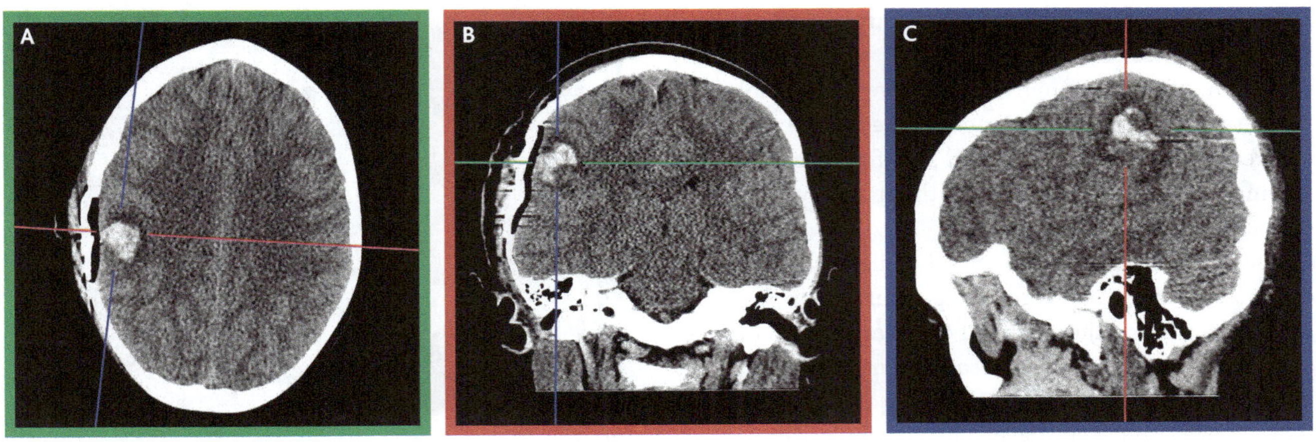

Figures 5-20A–C CT series taken 1 day after injury.

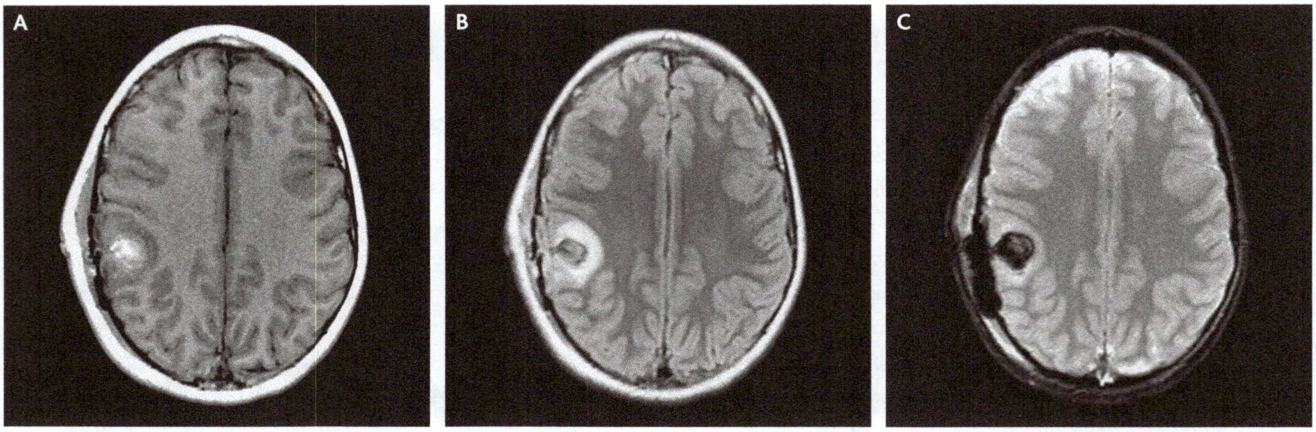

Figures 5-21A–C MRI series 4 days post-injury. **A:** T1. **B:** T2 FLAIR. **C:** GRE.

Contrecoup Injuries

Contusions are not always evident at the location of primary impact to the head. It is important to inspect the brain scan for contusions directly across from the region of impact. The region of impact is often evident by the soft-tissue scalp swelling or via skull fractures. The contusion at the site of direct impact is called the *coup* injury; the damage to the opposite side of the brain is called the *contrecoup* injury. Coup-contrecoup injuries are caused by the bouncing of the brain inside the skull resulting from the initial impact, or as a result of the head rapidly moving forward and back or side-to-side directly following an impact. As the soft brain bounces inside the cranium it contact the inner surface of the skull resulting in rapid deceleration at the site of impact (coup) and opposite the site of impact (contrecoup). Coup injuries may be easier to identify on imaging as the damage is often more focal and causes greater hemorrhagic contusion than contrecoup injuries. Contrecoup injuries may be more diffuse than direct coup injuries, and have less pathological markers evident on brain imaging. The diffuse nature of contrecoup injuries can result in significant loss of functioning for the patient, even without obvious signs of damage on imaging.

These three clinical examples highlight the relatively common finding that contrecoup injuries can be more severe than coup injuries. In all three cases, deficits were related primarily to the contrecoup injury, not to the coup injury. Of note, contrecoup injuries are often more diffuse than coup injuries, resulting in more generalized disruption of functioning. As a rule, it is important to avoid becoming so focused on brain tissue directly below the point of impact that you fail to investigate damage opposite the site of impact.

CLINICAL EXAMPLE

Kathryn: Contrecoup Injury

Kathryn slipped on some ice, hitting the back of her head. The direct impact was to her left parietal region, as evident by the soft tissue swelling of her scalp (Figure 5-22, arrow 1). Although her imaging studies indicated a small extra-axial left temporal-parietal hemorrhage (arrow 2) and right occipital low density (arrow 3), the most pronounced injury appeared to be within the right frontal and temporal lobe regions (arrow 4).

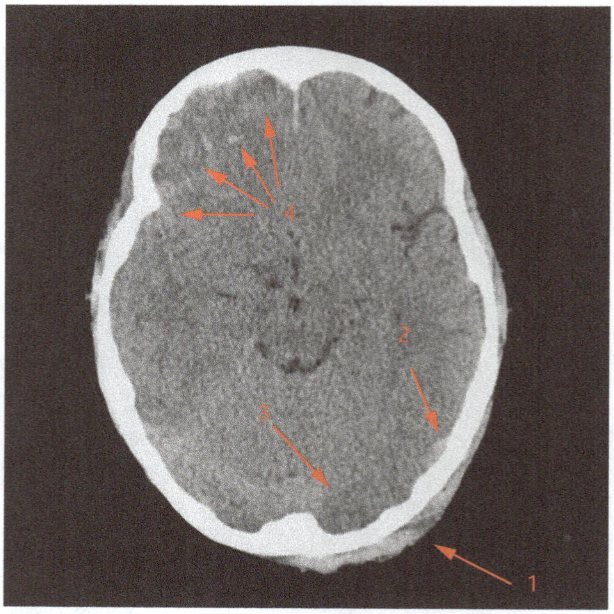

Figure 5-22 Clinical example Kathryn: contrecoup injury. Imaging taken on the day of the injury. Arrow 1 shows the area of direct impact. Arrow 2 shows a small extra-axial left temporal-parietal hemorrhage. Arrow 3 shows some right occipital low density from the direct impact (coup), and arrows 4 shows the right frontal and temporal injuries caused by the contrecoup.

Two days after the injury, T2 FLAIR imaging suggested significant edema and petechial hemorrhages within the right frontal lobe, with minimal peridural bleeding within the left temporal-parietal regions. Note the hyperintensity of the right frontal and anterior temporal lobes on T2 FLAIR imaging suggesting significant contusion (Figure 5-23).

On GRE sequences acquired 2 days following her injury, the petechial hemorrhages appear as black spots throughout the right frontal and right anterior temporal regions. On diffusion imaging, the contrecoup region appears hyperintense on DWI and hypointense on ADC, suggesting restricted diffusion. The images from 2 days post-injury clearly demonstrate that the contrecoup injury had a greater severity and extent of damage than that of the coup injury (Figures 5-24A–C).

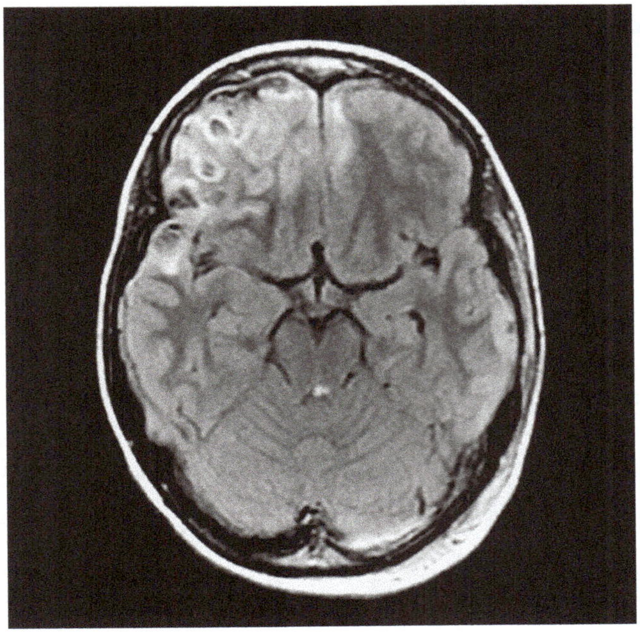

Figure 5-23 Clinical example Kathryn: T2 FLAIR imaging taken 2 days after injury showing significant edema and petechial hemorrhaging in the right frontal and temporal lobes, with less damage to the left temporal-parietal region.

Kathryn's deficits following the injury would not have made sense without the additional information provided by brain imaging. Although the physical trauma to her scalp and her described impact were on the back left side of her head, Kathryn's symptoms were more consistent with injury to the right frontal and anterior parts of her brain. During a follow-up appointment approximately three months after her injury, Kathryn underwent a full battery of neuropsychological tests. Although Kathryn's overall functioning had improved since discharge from the hospital, she continued to have difficulties with skills related to her frontal lobes. Kathryn was found to have verbal and nonverbal intelligence above the 99th percentile for her age. However, performance on measures of executive functioning involving mental flexibility and processing efficiency, rapid switching of mental concepts, and complex attention fell within the average range for her age. This is an example where "average" is not within the normal range for the patient; "average performance" represented a significant decline in functioning for Kathryn when compared to her premorbid abilities. Consistent with this finding, Kathryn indicated that complex cognitive tasks that were once simple for her had become much more challenging. Even though age-based norms indicated that Kathryn's functioning was within normal limits, this was indeed a deficit for her. Kathryn also underwent follow-up brain imaging approximately 3 months following her injury. On MRI T1 images (Figures 5-25A–C), atrophy of the right frontal and medial cortical lamina can be clearly seen on axial view, with loss of cortex within the frontal pole being clearly evident on sagittal view.

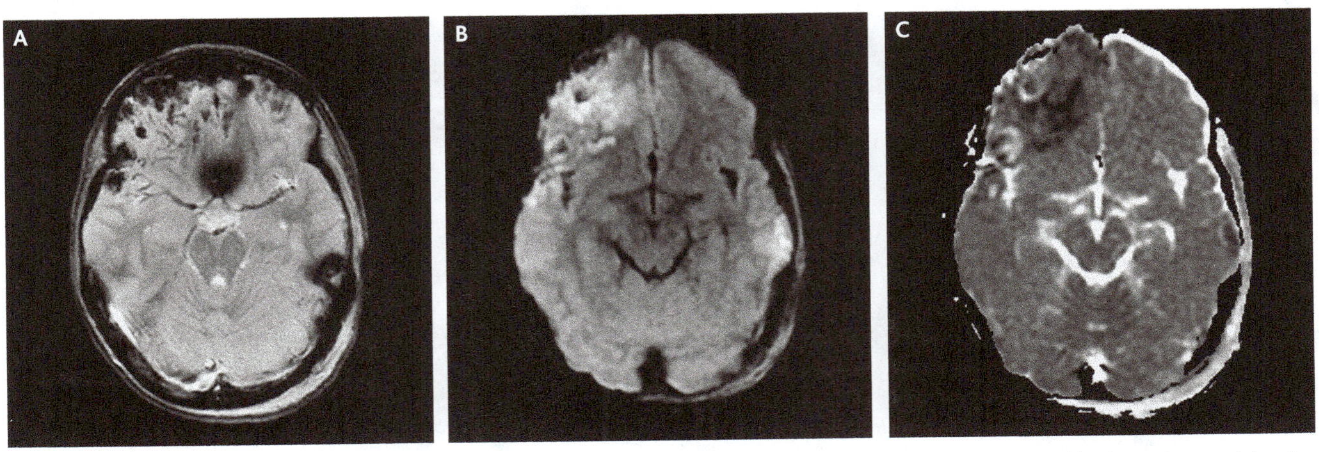

Figures 5-24A–C Clinical example Kathryn: MRI sequences 2 days following her injury, showing the extent of damage caused by the contrecoup injury to her right frontal and temporal lobes. The MRI images from 2 days post-injury clearly demonstrate that the contra-coup injury had a greater severity and extent of damage than that of the coup injury. **A:** GRE. **B:** DWI. **C:** ADC.

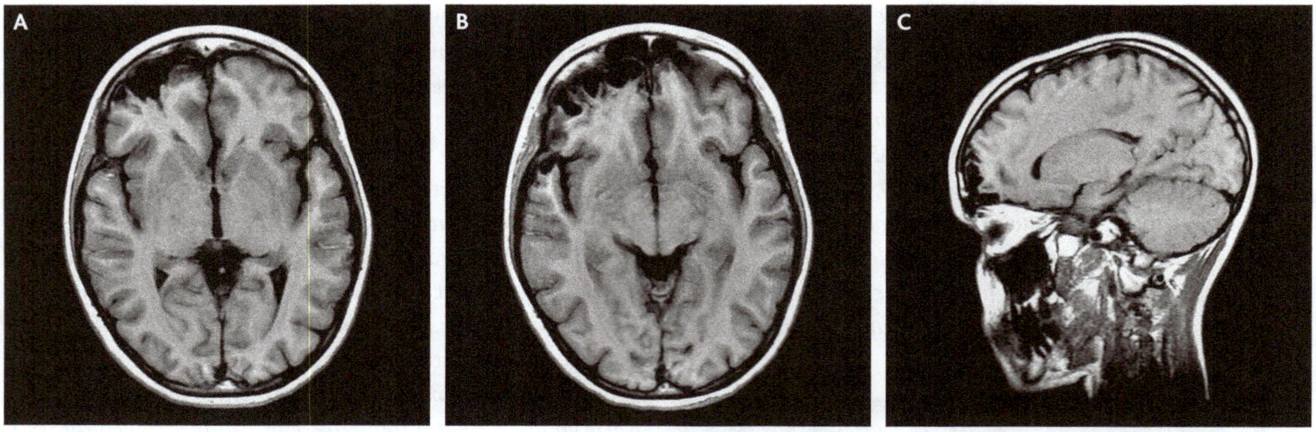

Figures 5-25A–C Clinical example Kathryn: MRI T1 series 3 months post-injury. Note atrophy of the right frontal cortical lamina on axial slices and loss of cortex within the frontal pole on sagittal view.

CLINICAL EXAMPLE
Ron: Contrecoup Injury

Ron was injured during a fall from a boulder while hiking in the mountains. Even though the left side of his forehead contacted the ground, the primary injury to his brain was within the right parietal lobe (Figure 5-26 arrows). With contact to the left frontal area, it was expected that Ron might have difficulty with motor functioning on his right side, with expressive language, and with executive functioning. However, his symptoms consisted primarily of difficulty with complex visual reasoning and a mild visual agnosia. His symptoms were related to his contrecoup injury, not to the area of brain directly below the region of contact with the ground.

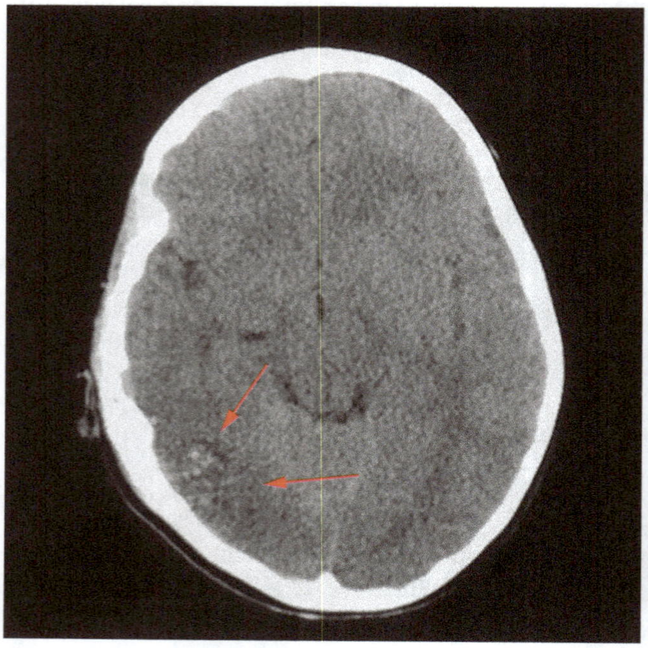

Figure 5-26 Clinical example Ron: contrecoup injury to right parietal lobe.

CLINICAL EXAMPLE
Jen: Contrecoup Injury

Jen's injury was similar to Ron's, described above. She was injured in a motor vehicle collision when her head hit the windshield of the car. The direct impact was to the right frontal-parietal area (Figure 5-27). Although she had some left-sided weakness relating to the area of direct impact, her primary symptoms were consistent with Wernicke's aphasia due to the contrecoup damage to her left parietal lobe.

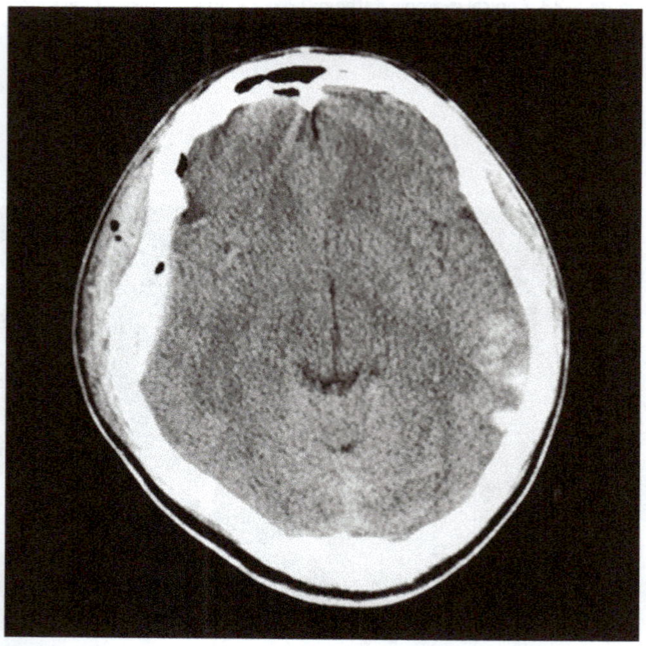

Figure 5-27 Clinical example Jen: contrecoup injury to left parietal lobe.

Common Locations for Hemorrhagic and Nonhemorrhagic Contusions

Contusions can be found in all lobes of the cortex and all regions of the brain. However, given the shape of the brain and cranium, there are some areas that are more prone to contusions than others. Contusions are most likely within the orbital and medial frontal, and anterior temporal lobes, areas surrounded by the bony ridges of the eye orbits and sphenoid and temporal bones. Figure 5-28 illustrates the primary areas of contusion; the orbital frontal region is identified in green, the medial frontal region in red and the anterior temporal lobes are identified in blue. Figures 5-29A–C provide 3D volume rendered images of the inside of the cranial vault showing the bony ridges of the eye orbits and sphenoid and temporal bones. Figures 5-30A–C provide bone windowed images and Figures 5-31A–C provide CT images showing the bony structures and ridges around the frontal and temporal lobes. Note how the soft brain parenchyma is surrounded by bone within the orbial and medial frontal lobes and temporal poles, evident on CT imaging. As physical forces act on the brain, the soft tissues of the orbital and medial frontal lobes and temporal poles becomes compressed against the rigid structures of the eye orbits and sphenoid and temporal bones, causing contusions of the soft brain parenchyma. Contusions are less common on the sides of the brain where the inner

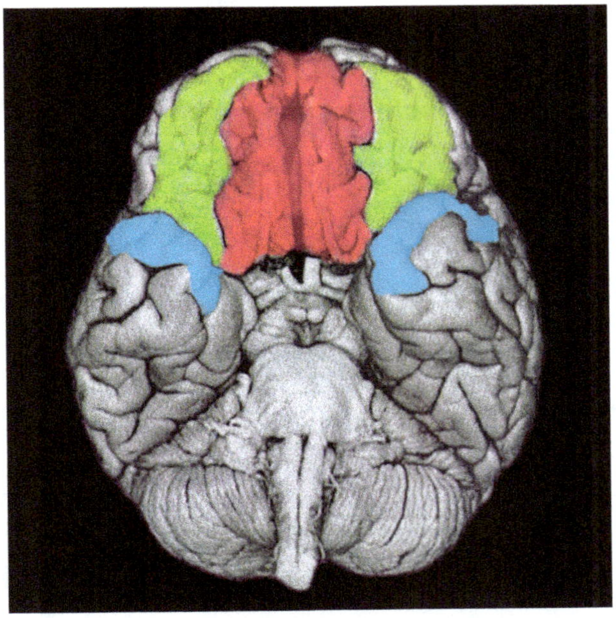

Figure 5-28 Common locations for hemorrhagic and non-hemorrhagic contusions. Red areas correspond with the medial frontal cortices, green areas correspond to the orbital frontal cortices, and blue areas correspond to the anterior and medial temporal poles.

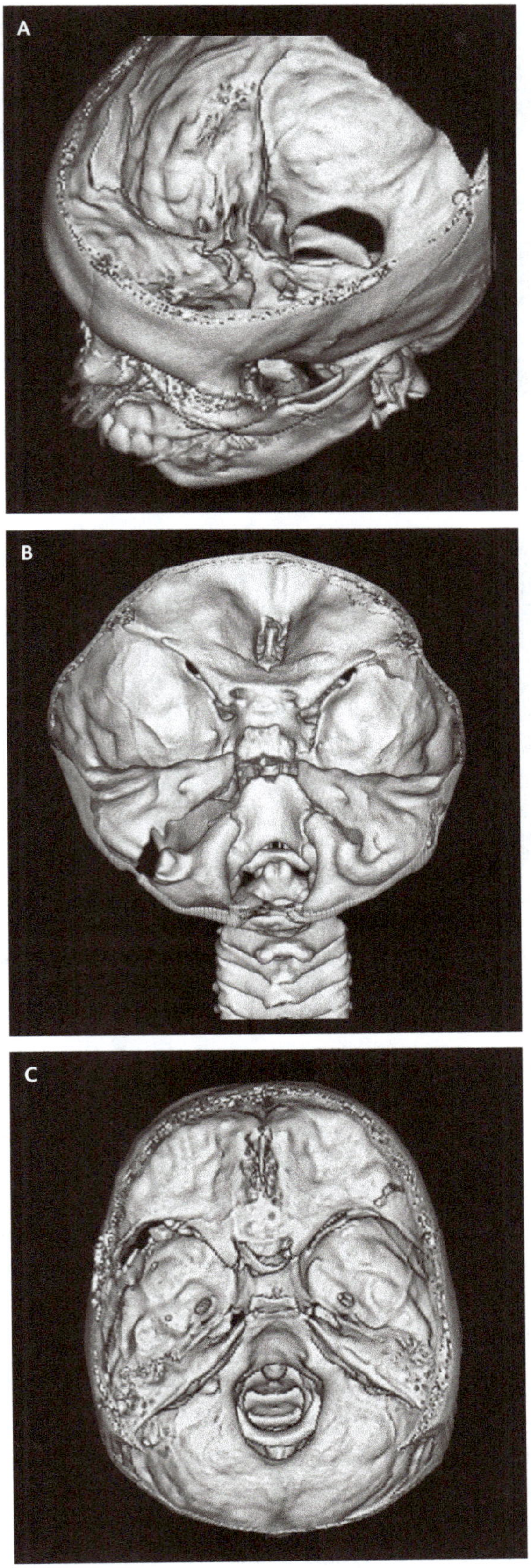

Figures 5-29A–C Bony structures around the eye orbits and anterior temporal lobes shown on 3D CT volume rendering. Note ridges and edges within these regions.

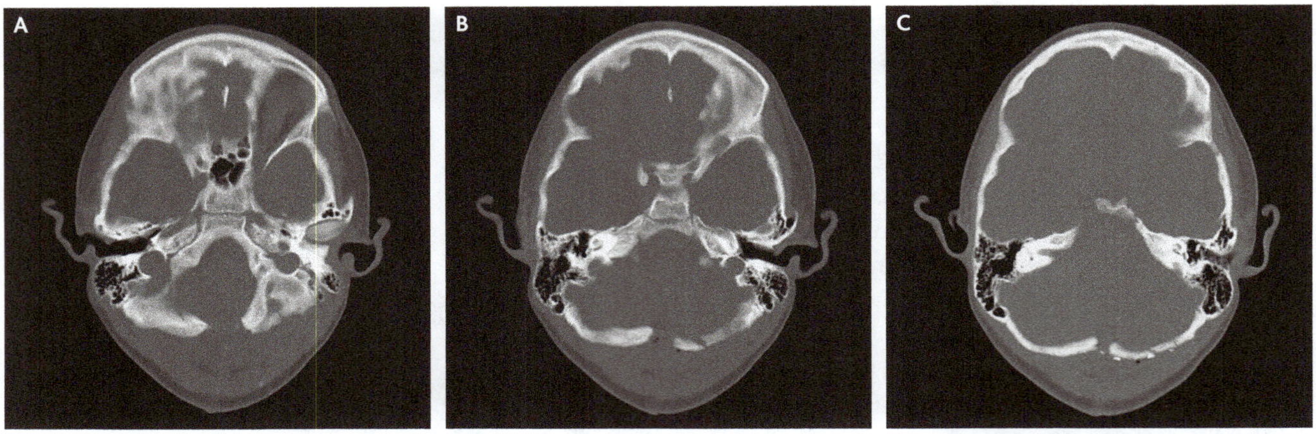

Figures 5-30A–C CT—bone window. Note bony structures directly above the eyes within the frontal and anterior temporal lobes. The images were chosen because of the asymmetry caused by the head being slightly tilted in the scanner. With the slice transecting tissue at different levels for the right and left sides of the cranium, a better appreciation of the boney ridges is possible.

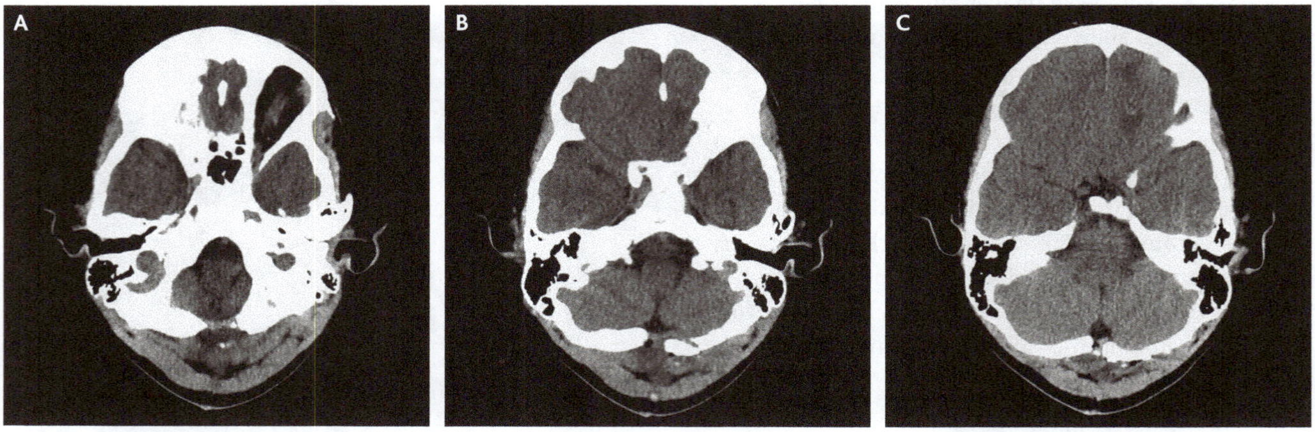

Figures 5-31A–C Standard CT imaging. Note the soft brain tissue surrounded by bone within the frontal lobes and anterior temporal lobes.

surface of the parietal bones are relatively flat and smooth (Figure 5-32).

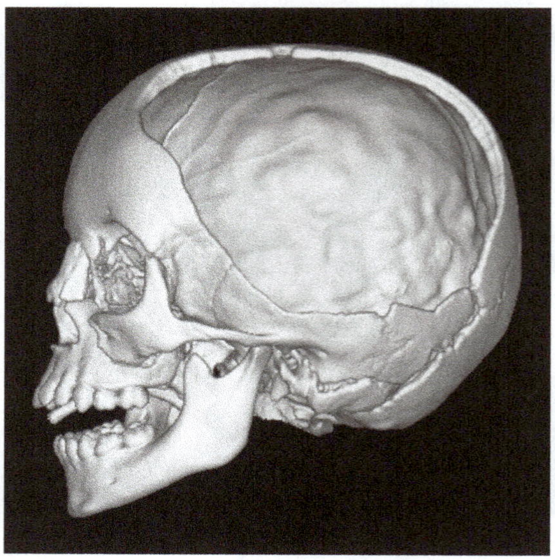

Figure 5-32 Inside of the skull showing the smooth sides of the calvarium, resulting in less contusions being evident along the sides of the brain compared to the front.

Injuries to the inferior frontal lobes, especially to the orbital and medial cortices, account for the most common symptoms of closed-head injuries. Damage to the orbital and medial frontal lobes results in disruption of emotional regulation and affect, in addition to behavioral inhibition. These patients may become disinhibited emotionally and behaviorally. If the damage involves more superior and lateral frontal-lobe structures, apathy and abulia, or the lack of goal-directed and self-motivated behaviors, may be evident. Damage to the temporal poles can result in an inability to store new memories, or *anterograde amnesia*, also a classic sign of a closed-head injury. Because the limbic structures, especially the amygdala bodies, are located within the anterior portion of the temporal lobes, disruption of more primitive emotions relating to fear and aggression may occur.

CLINICAL EXAMPLE

John: Orbital Frontal and Anterior Temporal Lobe Contusions

John was injured when his motorcycle left the road and he hit a fence post. Although he was wearing a helmet, the force of the impact resulted in hemorrhagic contusions within the inferior frontal lobes, especially the orbital and medial regions, and the temporal poles (Figures 5-33A–C and 5-34A–C).

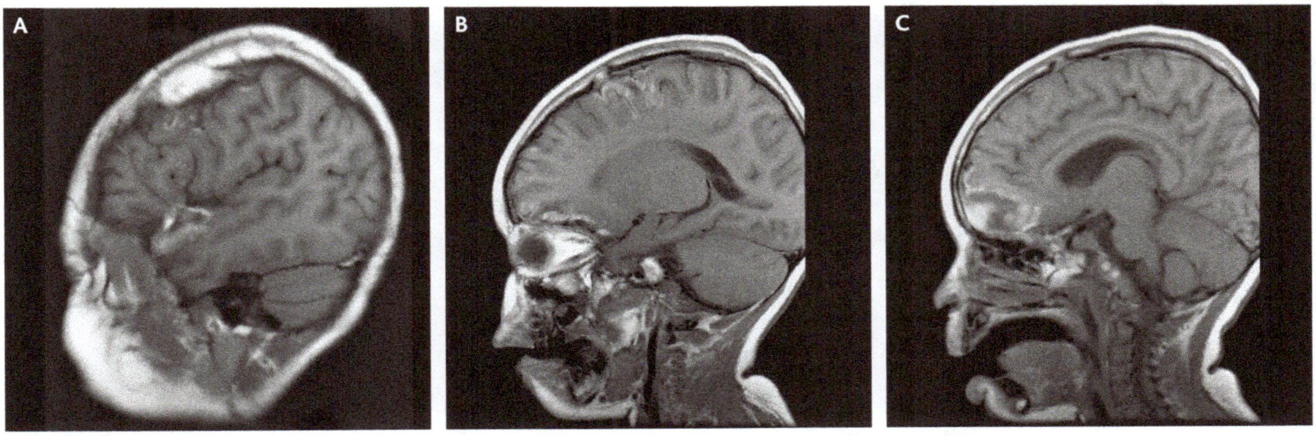

Figures 5-33A–C Clinical example John: T1 sagittal series of orbital frontal and anterior temporal lobe contusions. Note bright appearance of tissue on the anterior temporal lobes in 5-33A, orbital frontal lobe above the eye in 5-33B, and the medial frontal lobe in 5-33C.

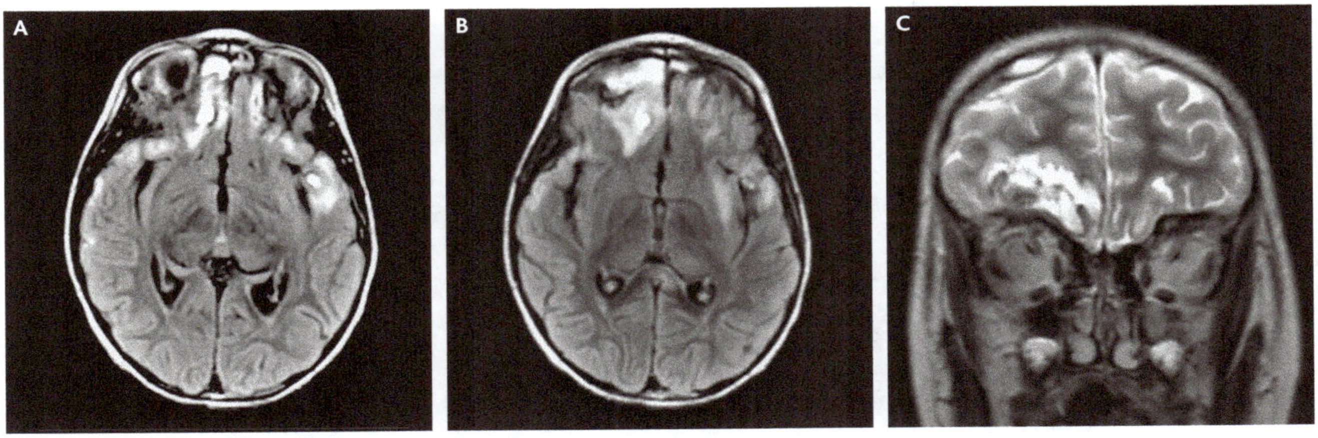

Figures 5-34A–C Clinical example John: T2 series of orbital frontal and anterior temporal lobe contusions. Note hyperintensity around the orbital and medial frontal lobes and temporal poles.

CLINICAL EXAMPLE

William: Multiple Frontal Contusions

Seemingly minor injuries can also result in damage to the orbital frontal and temporal lobe structures, especially with the cumulative effects of multiple concussions over a short period of time. William received several concussions over a period of less than a year while playing college-level ice hockey. He was eventually hospitalized after his head was pushed into the side of the rink and he experienced a loss of consciousness for several minutes. CT imaging (Figures 5-35A–C) revealed hemorrhagic contusions throughout his frontal lobes, with his right frontal lobe sustaining more injury than his left frontal lobe. Frontal hemorrhagic contusions were clearly evident on MRI imaging (Figures 5-36A–D). Note the bifrontal inflammation and petechial hemorrhages within the right orbital frontal and bilateral medial frontal lobes on T2 FLAIR (hyperintense) and GRE (hypointense-black), with restricted diffusion suggesting infarction on DWI (bright) and ADC (dark) sequences. Although he rapidly regained general cognitive faculties, he exhibited notable long-term deficits involving his anterograde memory (for new learning), executive functioning, mental-processing efficiency, and emotional regulation. His difficulties persisted for many months, resulting in significant disruption of his ability to tolerate college-level courses and demands. Even with intact intellect and understanding of the material, William was unable to organize his time or work, divide his attention during lectures, or complete assignments in the expected amount of time. For example, during lectures, he reported having difficulty writing notes while listening to the professor. He quickly fell behind because of the extra time it took him to process and record the information. Studying for exams was especially trying as his memory had deteriorated, and he would become frustrated at how difficult his college courses had become. Several years after his injury, William dropped out of college on account of failing grades and increasing frustration. William reported that he was never the same after the injury and was no longer able to keep up with the demands of college courses.

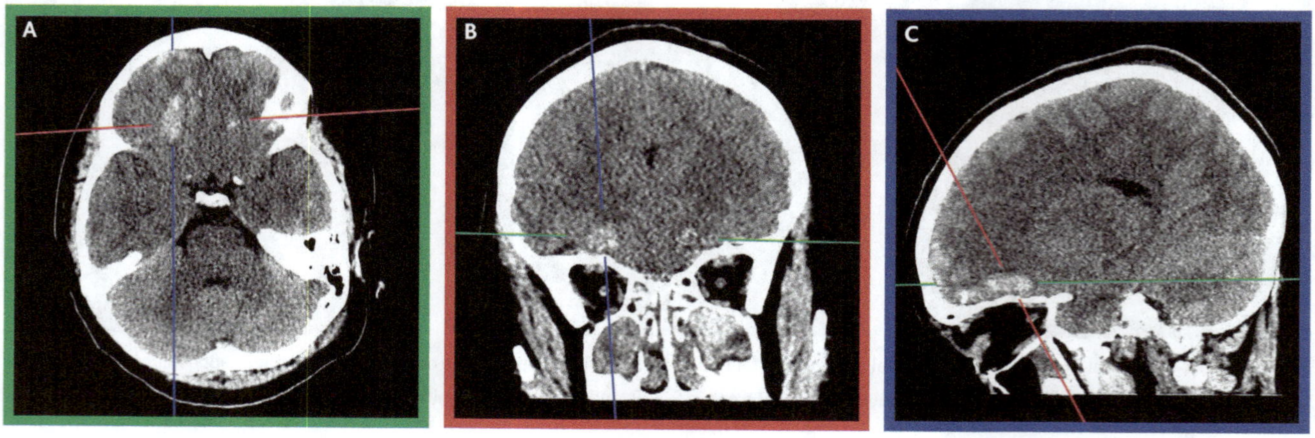

Figures 5-35A–C Clinical example William: CT series of multiple frontal contusions.

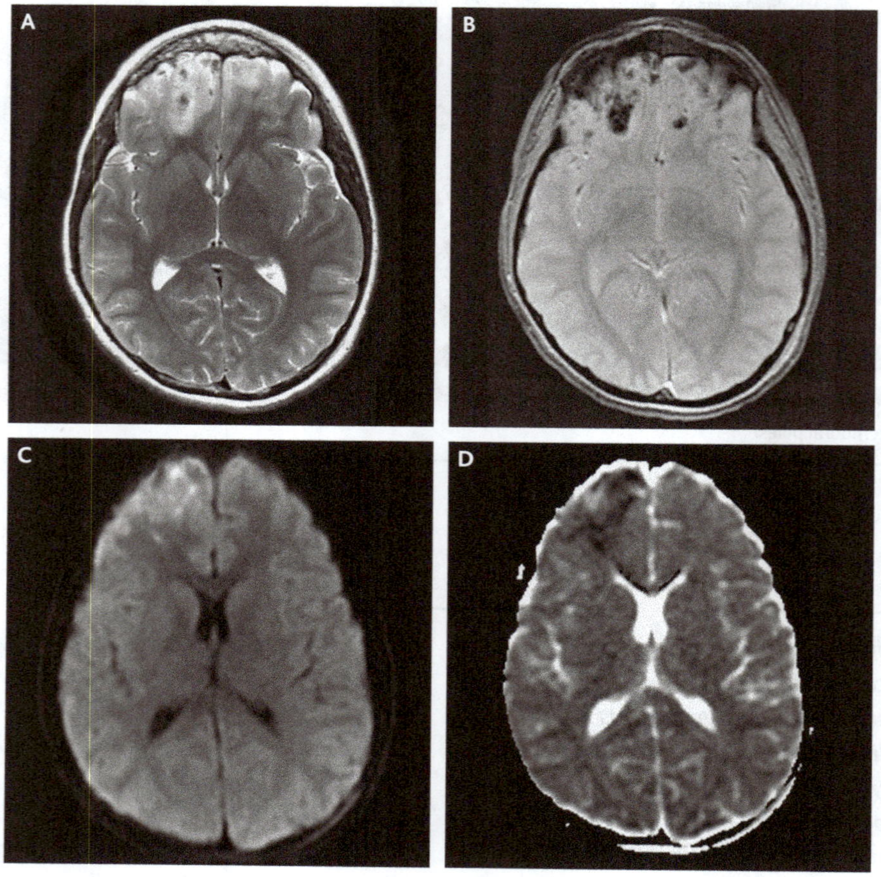

Figures 5-36A–D Clinical example William: MRI series of multiple frontal contusions. **A:** T2 FLAIR. **B:** GRE. **C:** DWI. **D:** ADC.

An interesting aspect of skull fractures is that quite marked damage to the cranium may not result in commensurate damage to soft brain tissues. In fact, some of the worst facial fractures may not result in notable deficits involving brain functioning. Car manufacturers build in "crumple zones," or structural regions designed to collapse in a collision. The collapse of the crumple zone reduces the forces acting on the occupants, who are protected by a more rigid structure. Fractures of the skull, especially those of the face, can act in the same manner as crumple zones, reducing the physical forces on the soft tissues of the brain. A remarkable example of this phenomenon involved Susan, who was involved in a severe automobile accident. Susan sustained profound crushing damage to the bones of her face. Susan's facial bones were crushed so badly that she lost sight in both eyes and required extensive facial reconstruction to rebuild her facial structure. Initial CT imaging revealed the crushing injury to her face (Figures 5-37A and B), but there was little to no subtantive damage to the soft tissues of her brain (Figure 5-37C). Given the severity of impact, it would be expected that she would have significant focal and diffuse injury to her brain, and hemorrhagic contusions within the frontal and temporal regions as described above. It was also expected that Susan would experience significant compromise to her cognitive and adaptive functioning, requiring lengthy rehabilitation following discharge from the intensive care unit. However, Susan regained basic cognitive functioning within a few weeks of her injury. By discharge from the hospital 2 months later, almost all of her cognitive abilities had returned to the normal range for her age, and she was mostly independent in her self-care. Mild limitations persisted for tasks requiring higher-level executive functioning, spatial awareness and memory functioning. Susan continued to experience mild difficulty with the formation of internal spatial representations and identification of object through touch, a condition called *astereognosis*. She also experienced visual hallucinations, a condition called *Charles Bonnet syndrome*, in which her brain formed complex visual sensations even though she was blind.

Upon follow-up examination, approximately 6 months after her injury, cognitive functioning was fully intact in all domains assessed. Performance ranged from average to high average, with quite marked improvements evident for tasks involving executive functioning, spatial reasoning, and memory. Although Susan continued to experience some phantom lights or sensations of bright spots in her visual fields, she no longer experienced the complex visual hallucinations consistent with Charles Bonnet syndrome. Susan was back in high school doing well with her studies, learning braille and walking with a cane.

Susan underwent cranioplasty (Figures 5-38A–C) and plastic surgery to reconstruct her face, and she quickly regained her previous appearance. The most remarkable aspect of Susan's recovery and facial reconstruction was the return of her smile and laugh, characteristics that exemplified the courage and spirit of this young woman. Susan was generous in allowing her case to be used within this guide in order to assist others in learning about neuroimaging and brain injury. Susan was elected to Homecoming Queen at her high school, demonstrating recognition from her peers for her bravery and courage, and also her positive attitude, love of life and willingness to mentor and help others in need.

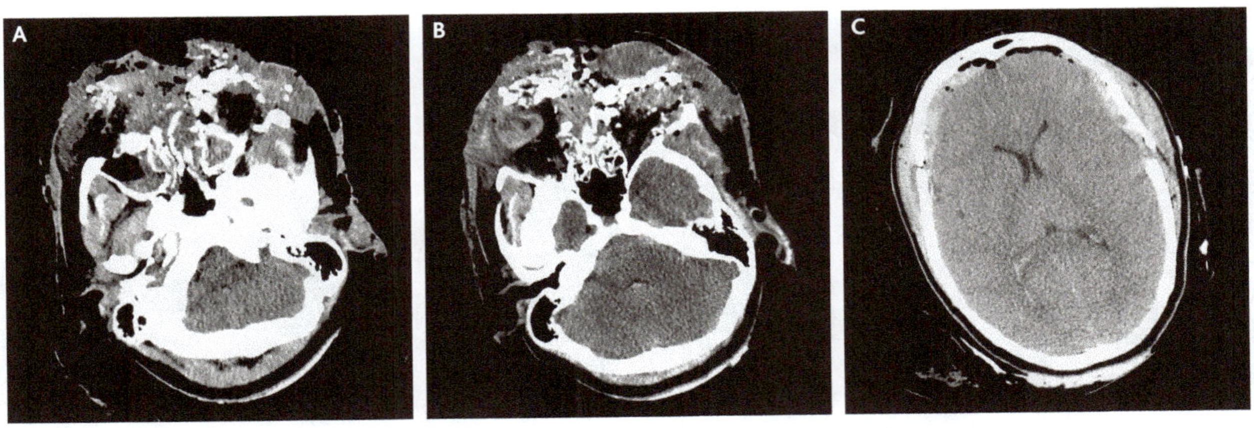

Figure 5-37A–C Clinical example Susan: CT series illustrating the crushing injury to Susan's face.

(*Continued*)

(*Continued*)

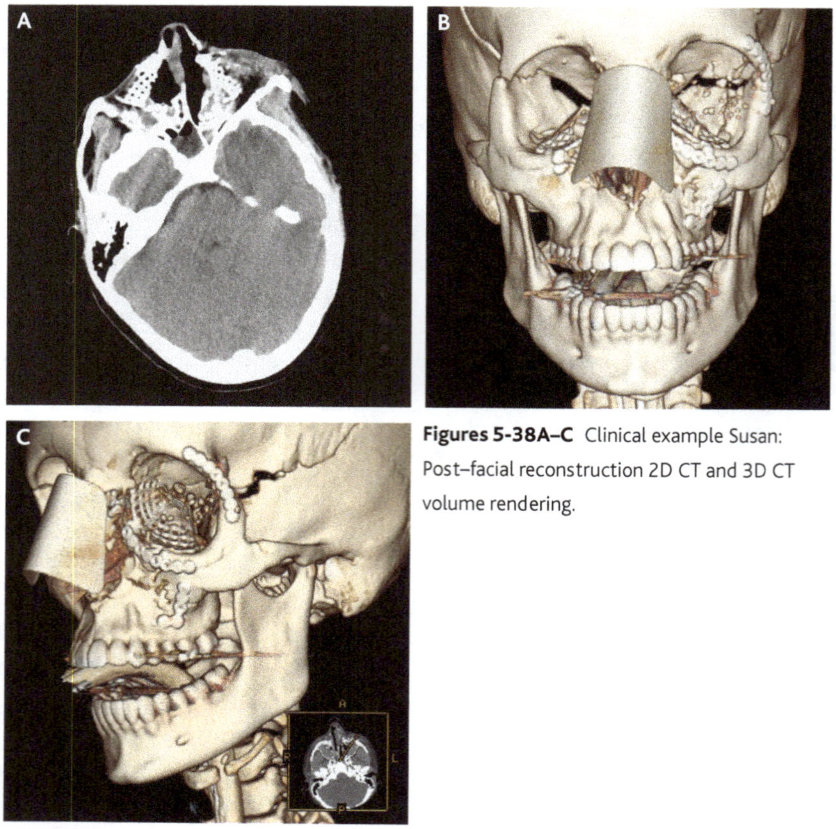

Figures 5-38A–C Clinical example Susan: Post–facial reconstruction 2D CT and 3D CT volume rendering.

Subcortical Hemorrhages

As a general rule, the deeper the hemorrhage in the brain, the more severe the injury and the worse the outcome. The deeper subcortical structures of the basal ganglia, thalamus, midbrain, and brain stem are protected from many physical injuries by the cortex, which acts as a shock absorber, receiving the greatest forces from an impact. Severe acceleration–deceleration or rotational injuries can result in damage to the cortex in addition to the deeper subcortical structures. The most common causes of deep subcortical damage are motor vehicle accidents, and nonaccidental traumas (NAT) in children.

When assessing brain scans following a severe injury, do not become so focused on the cortical areas that you fail to appreciate injury to the subcortical structures of the basal ganglia, thalamus, midbrain/pons, or brain stem. With severe brain injury, it is not unusual to discover subcortical hemorrhages on a variety of brain imaging sequences, with the bleeds ranging from large and obvious (Figures 5-39A–F) to small and easy to miss (5-40A–F).

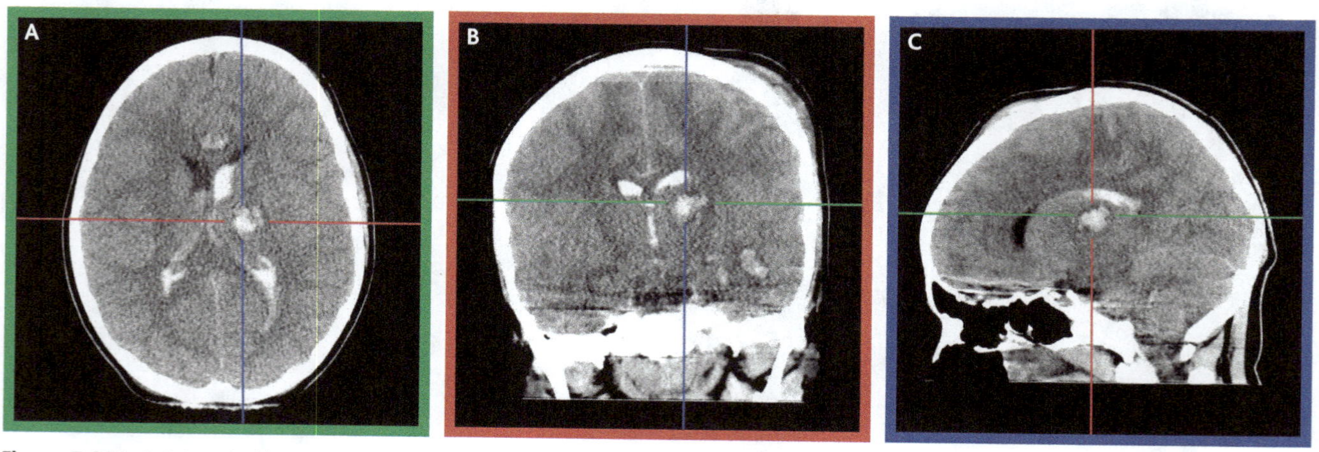

Figures 5-39A–C Subcortical hemorrhages on CT imaging.

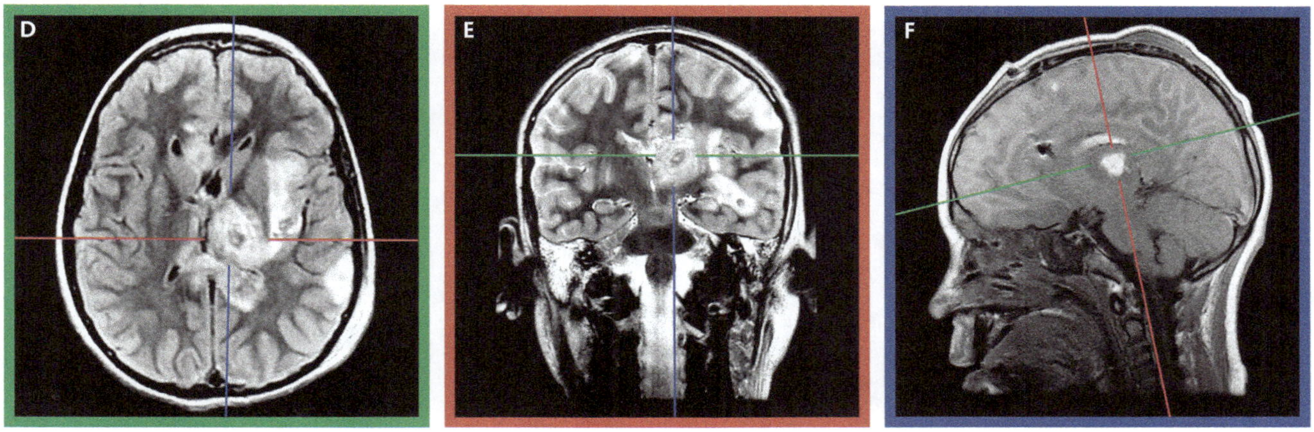

Figures 5-39D–F Subcortical hemorrhages on MRI imaging. **A:** T2 FLAIR **B:** T2 **C:** T1

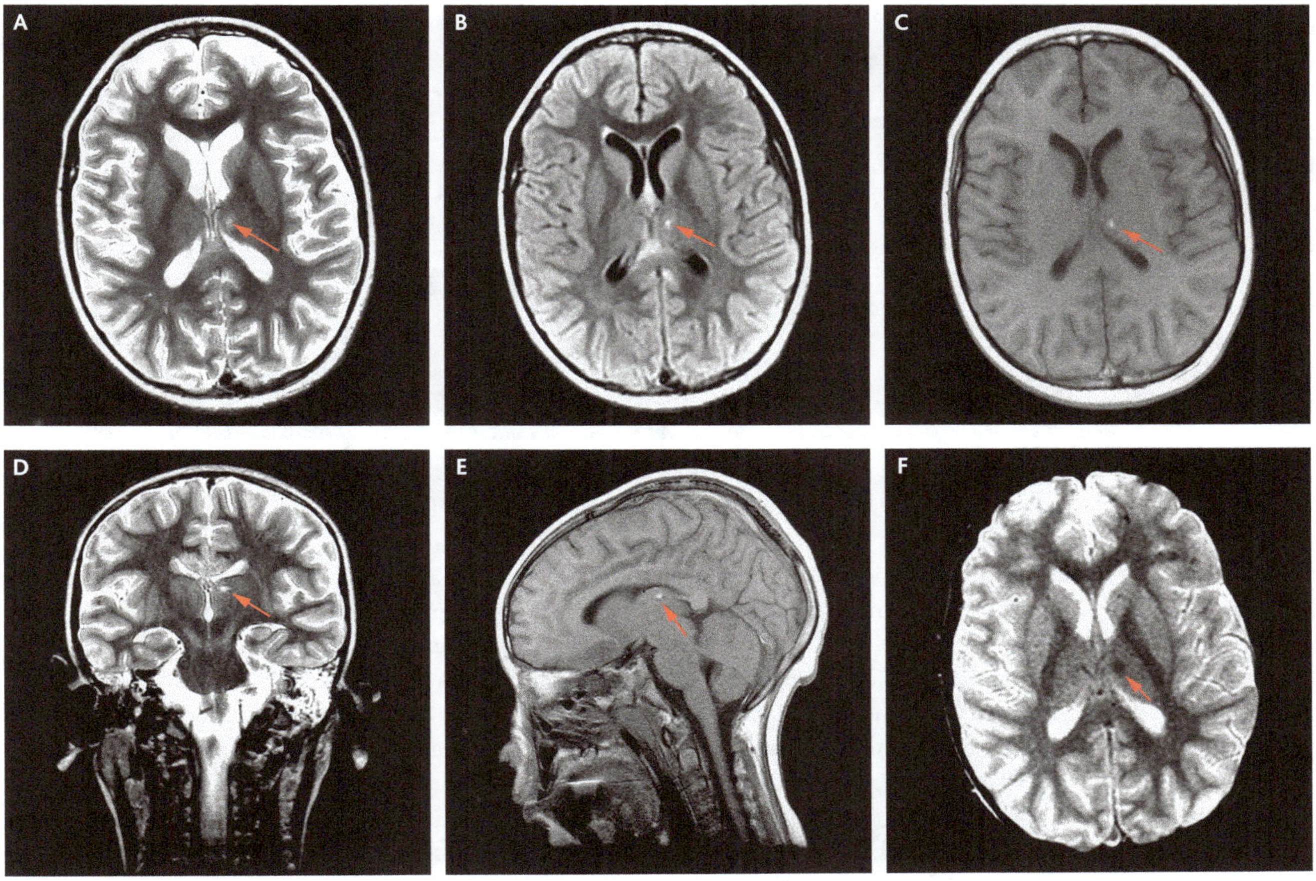

Figures 5-40A–F Less obvious, punctate thalamic hemorrhage on MRI series. **A:** T2. **B:** T2 FLAIR. **C:** T1. **D:** T2. **E:** T1. **F:** GRE.

POST-TRAUMATIC PNEUMOCEPHALUS

Post-traumatic pneumocephalus is a condition in which small pockets of air are located within the cranium. Pneumocephalus often accompanies skull fractures, especially those involving the frontal facial bones (Figures 5-41A–C arrows). Even without penetration of the skull, air can be seen inside the brain and cranium of patients after traumatic brain injury. Iatrogenic pneumocephalus is a frequent condition that occurs following surgical procedures to place intracranial pressure monitors, shunts, or external ventricular drains or to evacuate bleeds. Craniotomies to reduce pressure from swelling are also a source of pneumocephalus, especially along the extra-axial convexity between the scalp and dura, or dura and brain parenchyma (Figures 5-41D and E arrows). Projectile injuries such as gun shot wounds will frequently result in pneumocephalus along the bullet channel as air is drawn into the brain along with the projectile and bone fragments (Figure 5-41F arrow).

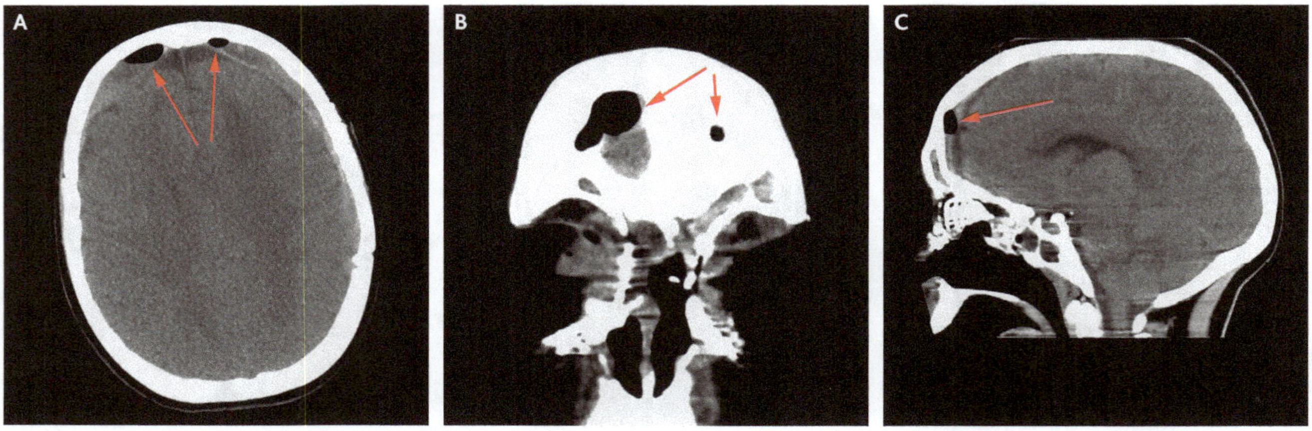

Figures 5-41A–C Examples of pneumocephalus from frontal skull fractures.

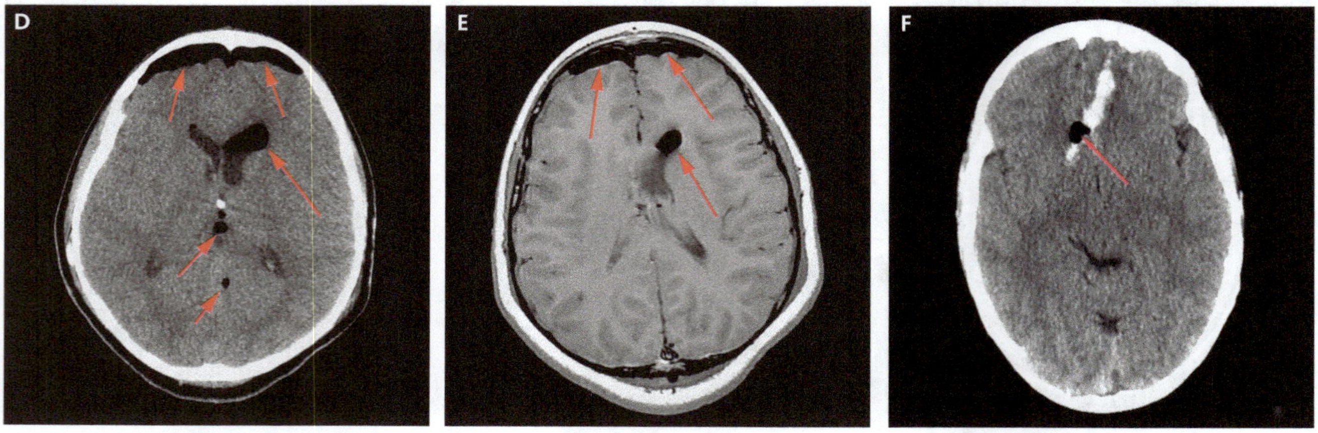

Figures 5-41D and E Examples of pneumocephalus from surgical intervention. **D**: CT. **E**: T1.

Figure 5-41F CT example of pneumocephalus due to air being pulled into a wound channel by a bullet (arrow).

On CT imaging, air appears black, as it is the least-dense material in the brain. On MRI there is an absence of signal, with air appearing black, similar to that on CT imaging. In general, given the extreme low density of air compared to that of other tissue in the brain, non-contrast CT imaging is the method of choice to assess for pneumocephalus.

Small amounts of air within the brain generally resolve spontaneously without complications. The morbidity for those with pneumocephalus is higher than for those without it; this is not so much due to the air in the brain as to the reasons for this air. Any openings in the skull or dura from penetrating or open head trauma or surgery increase infection risk, and pathologies that require surgical intervention are often more severe than those that do not.

POST-TRAUMATIC HYPOXIC ISCHEMIC ENCEPHALOPATHY

Most severe traumatic brain injuries result in some degree of hypoxic ischemic encephalopathy. Anoxia following a traumatic brain injury can result from a variety of secondary processes, such as respiratory arrest or airway compromise, post-traumatic seizures, hypotension, disrupted autoregulation, vascular spasm, hemorrhagic strokes, compression of blood vessels due to pressure from swelling, or chemical disruption of brain processes.

Anoxic ischemic infarction affects gray matter to a greater extent than white matter. It is frequently evident along the cortical mantle of the cerebrum and cerebellum and within the subcortical structures of the basal ganglia, amygdala, and hippocampus (Hutchison & Lebby, 2009). Hypoxic ischemic infarction along the cortical rim results in laminar necrosis, a condition that is relatively easy to visualize on a variety of brain scans.

REFERENCE

Hutchison, T., & Lebby, P. C. (2009). Traumatic encephalopathies. In R. B. David (Ed.), *Clinical pediatric neurology* (3rd ed.). New York: Demos Medical Publishing.

Ryan suffered bilateral basal ganglia hypoxic ischemic injury following prolonged status epilepticus that occurred a few minutes after a traumatic brain injury. Subcortical injury was evident within all structures of the basal ganglia. Damage to the caudate nuclei and putamena bilaterally was clearly evident on axial images, especially T2 FLAIR (Figure 5-42A). The coronal T2 sequences (Figure 5-42B) provided evidence of damage to all primary structures, including the caudate nuclei by the lateral ventricles; the putamena, just medial to the insular cortices; and the right and left globus pallidi, with evidence of lacuna infarctions. The hyperintensity of the three primary structures of the basal ganglia is evident bilaterally on the T2 coronal image. Diffusion-weighted imaging (DWI) (Figure 5-42C) suggests possible ischemic infarction, although the hyperintensity may be partial shine-through from the T2 weighting of the image. An apparent diffusion coefficient (ADC) sequence would have clarified the degree to which the hyperintensity on DWI is shine-through versus disrupted diffusion but unfortunately, an ADC sequence was not acquired for this patient. Given the degree of hyperintensity on DWI, in addition to the presence of lacuna infarctions medially within each globus pallidus, ischemic injury to the other structures is highly probable. The clinical presentation of this patient also suggested bilateral damage to his basal ganglia structures as he had an extrapyramidal choreiform movement disorder on examination.

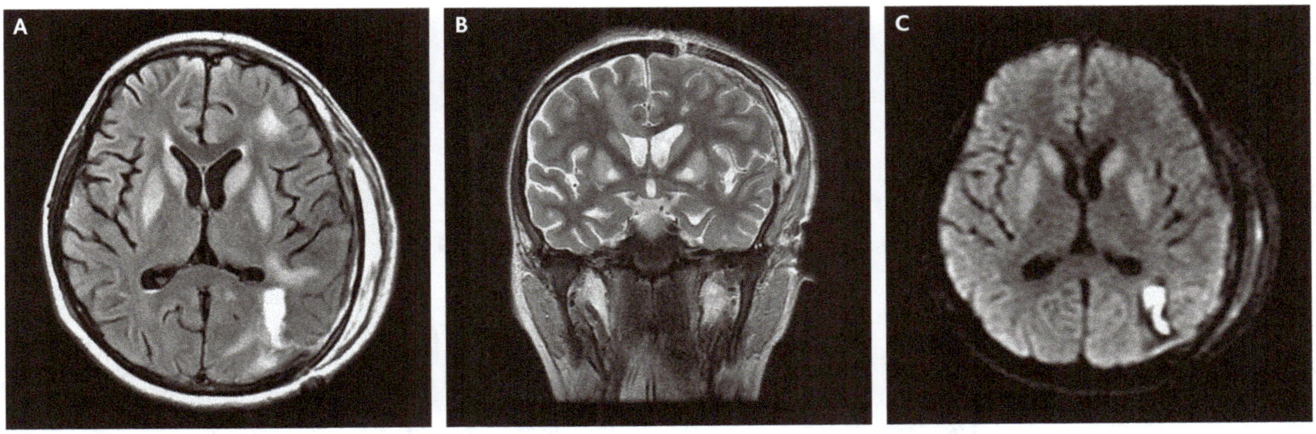

Figure 5-42A–C Clinical example Ryan: basal ganglia damage due to hypoxic ischemic injury. **A:** T2 FLAIR. **B:** T2. **C:** DWI.

Laminar Necrosis due to Hypoxic Ischemic Infarction

Anoxic ischemia can lead to lamina necrosis, or the breakdown of the cortical lamina. On CT, lamina necrosis is suggested by contours of hyperintensity following the gyral ridges (Figures 5-43A–C). Lamina necrosis is readily evident on T2 FLAIR sequences as a band of hyperintensity that follows the contours of the cortical gyri (Figure 5-44A). Lamina necrosis is also suggested by a bright appearance

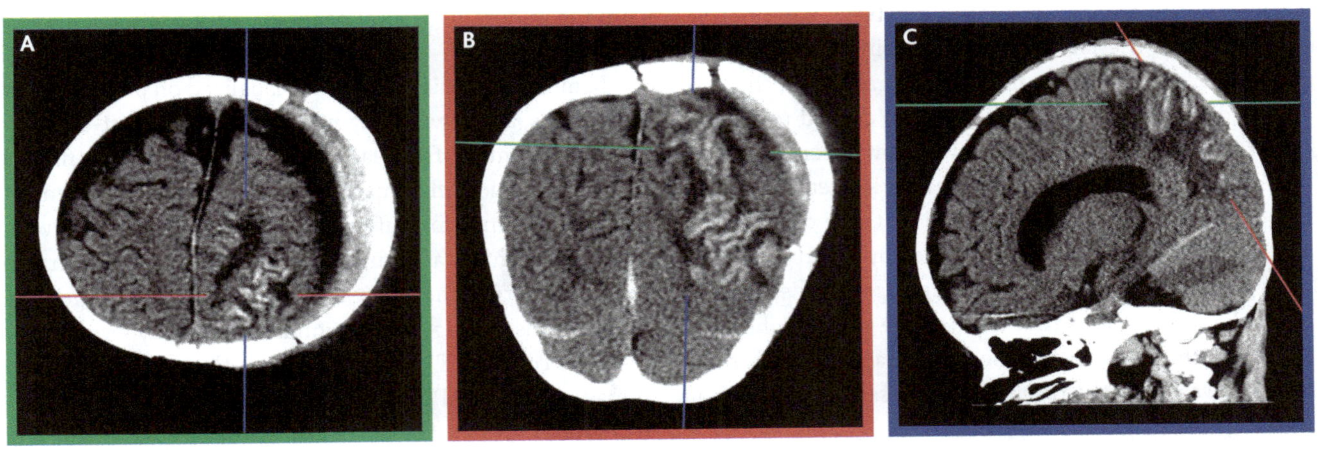

Figures 5-43A–C CT series. Laminar necrosis due to vascular compromise resulting from traumatic brain injury. Note bright appearance that follows contours of the cortical gyri, a sign of laminar necrosis.

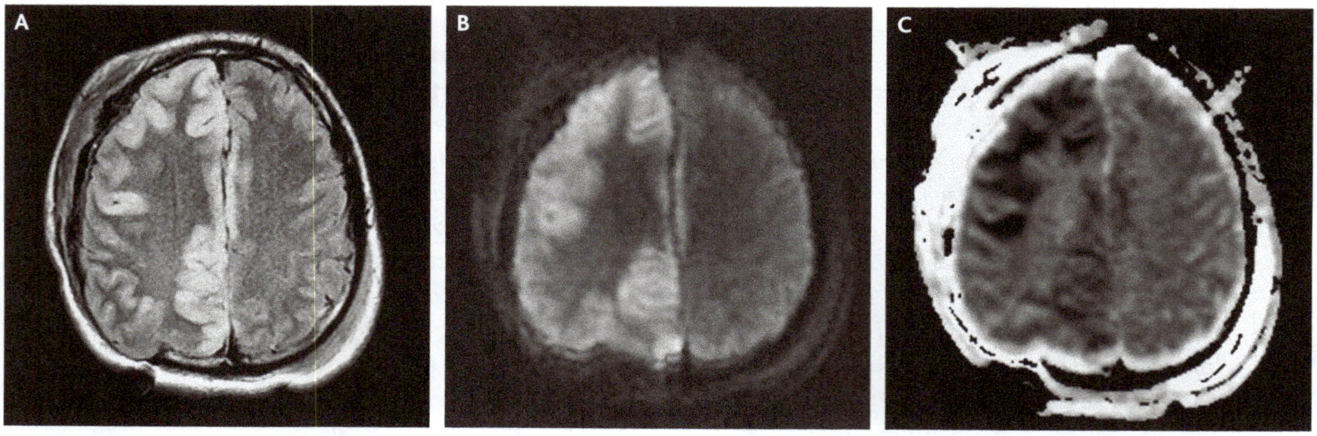

Figures 5-44A–C MRI axial series: Laminar necrosis due to hypoxic injury affecting the right hemisphere more than the left. Note hyperintensity around the cortical rim on T2 FLAIR, most evident in the right hemisphere and involving both the lateral and medial surfaces. Diffusion imaging suggests infarction of the cortical tissue. **A:** T2 FLAIR. **B:** DWI. **C:** ADC.

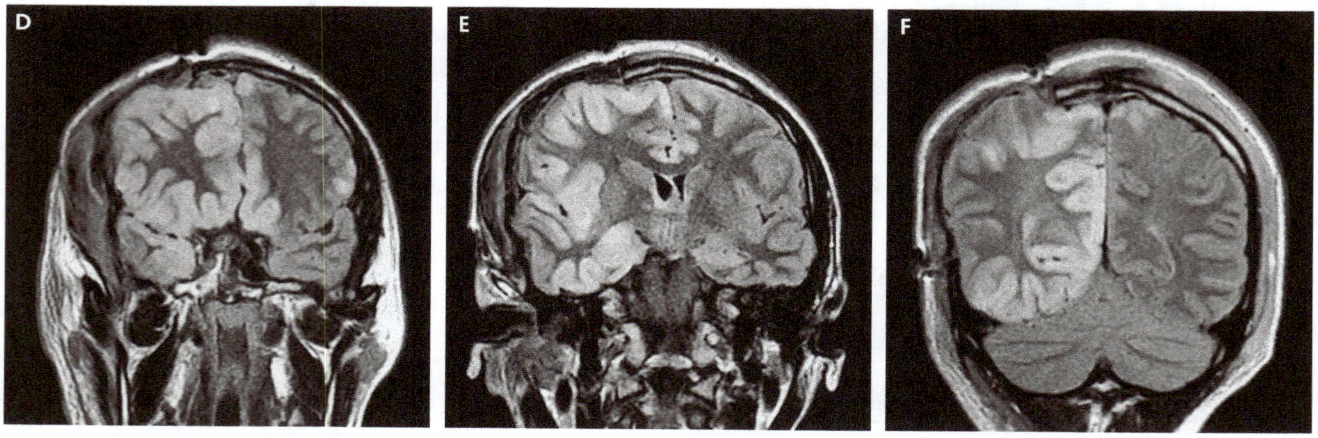

Figures 5-44D–F MRI T2 FLAIR coronal series showing extensive cortical laminar necrosis.

on DWI (Figure 5-44B) and a dark appearance on ADC (Figure 5-44C) sequences with a similar pattern of cortical involvement evident on T2 weighted imaging.

In assessment of the injury presented in Figures 5-44A–F, it-becomes apparent that multiple arterial distributions were affected. The lateral frontal and insular regions are supplied by the carotid to middle cerebral artery, the anterior medial cortices are supplied by the carotid to anterior cerebral artery, and the medial occipital cortex is supplied by the vertebral-basilar to posterior cerebral artery. Hypoxia involving tissue within all of these distributions suggests that the ischemia was caused by a diffuse process, not a post-traumatic stroke affecting a specific distribution. In this case, it appears that the damage to the right hemisphere, with injury to the medial surfaces of both hemispheres, was likely the result of compression of tissue from swelling of the right hemisphere.

Evidence for hypoxia being the result of compression of tissue from the right to left hemispheres comes from the hypothetical axis of compression shown in Figures 5-45A–C. The axis of compression is suggested by the injury, with most of the pressure being exerted against the medial border of the right and left hemispheres (double arrows) and the midbrain cerebral peduncle on the left side (single arrow).

Laminar necrosis can also be visualized on post-contrast T1 images, as shown in Figures 5-46A and B. Post-contrast T1 enhancement from laminar necrosis can be confused with arachnoid inflammation. With careful assessment of the images one can differentiate the two processes, with laminar necrosis affecting the cortical layers and arachnoiditis sparing the cortical tissue. T2 FLAIR images can assist in discerning the two conditions: the hyperintensity on post-contrast T1 images matches the cortical hyperintensity on T2 FLAIR. Figures 5-46B and C show a clear concordance between the post-contrast T1 enhancement and T2 hyperintensity of the cortical lamina, which is evident along the central sulcus (arrows).

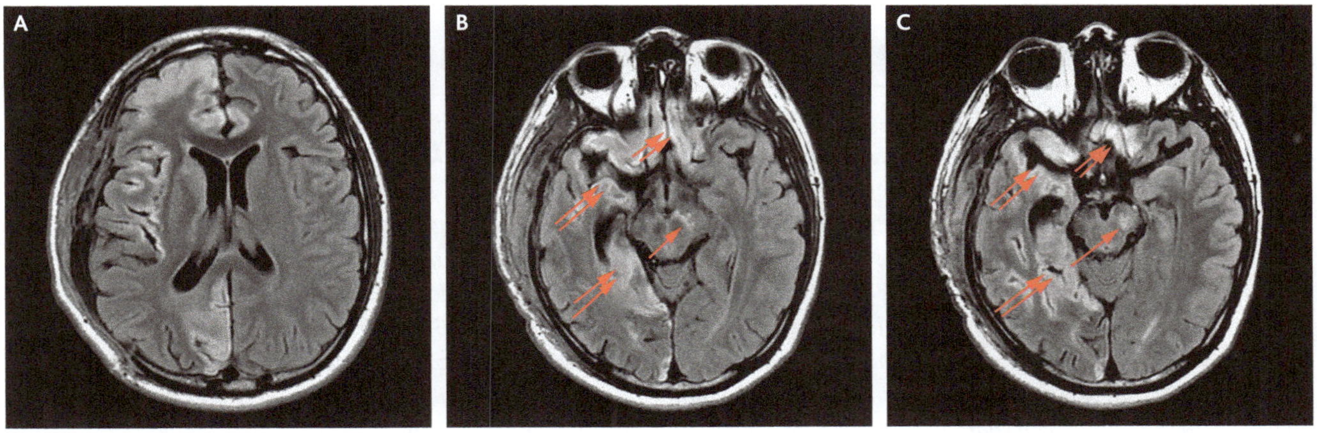

Figure 5-45A–C MRI T2 FLAIR axial series showing extensive cortical laminar necrosis (arrows), resulting from compression of the right hemisphere cortex and medial left hemisphere subcortical and cortical structures due to swelling of the right hemisphere.

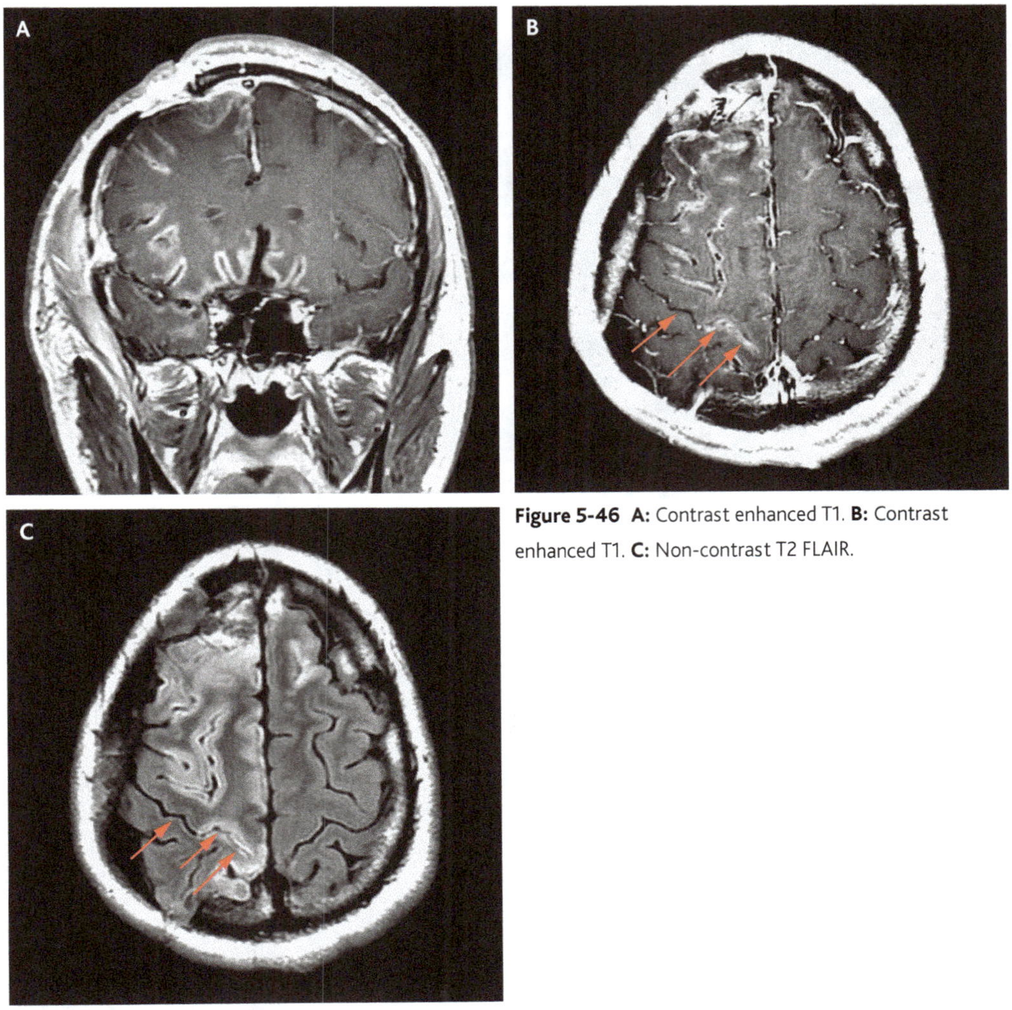

Figure 5-46 **A:** Contrast enhanced T1. **B:** Contrast enhanced T1. **C:** Non-contrast T2 FLAIR.

SECOND-IMPACT SYNDROME

Second-impact syndrome is a condition in which an impact to the brain during the acute stages of recovery following a previous injury can result in extensive damage to the brain. The damage from the second injury is greater than expected for the severity of the second impact or even the cumulative effects of the previous injury and the second injury. Damage can be profound and clearly out of proportion to the physical forces involved. Athletes who experience multiple, repetitive concussions over a short period of time are at greatest risk of sustaining second-impact syndrome.

CLINICAL EXAMPLE
Jeff: Second-Impact Syndrome

During summer break from school, Jeff spent much of his time practicing tricks on his skateboard. While skating at a new skate park, Jeff fell several times over a period of a few days. A subsequent, relatively minor fall resulted in Jeff being hospitalized, where his friends reported him having had symptoms of concussion on more than one occasion. After the fall, Jeff had joked with his friends before experiencing rapid deterioration of mental status and loss of consciousness within just a few minutes. Even though this fall was minor, Jeff had suffered a severe brain injury due to second-impact syndrome. Note the appearance of blood (hyperdense or bright) surrounded by edema (hypodense or dark) on CT imaging (Figures 5-47A–C). On standard and contrast-enhanced MRI imaging, the extent of injury can be appreciated by the heterogeneous (hyper and hypointensity) on T2 weighted images (5-48A and B), black appearance of blood on GRE imaging (5-48C) and hyperintensity suggesting breakdown of the blood-brain barrier on contrast-enhanced T1 weighted imaging (5-48D–F).

Although Jeff recovered much of his general cognitive ability, he continued to exhibit deficits involving executive functioning, mental flexibility, and attentional functioning several years after his injury.

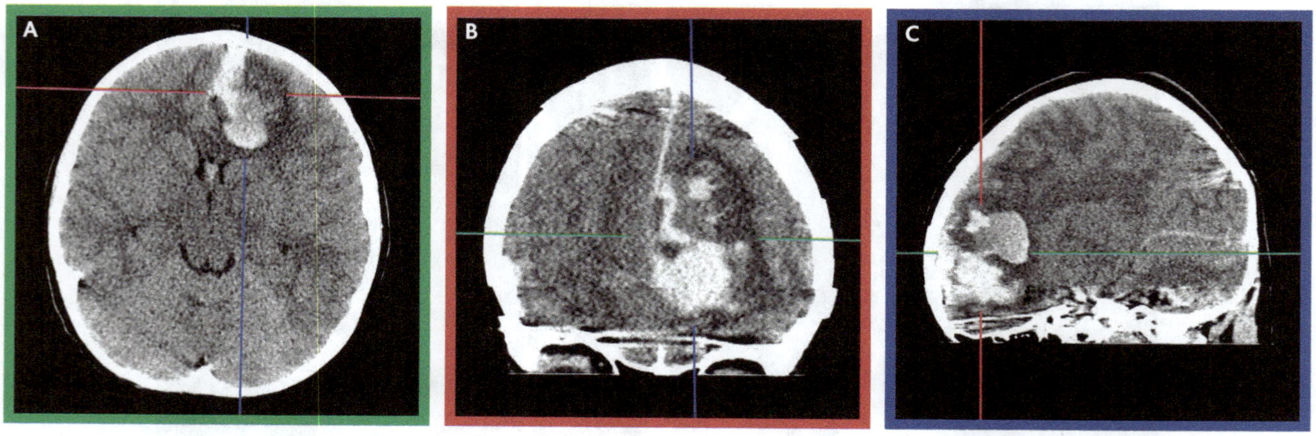

Figures 5-47A–C Clinical example Jeff: second-impact syndrome, CT series. Note appearance of blood (bright area) surrounded by edema (dark gray), suggesting significant intraparenchymal hemorrhage.

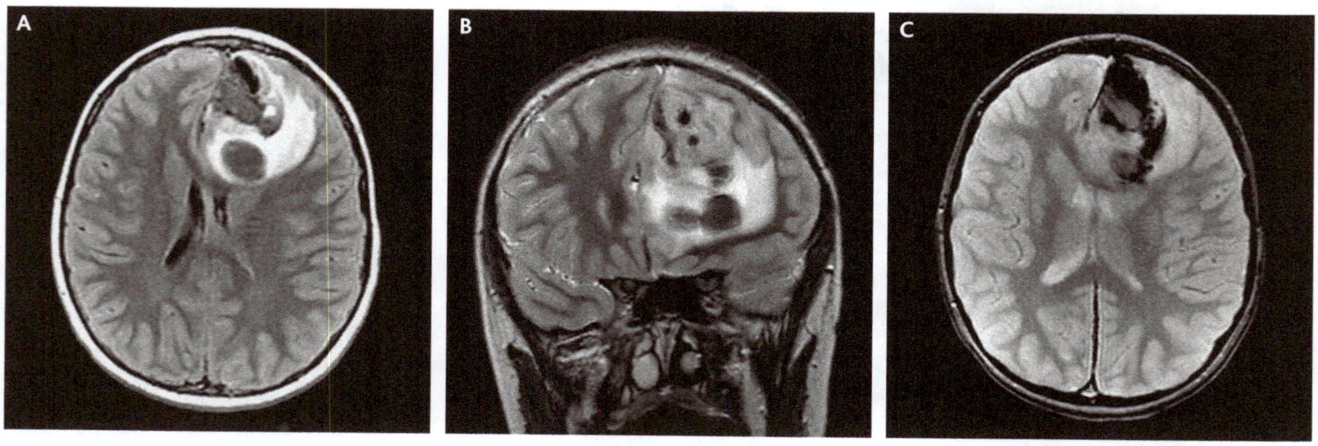

Figures 5-48A–C Clinical example Jeff: second-impact syndrome, MRI non-contrast series. The extent and severity of damage are clearly evident on the non-contrast T2 and T2 FLAIR images. On GRE, the blood is shown by the black region within the area of hemorrhagic contusion. **A:** T2 FLAIR **B:** T2 **C:** GRE.

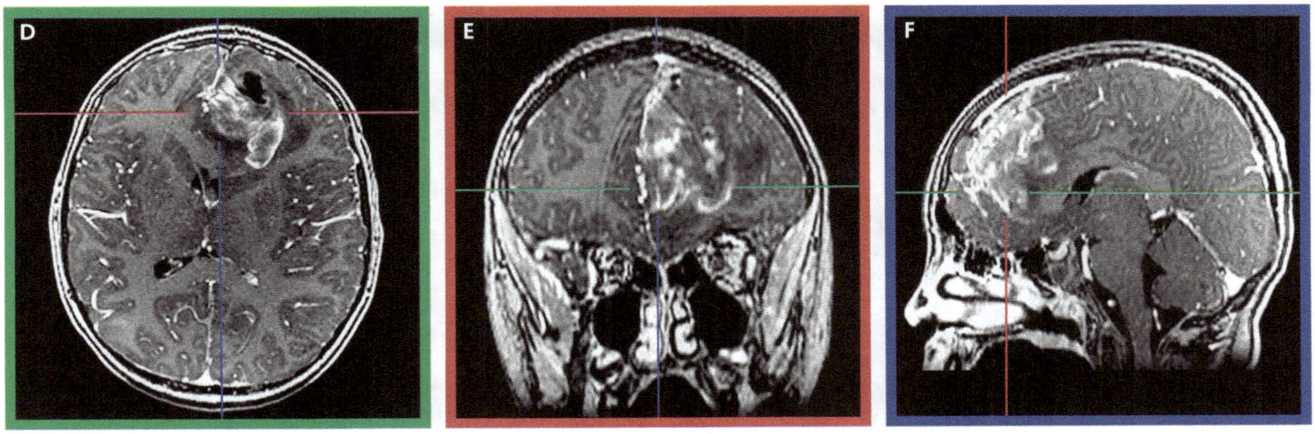

Figures 5-48D–F Clinical example Jeff: second-impact syndrome, contrast-enhanced 3D T1 FSPGR series. Contrast imaging suggests significant breakdown of the blood–brain barrier within the region of interest.

CLINICAL EXAMPLE
Julianne: Second Impact Syndrome

Julianne suffered from second-impact syndrome with symptoms and course being similar to that experienced by Jeff (see previous clinical example). After her second injury, which occurred shortly after her first injury, Julianne had a brief period of lucidity followed by rapid decline in mental status and prolonged loss of consciousness. Julianne was an accomplished gymnast who competed at a high level of competition. During practice, Julianne fell from the parallel bars, hitting her head hard enough to result in a concussion. She did not tell her coach about this, as she was training for an upcoming competition and did not want to be prevented from taking part in it. Less than 2 hours later she fell again, sustaining a second impact of the severity that would normally cause a relatively mild concussion. However, after the fall, she rapidly lost consciousness, with posturing and respiratory deterioration occurring by the time the first responders arrived. Julianne was intubated in the field and emergently transported to the nearest trauma center.

Neurosurgical craniotomy was required to treat severe swelling of her right hemisphere clearly evident on CT by the extensive midline shift of the lateral ventricles and falx cerebri (Figures 5-49A and B). Julianne remained in critical condition for several weeks due to difficulty controlling her intracranial pressure. A large, left-sided craniotomy was performed to prevent downward herniation of the brain; there was clear evidence of brain parenchyma herniating outside of the craniotomy hole (Figures 5-49C and D). Once stabilized, she was transported to the rehabilitation unit for intensive therapeutic intervention.

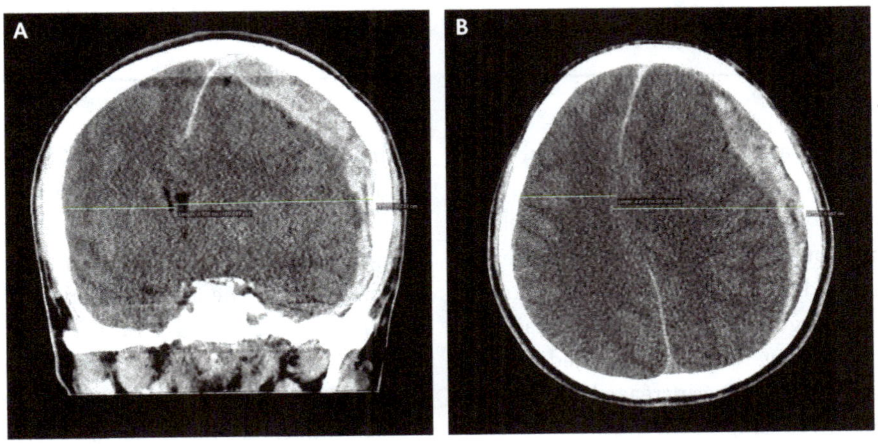

Figure 5-49A and B Clinical example Julianne: second-impact syndrome, CT series. Note extensive swelling and midline shift evident on Figures 5-49A (38 mm of shift) and 5-49B (45 mm of shift) acquired acutely. This CT series also provides evidence of left hemisphere extra-axial hemorrhage, with a swirl appearance suggesting either ongoing bleeding or mixing of blood and CSF. Following craniotomy to relieve intracranial pressure, almost complete resolution of the extensive midline shift was evident (5-49C and 5-49D). **A:** Midline shift 38 mm. **B:** Midline shift 45 mm.

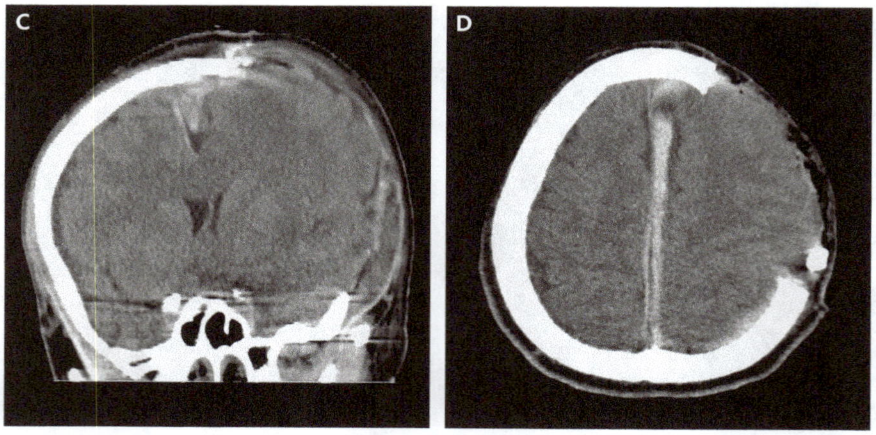

Figure 5-49C and D Clinical example Julianne: second-impact syndrome, CT series. **C:** Post-craniotomy with herniation and resolution of midline shift. **D:** Post-craniotomy with herniation and resolution of midline shift.

Follow-up MRI suggested global damage to her brain. Most of the pathology was within the left frontal and medial occipital regions (Figures 5-50A–C). Julianne never regained normal motor or cognitive functioning and will likely remain dependent on others for many years, if not her entire lifetime.

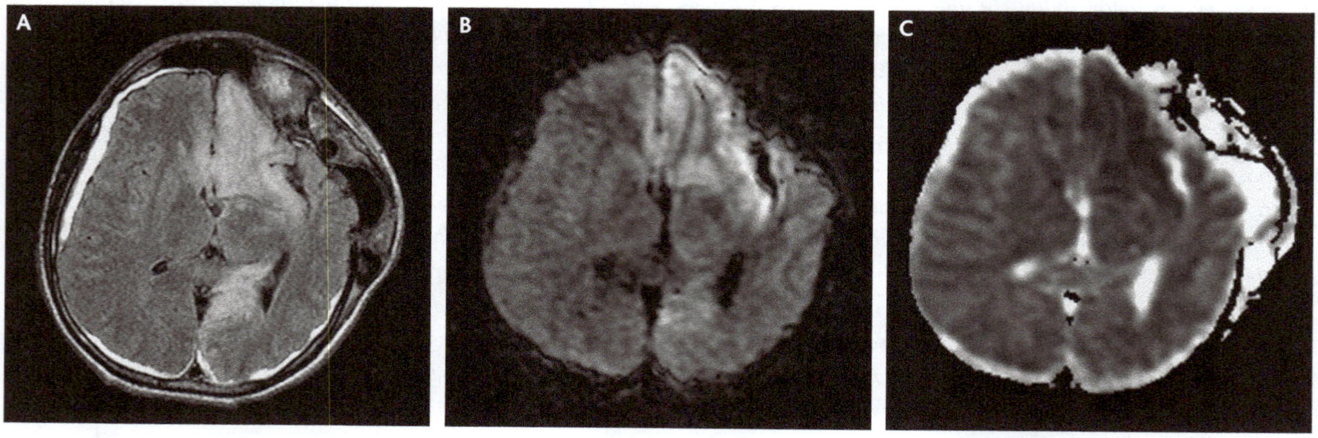

Figures 5-50A–C Clinical example Julianne: follow-up MRI series. Note left frontal and medial occipital damage most evident on T2 FLAIR and diffusion imaging. Restricted diffusion within these areas is suggested by the bright or hyperintense appearance on DWI and the dark or hypointense appearance on ADC. **A:** T2 FLAIR. **B:** DWI. **C:** ADC.

In the most severe cases, a second concussion during the period of recovery from a previous concussion can result in disrupted autoregulation of blood flow, severe swelling, and, ultimately, herniation of the brain if it is not treated within minutes. The rapid increase in cerebral blood volume due to loss of autoregulation can damage brain tissue, resulting in further injury due to extensive edema and increased intracranial pressure. The increased intracranial pressure can build rapidly, causing death in only a few minutes. In many cases, the condition is life threatening and responsible for severe disability or loss of life.

The incidence of second-impact syndrome is not well documented and is often combined with cases of "severe brain injury" (Bey & Ostick, 2009). The frequency of second-impact syndrome is difficult to assess, as many young athletes fail to report concussive injuries for fear of being benched for several weeks, not realizing the danger of returning to the athletic arena. This was the case with Julianne, a gymnast who did not report her first injury because she did not want to be prevented from competing in an upcoming event (see clinical example Julianne).

As expected, there is an increased incidence of second-impact syndrome in sports with a high risk of concussive injuries, such as boxing and football (Sullivan & Anderson, 2000). However, as was true for Julianne and Jeff in the clinical examples presented here, any activity in which a person is at risk of multiple concussions over a short period of time can result in second-impact injuries.

REFERENCE

Bey, T., & Ostick, B. (2009). Second impact syndrome. *Western Journal of Emergency Medicine, 10*(1), 6–10.

Sullivan, J. A., & Anderson, S. J. (Eds.). (2000). *Care of the young athlete.* Elk Grove Village, IL: American Academy of Pediatrics and American Academy of Orthopedic Surgeons.

INTRAVENTRICULAR HEMORRHAGES

Intraventricular hemorrhages form when blood collects within the ventricular system. Bleeds involving the ventricular system are often a sign of severe injury to the brain and usually have a poor outcome. At times, intraparenchymal bleeding may be delayed several hours or even days after an injury and, as such, will not be evident on acute brain scanning. The mechanism of this curious circumstance is unknown but may be related to clotting abnormalities or vascular responses to the trauma (Hutchison & Lebby, 2009).

REFERENCE

Hutchison, T., & Lebby, P. C. (2009). Traumatic encephalopathies. In R. B. David (Ed.), *Clinical pediatric neurology* (3rd ed.). New York: Demos Medical Publishing.

On CT, intraventricular hemorrhages are often easy to appreciate, as the blood within the ventricles will appear hyperdense or bright, in contrast to CSF, which is hypodense or dark (Figures 5-51A–C). The appearance of the hemorrhage on MRI is more dependent on the sequence being viewed. As is the case with other bleeds, it is important to take into account the age of the hemorrhage when assessing CT or MR images for intraventricular hemorrhages (see Table 2-4).

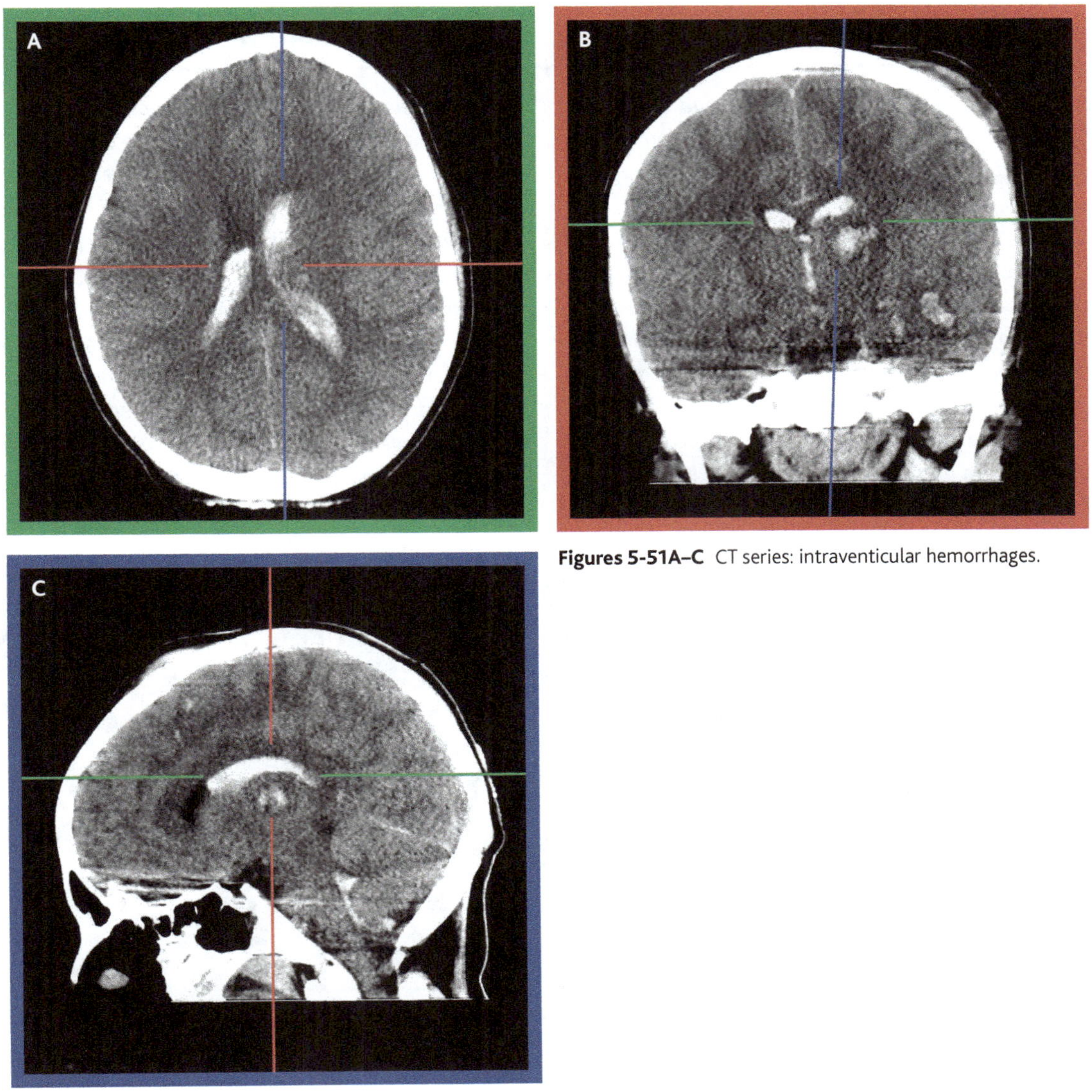

Figures 5-51A–C CT series: intraventicular hemorrhages.

POST-TRAUMATIC VASOSPASM

In addition to hemorrhages, it is important to evaluate for other vascular responses to physical trauma, such as vasospasm, as shown in the next clinical example.

INTRACEREBRAL EDEMA

CT is the method of choice to evaluate swelling in the emergency department or when imminent herniation is a concern. When there is little to no bleeding in the brain, swelling may be the only sign of traumatic injury, especially for mild closed-head injuries.

Because the brain is housed within the skull, a mostly closed container, any increase in CSF volume will result in either compensatory reduction of other fluids or tissue or an increase in intracranial pressure. In infants treated for intracerebral edema, before closure of the cranial sutures, enlargement of the cranial vault and head size may assist in compensating for mild increases in brain volume. Once the sutures are closed, increased pressure caused by swelling may result in downward herniation of the brain through the foramen magnum. If intracranial pressure rises to exceed perfusion pressure or systemic arterial blood pressure, there will be a rapid reduction of blood flow to the brain, a condition that can result in profound damage and imminent death unless treated.

Given the intracranial compliance curve (Figure 5-53), increased volume within the cranial vault due to brain swelling, hemorrhage, or ventricular dilation will not cause a large increase in intracranial pressure until the compensatory mechanisms of the brain become exhausted. Compensation for increased parenchymal volume can involve a variety of mechanisms, including but not

CLINICAL EXAMPLE
Marilyn: Post-traumatic Vasospasm

Marilyn was involved in a relatively minor head injury and was expected to make a good recovery, based on her grossly intact mental status while being examined in the emergency department. However, a few hours after her injury and while still in the emergency department, Marilyn's mental status began to deteriorate rapidly. She was rushed to the CT scanner, but imaging failed to provide an explanation for her deterioration. There was no swelling or evidence of hemorrhaging. Marilyn was then scanned using a variety of MRI sequences, including time-of-flight (TOF) magnetic resonance angiography (MRA), to assess vascular integrity. The circle of Willis TOF images suggested bilateral middle cerebral artery vasospasm. Although the vertebral, basilar, and internal carotid vessels appeared patent and visible on the image, there was less flow through the middle cerebral arteries (Figure 5-52A) than that expected (Figure 5-52B). Even with rapid treatment for the vasospasm, Marilyn suffered severe injury to her brain within the right and left middle cerebral artery distributions (Figure 5-52C).

Given her severe bilateral brain injury, Marilyn experienced profound loss of cognitive and functional abilities. She never regained independent functioning, and many years later, she was still dependent on others for all self-care and adaptive needs. Damage to her left perisylvian cortex also left her globally aphasic and unable to communicate verbally. Communication was achieved via behavioral and affective means.

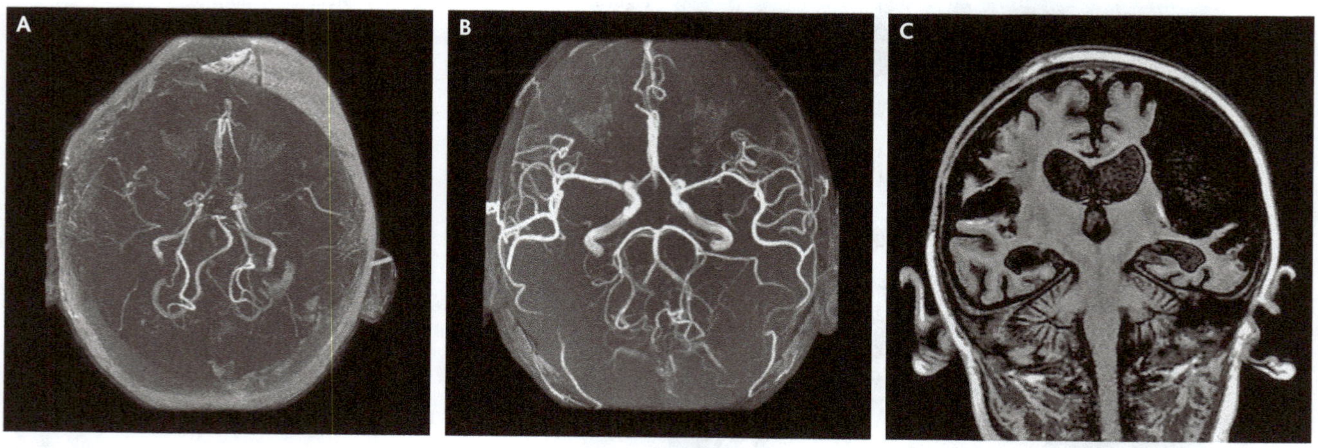

Figure 5-52 **A:** COW-TOF vasospasm affecting the bilateral middle cerebral arteries. **B:** COW-TOF normal showing patent bilateral middle cerebral arteries. **C:** Loss of tissue due to vasospasm within the bilateral middle cerebral artery distributions.

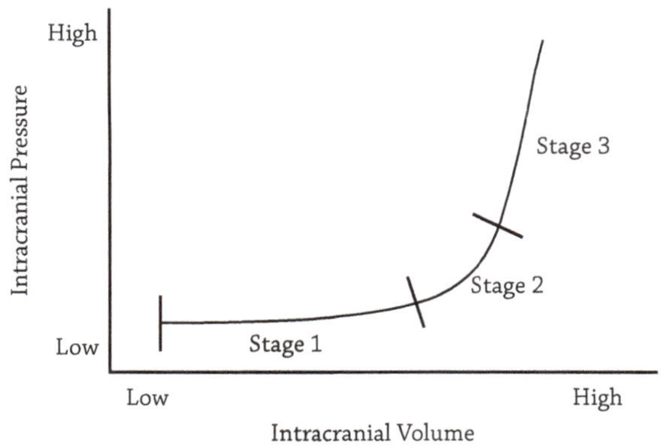

Figure 5-53 Intracranial compliance curve.

restricted to compression of the ventricles or cisterns, reduced blood volume, or even herniation of the brain outside the skull following decompressive craniectomy. Once these mechanisms are exhausted, there is often a rapid increase in intracranial pressure for each small increase in volume. Eventually, the soft brain parenchyma will become extruded through openings in the skull such as the foramen magnum, a life-threatening condition.

A simple way to conceptualize the change in pressure per unit increase in intracranial volume is to think of inflating a tractor inner tube inside the tractor tire. Until the inner tube fills the space inside the tire, it is easy to inflate. This corresponds to stage 1 of the compliance curve. However, once the inner tube fills the space within the tire and begins to push against the hard rubber, each additional, small increase in tube volume will result in a large increase in pressure within the tube. This corresponds to stage 2 of the compliance curve. Any further inflation of the tube will result in ever-increasing pressure per unit of volume, or an exponential increase in pressure per volume. This corresponds to stage 3 of the compliance curve.

On CT, diffuse swelling is easily appreciated by assessing for midline shift or compression of the ventricles or cisterns. Note the open appearance of the perimesencephalic or quadrigeminal cistern on Figures 5-54A–C, compared to the compressed cistern on Figures 5-54D–F. In addition, increased fluid within brain tissue will result in tissue appearing more hypodense or darker than nonedematous tissues. In addition, the increased fluid content in the brain parenchyma will result in attenuation of the gray–white

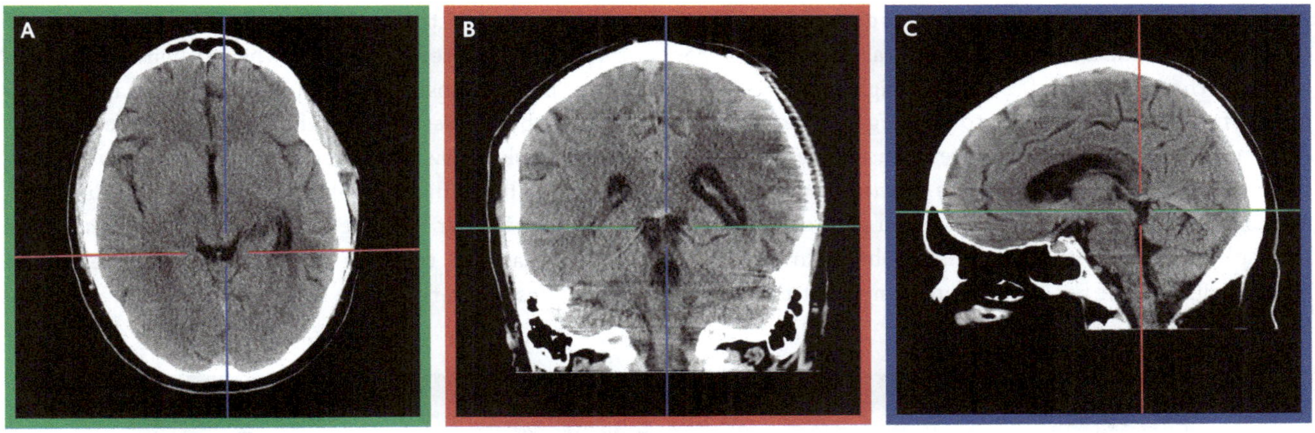

Figures 5-54A–C Open ventricles and cisterns. Note open perimesencephalic or quadrigeminal cistern identified by crosshairs.

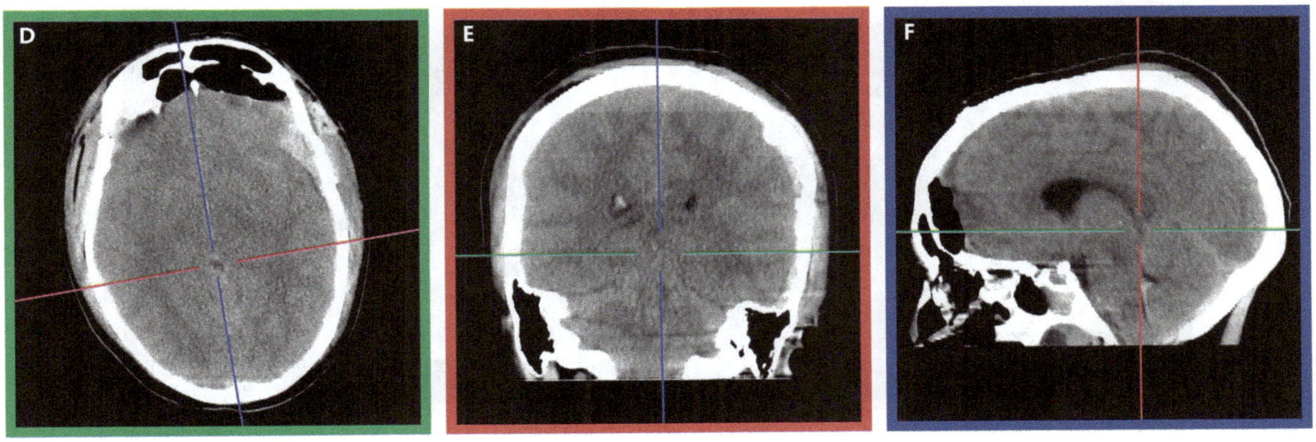

Figures 5-54D–F Compressed ventricles and cisterns. Note compressed perimesencephalic or quadrigeminal cistern identified by crosshairs.

density difference along the cortical and subcortical borders. Reduced size of the ventricles and cisterns, effacement of the sulci–gyri cortical pattern, and loss of gray–white cortical differentiation are all signs of increased pressure within the brain due to edema. Imminent herniation of the brain stem structures should be considered once the perimesencephalic cistern becomes so compressed that it is no longer visible on imaging.

Midline Shift and Asymmetrical Compression of the Ventricles

Prior to decompressive craniotomy, evidence of midline shift and asymmetrical compression of the ventricles provides clues about the primary area of pathology, and the degree to which each hemisphere is affected by edema. It is important to assess the brain parenchyma for evidence of focal or diffuse swelling, even if it does not appear to be the primary pathology for the patient. For example, a large extra-axial hemorrhage may be interpreted as a cause of midline shift, but the edema under the bleed may be responsible for much of the shift in midline structures. An assessment of the relative contribution of the bleed versus edema will provide a more accurate measure of injury. For example, the midline shift shown in Figures 5-55A and B may at first appear to be due to the large left hemisphere extra-axial hemorrhages. However, the degree of midline shift is greater than the thickness of the bleed; the thickness of the parenchymal tissue is much greater in the left hemisphere than in the right hemisphere. In this case, the contribution of the blood to midline shift is minimal compared to the contribution of the edematous brain parenchyma.

PEARL When assessing for post-traumatic edema, consider the thickness of brain tissue independent of any extra-axial hematoma (epidural or subdural). Bleeds are often so salient on brain scans that they become a distraction to the viewer. After assessing the effects of a bleed, spend some time considering other causes of a specific pathological presentation. As a rule, with any large epidural hematoma, there is a high probability of parenchymal swelling below the hemorrhage.

PERIL Large bleeds may lead the viewer to believe that any displacement of tissue is solely caused by the hematoma. This may result in the clinician failing to consider other causes of displacement, such as swelling of one hemisphere more than of the other.

Loss of Gray–White Differentiation

With increased fluid content in the soft tissues of the brain, the difference in density between gray matter and white matter becomes attenuated. Figure 5-56 shows a CT image of a patient with severe edema of the left hemisphere. This patient is status post-craniotomy, performed to allow swelling of the brain tissue outside the cranium in order to minimize the risk of downward herniation through the foramen magnum. The craniotomy also reduced the mid-line shift, although it is clear that the left hemisphere remains more swollen than the right on assessment of the respective thicknesses of the tissue.

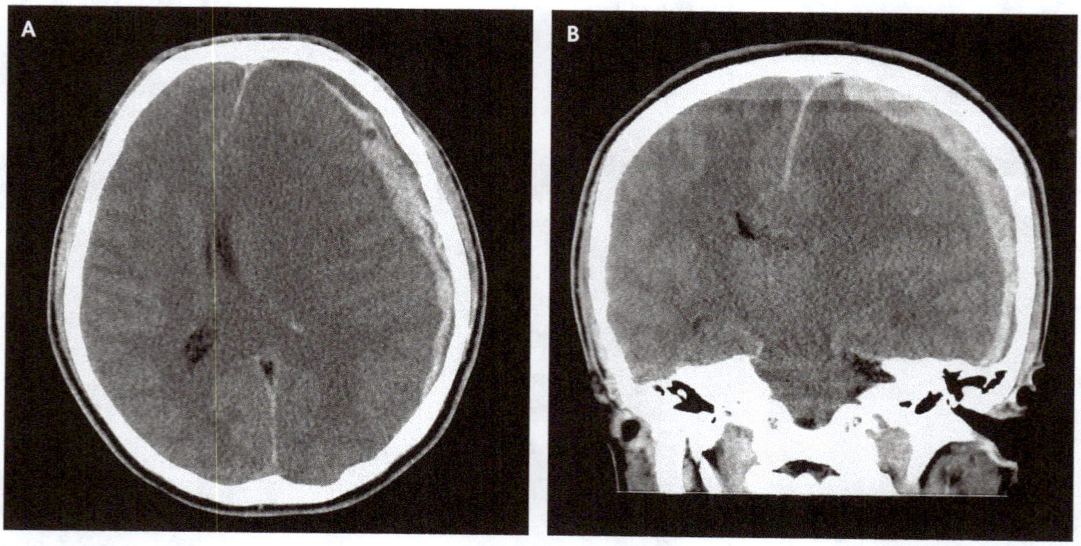

Figures 5-55A and B Midline shift. Note distance between midline of the ventricles and edge of the cortical mantle for the left and right hemispheres, respectively. This provides a measurement of brain swelling independent of the extra-axial hemorrhages.

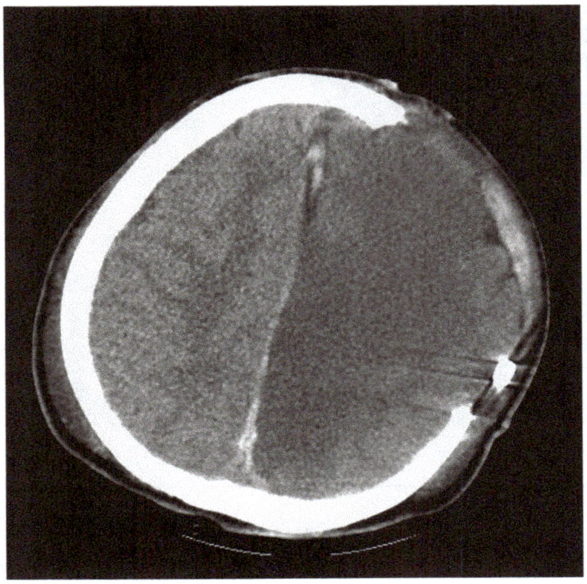

Figure 5-56 CT image of severe edema of the left hemisphere with herniation and loss of gray-white differentiation.

BLAST INJURIES

Blast injuries are unique in that they involve a pressure wave that travels through the soft tissue of the brain. Depending on the energy of the pressure wave, brain tissue may be severely damaged or even liquefied through cell-wall breakdown. One of the primary concerns in the treatment of blast injuries is that the often rapid, diffuse swelling of the brain can lead to herniation and loss of critical life-sustaining functions. The increased swelling can last for many weeks and require ongoing medical intervention to prevent secondary damage. With less severe blast injuries, a patient may go through stages of medical compromise due to extensive swelling, only to rapidly regain functioning following resolution of the edema. Long-term cognitive compromise is the norm for severe blast injuries, but for milder injuries with well-controlled edema and prevention of excessive intracranial pressure, a good recovery is possible.

CLINICAL EXAMPLE
Isaac: Blast Injury

Isaac was injured when a gas line exploded and he was thrown approximately 20 feet from the blast pressure wave. He experienced rapid onset of severe brain swelling necessitating medication and neurosurgical management, and his condition was critical for many weeks. Initial use of medications failed to reduce brain swelling. A large bilateral craniotomy was performed to allow his brain to swell outside of the bounds of his cranium (Figure 5-57A–C). Following resolution of edema, the bone flaps were replaced and Isaac demonstrated an excellent recovery (Figure 5-57D–F).

Isaac was fortunate that the rapid treatment for increased intracranial pressure prevented secondary injury to his brain. After the swelling had subsided, he was left with a relatively minor right parietal contusion where his head hit the ground after being thrown from the blast. A few months after his injury and after replacement of his bone flaps, Isaac was back at work functioning at premorbid levels.

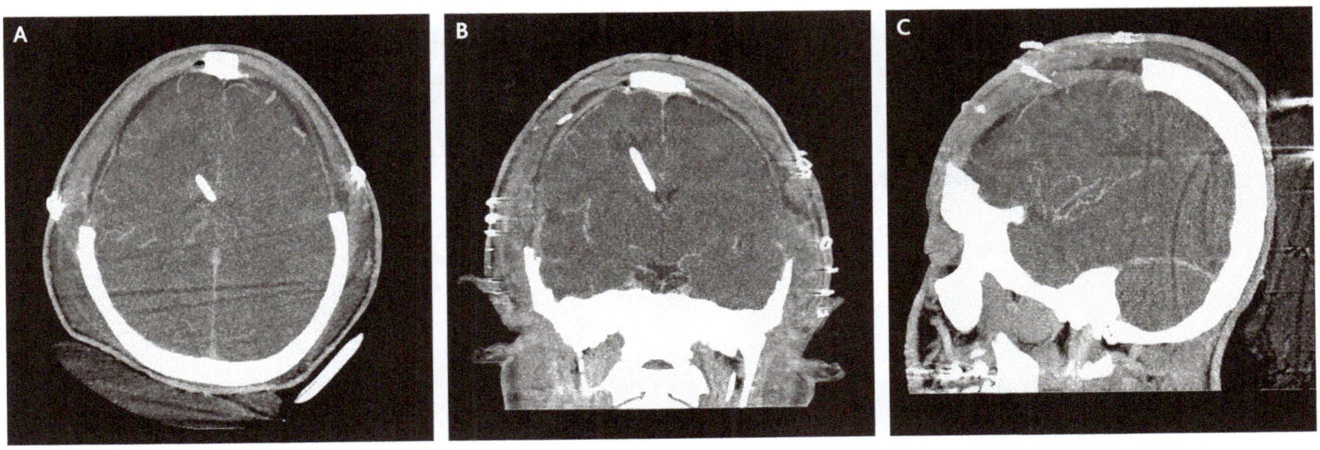

Figures 5-57A–C Clinical Example Isaac: Standard 2D CT showing bifrontal craniotomy.

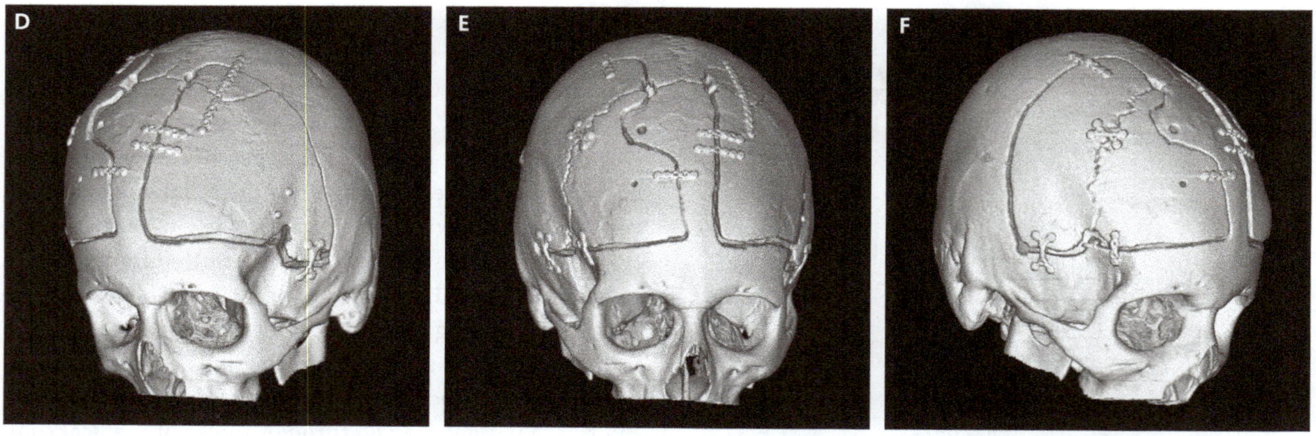

Figures 5-57D–F Clinical Example Isaac: 3D CT volume rendering acquired after replacement of bone flaps via cranioplasty.

Severe blast injuries from explosives can result in profound injury to the brain, with protracted periods of recovery and often devastating losses in functional abilities. Blast injuries from military explosions are often much more severe than those seen in the civilian arena.

IMAGING CHANGES OVER TIME AFTER SEVERE TRAUMATIC BRAIN INJURY

The appearance of post-traumatic pathology on brain imaging can change over time. Accordingly, it is critical to take into account the age of the injury when viewing brain scans. Many images acquired within a few hours of an injury may appear relatively normal, even when there is severe damage to the brain. For the first few hours following an injury, bleeds may appear isodense on CT and isointense on MRI, making them difficult to appreciate on imaging studies. Edema may not be evident, as it takes time to build, and microscopic damage to cells will not be visible because of the poor contrast and spatial resolution of current imaging techniques. Over the first few days, changes in brain pathophysiology and image appearance can be quite marked and, with time, provide a better indication of the severity and extent of injury.

Prior to formulating an opinion regarding the severity and extent of an injury, it is best to compare imaging studies over several days to weeks after an injury. In addition, the imaging findings should be correlated over time with changes in the patient's clinical presentation. Imaging that suggests relatively little cortical or subcortical damage at the time of injury but then suggests swelling for a few weeks, followed by resolution may explain changes in a patient's condition. Such a pattern may explain why the patient transitioned from a lucid period after impact to a state of low arousal for a few weeks and then returned to mostly normal levels of arousal as the edema subsided. Correlation of the changes in functioning with changes on brain imaging can assist in determining appropriate expectations, prognosis, and treatment plan.

It is not uncommon for early CT scans to appear relatively benign, except for a small area of contusion. However, serial assessment of the same patient can give critical information about the extent and severity of the injury. Information provided on follow-up imaging is often more informative than that from early scans, as most of the pathology may not be evident on scans acquired shortly after an injury.

Julia: Traumatic Brain Injury with Imaging Changes over Time

Julia was injured in a motor vehicle accident. Her initial CT suggested a relatively small area of contusion within the right orbital frontal region (Figure 5-58, arrows). The contusion was identified by the lighter area of blood close to the frontal bone. There was evidence of slight edema, with narrowing of the perimesencephalic or quadrigeminal cistern and ventricles.

If prognosis were based on the scan shown in Figure 5-58, the clinician might be inclined to report that a positive outcome was likely, with only minor disruption of functioning and possibly no significant long-term deficits. Julia was not so fortunate, however, and remained functionally compromised and dependent on others for adaptive and self-help skills for many years. If the initial CT sequences were the only ones available, it would be difficult to explain Julia's poor outcome and limited recovery. However, review of serial CT scans performed over several weeks indicates that her brain injury was more severe and extensive than suggested by the CT imaging conducted acutely.

By day 2 after her injury, Julia's CT scans began to suggest intraparenchymal hemorrhages within her right frontal and left temporal lobes (Figure 5-59). In addition, there was emerging evidence of injury to the right temporal pole close to the bony structure of the sphenoid wing and to the left frontal lobe, as indicated by the darker appearance of tissue in that area.

Axial T2 FLAIR sequences acquired 2 weeks after Julia's injury showed progression of tissue breakdown within the bilateral orbital and medial frontal lobes and temporal poles (Figure 5-60). Injury was so severe that lacuna infarcts were forming (arrows) as the tissue progressed through stages of encephalomalacia, or "softening of the brain," to atrophy.

Axial T2 FLAIR sequences acquired 7 weeks after Julia's injury revealed lacuna infarcts within both frontal lobes and temporal poles, with the greatest injury being to the right frontal and left temporal regions (Figure 5-61). Ongoing inflammation, encephalomalacia, and atrophy were evident, with areas or hyperintensity surrounding darker regions of lacuna infarction and atrophy, or holes, in the tissue (arrows). The comparison between Julia's initial CT (Figure 5-58) and her MRI seven weeks later (Figure 5-61) illustrates just how limited acute scans can be in assessing the extent and severity of an injury, and in predicting expected functional outcomes for the patient.

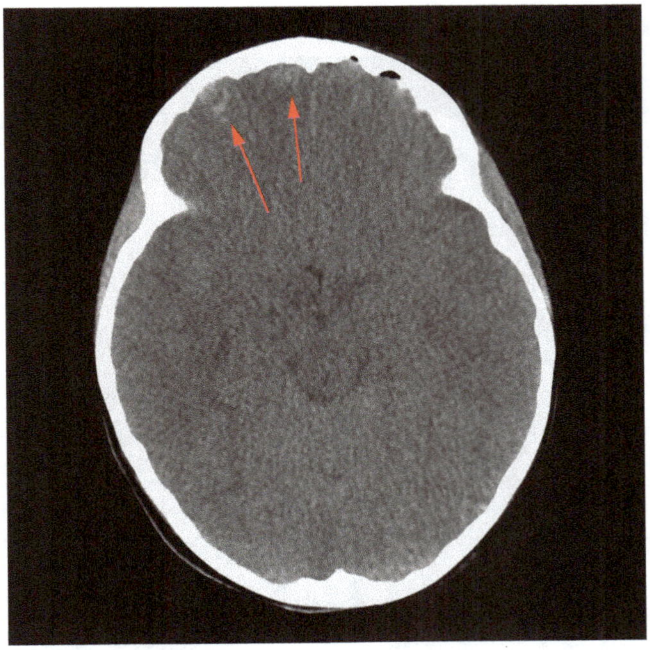

Figure 5-58 Clinical example Julia: initial CT scan of traumatic brain injury.

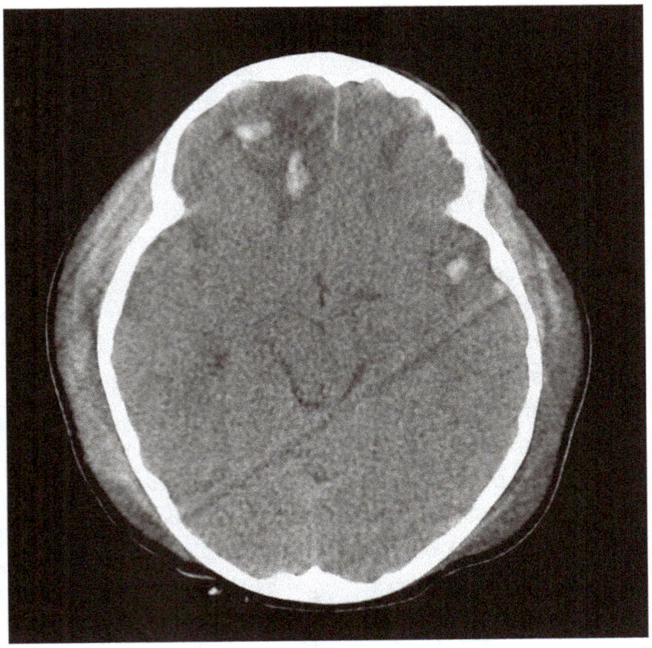

Figure 5-59 Clinical example Julia: CT scan of traumatic brain injury taken 2 days post-injury.

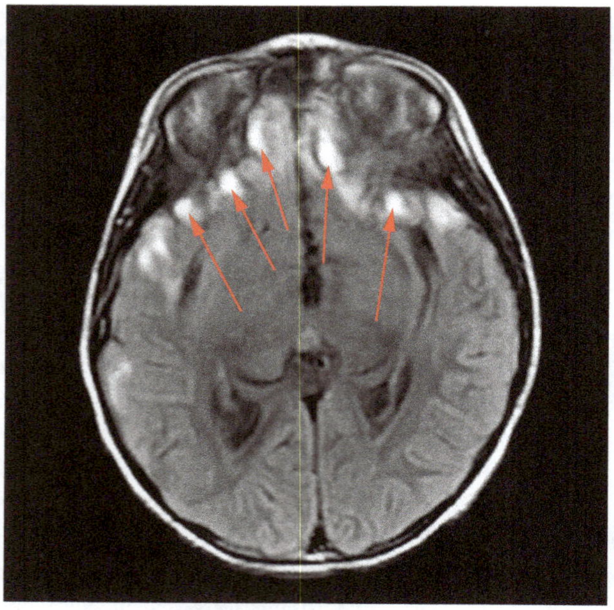

Figure 5-60 Clinical example Julia: axial T2 FLAIR sequence taken 2 weeks post-injury.

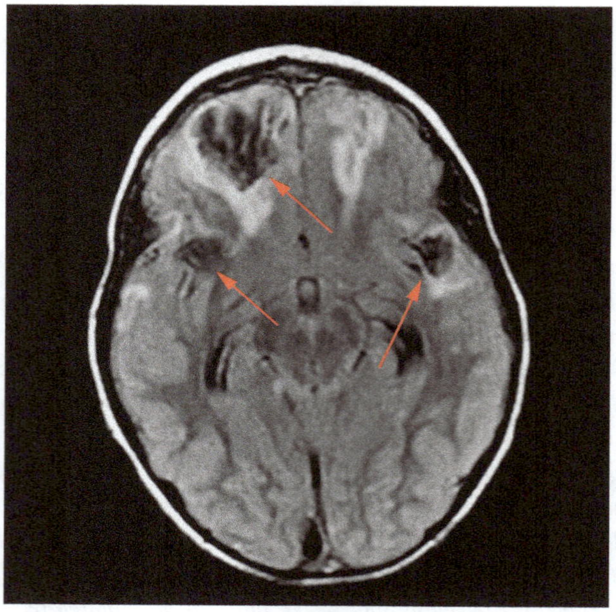

Figure 5-61 Clinical example Julia: axial T2 FLAIR sequence taken 7 weeks post-injury.

CLINICAL EXAMPLE
Hiroshi: Suspected Non-accidental Trauma with Imaging Changes over Time

Hiroshi, a delightful 4-year-old boy, was injured under suspicious circumstances believed to be nonaccidental abuse by a non-family member. As seen in Julia, Hiroshi's acute CT images taken the day of the trauma did not indicate the full extent of his injury. Most notable on the CT was a large subdural hemorrhage over the right frontal and temporal lobes, with some underlying edema of the right hemisphere (Figure 5-62). The midline shift was suggested by the bowing of the falx cerebri and asymmetrical compression of the ventricles. Extensive edema was not suggested as there was still clear gray–white differentiation in the right hemisphere.

By the second day after the injury, some of the midline shift had resolved through evacuation of the hematoma, although the right hemisphere continued to appear edematous compared to the left (Figure 5-63). Air (pneumocephalus) was evident in the right frontal extra-axial region as the black area between the skull and dural layer. The perimesencephalic or quadrigeminal cistern remained open, which suggested that there was no excessive-pressure effect caused by brain swelling. Put another way, there was still some CSF space within the brain to compensate for the mass effect of swelling, thus preventing catastrophic increases in intracranial pressure.

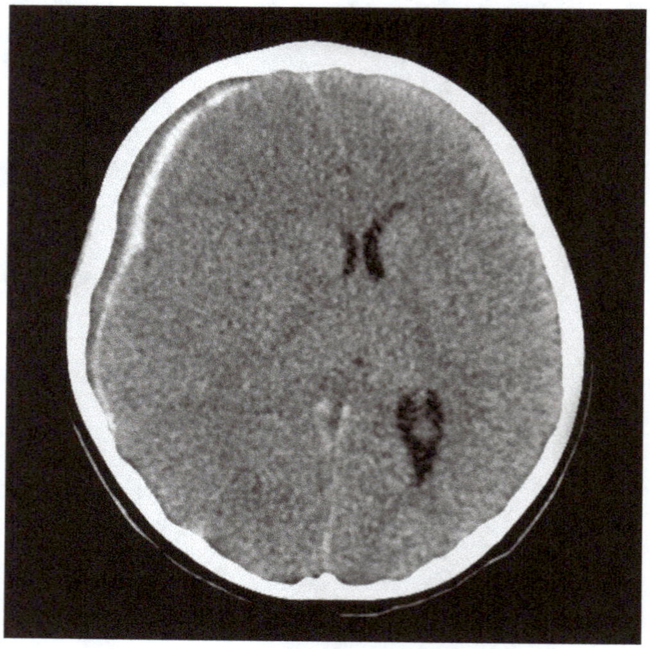

Figure 5-62 Clinical example Hiroshi: initial CT of suspected nonaccidental trauma.

By 4 days post-injury, Hiroshi's CT imaging (Figure 5-64) was beginning to suggest greater injury to the right hemisphere than that suggested by earlier scans. The loss of the gray–white differentiation and the diffuse hypodense appearance of the right hemisphere suggested that the tissue was edematous and possibly progressing to encephalomalacia and deterioration

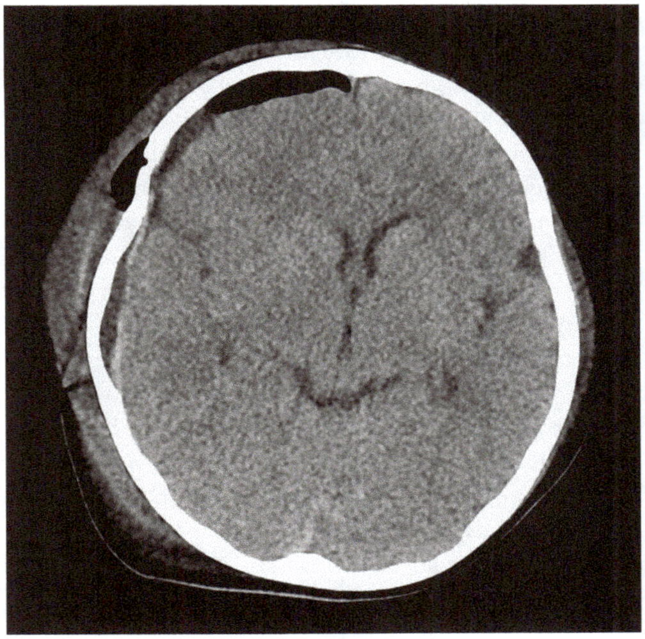

Figure 5-63 Clinical example Hiroshi: 2 days post-injury.

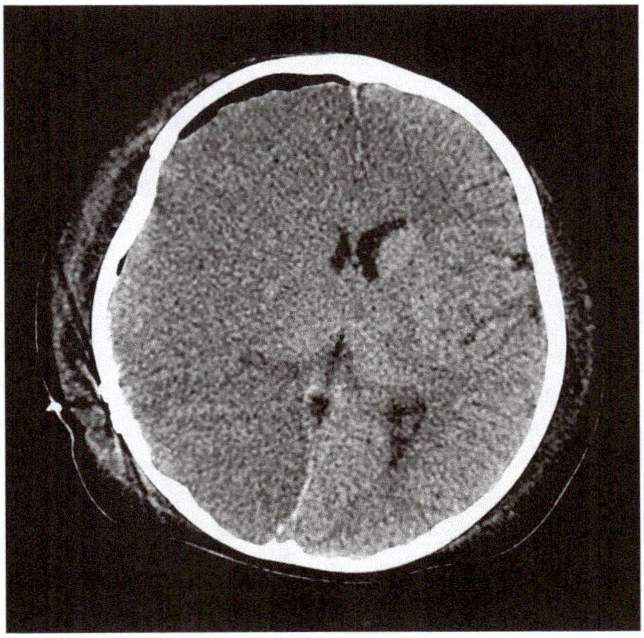

Figure 5-64 Clinical example Hiroshi: CT imaging 4 days post-injury.

of cellular structure. Compared with the left hemisphere, the right hemisphere showed effacement of the sulci–gyri pattern, which is consistent with significant pressure effect. In the left hemisphere, the difference between the gray matter density and white matter density was still evident, which suggested that the left hemisphere was less damaged than the right. In addition, there was emerging evidence of damage to the left medial frontal region, with the darker or hypodense appearance of this area matching that of the damaged right hemisphere.

At 8 days post-injury, CT scans became highly suggestive of the progression from edema to encephalomalacia within the right hemisphere. This was evident on CT as a darker appearance to the tissue through the loss of structural integrity and density (Figure 5-65), with the tissue becoming "softer." The left hemisphere remained relatively normal with the exception of the medial frontal region. The right hemisphere remained mildly edematous, as evidenced by the continuing midline shift, although it appeared that the edema was resolving to a mild degree.

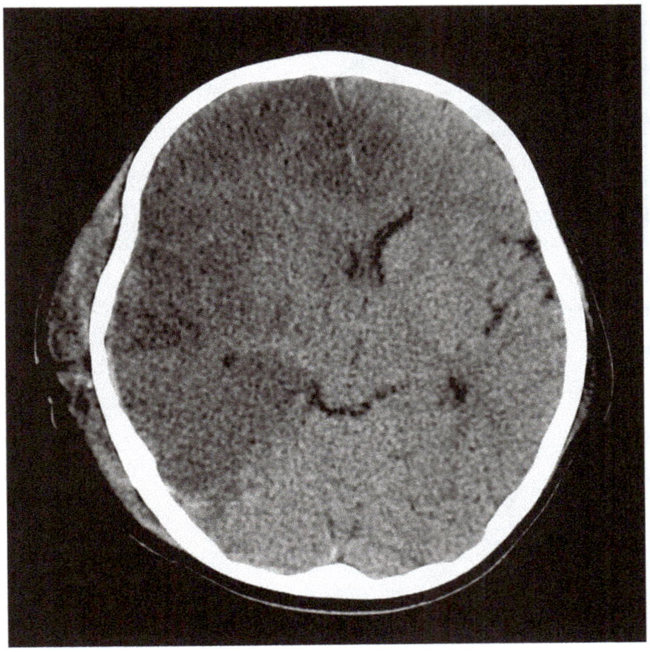

Figure 5-65 Clinical example Hiroshi: CT imaging 8 days post-injury.

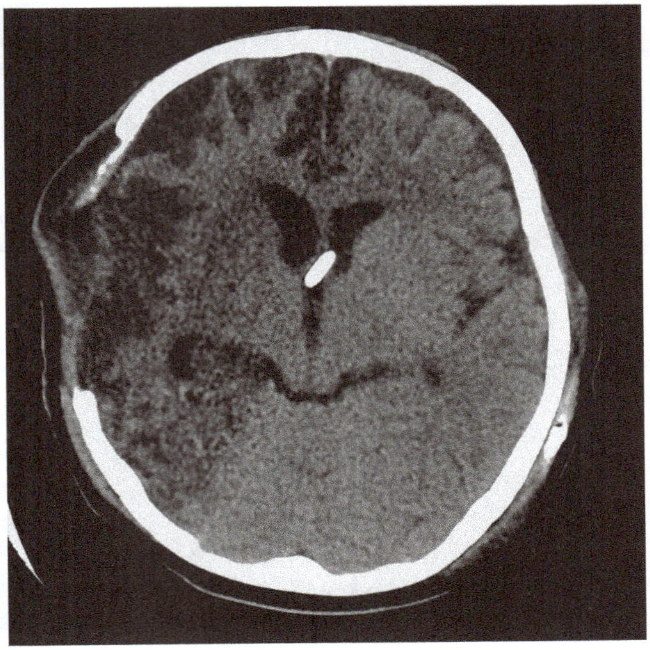

Figure 5-66 Clinical example Hiroshi: CT imaging 3 weeks post-injury.

Because of persistently increased intracranial pressure secondary to swelling of the right hemisphere, Hiroshi underwent craniotomy so that the risk of downward herniation of the brainstem woud be reduced. In Figure 5-66, the craniotomy is evident as the gap in the skull on left side of the image. The CT at 3 weeks (Figure 5-66) suggests resolution of midline shift, likely due to to the craniotomy and also to resolution of the right-hemisphere edema. Reduced edema is indicated by the prominence of the sulci and gyri in the right hemisphere without effacement, in addition to the patent appearance of the ventricles and cisterns (no compression). The edematous appearance of the right hemisphere had transitioned to one of encephalomalacia and atrophy. The tissue remained hypodense with significant atrophy of the cortical surface and even of some subcortical white matter, as suggested by the slight prominence of the right lateral ventricle and inferior horn compared to the left.

By 6 weeks after Hiroshi's injury, CT imaging (Figure 5-67A) suggested ongoing atrophy, with additional loss of tissue from both hemispheres, especially from the right side of the brain. Loss of tissue from the left frontal region was clearly evident and was expected, given the low-density appearance 3 weeks after his injury. Damage to the right occipital lobe appeared on this scan, but not on earlier images, because a different slice-acquisition angle was used. An area of low density became evident in the deep left temporal region just posterior to the insular cortex, suggesting damage to this region in addition to the more obvious damage to other brain tissues. Upon review of the image, there also appeared to be a subtle midline shift and effacement of the lateral convexity of the left hemisphere, conditions that are unexpected given the degree of atrophy. However, further review of the image confirms that the right hemisphere craniotomy hole has been replaced with the bone flap. The subtle right hemisphere pressure effect was likely the result of the cranioplasty 1 day before image acquisition for Figure 5-67A, and is not of significant clinical concern. Figure 5-67B provides a clear picture of the cranioplasty and bone-flap replacement on 3D volume rendered CT.

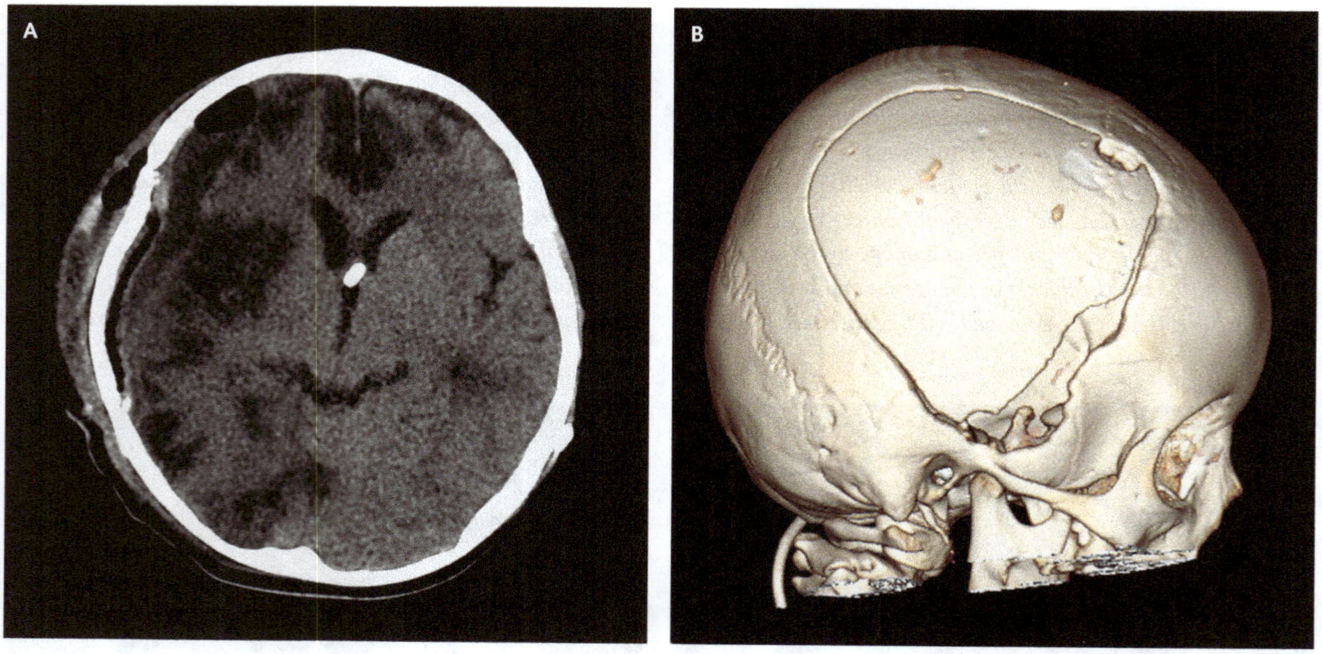

Figures 5-67A and B Clinical example Hiroshi: standard 2D CT and 3D CT volume rendering 6 weeks post-injury.

Edema, Encephalomalacia, and Atrophy

Following severe traumatic injury to the brain, damaged tissue will appear different on brain imaging, depending on the stage of tissue breakdown.

Edema

When edematous, brain parenchyma appears darker on CT and T1 images and brighter on T2 sequences than normal tissue. In addition, because of the increased parenchymal volume resulting from the higher water content, tissue can appear swollen and compressed. Edema will produce a mass effect on the brain, resulting in markers such as midline shift, compression of ventricles or cisterns, effacement of the sulci–gyri patterning, or even herniation.

Encephalomalacia

During the early stages of breakdown and decomposition, also known as *encephalomalacia*, the parenchyma may appear darker on CT and T1 images and brighter on T2 sequences than normal tissue. In addition, because encephalomalacia involves the breakdown of tissue, or "softening of the brain," often there is resolution of the mass effect seen with edema.

Atrophy

Following encephalomalacia there is often a thinning of the parenchyma, as the affected region can atrophy over several weeks to months. The total mass of tissue will decrease as cells are absorbed by the body. The outside of the brain becomes shriveled and the ventricles enlarge as CSF fills in space once occupied by brain tissue. With ongoing atrophy, the mass of tissue declines with compensatory expansion of the ventricles and cisterns (ventriculomegaly or cisternomegaly ex vacuo). Assess for excessive intraventricular pressure or high-pressure hydrocephalus, which can account for ventriculomegaly, before concluding that it is caused by atrophy. Cortically, the gyri become thinner and the sulci expand, giving a more wrinkled appearance to the cortex.

PEARL The extent and severity of a traumatic brain injury can become evident on brain imaging over a long period of time. The initial scans may be misleading and may suggest less injury than was actually sustained by the patient. Follow-up imaging several weeks after an injury may be more representative of the true extent and severity of damage.

PERIL Be cautious about making predictions about recovery based on neuroimaging obtained in the emergency room or within a few hours following an injury. A review of scans over a longer period of time is often necessary to fully appreciate the extent and severity of a traumatic brain injury.

PENETRATING INJURIES

Penetrating injuries are caused by an object passing through the cranium and into the soft brain tissue. The extent and severity of injury to brain parenchyma are primarily dependent on the size and velocity of the penetrating object. Sometimes bone fragments or debris such as glass will penetrate the brain after physical trauma to the head. Other times the projectile is a metal rod, knife, or bullet. Most projectile injuries involve BBs, pellets, bullets, or shrapnel from explosives, with varying diameters (calibers) and penetration speeds.

Penetration by Bone or Debris

CT imaging is the technique of choice for most penetrating injuries. CT provides high contrast and spatial resolution for bone and dense objects. In addition, CT does not carry the same risks as MRI of dislodging ferromagnetic objects and causing further injury to the brain.

CLINICAL EXAMPLE

Frank: Penetration by Bone

Frank was injured when he walked into a busy road while texting someone on his phone. He sustained a frontal skull fracture with a piece of bone becoming displaced into the orbital-medial area of his frontal lobe (Figures 5-68A–C, arrows). Frank required cranioplasty to repair his skull and inpatient rehabilitation to facilitate recovery. Shortly after this injury, neuropsychological assessment revealed grossly intact basic intellect and reasoning skills but with notable deficits involving executive functioning, affect regulation, and behavioral control. Several years after the injury, Frank continued to be impulsive, became easily angered, and was described as having a low frustration tolerance. He was also noted to express inappropriate comments in public and have difficulty adapting his behavior to the social context and environment.

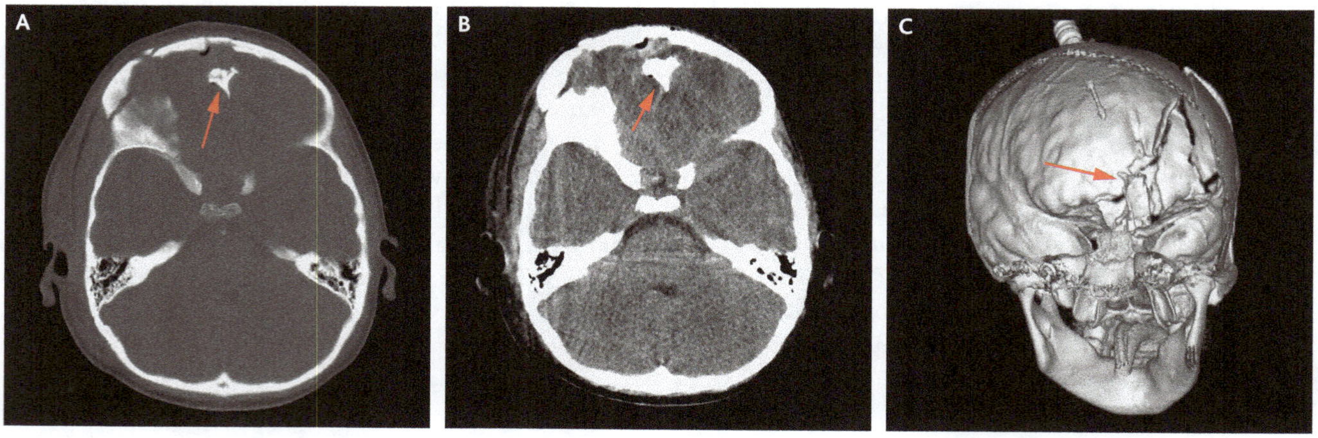

Figure 5-68A–C Clinical example Frank: penetration by bone. **A:** CT bone window. **B:** CT. **C:** 3D CT volume rendering.

CLINICAL EXAMPLE

Fred: Penetration by Bone due to Orbital–Facial Fractures

Given the high incidence of frontal-impact injuries caused by unrestrained motor vehicle accidents, it is not uncommon to have cases of bone penetration around the frontal and temporal lobes. Fred sustained a depressed fracture to his left frontal bone, including the supraorbital structures, with penetration of brain parenchyma (Figures 5-69A–C). Neurosurgical intervention was required to debride the wound and to repair the skull fracture.

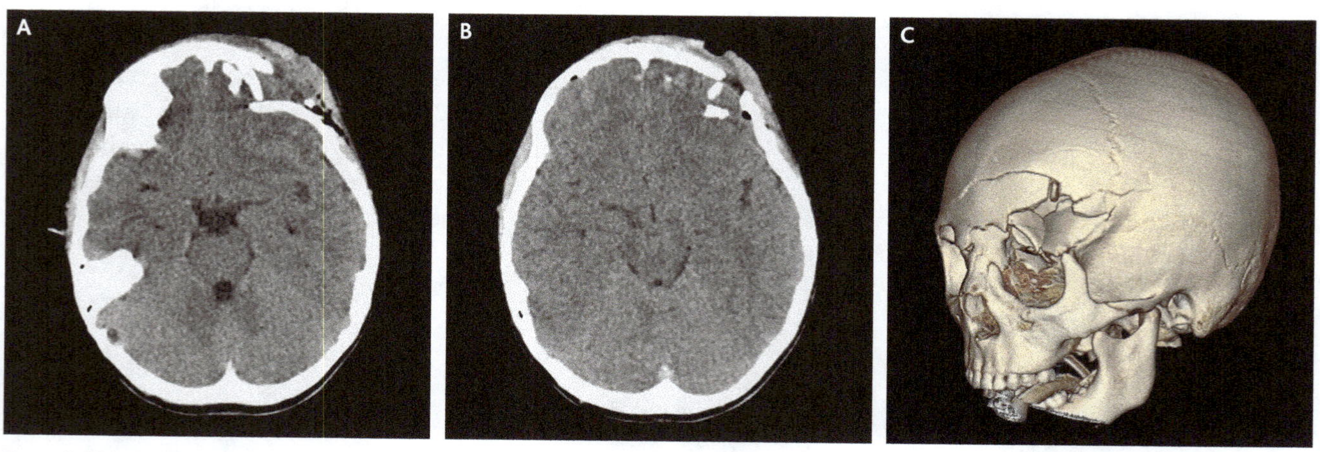

Figure 5-69A–C Clinical example Fred: penetration by bone due to orbital—facial fractures on standard 2D CT imaging (A and B) and 3D CT volume rendering.

Susan was injured in an automobile accident, as described earlier in the section on facial injuries. In addition to the facial trauma, she sustained injury to her face and brain by penetration of glass. Most of the glass remained outside of the brain, although a few pieces penetrated the skull and caused injury to the brain. One piece in particular came to rest just above the pituitary, at the location of the infundibulum or pituitary stalk. It was not possible to determine whether the piece of glass damaged the pituitary or the stalk, although this is suspected, given the disruption to her endocrine functioning after the injury. On 3D CT volume rendering of her cranium (Figure 5-70), several pieces of glass are visible (arrows), with one close to the center of the image in the vicinity of the pituitary. The piece of glass close to the pituitary and infundibulum is identified in bone windowed and standard CT images (Figures 5-71A–D).

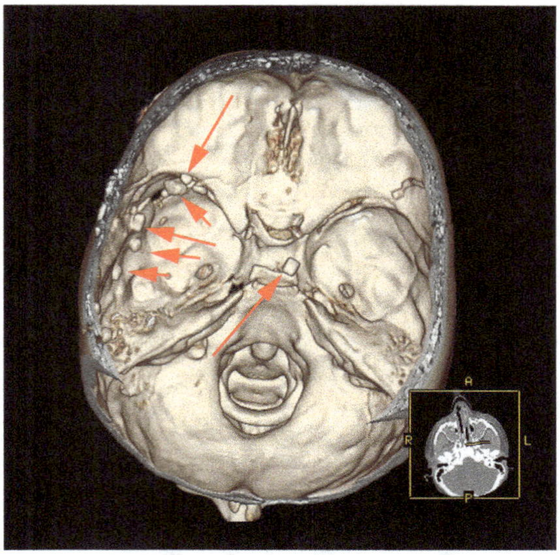

Figure 5-70 Clinical example Susan: penetration by glass. The glass within her cranium is shown on 3D volume rendering by the arrows.

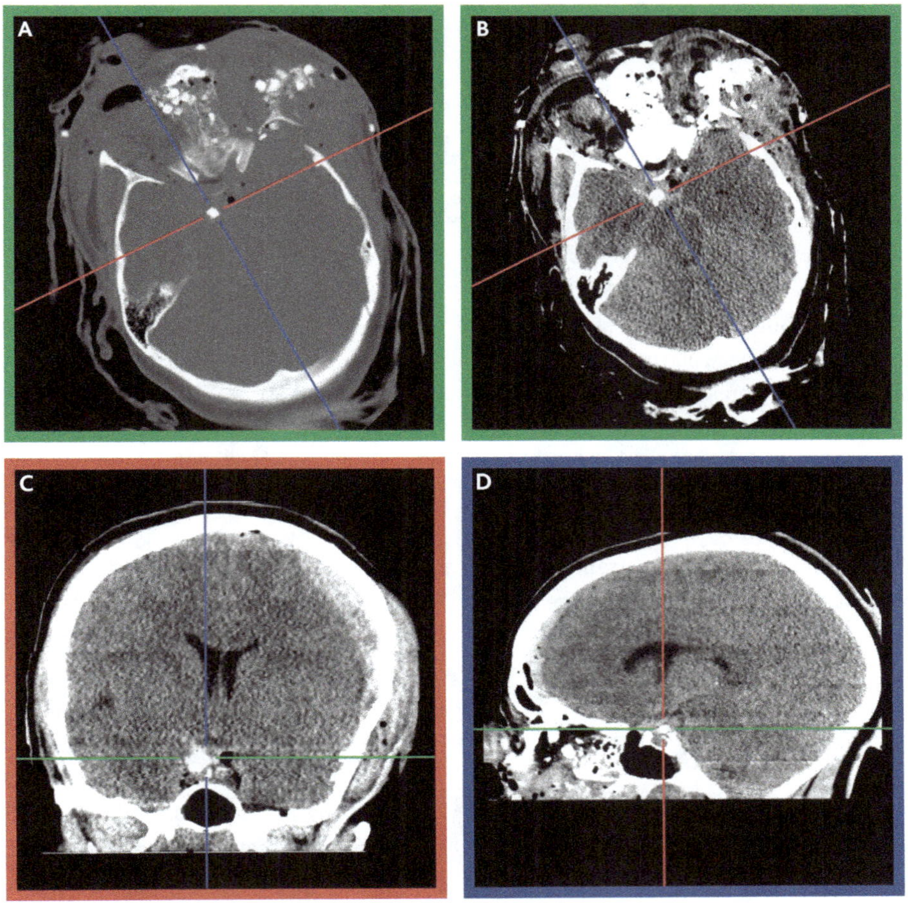

Figures 5-71A–D Clinical example Susan: CT bone window (A) and standard imaging (B–D) identifying piece of glass close to the pituitary and infundibulum (pituitary stalk).

Gunshot Wounds

Given the metallic nature of gunshot projectiles, it is not surprising that CT is the scanning method of choice for such injuries. Although MRI offers more choices of available sequences and may provide higher resolution, the metallic nature of most projectiles precludes the use of MRI. Without information on the ferromagnetic nature of a projectile (BB, pellet, or bullet), the risk of dislodging or moving the object through the effects of the magnetic field outweigh any gains in image quality. CT imaging provides clinically useful images of the skull, bone fragments within the brain, blood products, and soft-tissue damage. Skull fragments appear hyperdense, with a brightness level equivalent to that of the calvarium. Blood can have a different appearance depending on the age of the injury, although in most scans produced after a gunshot wound, blood appears hyperdense but not as bright as bone. Bone is often displayed with well-defined margins, while blood usually appears with less-defined margins or blotchy. Torn and edematous tissue surrounding the wound channel often appears darker than surrounding tissue but not as dark as CSF. Within the wound channel, the appearance can be similar to that of CSF.

Low-Velocity Penetrating Injuries

Small objects traveling at a low velocity may cause very little damage to the brain; the injury may be restricted to the path of the object as it tears nerve fibers, blood vessels, and other brain tissues. Larger objects tend to cause more extensive damage, although if they are slow moving, they can also produce focal injuries relating to the wound channel. As slow-moving objects push through brain tissue, additional injury may be caused by bone displaced into tissue a short distance from the channel. With low-velocity projectile injuries, the patient may not experience a loss of consciousness, but there is a high risk of hemorrhage, infection, or seizures. Clinical sequalae often relate to disrupted functioning of the tissue within or close to the wound channel.

Low-Velocity, Small-Caliber Gunshot Wounds

Low-velocity, small-caliber injuries are frequently the result of accidents involving BB or pellet guns and rifles. Although air pressure is used to propel the BB or pellet, velocities are high enough to produce penetration of the skull and soft tissue of the brain. Figure 5-72A provides a clear view of the projectile path from the right frontal lobe across the midline and the BB coming to rest within the left lobe of the cerebellum. CT imaging suggested focal damage along the path of the pellet but without obvious damage to other areas of the brain. Along the path of the BB, there is evidence of blood and bone that was pushed into the channel. The metallic nature of the BB results in a starburst artifact on CT, visible within the cerebellum. Following the pellet injury, the patient experienced minimal functional deficit. Cognitive abilities were retained, although a mild left-sided hemiparesis persisted after discharge from the hospital. Disruption of endocrine function was also evident and likely due to damage of the pituitary or infundibulum (pituitary stalk), given their location in the path of the projectile.

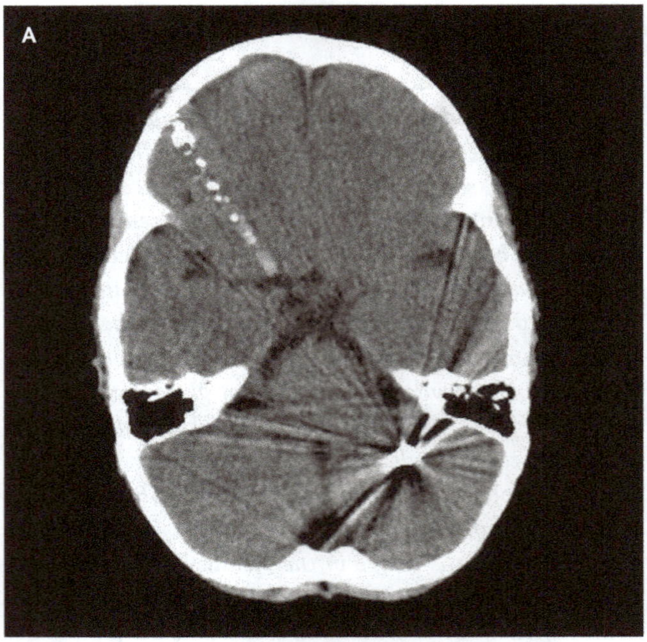

Figure 5-72A Projectile path of pellet in low-velocity, small-caliber BB injury.

If the pellet or BB transects a major blood vessel, the outcome may not be as good as it was for the patient described above. Figures 5-72B–D are from a patient who was also shot with a BB gun, although the BB transected his left middle cerebral artery. AP angiography of his vessels (Figure 5-72B) shows intact flow through the left anterior cerebral artery, but no flow through the transected left middle cerebral artery. Follow-up CT imaging 2 months after his injury indicated that the loss of blood flow through the transected left middle cerebral artery had resulted in severe damage to his left hemisphere, with almost complete atrophy of the tissue around the Sylvian fissure (Figures 5-72C and D).

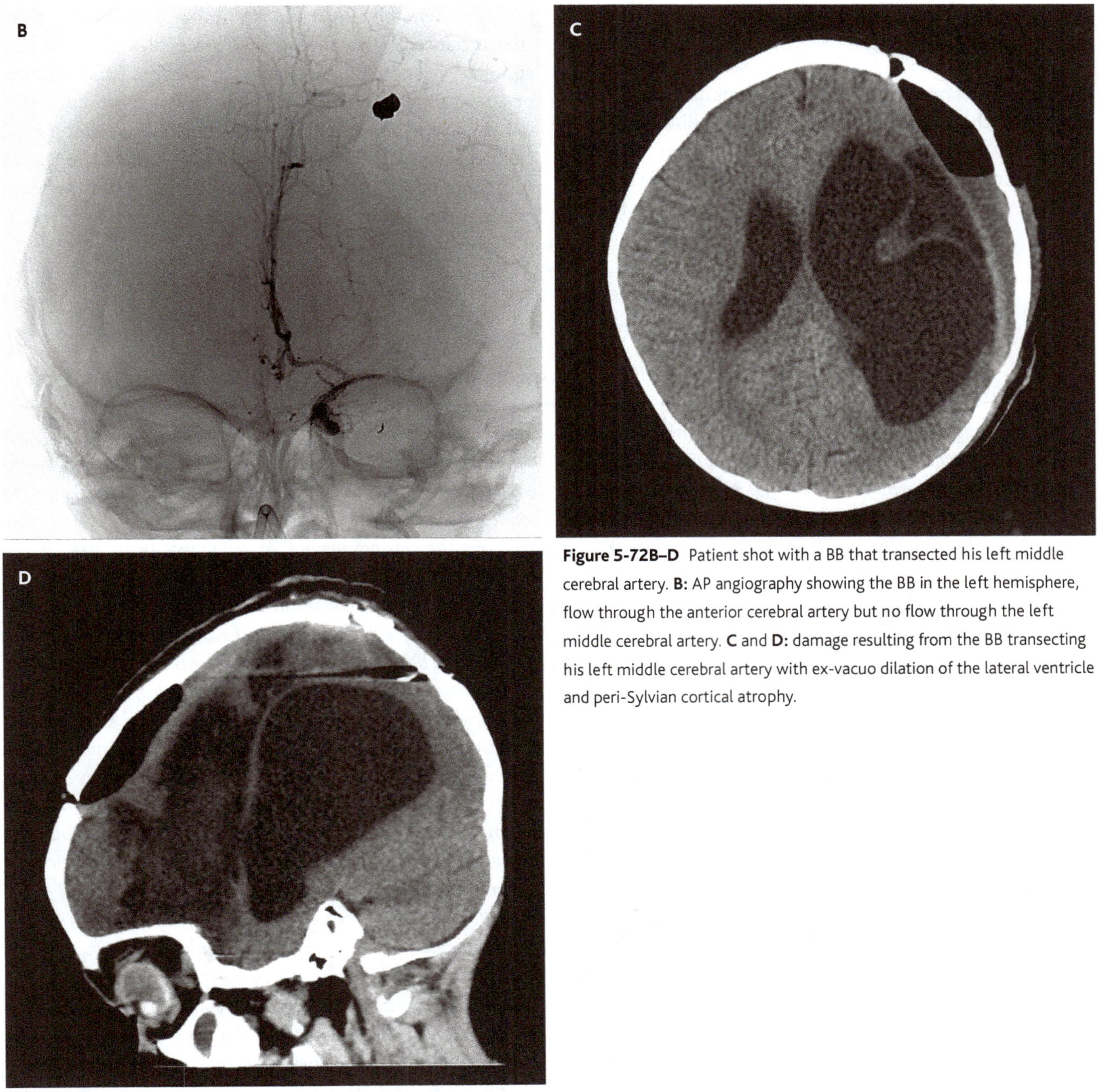

Figure 5-72B–D Patient shot with a BB that transected his left middle cerebral artery. **B:** AP angiography showing the BB in the left hemisphere, flow through the anterior cerebral artery but no flow through the left middle cerebral artery. **C** and **D:** damage resulting from the BB transecting his left middle cerebral artery with ex-vacuo dilation of the lateral ventricle and peri-Sylvian cortical atrophy.

Low-Velocity, Large-Caliber Gunshot Wounds

Low-velocity, large-caliber gunshot wounds tend to be similar to those of low-velocity, small-caliber projectile injuries. There is focal damage within the channel but little injury to other parts of the brain. As larger projectiles displace more tissue, they cause more extensive tearing of axon fibers, blood vessels, and other brain tissues than that produced by smaller-caliber projectiles. For this reason, low-velocity injuries caused by a 9-mm (0.308), 0.40, or 0.45 caliber projectile will cause a larger wound channel and more damage than a low-velocity BB, pellet, or .22 caliber bullet. Clinical symptoms are related to the loss of functioning for the structures within or close to the wound channel.

CLINICAL EXAMPLE

Angelino: Low-Velocity, Large-Caliber Gunshot Wound

Angelino, a delightful 17-year-old high school senior, and innocent bystander, was injured when a stray 9-mm bullet hit him in the head from a nearby gang shooting. By the time the bullet entered Angelino's brain, it had slowed significantly and thus did not produce a large shock wave (see High-Velocity Penetrating Projectiles, below). The damage to Angelino's brain was isolated to the wound channel and a small border of hemorrhagic and edematous brain tissue (Figure 5-73).

Follow-up CT imaging of Angelino's brain showed a well-circumscribed channel from his left frontal lobe to his right parietal-occipital region, with little damage to other brain structures (Figures 5-74A–I). Given the relatively narrow wound channel, with minimal damage to surrounding tissue, Angelino made a good recovery from his injury. Only a few weeks after receiving the gunshot wound, Angelino was transferred to the medical rehabilitation unit where he progressed in all areas of functioning. On the rehabilitation unit, his cognition returned to premorbid baseline levels, as did his affect and emotional disposition and behavior. Some minor motor limitations on the left side persisted, likely owing to partial shearing of the right internal capsule, but improvements were evident and Angelino was independent in his mobility and self-help and adaptive skills. Angelino, a happy young man who was fully cooperative, gave a good effort to all tasks asked of him and was pleased by his rapid progress. He was discharged home and he returned to full-time schooling without the need for special education services or accommodations.

Unfortunately, as noted above, penetrating injuries significantly increase one's risk of infection along the wound channel. Shortly after his acute recovery, Angelino began to exhibit flu-like symptoms suggesting an infection. He experienced a rapid decline in mental status and quickly became unresponsive. Follow-up imaging revealed extensive abscess and edema within his frontal lobes refractory to intensive critical-care management (Figures 5-75A–C). The abscess was located along the wound channel and spread from his left frontal lobe where the bullet entered his skull to the right parietal lobe where the bullet remained. Only a few days after hospitalization for the infection, Angelino's conditions deteriorated to the point of brain death and he was sadly removed from life support.

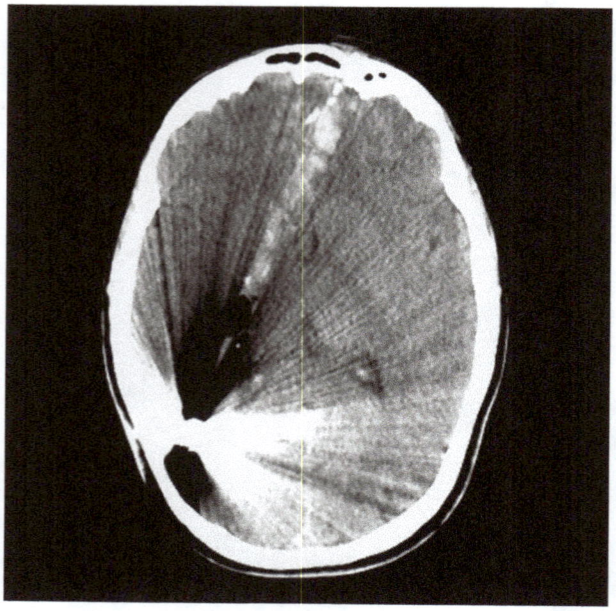

Figure 5-73 Clinical example Angelino: low-velocity, large-caliber gunshot wound. Acute CT showing blood along the bullet track and metallic artifact where the bullet came to rest in Angelino's right parietal-occipital region.

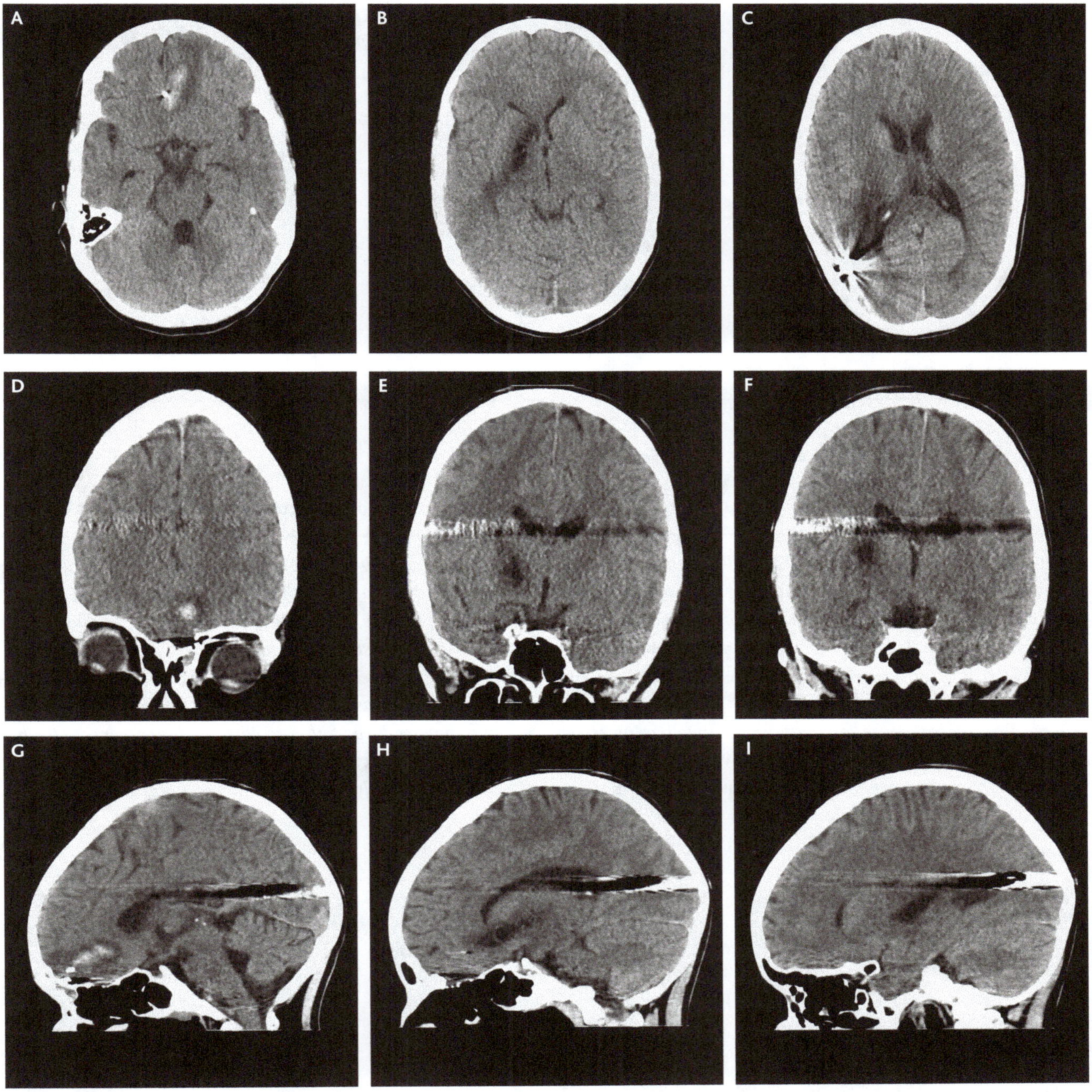

Figures 5-74A–F Clinical example Angelino: follow-up CT series showing the wound channel on axial, coronal, and sagittal sequences. Other than within and close to the wound channel, the brain appears mostly undamaged. Note metallic artifact radiating from the bullet, giving an appearance of more damage than in actuality.

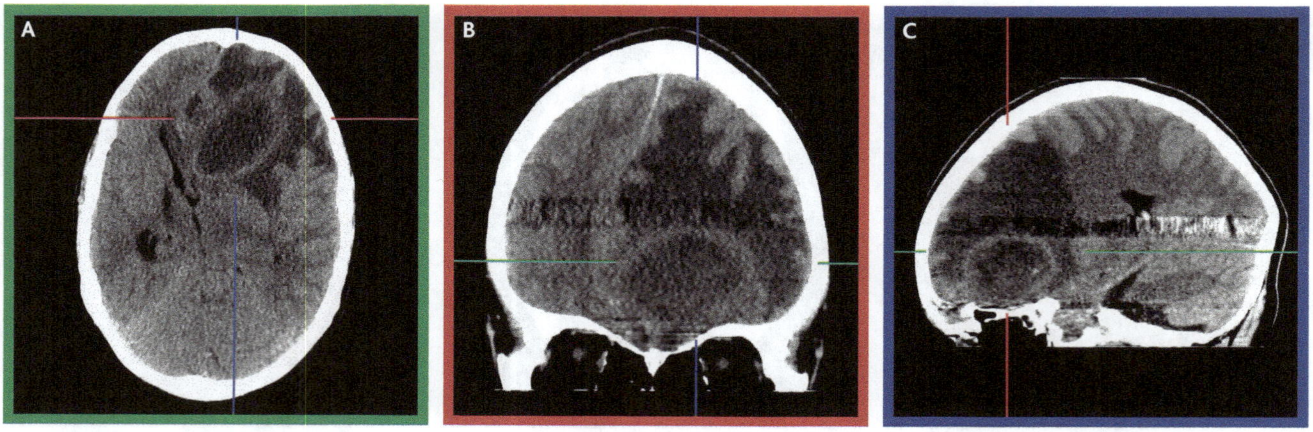

Figures 5-75A–C Clinical example Angelino: CT series showing Angelino's frontal abscess.

CLINICAL EXAMPLE

Barclay: Low-Velocity, Large-Caliber Gunshot Wound

Barclay suffered a low-velocity, large-caliber gunshot wound from a stray bullet shot into the air during New Year's Eve celebrations. Because of the slow speed of the bullet when it penetrated his skull, he sustained relatively minor damage to the superior left frontal lobe (Figures 5-76A–C). Like Angelino, Barclay recovered rapidly with only minor disruption to functioning. Barclay was more fortunate than Angelino, however, in that he did not develop any secondary medical complications such as infection, seizures, or excessive swelling. Barclay returned to his previous work as a professional photographer, only a few months after discharge from rehabilitation. Barclay was fortunate to be left-handed, as the minor residual motor limitations were restricted to his nondominant right arm and hand. During landscape photography, the use of a tripod and a remote shutter release allowed for rapid return to his work. The use of a monopod was found to adequately compensate for his right upper extremity weakness during portrait sessions, allowing Barclay to quickly return to all of his professional duties.

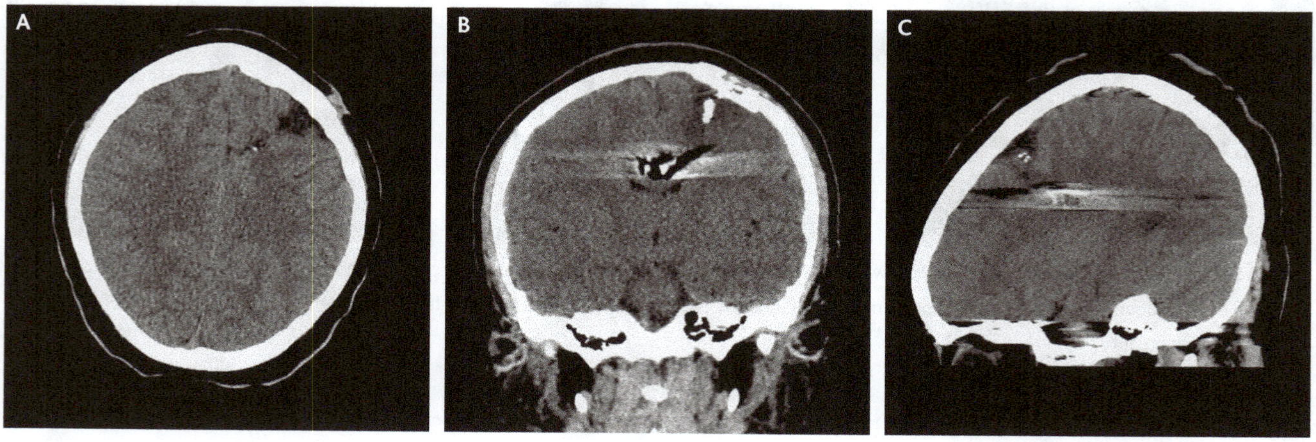

Figures 5-76A–C Clinical example Barclay: CT series of low-velocity, large-caliber gunshot wound, showing damage to the left superior frontal lobe. Note metallic artifact, most evident on coronal and sagittal sequences.

High-Velocity Penetrating Injuries

The effects of high-velocity penetrating objects on the brain are markedly different from those of low-velocity objects and often result in severe to profound injury. Based on the law of conservation of energy, the total amount of energy in a system remains constant over time. This means that energy cannot be created nor be destroyed; energy can only be transformed from one state to another. In low-velocity penetrating injuries, the small amount of energy contained within the projectile pushes through the skull and soft tissue but does not have enough energy to cause further injury. However, high-velocity projectiles contain significant amounts of energy, measured in foot-pounds. For example, a .223 caliber 55 grain round traveling at 3240 feet per second has approximately 1281 foot-pounds of energy, and a .45 caliber 125 grain round traveling at 1225 feet per second has approximately 616 foot-pounds of energy. From these values it is evident that small-caliber projectiles traveling at high velocities can carry more energy than larger-caliber projectiles at slower velocities.

When a bullet penetrates the brain and comes to rest within the cranial vault, the energy of the projectile has to go somewhere. Upon impact, a large amount of energy from high-velocity projectiles is rapidly converted into a pressure wave and heat. The pressure wave can cause severe damage to tissue some distance from the wound channel, in a manner similar to the shock wave seen in high-speed closed-head injuries. Pressure waves result in severe focal damage close to the wound track and diffuse damage throughout the rest of the brain. The heat generated by the dissipation of energy can be so extreme that the fluid in the brain turns into steam, creating a rapid increase in pressure and a large wound cavity. The rapid transfer of energy, the pressure wave, and the production of heat are greater if the bullet is designed to stop rapidly by mushrooming or fragmenting upon impact with body tissue. For this reason, injuries by hollow-point rounds can be more devastating than those with a full metal jacket.

High-Velocity, Small-Caliber Gunshot Wounds

Small-caliber bullets traveling at high speed contain enough energy to cause profound damage to brain tissue, irrespective of the relatively small diameter of the projectile.

CLINICAL EXAMPLE

Jennifer: High-Velocity, Small-Caliber Gunshot Wound

Jennifer, an army captain, was injured during a military campaign. She sustained a gunshot wound to the head from a .223 bullet, a common military round. Although the bullet passed through two sheets of plasterboard before hitting her, it had enough retained energy to cause significant injury to her brain. The bullet fragments are best visualized on CT bone windowing (Figures 5-77A–C), as the contrast range is more appropriate for high-density substances. Brain imaging revealed a large cavity with surrounding damage severe enough to result in encephalomalacia and atrophy of much of her right hemisphere. On standard CT imaging, the cavity is evident as the hypodense region in the right hemisphere, and the bullet fragments are visible as bright spots due to their high density, and metallic artifacts radiating from the fragments (Figures 5-78A–C). Note the size

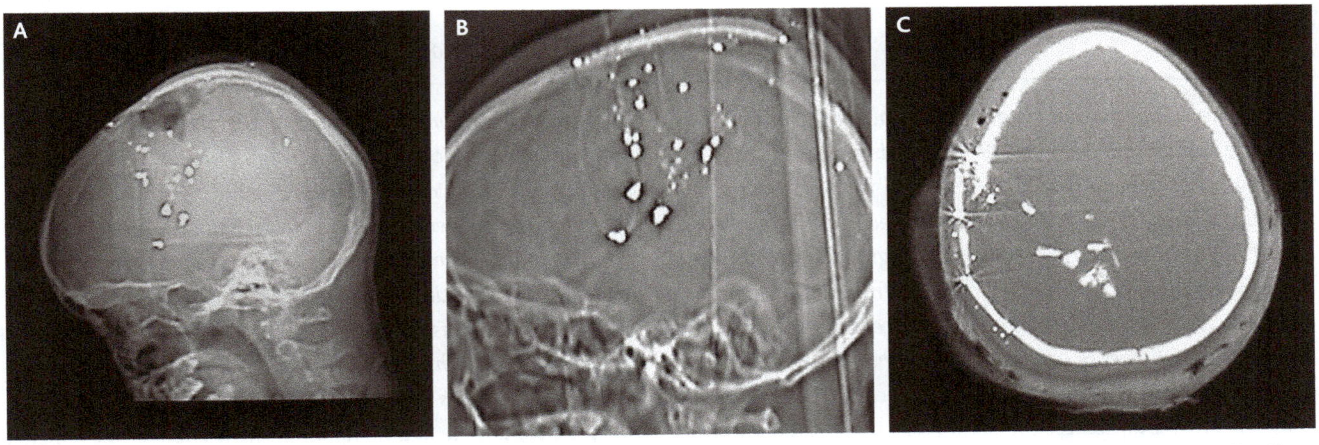

Figures 5-77A–C Clinical example Jennifer: x-ray, sagittal and axial bone window CT images showing bullet fragments from a high-velocity, small-caliber gunshot wound. **A:** X-ray. **B:** Sagittal CT bone window. **C:** Axial CT bone window.

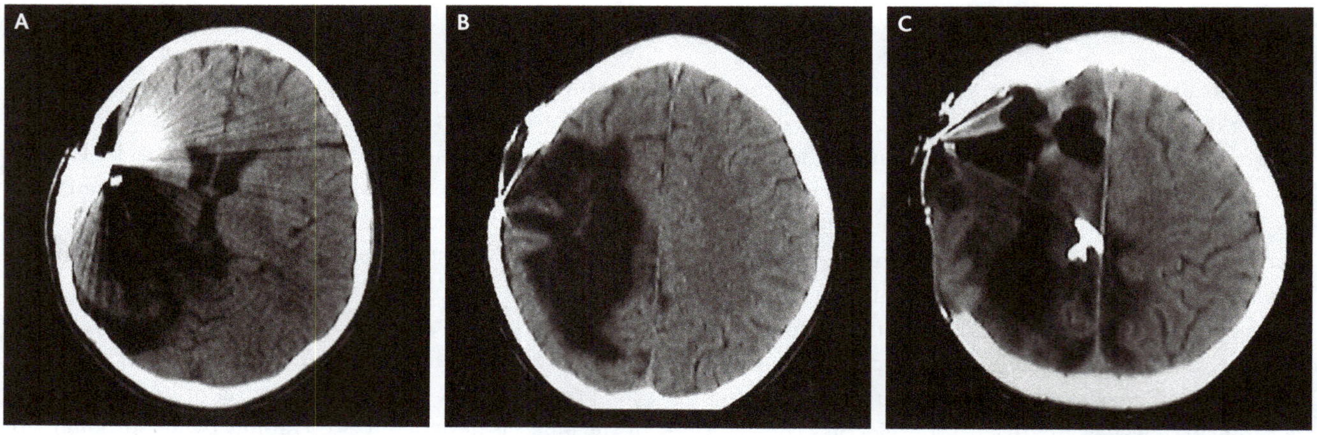

Figures 5-78A–C Clinical example Jennifer: CT series showing the large cavity within the right hemisphere (dark) and bullet fragments shown in white with radiating metallic artifacts.

of the wound cavity within the right hemisphere, caused by the sudden transfer of energy from the projectile to the tissue. The transfer of energy resulted in a pressure wave exerting extreme physical forces on the soft parenchyma, in addition to the rapid increase in heat, and resultant expansion of gases.

Jennifer was fortunate to have all of her language and verbal skills lateralized to her less injured left hemisphere. She retained her language skills but was left with some notable cognitive and motor deficits. After several years of recovery, Jennifer continued to experience left sensory hemineglect and left visual-field hemianopia. In addition, she had visual agnosia and prosopagnosia, deficits involving the visual recognition of objects and faces. As expected, given the extent of right-hemisphere damage, Jennifer also experienced left-sided upper- and lower-extremity hemiparesis, although she was able to walk using a brace for her ankle and a special cane.

High-Velocity, Large-Caliber Gunshot Wounds

Similar to that seen in high-velocity, small-caliber projectiles, the amount of brain trauma caused by large-caliber projectiles is frequently a function of velocity. The following two clinical cases represent injuries sustained by large-caliber bullets traveling at high velocities, although at slower speeds than was the case for Jennifer (see case example above). Although widespread damage occurred from the pressure wave, there was no large cavity as seen with Jennifer, likely because the speed of the bullet was insufficient to cause excessive heat, steam, and rapid expansion of gases.

CLINICAL EXAMPLE

Dan: High-Velocity, Large-Caliber Gunshot Wound

Dan received a head wound from a large-caliber bullet that was traveling rapidly but was slowed by passing through the side window of his vehicle. The bullet traveled through both of his frontal lobes (Figures 5-79A–D) and resulted in almost complete loss of his frontal lobe functioning. On Figures 5-79A–D, note the hypodense areas within the bilateral frontal and temporal lobes, but without the appearance of increased pressure. This suggests that the acute edema has resolved and the process of encephalomalacia and atrophy is taking place. The most superior image (5-79D) is difficult to interpret given the metallic artifacts from the bullet, although careful review suggests severe bilateral frontal lobe damage. The temporal lobe structures are not visible on the most superior slice because of the artifact. Dan became profoundly apathetic and abulic, losing self-drive, initiation, and goal-directed behaviors. He could respond to simple questions or commands but was unable to independently perform basic activities of daily living without prompts from others. He spent most of his time sitting in a chair producing different nonverbal sounds, smacking his lips, and smiling. When asked a question, he responded in a highly perseverative fashion, repeating the answer many times before stopping. His affect was perpetually positive, and he had no apparent awareness of his deficits, dependent condition, or appearance to others. Put simply, Dan took on the presentation of someone who had been lobotomized.

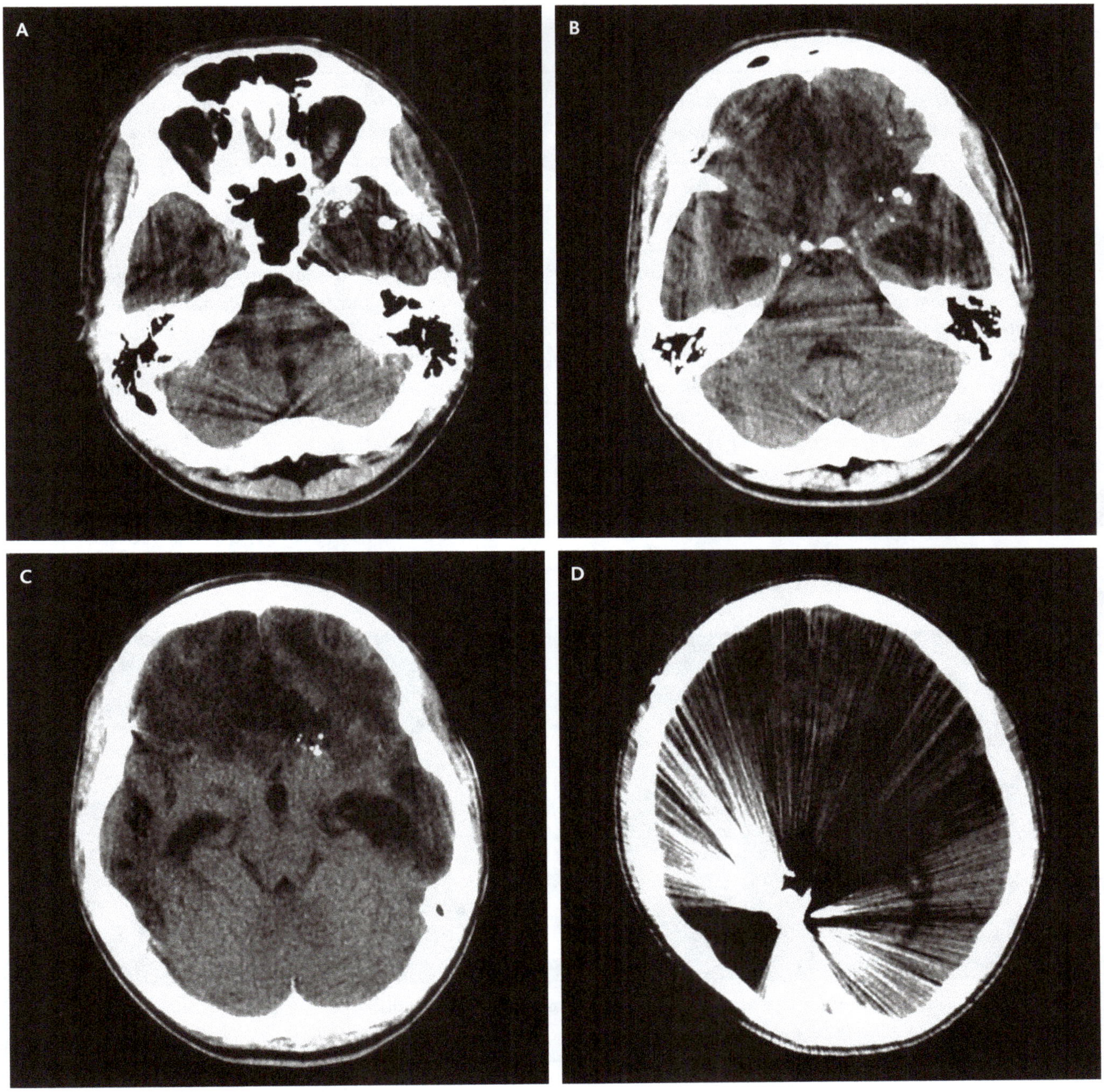

Figures 5-79A–D Clinical example Dan: CT series of high-velocity, large-caliber gunshot wound showing severe bilateral frontal and temporal lobe damage. The bullet is identified by the white areas with radiating metallic artifact on Figure 5-79D.

Oscar: High-Velocity, Large-Caliber Gunshot Wound

Oscar was injured by a large-caliber bullet traveling at high velocity. The bullet entered the left parietal lobe and excited through the left frontal lobe. As the bullet traveled across his left hemisphere, it caused damage to most of the tissue around the Sylvian fissure. For most people, the left peri-Sylvian region is responsible for language and verbal skills, with the three primary language structures being located within that area. Oscar sustained severe damage to Broca's area, Wernicke's area, and the arcuate fasciculus, or the band of axons that connects the two regions.

Blood, bone, and edema are evident within the wound channel on Figures 5-80A–C. Blood is evident at the temporal-parietal junction as brighter areas without well-defined margins. The blood is best viewed in Figure 5-80A and is identified by the arrows. Bone appears bright with well-defined margins and is best viewed in Figure 5-80B (arrows). The darker areas on all images represent edema, with one cavity being evident in Figure 5-80C (arrows 1). The peri-Sylvian injury resulted in profound global or mixed receptive-expressive aphasia with oral-motor apraxia and alexia. Even years after his injury, Oscar remained functionally mute, without the ability to understand verbal communication. Although he was able to speak a handful of words and would respond to his name, he had no ability to use language in any meaningful manner. In addition to Oscar's language disorder, he also experienced deficits with his motor functioning on the right side as expected given the extent of damage to his left frontal lobe. Oscar also experienced disruption to his vision as a result of the injury. When the bullet entered Oscar's brain, a large piece of bone was pushed into the left hemisphere optic radiations, severing connections between the lateral geniculate nucleus and the visual cortex of the left side (Figure 5-80C arrow 2). This resulted in Oscar experiencing a dense right visual-field hemianopia.

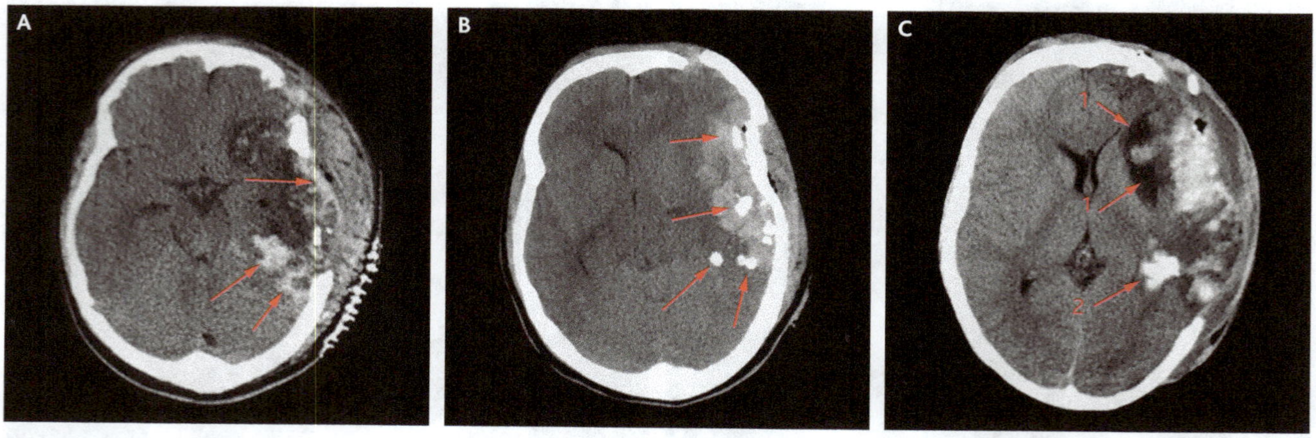

Figures 5-80A–C Clinical example Oscar: CT series of high-velocity, large-caliber gunshot wound showing blood (Figure 5-80A arrows), bone fragments (Figure 5-80B arrows, and 5-80C arrow 2) and a cavity within the brain parenchyma (Figure 5-80C arrow 1).

Shotgun Injuries

Unlike other firearms or pneumatic-based pellet and BB guns, shotguns shoot many small, round projectiles, called shot. The effective range of shotguns is quite small, with the shot rapidly losing velocity after leaving the shotgun barrel. Unless shot at close range, the velocity of the shot is relatively slow compared to projectiles from other firearms. However, with the high number of shot leaving the barrel, damage to the brain can be quite extensive. Even low-velocity shot can penetrate the skull and soft brain tissue, similar to penetration seen in injuries from pellet or BB guns.

Steven was shot in the face by a shotgun during an incident of gang retaliation. The shot caused irreversible damage to the globes of his eyes, rendering him blind. Some of the shot penetrated the skull, resulting in damage to his brain. Most of the damage was localized to the frontal lobes, although some of the shot penetrated to the parietal and occipital lobes (Figures 5-81A–F). Steven recovered relatively quickly but continued to exhibit deficits involving executive functioning, insight, and spatial awareness many years after the injury. The most remarkable aspect of Steven's impairment was his almost complete lack of spatial awareness. Even with practice, Steven was unable to learn the route from his room to the nurse's station or the therapy gym. On neuropsychological examination, Steven was unable to recognize the shapes of objects placed in his hands (astereognosis), was unable to recognize the shapes of holes with his fingers, and was unable to describe the location of items in his room, after many weeks of occupancy.

Steven's lack of spatial awareness made it extremely difficult for him to navigate with a cane; years after the injury he continued to rely on others for navigation and mobility. In addition, Steven was left with an almost complete lack of insight into his condition, frequently acting as if he had intact vision. When asked what he wanted to do after leaving the hospital, Steven reported, "I would like to be a pilot." When questioned about being a pilot without the ability to see, he responded, "Oh yeah, I forgot that I can't see." Steven's lack of insight was not a function of dementia or global cognitive impairment, as his general intellectual functioning for verbally based tasks was intact and unremarkable. His deficits were specific to the areas of damage caused by the many pieces of shot penetrating his brain.

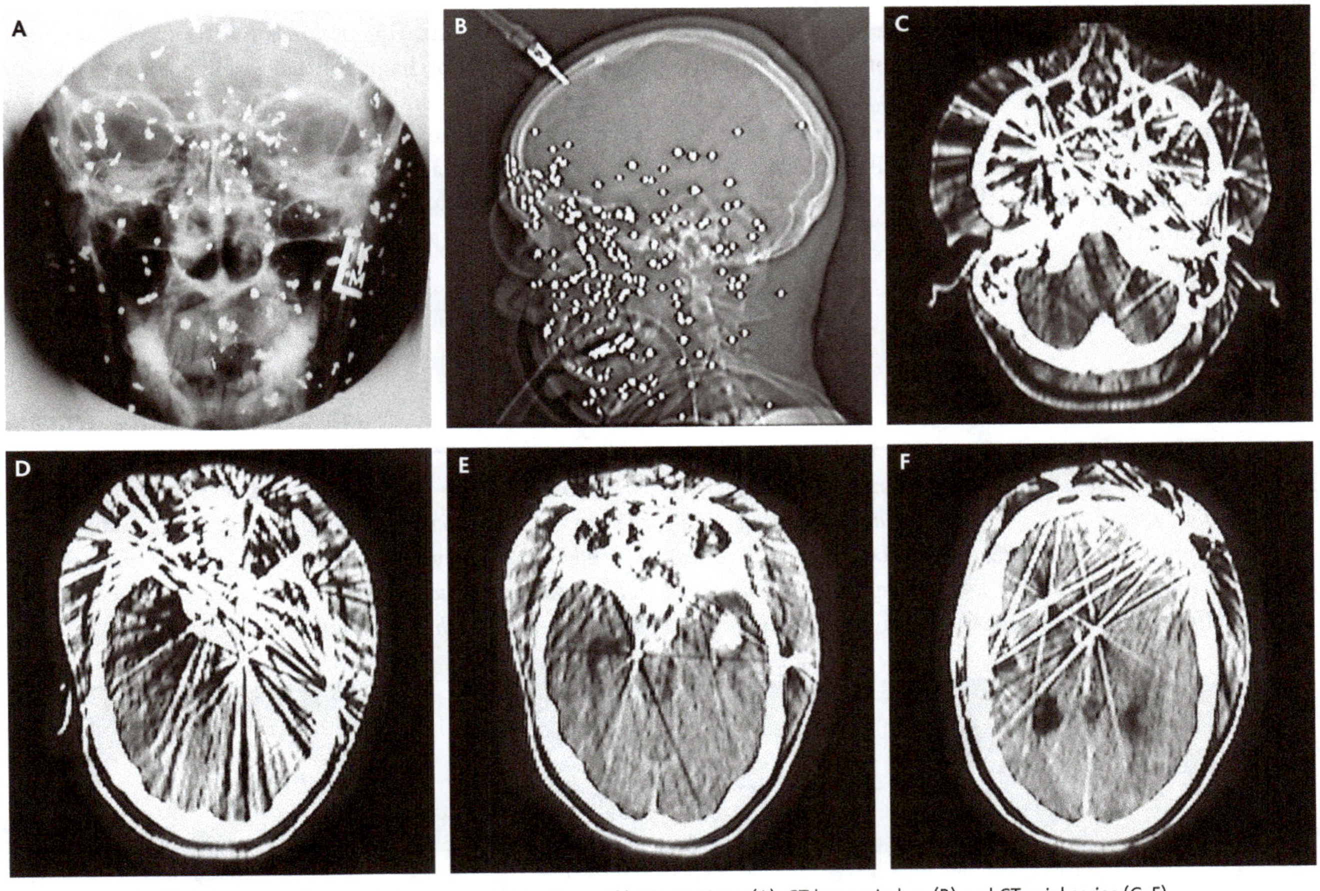

Figure 5-81A–F Clinical example Steven: shotgun injury to the face and brain on X-ray (A), CT bone window (B) and CT axial series (C–F).

NONACCIDENTAL TRAUMA (NAT)

Some of the worst brain damage and appearance on brain imaging stems from nonaccidental traumas (NAT). Although the term *nonaccidental trauma* can be applied to deliberately inflicted gunshot wounds, stabbings, poisonings, and such, it is predominantly reserved for injuries deliberately inflicted on babies, infants, and children through a variety of physical forces. Many terms have been used to describe NAT; some of the earliest descriptions of "battered child syndrome" were coined by C. Henry Kempe, M.D. Following Kempe's descriptions of the syndrome, the term *Kempe's baby*, describing a baby who had been abused, or *Kempe's series*, describing a workup for child abuse, became the norm. Later, *shaken baby syndrome* became more common, but the term failed to fully describe all of the injuries seen in abused children (Hutchison & Lebby, 2009). It has been argued that the sole act of shaking an infant does not produce sufficient force to cause severe diffuse axonal injury and hemorrhagic contusions often seen in these cases, and that impact against a hard surface may account for some of the more severe injuries seen in abused children. Alexander et al. (1990) suggested that shaking alone is sufficient to cause severe or fatal intracranial injury, although there is a wide range of etiologies for such injuries. The term *shaken-impact syndrome* was coined to suggest the role of an impact in many cases of nonaccidental brain trauma, even though impact may not have been a component of the specific case in question. *Nonaccidental trauma*, or *NAT*, will be used in this text, as it is the most general of terms and does not imply a specific etiology, something that is often not available or completely known. It is important to note that severe brain injuries rarely occur in infants who fall from a height less than that of an adult (Chadwick et al., 1991), making many explanations for severe brain injuries in infants untenable.

REFERENCES

Alexander, R., Sato, Y., Smith, W., & Bennett, T. 1990. Incidence of impact trauma with cranial injuries ascribed to shaking. *American Journal of Diseases of Children, 144,* 724–726.

Chadwick, D. L., Chin, S., Salerno, C., Landsverk, J., & Kitchen, L. 1991. Deaths from falls in children: How far is fatal? *Journal of Trauma 30,* 1353–1355.

Hutchison, T., & Lebby, P. C. (2009). Traumatic encephalopathies. In R. B. David (Ed.), *Clinical pediatric neurology* (3rd ed.). New York: Demos Medical Publishing.

In general, evidence of NAT on brain imaging can range from no obvious signs of injury to profound indications of brain trauma. The appearance of brain imaging depends on the severity and extent of the injury and on the various physical forces acting on the brain tissue. Respiratory arrest or the introduction of toxic substances can also influence how injuries appear on neuroimaging. Because NAT involves a variety of forces acting on soft brain tissues, injuries can involve a variety of pathological processes such as tearing of blood vessels, shearing of white-matter tracts, nonhemorrhagic and hemorrhagic contusions, hypoxic ischemia, or diffuse swelling. Shortly after an injury, images may appear relatively benign and may fail to show the full extent of damage. Hemorrhages and swelling are frequently evident soon after the injury, although the magnitude of damage may be difficult to assess.

CLINICAL EXAMPLE
Jaime: Nonaccidental Trauma

Jaime was a 6-month-old child who sustinaed injuries attributed to nonaccidental trauma (NAT). Figure 5-82 shows a CT series shortly after injury and Figures 5-82D–F show a CT series acquired 1 month post injury. Even though the initial scans suggest diffuse edema, much of the brain parenchyma is still present. One month later, the extent and severity of the injury is more easily appreciated, given the highly atrophic appearance of the brain. Atrophy would be expected for some time after the CT images were acquired in Figures 5-82D–F, and so even these scans fail to reveal the full extent of the damage.

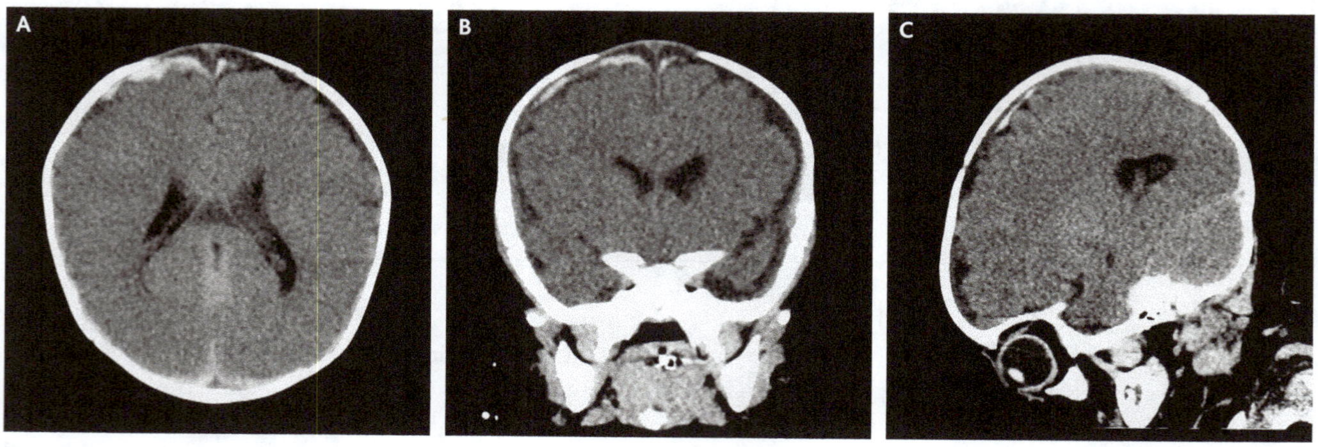

Figures 5-82A–C Clinical example Jaime: CT series shortly following NAT in a 6-month old child.

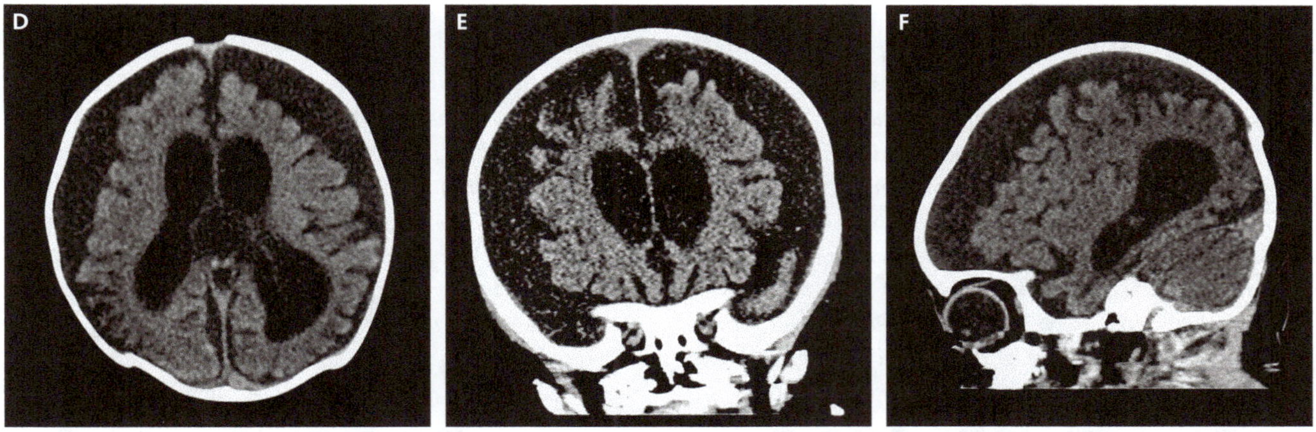

Figures 5-82A–F Clinical example Jaime: CT series taken 1 month after NAT. To facilitate comparison with the images taken shortly after the injury, slices of similar locations and angles are displayed. Compare the acute images taken shortly after the injury with those acquired 1 month later.

Although brain plasticity in a baby or infant allows for some recovery after a severe NAT, if significant amounts of tissue become damaged, the child will likely have disrupted functioning for the rest of his or her life. While atrophy to the brain can stabilize after a few months and compensatory mechanisms may enable some recovery of functioning, brain scans many years later may appear similar to those acquired acutely. In the clinical example presented below, Jolie was injured during a NAT incident and received CT imaging shortly after injury, 1 month post-injury, 5 years post-injury, and again at 10 years post-injury. The lack of significant change in the brain images demonstrates the limits of brain recovery following such an injury.

CLINICAL EXAMPLE
Jolie: Nonaccidental Trauma in a 7-Month-Old with Follow-up Imaging for 10 Years

Jolie was 7 months old when she was injured by nonaccidental trauma. Follow-up imaging was acquired for a little over 10 years, allowing for comparison over an extended period of time (Figures 5-83A–H). Two weeks following her injury, CT imaging revealed hypodense areas within white matter and hyperdense ridges along gyral contours, suggesting onset of

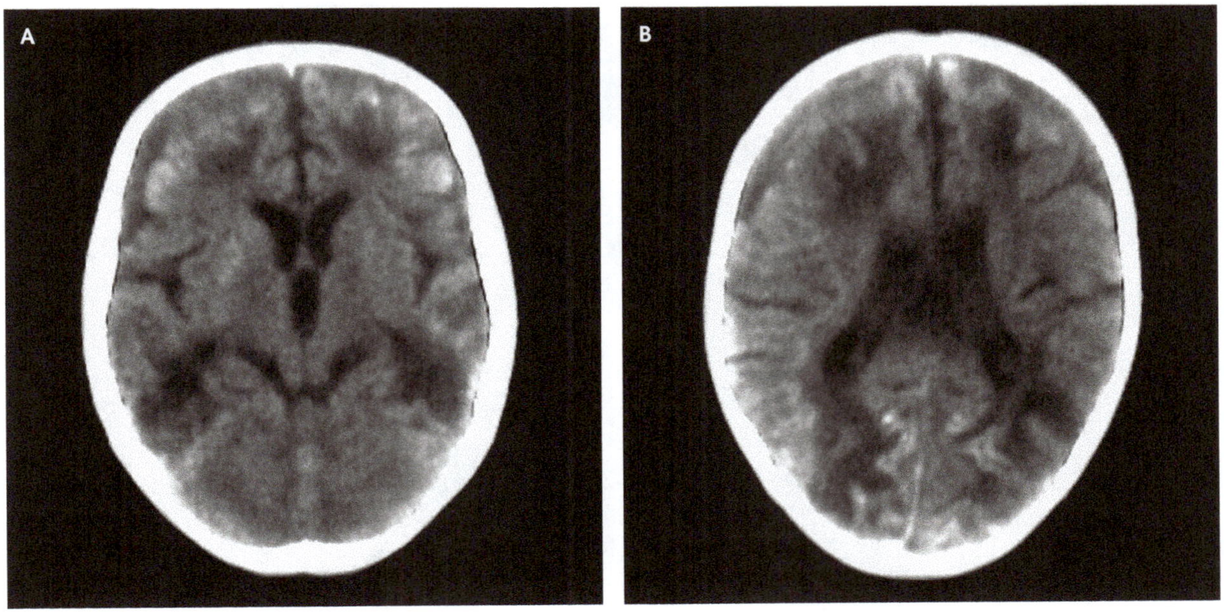

Figures 5-83A and B CT imaging of Jolie, taken 2 weeks after sustaining NAT, suggesting severe bilateral damage.

encephalomalacia and laminar necrosis. Edema had mostly resolved, as evident by the prominence of sulci–gyri patterning and relatively large ventricles and cisterns (Figures 5-83A and B). Six weeks after the injury, substantial bifrontal and biparietal-occipital encephalomalacia and atrophy was evident (Figures 5-83C and D). CT imaging 5 years (Figures 5-83E and F) and 10 years following her NAT (Figures 5-83G and H) revealed the pattern of damage had remained mostly unchanged over the 10 years of ongoing brain development. The images acquired 10 years following her injury continued to suggest primary damage to the frontal and parietal lobes; the general pattern of damage was moltly unchanged over the 10-year period.

Unfortunately, as would be expected given the initial CT evidence of permanent brain injury, Jolie experienced severe developmental difficulties as she matured. On follow-up neuropsychological assessment at 10 years of age, she performed well below the first percentile for her age on measures of cognition and adaptive functioning. Although the brain is capable of compensating to a small degree after injury in infancy, the benefits of plasticity are limited. Severe injuries to the brain often cause lifelong deficits, even if the injury took place in infancy (Lebby & Asbell, 2007).

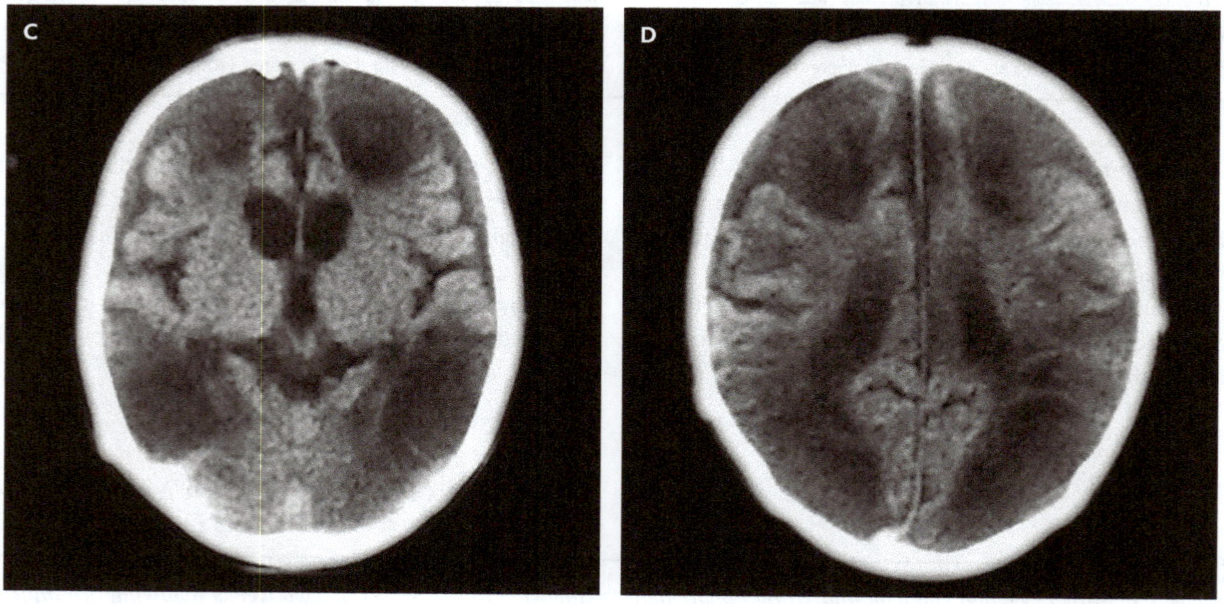

Figures 5-83C and D CT imaging of Jolie at 6 weeks. Note the substantial bifrontal and biparietal-occipital encephalomalacia and atrophy with ventriculomegaly ex vacuo.

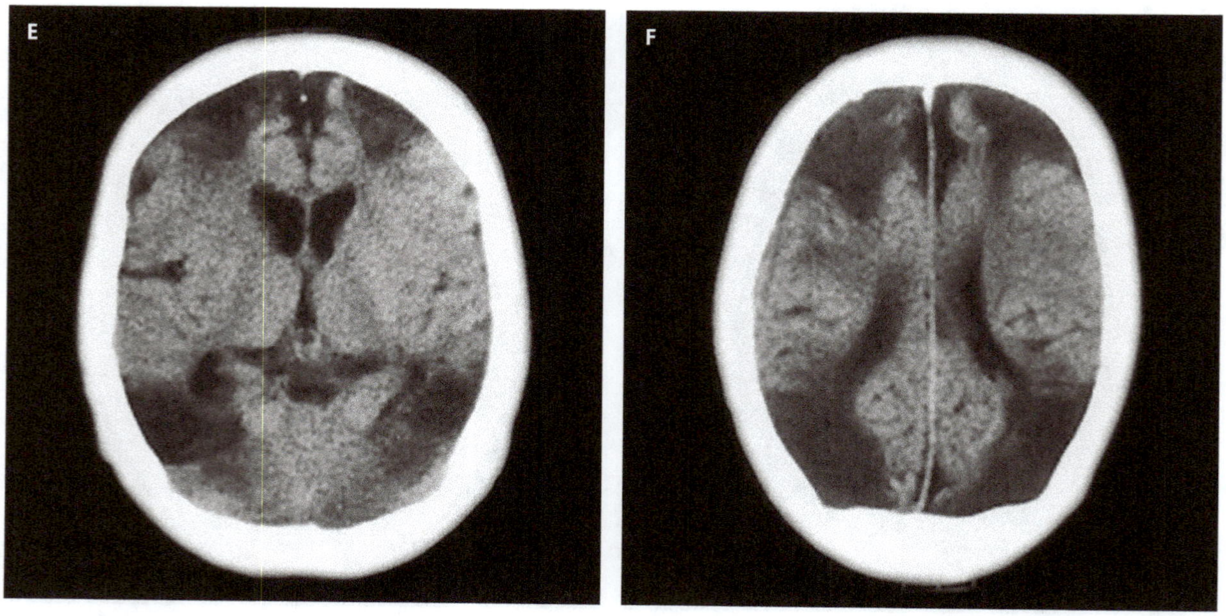

Figures 5-83E and F CT imaging of Jolie at 5 years post-injury showing little change in the pattern of damage over the previous five years of development.

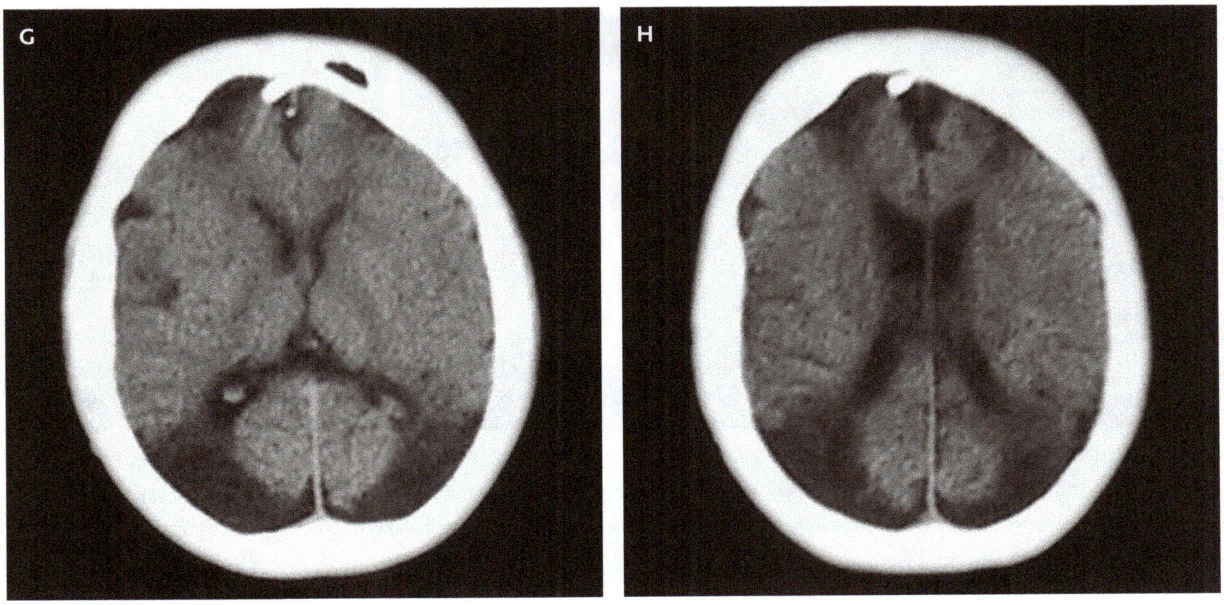

Figures 5-83G and H CT imaging of Jolie at 10 years post-injury showing little change in the pattern of damage over the previous 10 years of development.

REFERENCE

Lebby, P. C., & Asbell, S. J. (2007). *The source for TBI: Children and adolescents*. East Moline, IL: LinguiSystems, Inc.

Suspected Nonaccidental Trauma, but Not Nonaccidental Trauma

When viewing brain scans for evidence of NAT, it is important to consider the possibility that severe to profound injuries can result from relatively benign accidents unrelated to abuse. Infants and children with vascular anomalies such as arteriovenous malformations (AVMs) or aneurysms are at risk of significant damage to brain tissue from bleeds and swelling following a relatively small impact to the head. Sometimes small impacts can tear immature blood vessels in infants, resulting in an appearance on imaging suggestive of NAT, even when this is not a factor. It is important to take into consideration all available information and possible etiologies before concluding that the damage suggested by brain imaging is the result of NAT.

CLINICAL EXAMPLE

Lucius: Injury that Appeared to be NAT but Was Not NAT

Lucius, the same child from the clinical example on subdural hematomas, presented to the emergency department with severe and rapid neurological deterioration. Remember that he had fallen only a short distance onto a carpeted floor while pulling to stand using the side of a sofa. Initial CT studies suggested NAT because of the degree of parenchymal swelling and extensive subdural hemorrhage surrounding most of the left hemisphere (Figures 5-84A–C). Assessment by child abuse specialists quickly determined that this was not a case of NAT but instead an unfortunate accident. Further studies revealed that the fall tore a vein leading to the superior sagittal sinus, resulting in extensive bleeding into the subdural space. Even though the severity of brain injury was inconsistent with a fall to the carpet by a standing toddler, the medical team was cautious in their evaluation. Clues suggesting that this was not NAT came from a parental interview, in addition to the appearance of brain imaging and other medical tests. For example, on CT, other than the swelling and subdural hemorrhage in the left hemisphere, there was little evidence of injury to the rest of the brain. In addition, there was no evidence of diffuse physical trauma to the left hemisphere, such as petechial hemorrhaging, that would indicate an impact or shearing type injury. The edema appeared secondary to the hemorrhage and loss of oxygenated blood to the left

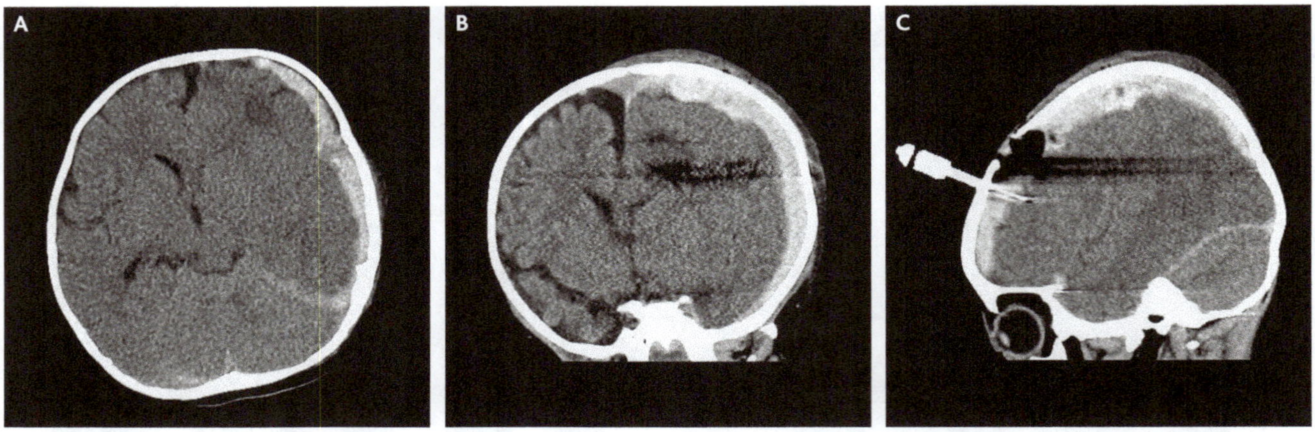

Figures 5-84A–C Clinical example Lucius: injury that appeared to be NAT but was not NAT. CT scans acquired shortly after injury. Note left-hemisphere swelling with midline shift, left frontal areas of low-density, subarachnoid blood along the tentorium, and extensive subdural bleed along the lateral convexity of the left hemisphere. Also note the relatively intact right hemisphere and lack of petechial bleeds that would be expected diffusely across a brain following a NAT incident.

hemisphere, not physical trauma per se. By careful review of Lucius's brain scans, in addition to a solid clinical evaluation, his parents were not inappropriately accused of hurting him, and significant social and emotional distress to Lucius and his family was avoided.

Over time, brain imaging suggested relatively localized damage to the left hemisphere resulting from Lucius's vascular injury, not diffuse damage to the brain as would be expected in NAT (Figure 5-85). Follow-up developmental assessment of Lucius revealed remarkable functioning given the severity and extent of his left hemisphere injury. Although he had a right sided hemiparesis, he was fully ambulatory and could run and jump. His cognitive abilities 3 years after his injury, at the age of 4, fell within normal limits for verbal and visual reasoning and pre-academic skills. Given the extent of his injury and young age, his parents were cautioned that his early injury will likely disrupt future development, and he may have increasing difficulties as he matures and is faced with higher expectations for complex cognitive functioning and sustained attention. Even with intact reasoning skills, at 4 years, Lucius was already exhibiting high levels of hyperactivity, impulsivity and difficulties focusing his attention for more than a few seconds at a time.

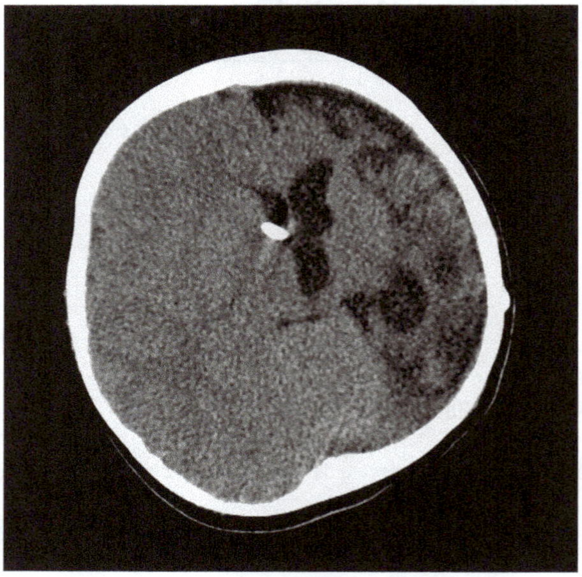

Figure 5-85 Follow-up CT of Lucius, acquired at 18-months post-injury, to assess integrity of the shunt and to rule out any hydrocephalus. Note localized damage and atrophy to the left hemisphere, with preservation of the right hemisphere. The left-to-right midline shift is a function of the asymmetric atrophy, not right-hemisphere swelling, and the enlarged ventricles in the left hemisphere represent hydrocephalus ex vacuo.

PEARL When reviewing brain scans, consider all information available to you before concluding a specific etiology. In the case of Lucius, consultation with his parents suggested that his injury was not a result of NAT. Further tests confirmed this, allowing Lucius to remain with his parents during his hospitalization. Information from brain scans should always be correlated with the medical history and your clinical examination in order to provide adequate context for facilitating accurate image interpretation.

PERIL It is easy to jump to conclusions upon review of a patient's brain scans, especially if the images appear normal or markedly abnormal. Normal scans can suggest that the brain was not damaged, even with notable injury. Clearly abnormal scans can suggest injury due to excessive physical forces or abuse, even when the damage was unrelated to this. In Lucius's case, the highly abnormal scans in a infant could lead one to conclude that his injury was the result of abuse or excessive physical forces acting on his brain. However, only a light impact with a carpeted floor resulted in rupture of a blood vessel, a conclusion not readily apparent on initial review of his imaging.

CONCLUDING REMARKS

This chapter provided clinical examples and information relating to the use of brain imaging for patients with traumatic injuries to the brain. Chapter 6 provides clinical examples and information relating to nontraumatic injuries to the brain, such as infections, strokes, and hypoxemia. It is important to consider the considerable overlap of conditions presented in this chapter and those in the next chapter. For example, physical trauma to the brain and skull can result in strokes and hypoxic-ischemic injuries, in addition to infections of the meninges or brain parenchyma via skull fractures. Both traumatic and nontraumatic injuries to the brain can result in edema and increased intracranial pressure or herniation, or vascular compromise due to vasospasm or loss of autoregulation. As you progress through Chapter 6, consider how some of the conditions can also be caused by physical trauma. In addition, consider how the conditions in this chapter can lead to secondary damage unrelated to the physical trauma per se, but more to the effects of injury to brain tissues.

6

NONTRAUMATIC BRAIN INJURIES

The previous chapter provided clinical examples of traumatic brain injuries. Damage to the brain is often caused by nontraumatic events such as infections, vascular disorders, demyelinating conditions, hypoxic events, and neoplasms. This chapter will provide clinical examples and information pertaining to the use of brain imaging for a variety of nontraumatic conditions affecting the brain.

INFECTIONS OF THE BRAIN

Infections of the brain are labeled according to the brain structures most influenced. For example, infection of the meningeal layers is considered *meningitis*, infection of the brain parenchyma is called *encephalitis*, and of the combination of both is called *meningoencephalitis*. Finer distinctions in labeling apply to inflammation of specific tissues, such as the arachnoid layer; this condition is called *arachnoiditis*. Infections can also result in *abscesses*, or encapsulated pockets of pus within the brain. When the pus is not encapsulated, it is called *empyema*.

Meningitis

On brain imaging, meningitis is most easily identified by the inflammatory infiltration of the pia and subarachnoid spaces, resulting in sulcal or arachnoid cistern contrast enhancement. Early imaging may be unremarkable; later imaging is more useful in determining the extent and severity of postinfectious damage to the brain. Early markers of infection can include hydrocephalus, abscess or empyema, and inflammation. Later markers may include the presence of cellular breakdown secondary to ischemic infarction.

On nonenhanced CT, meningitis may not be evident. However, the primary markers of infection, such as ventricular enlargement, edema, and effacement of the sulci–gyri pattern, may be visible. Contrast CT imaging may show enhancement of the arachnoid cisterns and sulci. MRI can be more useful than CT given the larger number of sequences available. T2 imaging may show general hyperintensity, and T2 FLAIR imaging may show hyperintensity specific to the sulci and arachnoid cisterns. T1 post-contrast imaging may show enhancement along the brain surface due to involvement of the pial layer. Complications such as abscess or empyema may be evident on diffusion-weighted imaging (DWI) sequences.

Because the imaging of meningitis can be nonspecific and similar to that of other conditions such as subarachnoid hemorrhaging, clinical examination with correlation between symptoms and imaging is important.

Encephalitis and Cerebritis

Encephalitis and cerebritis involve infections of brain parenchyma that are caused by a variety of different pathogens. One of the primary markers of encephalitis or cerebritis is diffuse parenchymal inflammation with T2 hyperintensity involving either gray or white matter and sometimes both. Because the inflammation is generally nonspecific, the effects of encephalitis or cerebritis can appear similar to those of other conditions, such as hypoxic ischemia, infiltrating neoplasms, diffuse axonal injury, or even toxic or metabolic injuries.

Standard nonenhanced CT imaging may not show the effects of mild infections, although it may show the secondary effects of the illness, such as hemorrhages or infarctions. MRI is considered the best choice for imaging encephalitis or cerebritis because of the number of sequences available. FLAIR, DWI, and post-contrast imaging may be useful in determining the extent of infection. Post-contrast T2 FLAIR imaging is often the most revealing, although this can vary. Meningeal post-contrast enhancement may be present in cases of encephalitis or cerebritis.

The following examples of encephalitis resulted in relatively localized or focal damage to the brain. However, some forms of encephalitis can lead to severe to profound global encephalopathy that is sometimes fatal. If the patient survives, he or she may experience profound neurological and functional compromise. Herpes encephalitis often results in severe damage to the brain, especially to the entorhinal cortex and subcortical structures of the limbic system. Other pathogens can also produce severe bilateral cortical and white-matter inflammation and infarction, with eventual

CLINICAL EXAMPLE
Viral Meningitis

Figure 6-1 shows an example of viral meningitis on non-contrast MRI and contrast-enhanced MRI. On non-contrast imaging (Figures 6-1A–C), the areas of post-infections meningeal inflammation are identified on T2 FLAIR sequences by hyperintensity and on DWI and ADC sequences by hyperintensity and hypointensity respectively, suggesting restricted diffusion over the meningeal layers. This is most evident on Figures 6-1A–C (arrows) surrounding the medial and anterior right temporal lobe and inferior surface of the right frontal lobe adjacent to the temporal pole. Close inspection of the images also reveals slight meningeal hyperintensity within the analogous areas of the left hemisphere, although not to the same degree. On contrast-enhanced MRI (Figures 6-1A–F), the areas of meningeal inflammation enhance, making it easier to appreciate the severity and extent of infection. Note that contrast-enhanced T2 FLAIR (6-1D) provides the best visualization of the meningeal infection on this series of MRI images.

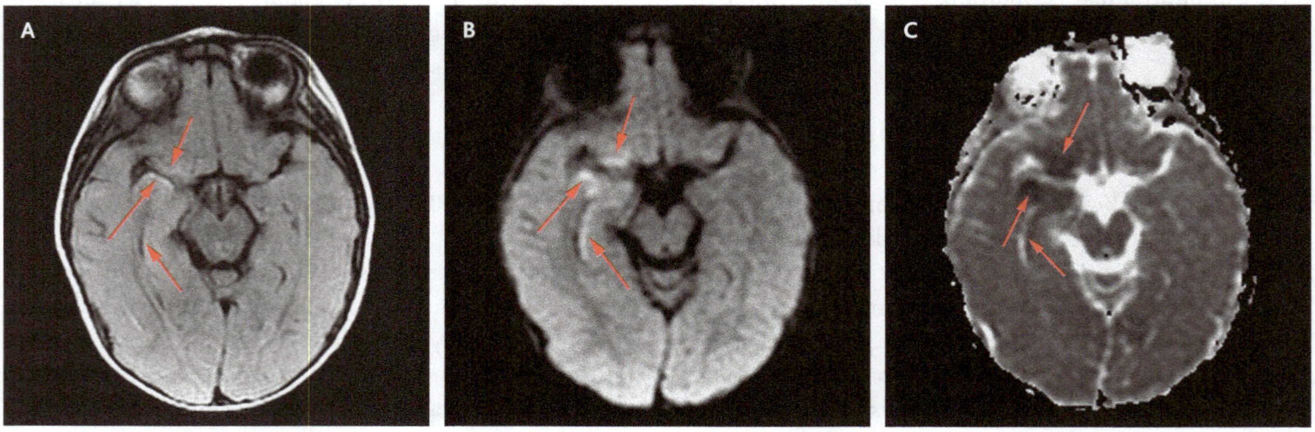

Figures 6-1A–C Non-contrast MRI series showing evidence of viral meningitis (arrows). **A:** T2 FLAIR. **B:** DWI. **C:** ADC.

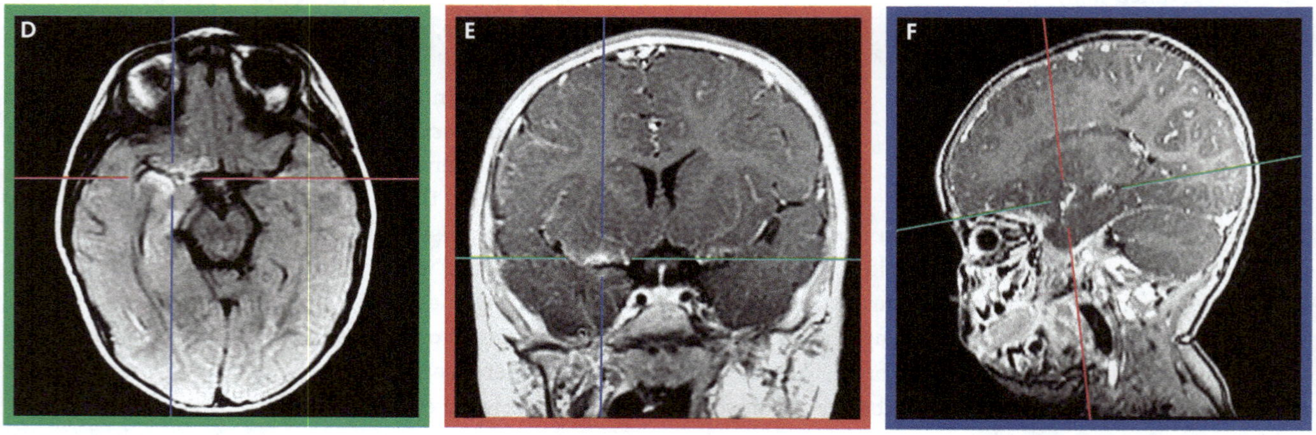

Figures 6-1A–F Contrast-enhanced MRI series showing evidence of viral meningitis. **A:** CE T2 FLAIR. **B:** CE T1 **C:** CE T1.

CLINICAL EXAMPLE
Tatum: Encephalitis

Tatum contracted encephalitis, resulting in damage to several regions of her brain. Most of the damage was localized to the medial cortical and subcortical right occipital lobe, with additional injury to her left occipital lobe and bilateral hippocampi. On acute CT imaging (Figure 6-2), there was evidence of low density just posterior to the splenium of the corpus callosum on either side of the longitudinal fissure (arrows).

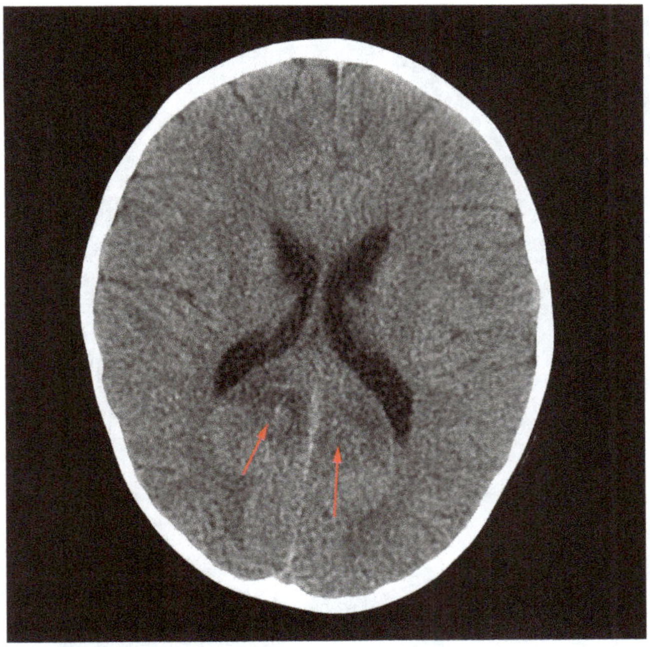

Figure 6-2 Clinical example Tatum: acute CT showing encephalitis, with damage most evident just posterior to the splenium of the corpus callosum (arrows).

Those same regions appeared mildly hyperintense on T2 and T2 FLAIR imaging, suggesting inflammation. Also on T2 and T2 FLAIR imaging, hyperintensity was evident within the optic radiations and in the lateral cortical rim and subcortical white matter (Figures 6-3A and B). The areas became even more pronounced or hyperintense on contrast-enhanced T2 FLAIR sequences (Figures 6-3C and D). Diffusion imaging clearly indicated disrupted diffusion within the same regions identified on CT and T2-weighted non-contrast and contrast imaging, with a bright appearance on DWI (Figure 6-3E) and dark appearance on the apparent diffusion coefficient (ADC) map (Figure 6-3F).

Two months after her infection, the damage to the occipital lobes was even more evident on MRI sequences. The T2 and T2 FLAIR white-matter hyperintensity (Figures 6-4A and B) was likely the result of either posterior reversible encephalopathy syndrome (PRES) or Wallerian degeneration (see box on Wallerian degeneration) and unlikely due to ongoing inflammation caused by the infection. The slightly brighter appearance of the white matter on T2 weighted imaging (Figure 6-4A and B), DWI (Figure 6-4C), and the ADC sequence (Figure 6-4D) suggests vasogenic edema.

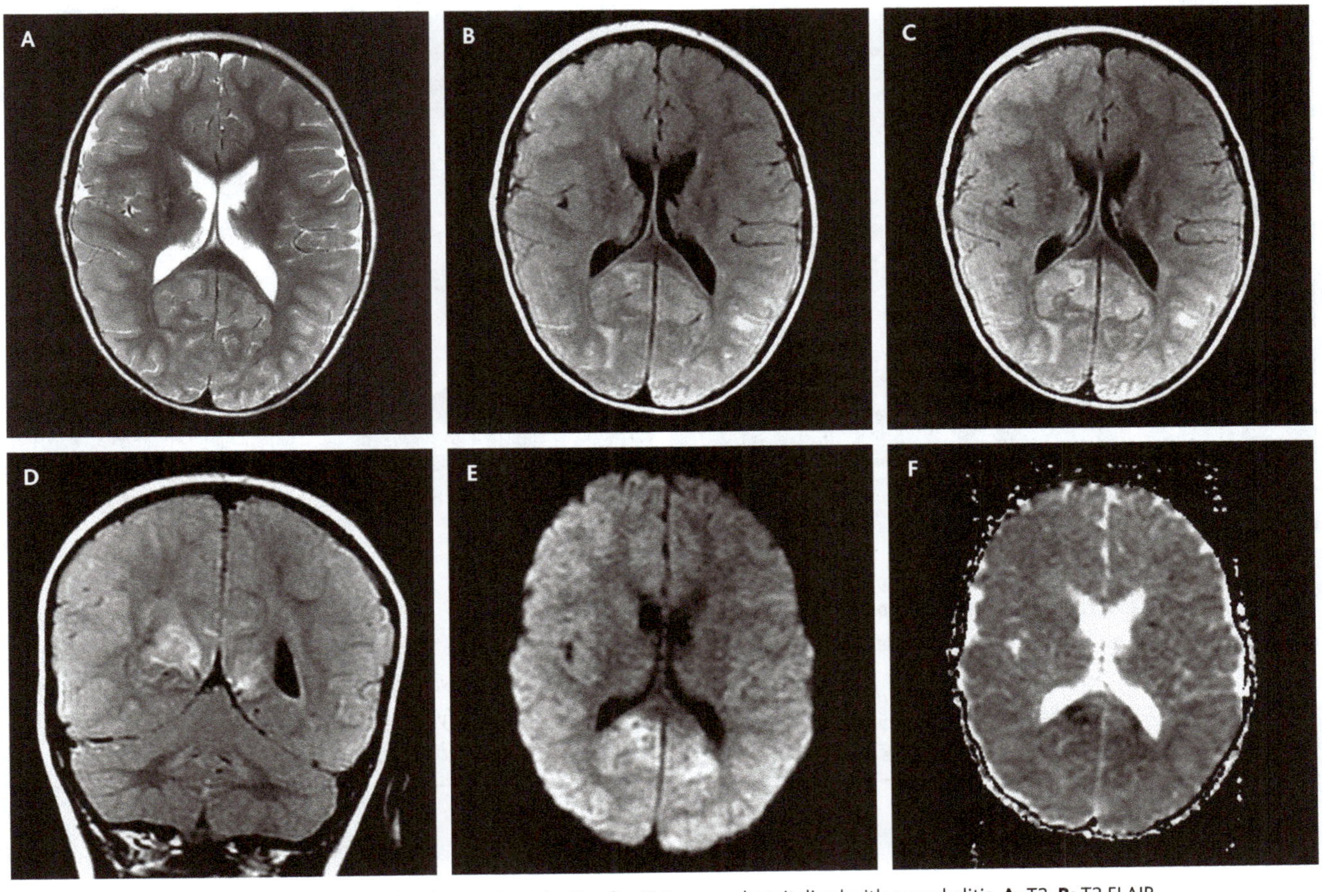

Figures 6-3A–F Clinical example Tatum: MRI series acquired shortly after Tatum was hospitalized with encephalitis. **A:** T2. **B:** T2 FLAIR. **C:** Contrast-enhanced T2 FLAIR. **D:** Contrast-enhanced T2 FLAIR. **E:** DWI. **F:** ADC.

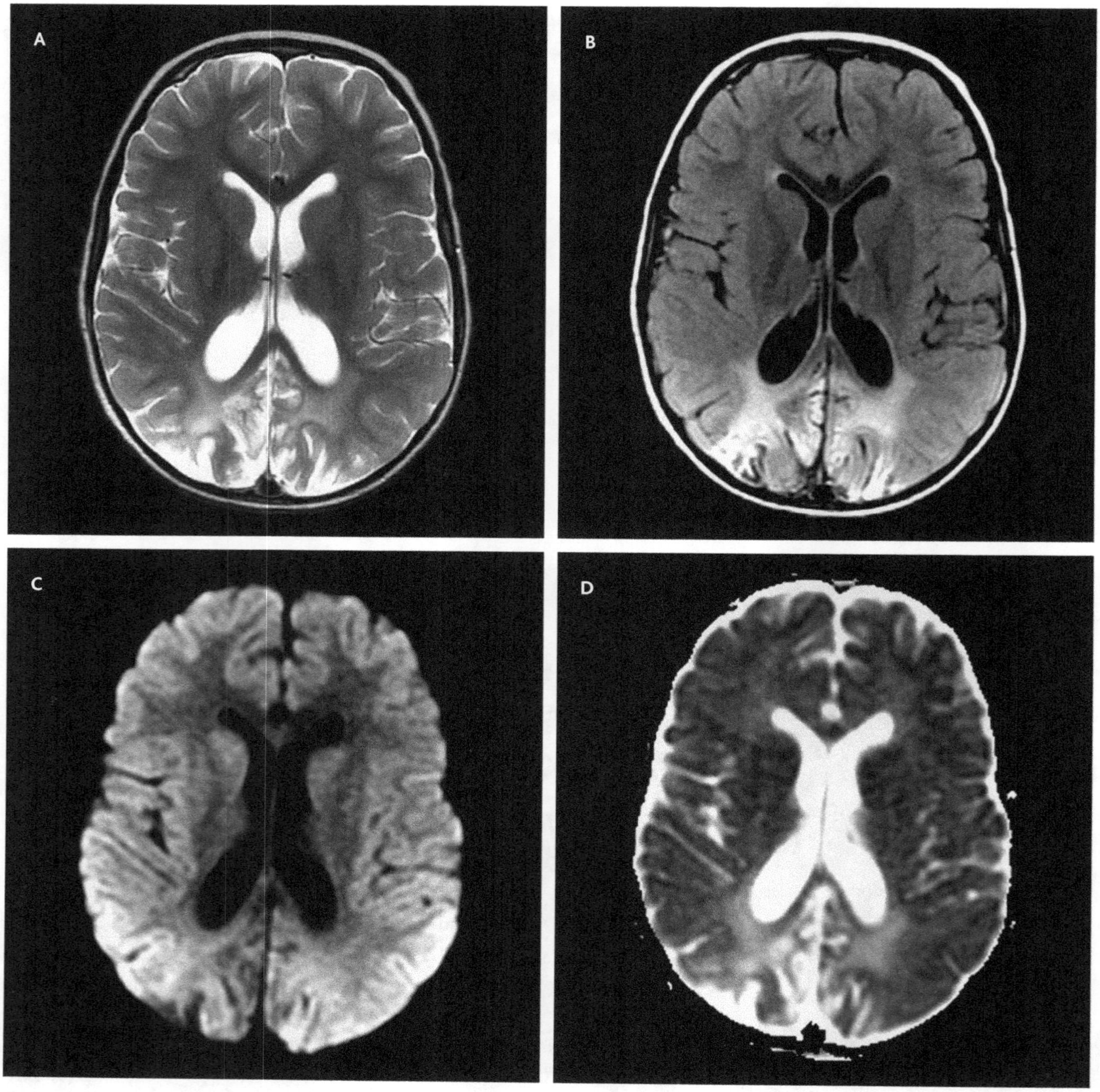

Figures 6-4A–D Clinical example Tatum: MRI series taken 2 months after Tatum's discharge from the hospital suggesting either Wallerian degeneration or PRES. **A:** T2. **B:** T2 FLAIR. **C:** DWI. **D:** ADC.

The occipital pole atrophy is indicative of permanent damage, which is more suggestive of Wallerian degeneration than PRES.

With damage to her secondary and tertiary visual cortices, Tatum experienced visual-processing deficits unrelated to sensation per se but related to higher-order processing of visual information. Tatum developed Balint's syndrome, a visual-processing disorder affecting her spatial awareness, ability to simultaneously attend to multiple visual stimuli, and ability to track and localize objects in space.

Wallerian Degeneration

Wallerian degeneration refers to the gradual process of white-matter demyelination and atrophy due to death of either distal axon segments or proximally at the neuronal body. Wallerian degeneration can result from a variety of pathological processes, such as physical trauma, hemorrhages, hypoxic ischemic infarction, encephalitis, chemotherapy, radiation therapy/necrosis, leukoencephalopathies, or focal demyelination. Because of the gradual process of Wallerian degeneration and the various metabolic and histological changes that take place, the appearance on neuroimaging changes over time. Wallerian degeneration may not become evident on brain scans until the post-acute stages or even later.

The first stage of Wallerian degeneration involves demyelination of the axon, which can take several weeks. No specific changes on T1 or T2 sequences may be evident during stage 1, although in some patients, DWI and ADC images may show changes during this stage. New techniques involving diffusion tensor imaging (DTI) are being studied as options to assess the early stages of Wallerian degeneration, even within days of the insult. Rapid breakdown of the remaining fragments of myelin takes place during the second stage of degeneration, approximately 1 to 3 months after injury. Imaging completed during stage 2 of Wallerian degeneration may show T2 hypointensities. After several months, during the third stage, the myelin sheath has almost completely atrophied, with gliosis becoming more evident. T2 and T2 FLAIR sequences show increasing hyperintensity. Volume loss becomes most prominent during the fourth stage, following final atrophy of the white-matter pathways. During stage 4, the most obvious signs on brain imaging involve volume loss within the affected area or within pathways connected to that area, such as the corpus callosum, brain stem, and corticospinal tract.

CLINICAL EXAMPLE

Andy: Encephalitis with Damage to the Basal Ganglia

Andy contracted encephalitis, resulting in damage to his basal ganglia structures bilaterally. Motor functional was compromised, as was general cognition and his ability to perform normal activities of daily living. Imaging conducted while Andy was in the intensive care unit (Figures 6-5A–C) showed only subtle hyperintensity of the bilateral caudate and putamen structures and was not of the magnitude to suggest significant involvement of these structures. Diffusion imaging acquired while Andy was in the intensive care unit also suggested only subtle restriction of diffusion within the bilateral basal ganglia structures (Figures 6-6A and B). Note the slightly brighter appearance on DWI and slightly darker appearance on ADC. The hypointensity on ADC suggests restricted diffusion and not T2 shine-through. Three weeks after contracting encephalitis, restricted diffusion was much easier to appreciate within the bilateral basal ganglia structures, likely due to some ongoing damage.

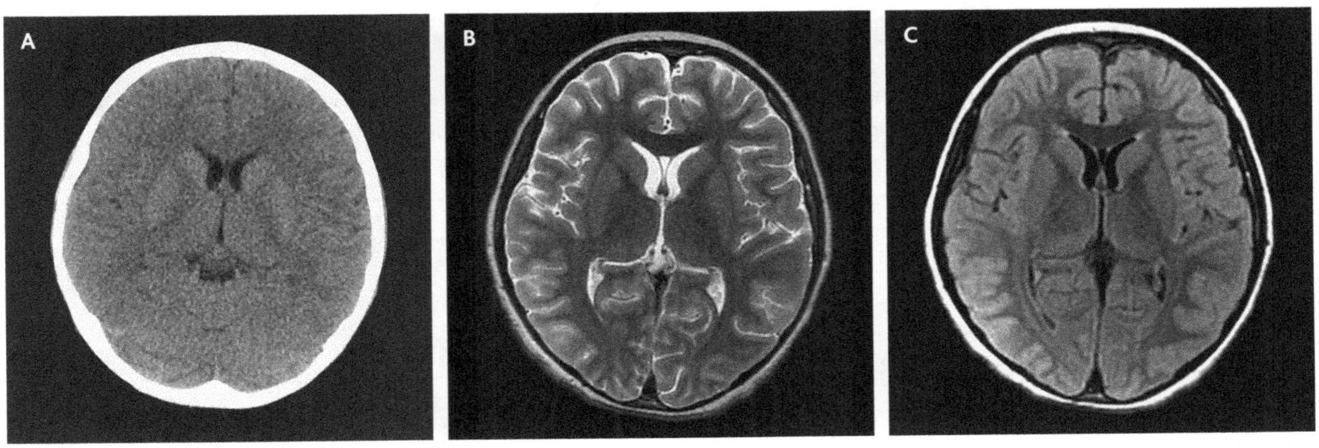

Figures 6-5A–C Clinical example Andy: imaging conducted while Andy was in the intensive care unit showed only subtle hyperintensity of the bilateral caudate and putamen structures. **A:** CT. **B:** T2. **C:** T2 FLAIR.

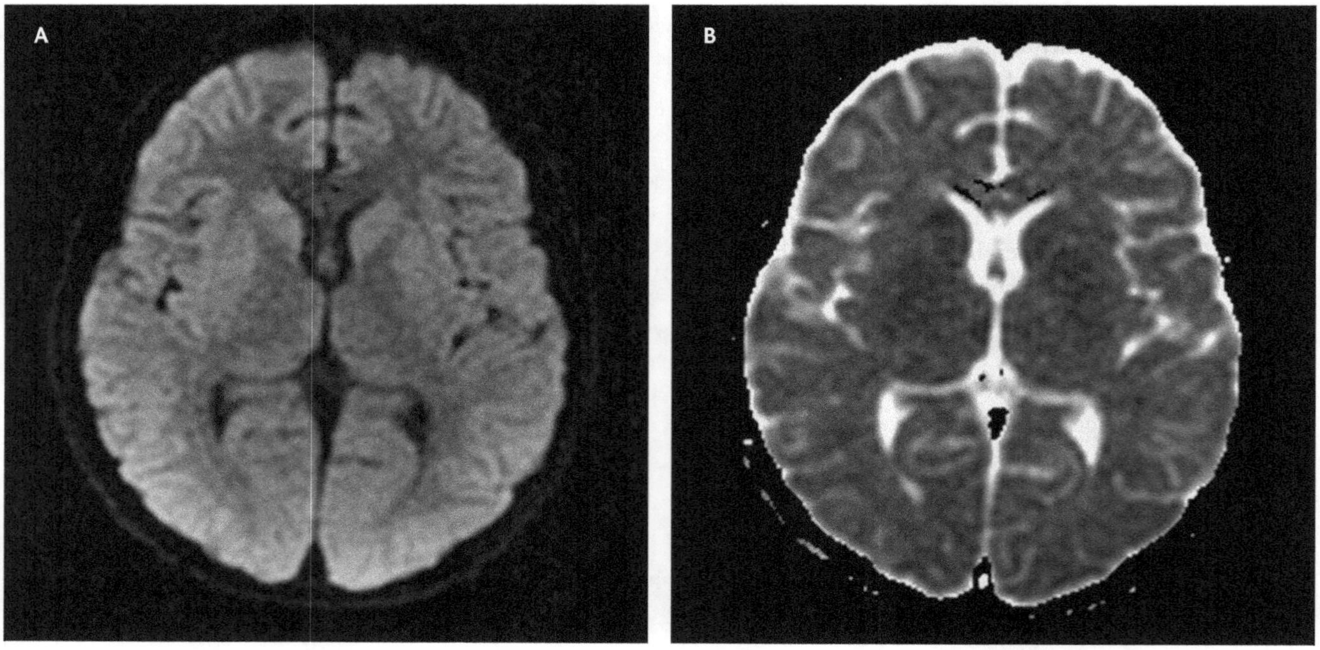

Figures 6-6A and B Clinical example Andy: diffusion series taken while Andy was in the intensive care unit. **A:** DWI. **B:** ADC.

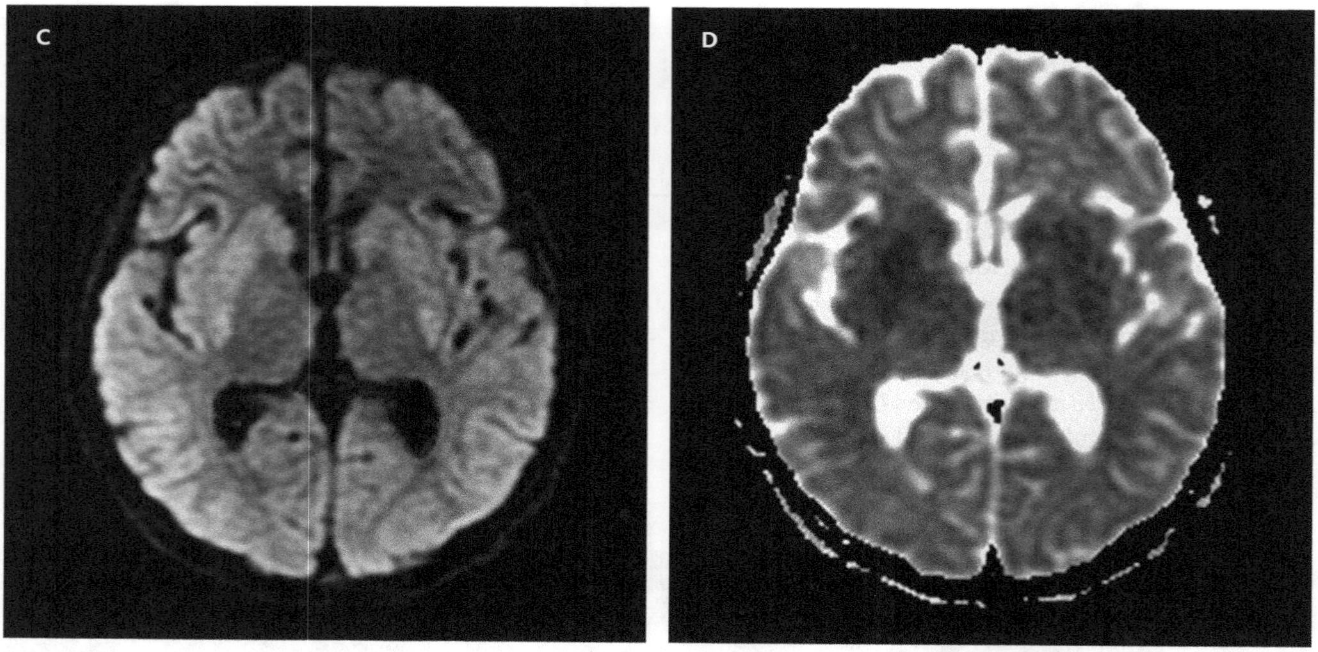

Figures 6-6C and D Clinical example Andy: diffusion series taken 3 weeks after contracting encephalitis with evidence of restricted diffusion within the bilateral basal ganglia structures. **C:** DWI. **D:** ADC.

encephalomalacia and global parenchymal atrophy. Given the severity of some cases of encephalitis, many patients fail to survive the initial stages, with malignant intracranial hypertension from edema or severe damage to the deeper brain structures resulting in death. Other patients with severe diffuse encephalitis may survive the acute stages of the illness, only to be left with profound neurological deficits and functional compromise. It is important to understand that encephalitis can range from very mild and localized to severe and diffuse, with outcomes being highly dependent on the extent and severity of brain injury and on the areas of the brain most affected.

Meningoencephalitis

Meningoencephalitis is a condition in which there is infection of the meningeal layers (meningitis) and the brain parenchyma (encephalitis).

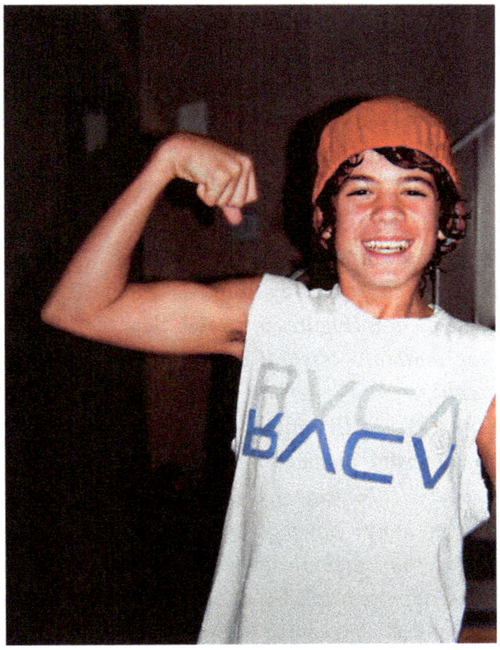

Figure 6-7 Clinical example Tyler: photograph of Tyler taken shortly before onset of meningoencephalitis due to disseminated coccidioidomycosis (Valley Fever).

CLINICAL EXAMPLE

Tyler: Meningoencephalitis due to disseminated coccidioidomycosis (Valley Fever)

Tyler, a delightful 12-year-old young man (Figure 6-7), contracted disseminated coccidioidomycosis, an infection of the brain by spores of the fungus Coccidioides immitis. The infection affected his meninges and brain tissue, resulting in significant medical and functional compromise. In addition to the effects of the fungus on the meninges and brain tissue, the antifungal medications resulted in increased inflammation of the arachnoid layer, a condition called arachnoiditis. Over a period of several weeks, Tyler went through cyclic stages of recovery and relapse, but with the effects of the infection and medications gradually damaging more and more of his brain. The infection of his meninges and fungal growth began to disrupt flow through the blood vessels within the meningeal layers, resulting in microstrokes. Most microstrokes appeared within the deep subcortical gray matter of the basal ganglia.

Proteins in Tyler's cerebrospinal fluid (CSF) increased the viscosity of the fluid to the point that flow through the smaller channels such as the cerebral aqueduct of Sylvius became restricted, necessitating many surgeries to shunt the fluid from the ventricles and cisterns. Eventually, Tyler's functioning deteriorated to being in a state of constant discomfort and confusion; insight and awareness of his environment declined over time.

Throughout his ordeal, Tyler remained strong, and a couple of weeks before succumbing to his illness, he apologized to his parents for getting sick and putting them through the pain of his dying. It is always amazing how children can be so compassionate and giving to others, even in times of severe discomfort and trauma. Tyler's parents kindly gave permission to use his case as an example within this guide so that others might learn from it.

Of the many scans taken of Tyler, those presented here are examples that highlight some of his more salient neurological conditions (Figures 6-8 through 6-13). Ongoing meningeal inflammation with involvement of the subcortical basal ganglia and thalamic structures became evident with progression of Tyler's illness. Imaging findings changed commensurate with adjustments to his treatment regimen and progression of his illness. At times, Tyler experienced improved functioning through the use of antifungal medications, then suffered deterioration due to arachnoiditis. When this occurred his medications were adjusted to improve functioning until the fungal load increased once again. Over time, it became increasingly more difficult to introduce the medications to the areas of greatest fungal load, and Tyler ultimately died from the illness.

The radiology series presented in Figures 6-8 through 6-13 are arranged by date, to highlight the progression of the illness and the changing pathology over the almost 3 months of his hospitalization. Even though the images from December appear less involved than earlier images, it is important to understand the different processes taking place and being highlighted in the images. For example, some of the earlier scans appear worse because of the extensive inflammation, although there was little infarction of tissue or deeper structures. Later images appear better but show lacuna infarctions to the deeper structure. Scans were not obtained close to his death; if they had been, it is likely they would have shown greater inflammation than that in Figures 6-8 through 6-13.

Shortly after Tyler's onset of symptoms in late October, meningeal hyperintensity was evident on CT imaging, most notable within the arachnoid layer around the perimesencephalic cistern, indicated by crosshairs on Figures 6-8A–C. The meningeal hyperintensity is more easily appreciated on MRI T2-weighted imaging than on CT, especially T2 FLAIR and contrast-enhanced T2 FLAIR sequences (Figures 6-9A–C). Note the hyperintensity around the midbrain cerebral peduncles and perimesencephalic or quadrigeminal cistern at the back of the midbrain. On post-contrast T2 FLAIR imaging, notable enhancement around the optic chiasm and medial temporal lobes is evident.

By the middle of November, Tyler's CSF had become so viscous that it was no longer flowing through the ventricular system, especially the thin cerebral aqueduct of Sylvius. On ventriculograms and cisternograms, it was clear that the radio-opaque tracer (white) was not flowing from the lateral ventricles down through the cerebral aqueduct of Sylvius to the fourth ventricle and arachnoid cisterns. The crosshairs are centered over the fourth ventricle on Figures 6-10A–C showing a lack of contrast agent in the fourth ventricle, even though there is contrast agent in the lateral and third ventricles. MRI with and without contrast suggested inflammation of the basal ganglia and thalami structures that was so severe that it was becoming difficult to appreciate the structures on MRI T2 sequences (Figures 11A–C). In addition, prominent meningeal inflammation caused by the fungal infection and antifungal medications was clearly evident on Tyler's post-contrast MRI sequences (Figures 6-12A–C).

By the end of December, the extensive inflammation noted in Figures 6-11A–C had resolved somewhat, allowing for improved visualization of the basal ganglia structures (Figures 6-13A–F). With improved ability to see the basal ganglia and thalamic regions, it became clear that lacuna infarcts or small holes were forming in the subcortical structures (arrows), with some smaller infarcts becoming evident within the white matter, most evident on T2 FLAIR (arrows).

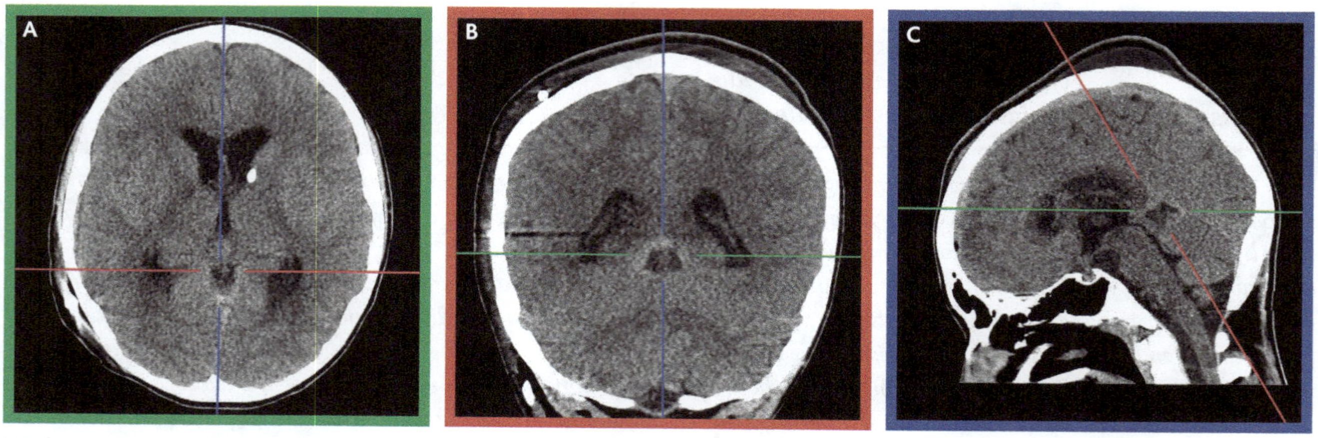

Figures 6-8A–C Clinical example Tyler: CT series acquired shortly after Tyler's onset of symptoms in late October, showing hyperdensity of the arachnoid layer.

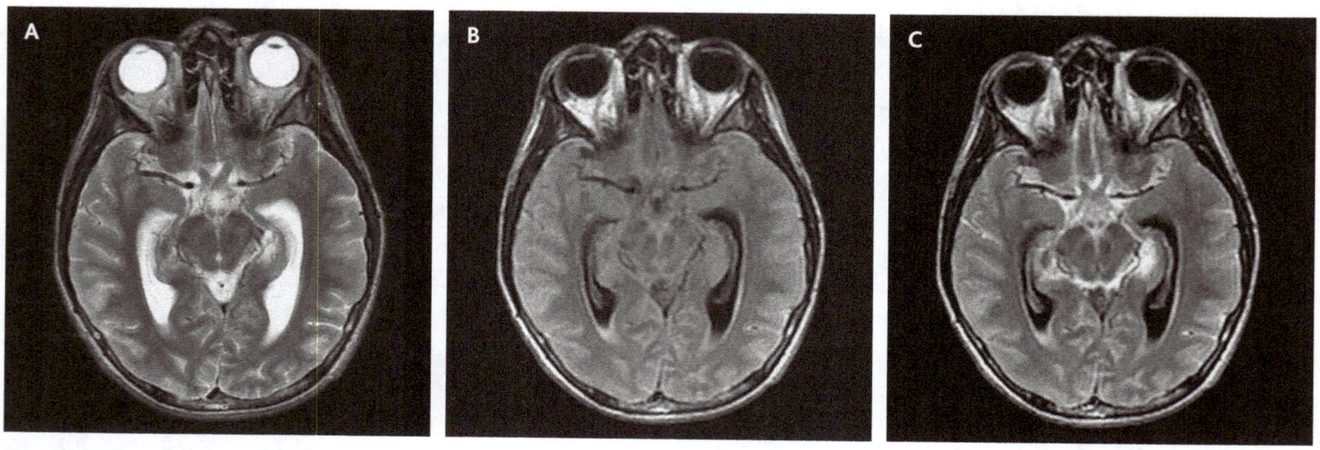

Figures 6-9A–C Clinical example Tyler: MRI series with, and without contrast, showing the hyperintensity of the meningeal layers, most evident on contrast imaging. **A:** T2. **B:** T2 FLAIR. **C:** Contrast-enhanced T2 FLAIR.

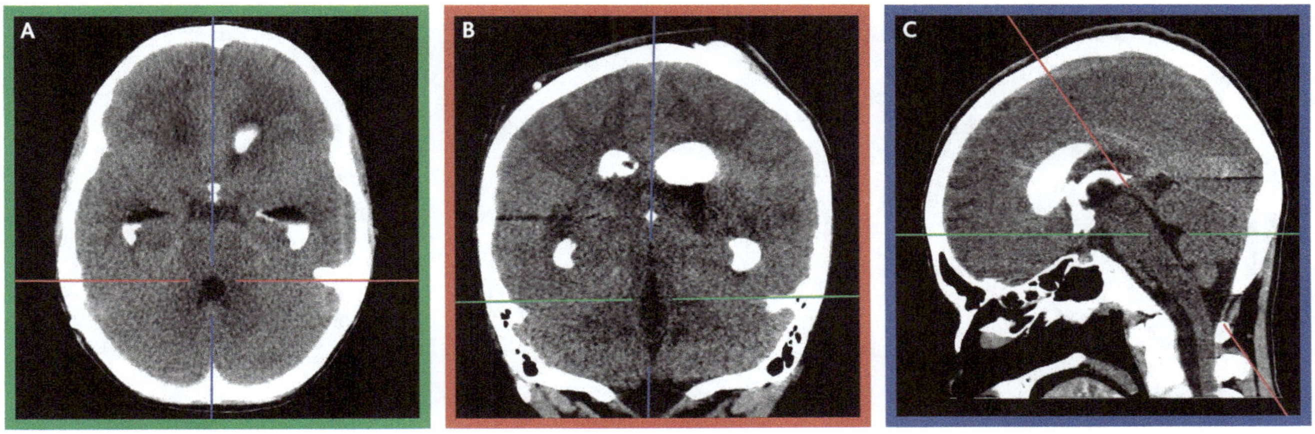

Figures 6-10A–C Clinical example Tyler: ventriculograms and cisternograms showing a lack of CSF flow through the cerebral aqueduct of Sylvius to the fourth ventricle and arachnoid cisterns.

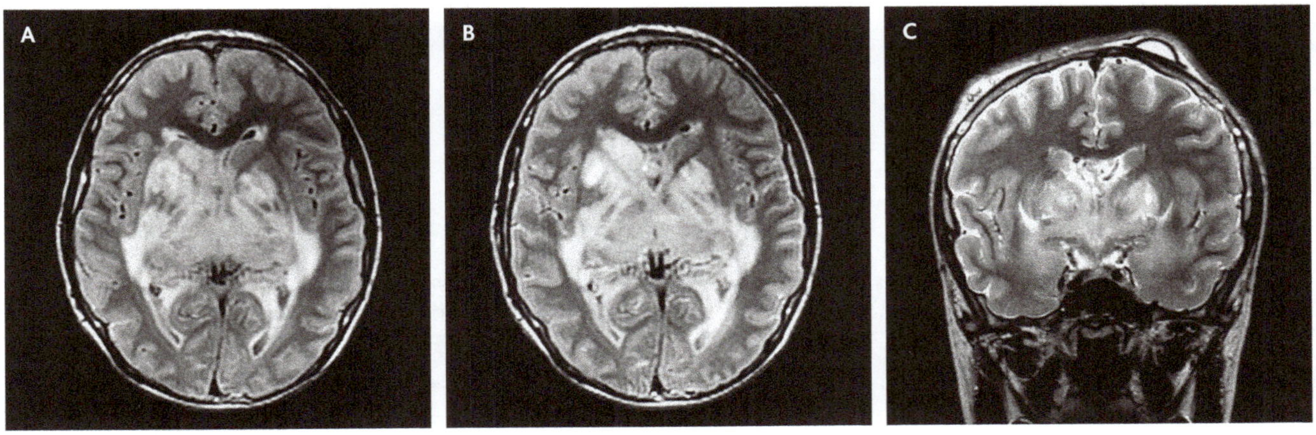

Figures 6-11A–C Clinical example Tyler: T2 MRI series with, and without contrast, acquired in mid-November, showing extensive inflammation of the basal ganglia and thalami. **A:** T2 FLAIR. **B:** Contrast-enhanced T2 FLAIR. **C:** T2.

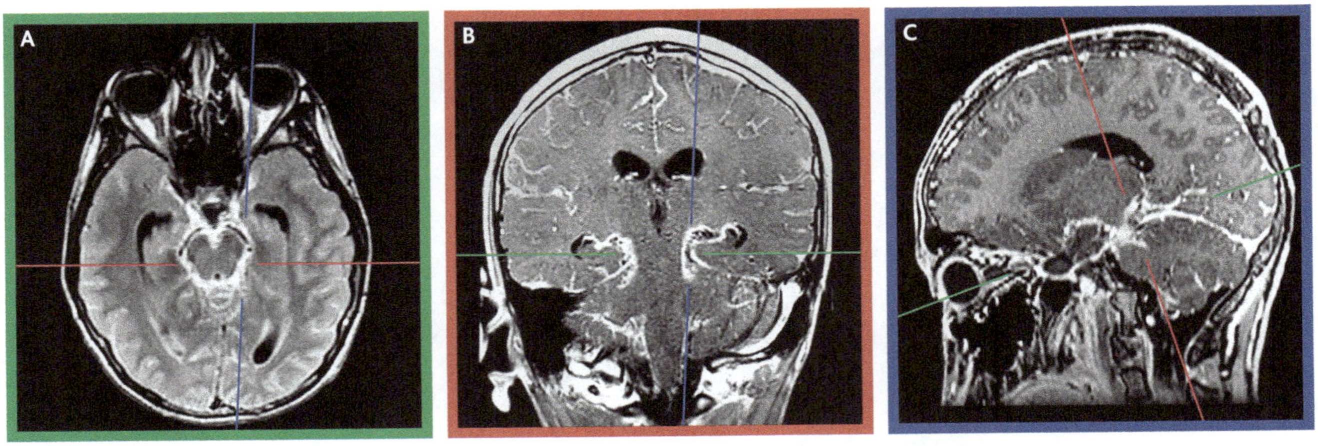

Figures 6-12A–C Clinical example Tyler: contrast-enhanced T2 and T1 images acquired in mid-November, showing prominent meningeal inflammation. **A:** CE T2 FLAIR. **B:** CE T1. **C:** CE 3D T1 FSPGR.

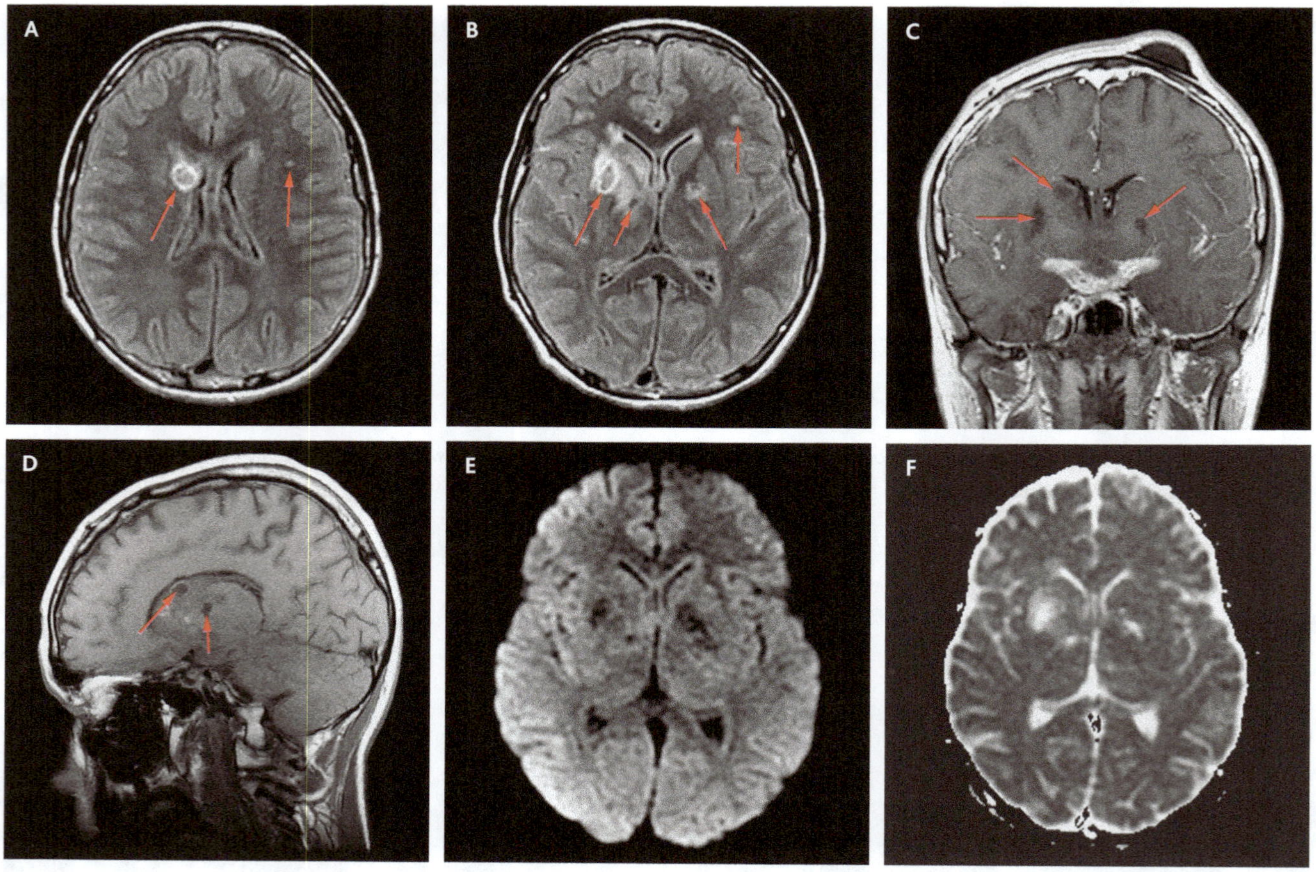

Figures 6-13A–F Clinical example Tyler: MRI series acquired late December, showing lacuna infarcts mostly within Tyler's basal ganglia and thalamic regions, but alsow within his white matter (arrows). **A:** T2 FLAIR. **B:** T2 FLAIR. **C:** T1. **D:** T1. **E:** DWI. **F:** ADC.

Abscess

Brain abscesses form over time. The abscess will start as cerebritis and eventually become encapsulated within a defined collagen and reticulin wall. Inside the wall there is a core of necrotic and inflammatory substances, and outside the wall, there is often edema. The capsule wall often shows enhancement with the use of contrast agents. Brain abscesses can easily be confused with high-grade tumors that also have edema surrounding a ring-enhancing lesion. As an abscess forms and matures, the appearance on brain imaging can change.

Non-contrast CT may show the hypodense edema and lesion, in addition to any mass effect. The rim of the capsule may appear slightly hyperdense on non-contrast CT. Figures 6-14A–C illustrate the appearance of a large left frontal abscess with extensive edema covering most of the left frontal lobe. The abscess capsule is identified by the hyperdense ring surrounding the hypodense center. Midline

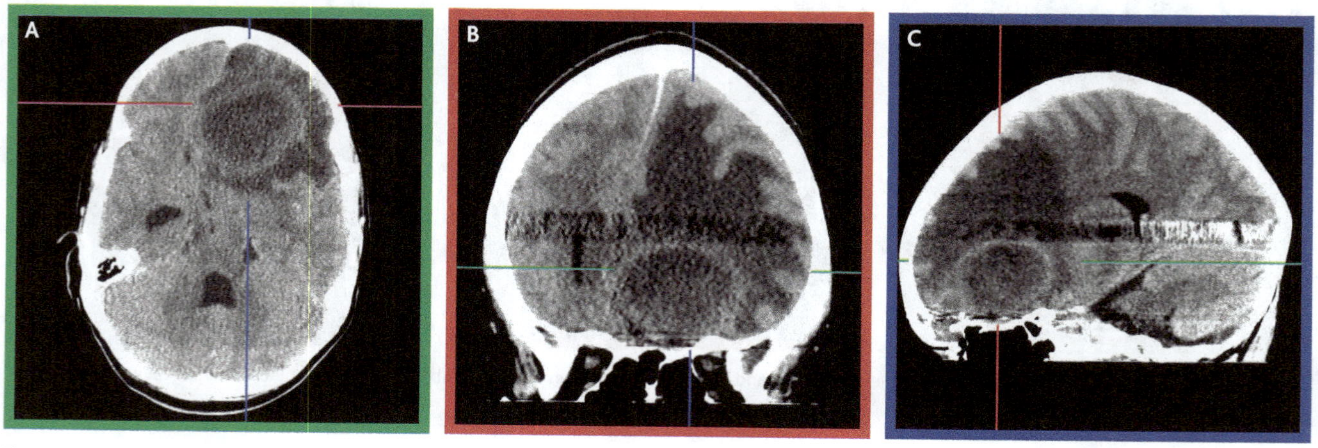

Figures 6-14A–C CT series showing a large left frontal abscess with extensive edema covering most of the left frontal lobe.

shift from the mass effect of the abscess is also readily evident. Rim enhancement may be seen on post-contrast CT, with a low-density core inside the capsule. On MRI, T2 and contrast-enhanced T1 sequences combined with DWI and ADC may be most useful. T2 images often show a hyperintense mass early in abscess formation and later a hyperintense mass surrounded by the hypointense rim. Edema surrounding the abscess will be hyperintense on T2-weighted sequences. T1 contrast-enhanced sequences may show a hyperintense, well-defined ring surrounding the abscess. Sometimes, contrast enhancement appears greater on the ventricle side of an abscess than on the side away from the ventricles. Diffusion imaging can show increased signal on DWI and decreased signal on ADC because of restricted diffusion within the abscess.

Empyema

Empyema is a collection of pus that is not encapsulated, as is true with an abscess. Empyema is generally found within the extra-axial space above the dura (epidural), below the dura (subdural), or within both cavities.

On imaging, the inflammatory component is often evident on contrast sequences as an enhancing border between the empyema and other tissue. Displacement of the dura by the extra-axial fluid may also suggest empyema. Similar to bleeds within the extra-axial space, the shape of the pus cavity differs depending on the location of the empyema. Epidural empyema often takes on a lenticular shape, similar to that of an epidural hematoma. Subdural empyema often takes on a crescent shape, similar to that of a subdural hematoma.

On non-contrast CT, the fluid collection may appear isodense to hyperdense compared to CSF. The border of the fluid is enhanced on contrast CT, similar to that on MRI. Non-contrast T1 imaging may show empyema as hyperintense to CSF, with notable margin enhancement on contrast T1 sequences. On T2 imaging, empyema may appear isointense to hyperintense compared to CSF, with the dura appearing hypointense or as a darker line. Given the inflammatory nature of empyema, T2 FLAIR imaging can appear hyperintense. Diffusion imaging may show restricted diffusion or a lighter appearance on DWI and a darker appearance on ADC.

Sometimes a patient will present with a combination of abscess and empyema, a condition that can produce significant long-term damage to the brain, as in the patient Jeanette (see clinical example).

CLINICAL EXAMPLE

Jeanette: Right Frontal Lobe Infection with Abscess and Empyema

Jeanette was hospitalized with an infection of her brain, mostly within the right frontal lobe. On imaging, she had evidence of both abscess and empyema within the epidural and subdural spaces. The abscess is best visualized on the contrast enhanced CT series (Figures 6-15A and B), as low-density edema surrounding the bright enhancing circular shaped capsule of the abscess. The epidural empyema is seen on standard and contrast enhanced CT within the longitudinal fissure, and involves the superior and frontal portions of the falx cerebri (Figures 6-16A–D). Subdural empyema is seen within the frontal lobe and between the tentorium and occipital lobe on Figures 6-17A and B (arrows).

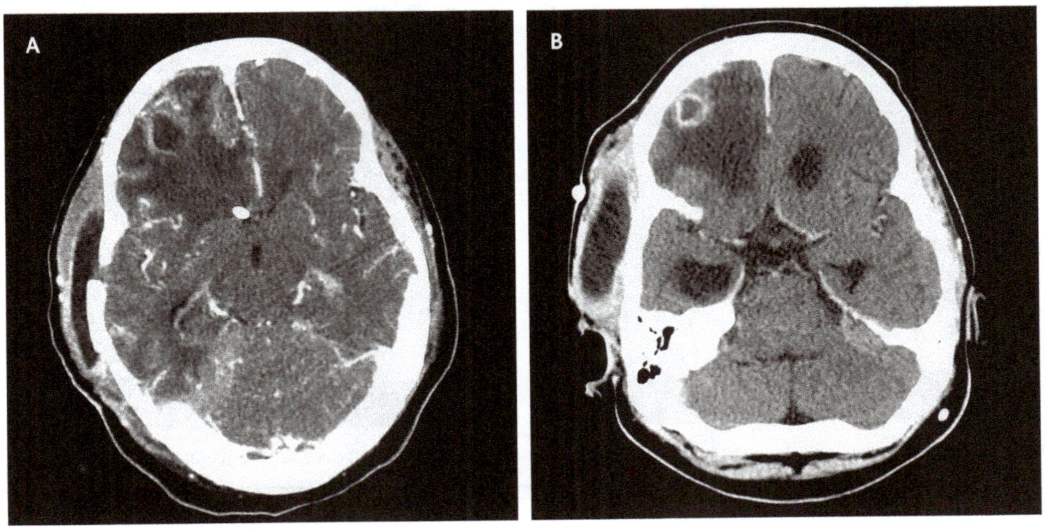

Figures 6-15A and B Clinical example Jeanette: CT series showing small right frontal abscess.

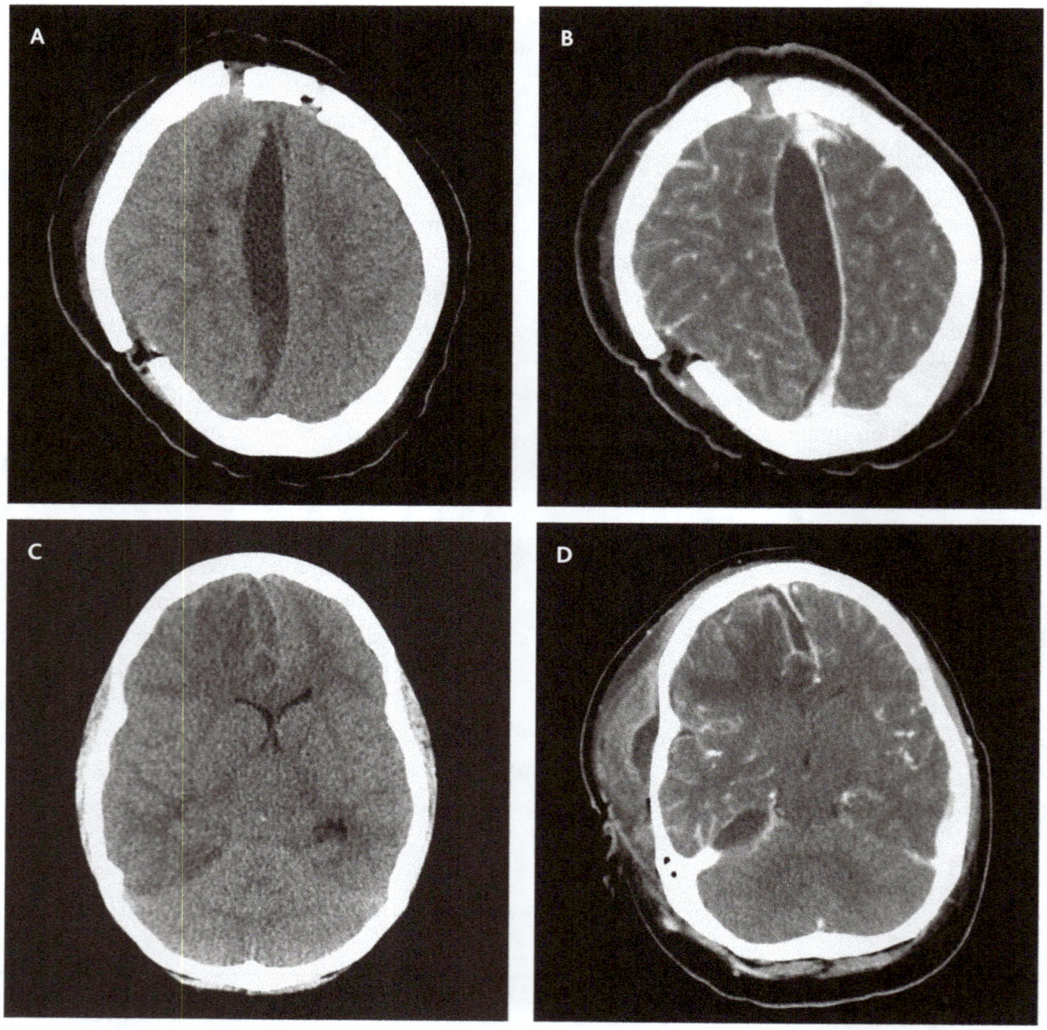

Figures 6-16A–D Clinical example Jeanette: epidural empyema within the longitudinal fissure involving the superior and frontal falx cerebri. **A:** CT. **B:** Contrast-enhanced CT. **C:** CT. **D:** Contrast-enhanced CT.

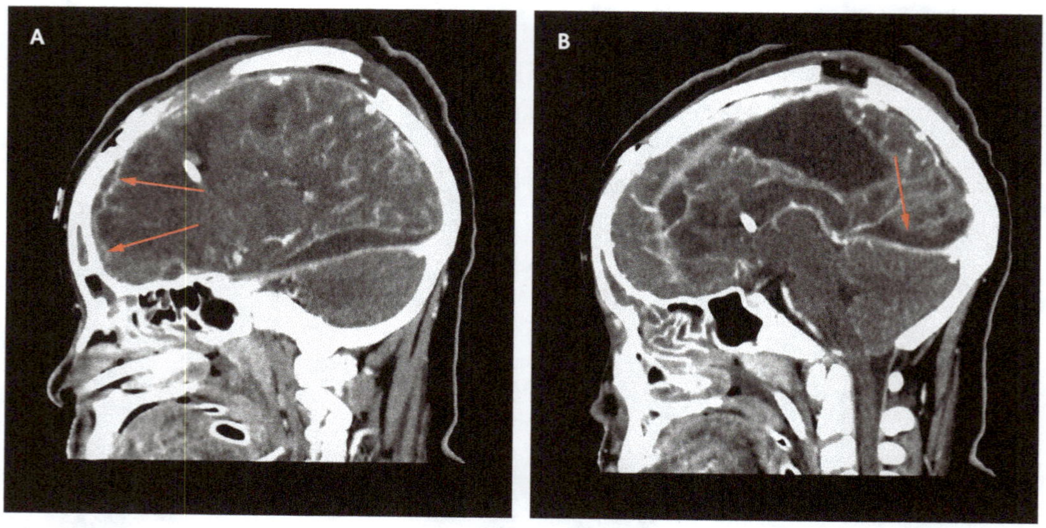

Figures 6-17A and B Clinical example Jeanette: contrast-enhanced CT series showing areas of subdural empyema (arrows).

STROKE AND VASCULAR PATHOLOGIES

Stroke is a general term referring to a cerebral vascular accident (CVA) resulting from either reduced blood flow or uncontrolled release of blood caused by damage to a vessel wall, surgical procedures, or clotting disorders. Reduced blood flow can be caused by a variety of processes, including but not limited to embolic blockage, vascular spasm, and pressure against a blood vessel reducing the inner lumen diameter. Clinically, the term *stroke* can result in confusion because of its many causes and because a stroke can involve either reduced blood flow or bleeding into the brain, depending on the specific pathological condition.

Nontraumatic strokes can result in damage ranging from small petechial infarctions, when tiny vessels are involved, to large ischemic infarction involving one or more vessel territories. Some of the images from the clinical example of Tyler described above show lacunar infarctions from occlusion of the lenticulostriate arteries leading from the middle cerebral artery to the basal ganglia. Like that seen in Tyler, lacuna infarctions due to vascular compromise are most commonly seen within the deep subcortical nuclei of the basal ganglia and thalami.

Nontraumatic vascular pathologies frequently result in reduced flow of oxygenated blood to brain parenchyma, leading to ischemic infarction. As noted in previous chapters, the appearance of blood on brain imaging changes over time as it passes through hyperacute, acute, subacute, and chronic stages. Any evaluation of bleeds within the brain should take into account the expected appearance of blood given the age of the bleed (see Table 2-4). Spontaneous hemorrhaging is more common in older patients with hypertension, although it is also seen in patients with vascular anomalies such as arteriovenous malformations (AVMs), aneurysms, or cavernomas.

Imaging Nontraumatic Hemorrhagic Strokes—Cerebral Vascular Accident

Non-contrast CT imaging is often the technique of choice for assessing hemorrhagic strokes, although the earliest CVAs may not be evident on CT imaging. Hyperacute and acute bleeds can initially look isodense or heterogeneous, with the brightness of the hemorrhage increasing over the first few hours and becoming hyperdense up to a few days following the hemorrhage. Commensurate with the changes over the first few hours to days, there is often an increase in edema and mass effect of the surrounding parenchyma. As seen in post-traumatic hemorrhages, a swirl sign may suggest ongoing bleeding. After several days, the bright appearance of the blood may decline, with the hemorrhage becoming isodense over the next month or so. Contrast-enhanced CT may be helpful during active bleeding and after a few days, with the appearance of a hyperdense rim to the bleed.

MR imaging has improved our ability to appreciate hemorrhagic stokes, especially with the addition of gradient echo (GRE), susceptibility-weighted imaging (SWI), DWI, ADC, and perfusion-weighted imaging (PWI) sequences. Diffusion sequences are often the first to become abnormal shortly following a CVA, with evidence of restricted diffusion. The combination of DWI and ADC is useful for identifying an ischemic area, although it is important to rule out T2 shine-through from edema. Comparison of DWI and ADC images can be useful in differentiating ischemia from T2 shine-through. A combination of DWI and PWI sequences may indicate an ischemic penumbra, with a salvageable noninfarcted border zone where diffusion is still intact but perfusion is reduced. On non-contrast T1-weighted imaging, bleeds may appear hypointense to isointense, with a hyperintense border forming over a few days to weeks. T2-weighted imaging is often more revealing: recent hemorrhages appear bright, and the blood changes to hypointense and the surrounding edema to hyperintense over the first few hours to days. FLAIR sequences follow a similar course, although they may be easier to interpret given the attenuation of CSF. GRE and SWI sequences are useful for isolating blood: the susceptibility artifact of the hemorrhage results in dark, hypointense blooming on the images.

CLINICAL EXAMPLE

Erin: Spontaneous Hemorrhagic Stroke due to Ruptured Arteriovenous Malformation

Erin was hospitalized following rupture of a large left parietal arteriovenous malformation (AVM), resulting in significant hemorrhagic stroke. Angiography prior to coiling, embolizing, and surgical clipping reveals the tangle of vessels that form the AVM within Erin's left parietal lobe (Figures 6-18A–D). The appearance of an AVM on angiography is often described as being like a pile of worms, as is evident on Erin's scans. Erin underwent interventional radiologic treatment with coiling and embolization, followed by surgical clipping. On CT (Figures 6-19A–C), the left parietal bright spot with starburst radiations is the coil. The poorly defined white patches are blood, with the darker surround being edema with some likely encephalomalacia. The right frontal white spot is from an external ventricular drain. There is subtle mass effect causing midline shift evident in left-hemisphere to right-hemisphere bowing of the falx cerebri.

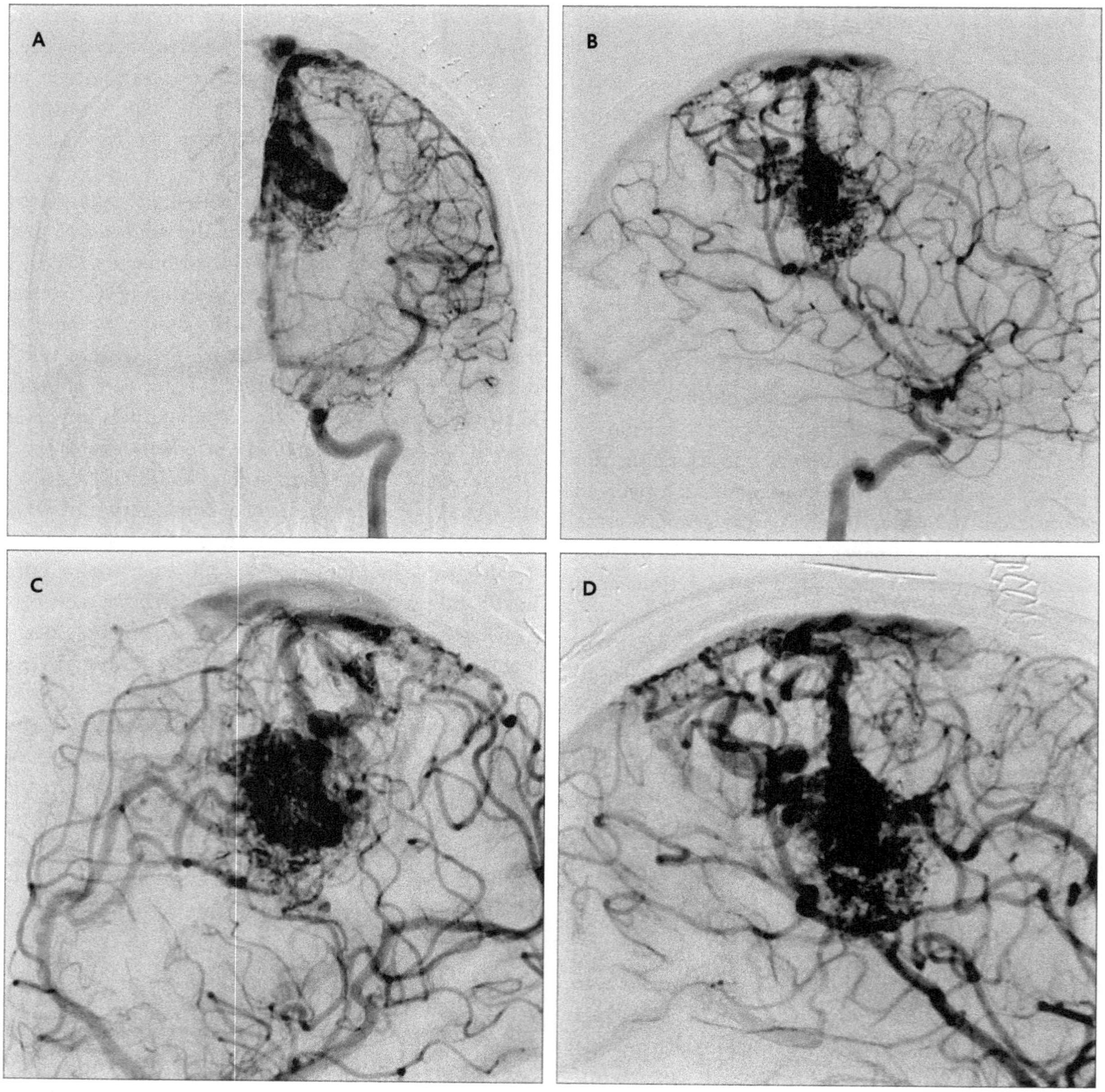

Figures 6-18A–D Clinical example Erin: spontaneous hemorrhagic stroke due to a ruptured arteriovenous malformation.

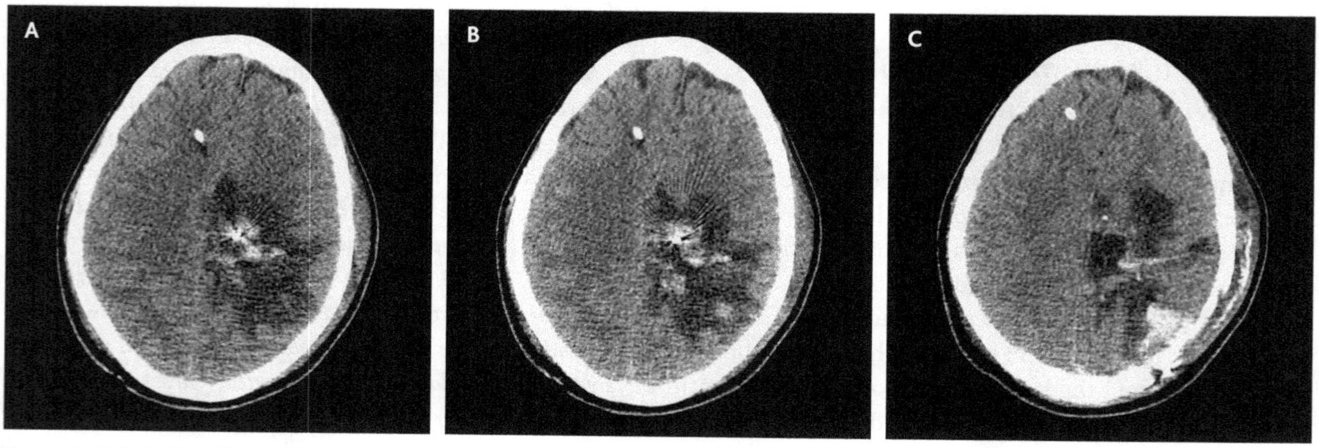

Figures 6-19A–C Clinical example Erin: CT series after coiling and embolization.

CLINICAL EXAMPLE

Pilar: Ruptured Arteriovenous Malformation

Pilar was hospitalized secondary to a ruptured AVM. However, in this case, there was only minimal parenchymal disruption; the hemorrhage was predominantly intraventricular. On contrast-enhanced CT imaging (Figures 6-20A–C) the intraventricular blood takes on a light gray appearance within the ventricular system.

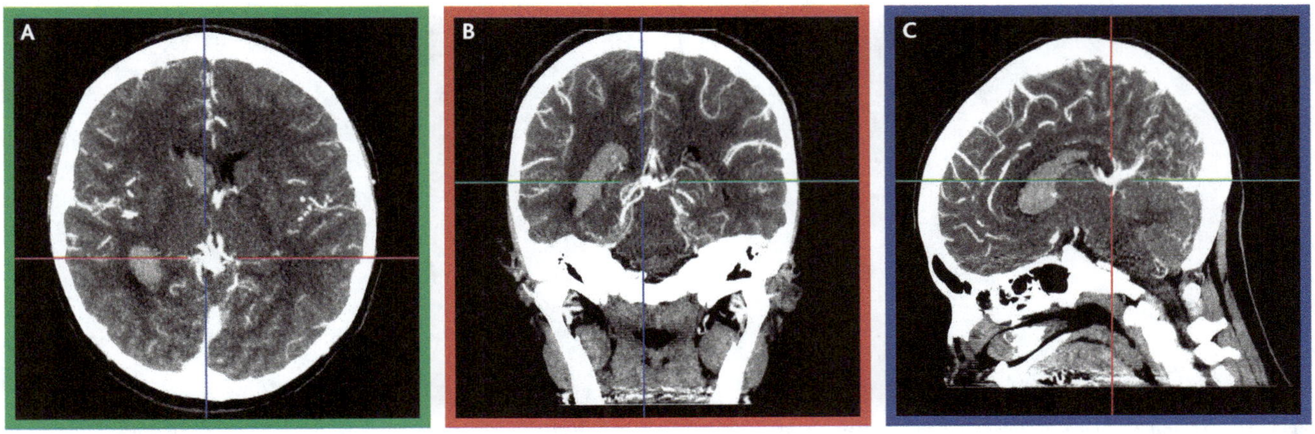

Figures 6-20A–C Clinical example Pilar: contrast-enhanced CT series showing ruptured AVM resulting in an intraventricular hemorrhage.

Hemorrhagic Cavernomas

Cavernomas are also called cavernous malformations or cavernous angiomas. Cavernomas are formed from tiny vascular lobules, their appearance often described as being similar to a mulberry, raspberry, or popcorn with a hemosiderin ring. They are similar in size to a small table grape. The lobules are filled with blood at various stages of decomposition, and unlike AVMs, there may be no significant blood flow through the lesion. Unless there is notable hemorrhage of the cavernoma, it generally will not show enhancement on contrast imaging. Given the lack of blood flow through the lesion, a cavernoma does not show up on standard angiography unless there is an active bleed. Because cavernomas are generally not visible on an angiogram, they are sometimes referred to as angiographically occult vascular malformations (AOVMs). Time-of-flight (TOF) imaging may show cavernomas, although they can appear relatively faint because of the lack of significant blood flow through the lesion.

Some patients have multiple cavernomas, resulting in significant disruption of neurological functioning, as was true of Leone who underwent a long history of surgical interventions to treat multiple cavernous malformations (see clinical example Leone).

CLINICAL EXAMPLE

Christopher: New-Onset Seizures Caused by a Small Cavernoma

Christopher experienced new-onset siezures at the age of 25 that were caused by a small cavernoma. The cavernoma was not visible on AP or lateral angiography conducted as part of a pre-surgical assessment (Figures 6-21A and B). Cavernomas are best viewed using a combination of non-contrast and contrast-enhanced sequences in addition to GRE or SWI. On T2 imaging (Figures 6-22A–C) the cavernoma can take on a dappled form, sometimes referred to as a "popcorn" appearance. On standard T1 imaging without contrast, the lobular structure of the cavernoma may be visible and appear slightly hypointense (Figures 6-22D–F), and on contrast T1 and T2 sequences the cavernoma may enhance to provide a hyperintense appearance (Figures 6-22G–I). Because cavernomas contain blood products at various stages of breakdown and can seep small quantities of blood, they are often evident on GRE or SWI sequences. On GRE and SWI, cavernomas take on a blotchy or black-blooming appearance, especially around the border.

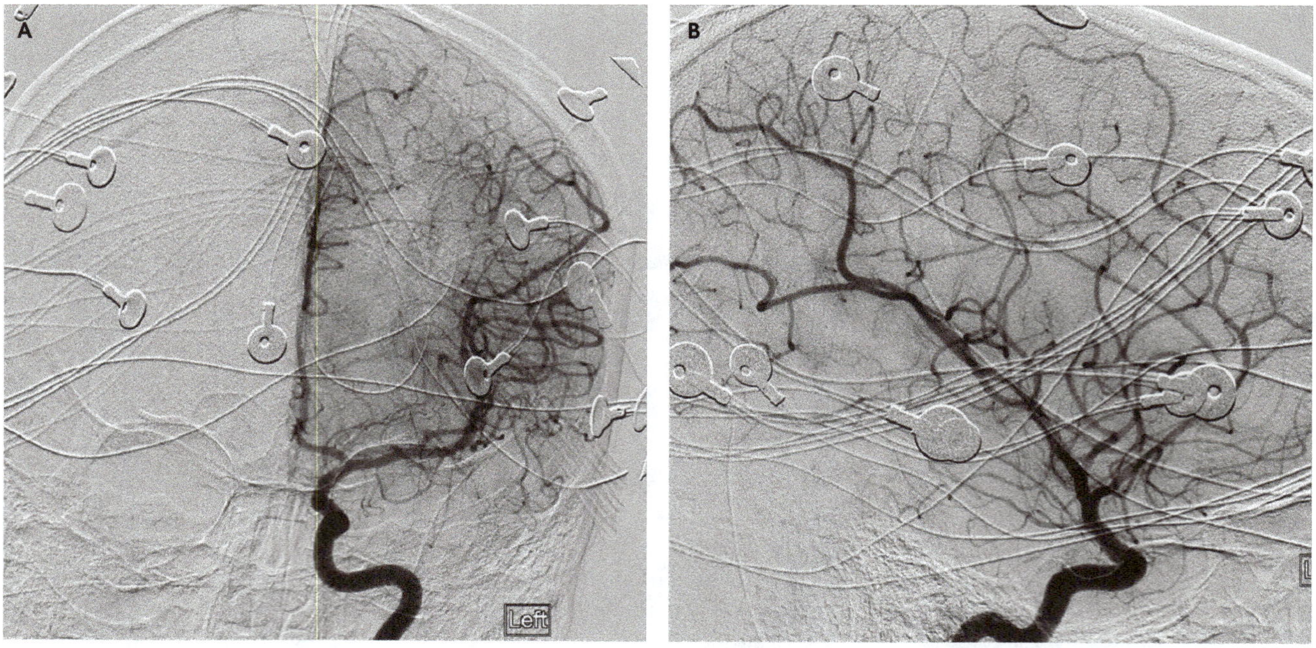

Figures 6-21A and B Clinical example Christopher: new-onset seizures caused by a small cavernoma not visible on angiography. **A:** AP angiography. **B:** Lateral angiography.

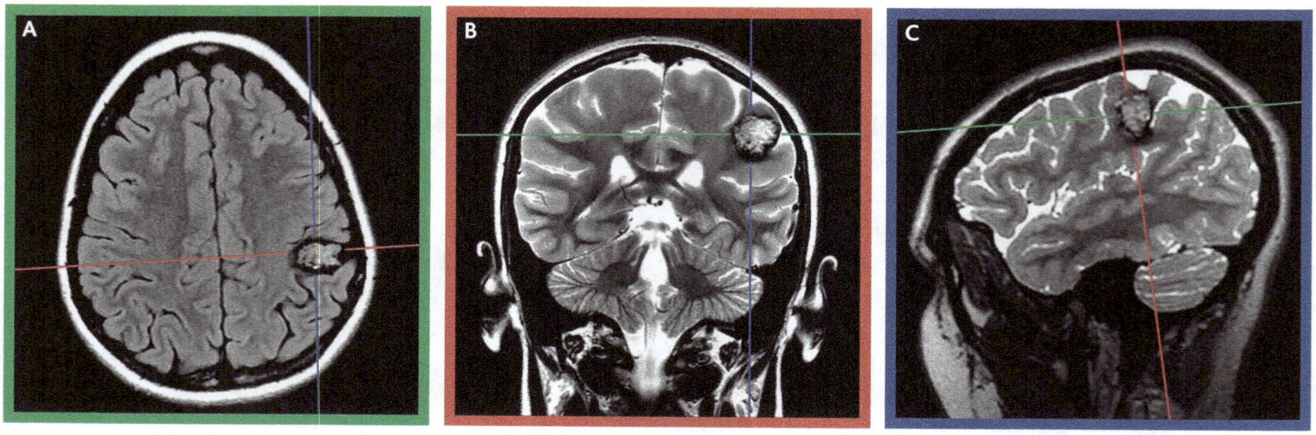

Figures 6-22A–C Clinical example Christopher: T2 series of cavernoma. **A:** T2 FLAIR. **B:** T2. **C:** T2 cube.

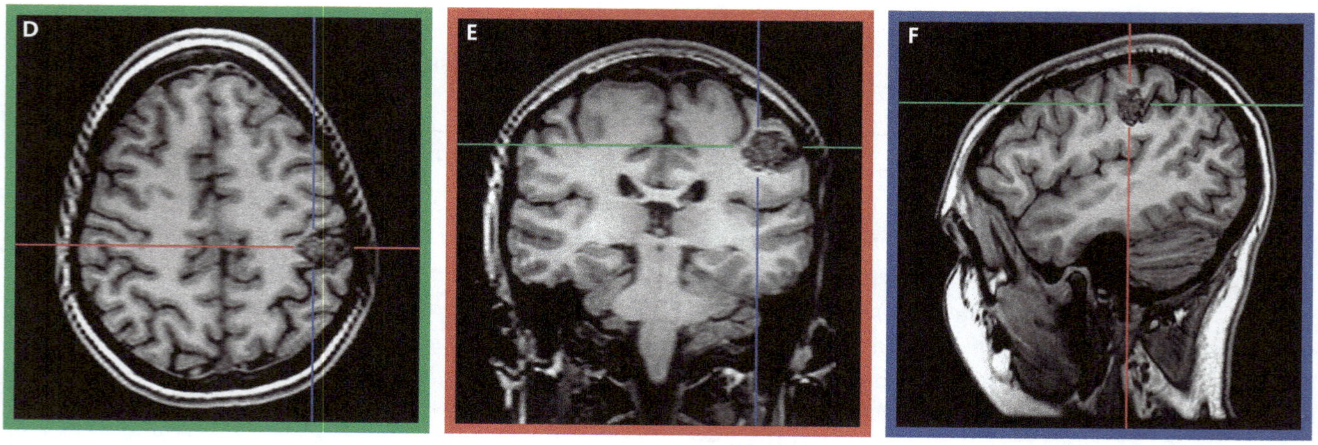

Figures 6-22D–F Clinical example Christopher: non-contrast T1 BRAVO series of cavernoma.

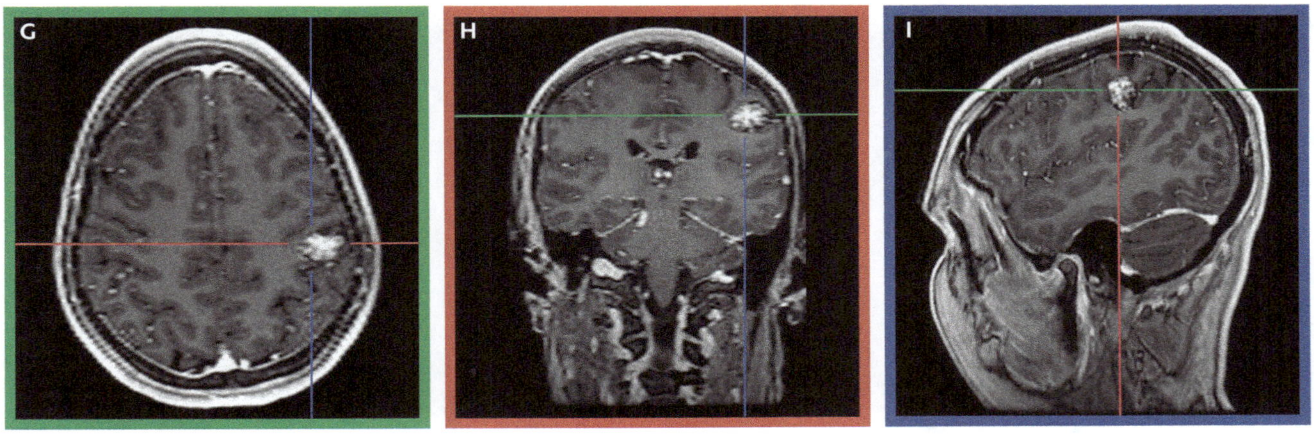

Figures 6-22G–I Clinical example Christopher: post-contrast T1 series of cavernoma showing clear enhancement of the lesion.

CLINICAL EXAMPLE

Leone: Multiple Cavernomas—the Largest Within the Left Basal Ganglia and Thalamic Region

Leone's largest cavernoma was within the left subcortical basal ganglia and thalamic region. It resulted in a right hemiparesis and compromise to cognition, likely because of the direct effects of the lesion in addition to the secondary hydrocephalus resulting from compression of the third ventricle and cerebral aqueduct. Shunt placement was necessary to control CSF pressure, which resulted in partial resolution of the cognitive difficulties. As small amounts of blood can seep out of cavernomas, small lesions may be visible on GRE (Figures 6-23A–C) or SWI, even if they do not appear on other sequences.

The primary lesion increased in size over a several-year period, leading to gradual deterioration of Leone's motor functioning until eventually he experienced full paralysis on the right side. The primary cavernoma extended to an area normally occupied by the internal capsule, including the posterior limb and cerebral peduncle containing both motor and sensory fibers.

Surgical excision of the largest cavernoma in the left basal ganglia region was performed in order to relieve some of the disruption to the internal capsule and cerebral peduncle pathways (corticospinal tract). To provide a measure of internal capsule axon integrity, DTI fractional anisotropy (FA) maps and tractography was used before and after surgery (see Chapter 4 for examples of these technologies). Interestingly, prior to surgery, on FA imaging and tractography there was complete disruption of diffusion within the internal capsule on the left side, likely due to growth of the primary cavernoma (Figures 6-23D–F). However, after surgery, FA imaging and tractography demonstrated diffusion within a small region of the corticospinal

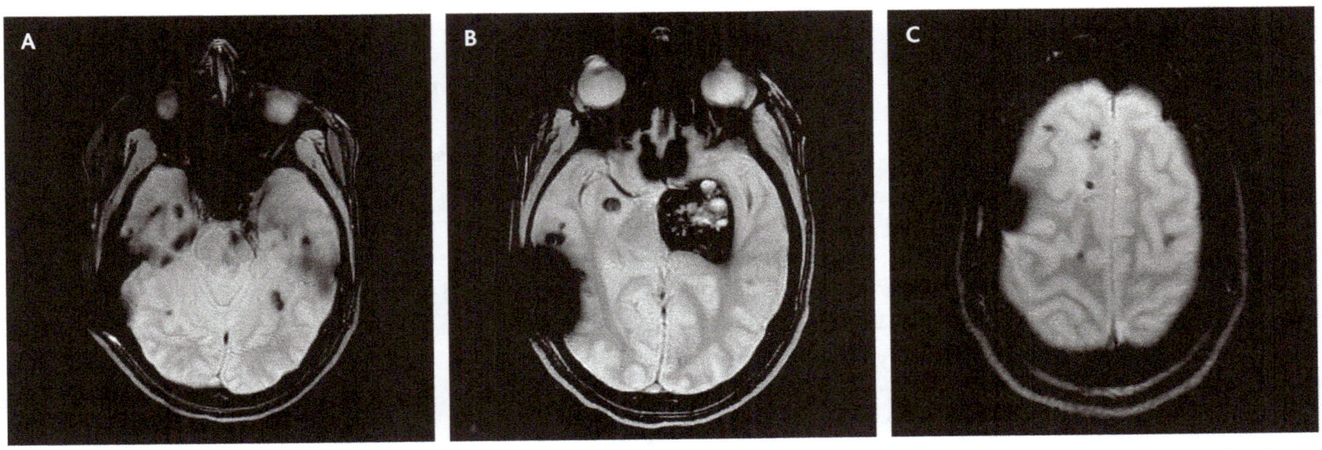

Figures 6-23A–C Clinical example Leone: GRE series of multiple cavernomas, easily visualized due to the black appearance of blooming caused by the magnetic susceptibility of blood products seeping out of cavernomas.

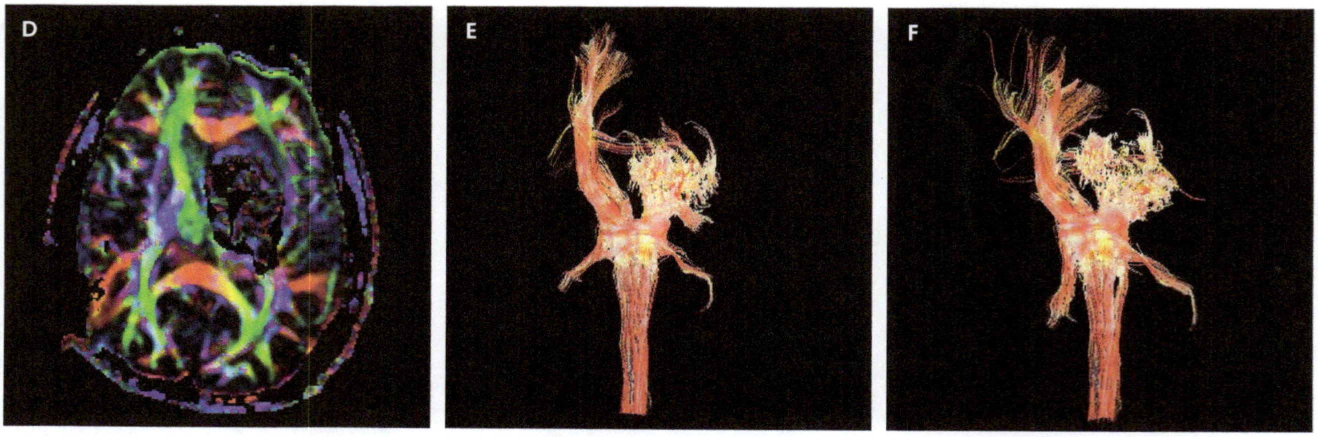

Figures 6-23D–F Clinical example Leone: FA map and tractography acquired prior to Leone's surgery to resect the largest cavernoma within the left subcortical and thalamic region. **D:** FA map. **E:** DTI tractography. **F:** DTI tractography.

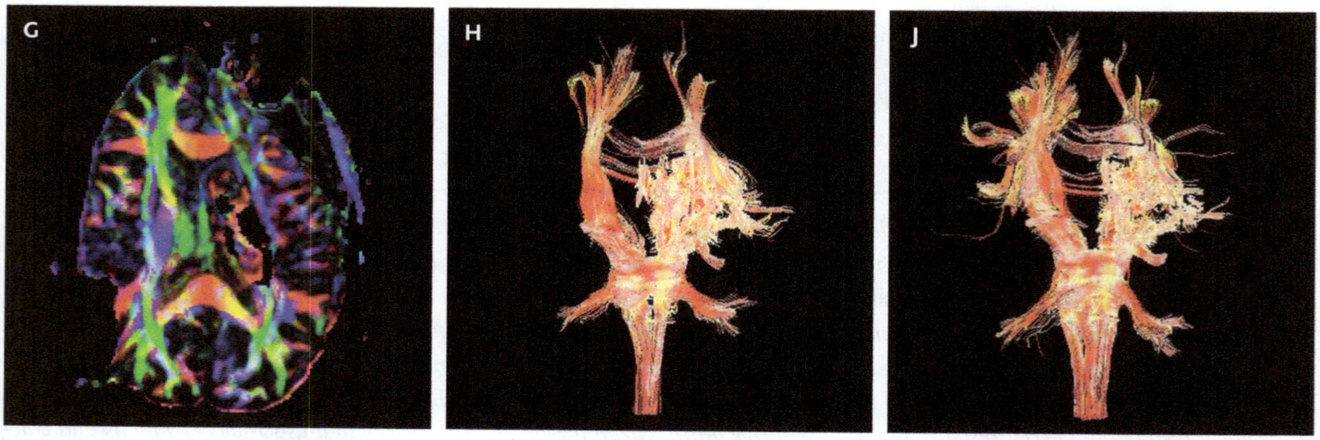

Figures 6-23G–I Clinical example Leone: FA map and tractography following Leone's surgery to resect the largest cavernoma within the left subcortical and thalamic region. **G:** FA map. **H:** DTI tractography. **I:** DTI tractography.

tract, likely due to recovery of functioning within parts of the internal capsule (Figures 6-23G–I). Most pathways through the region of the primary cavernoma were highly disorganized, accounting for the persistence of Leone's right-sided paralysis following surgery. While mild recovery of motor strength on the right side was noted post-surgery, it was not of the magnitude to enable full motor functioning, especially with the right upper extremity.

Bleeding Disorders Resulting in Spontaneous Hemorrhage

Bleeding disorders can result in spontaneous hemorrhaging into the brain. Symptoms are varied and depend on the location of the bleeds.

CLINICAL EXAMPLE

Ambros: Idiopathic Thrombocytopenic Purpura

Ambros suffered from idiopathic thrombocytopenic purpura (ITP), a condition that can lead to spontaneous hemorrhaging in the brain. Review of brain imaging suggested that Ambros had suffered from multiple intraparenchymal bleeds, the largest being in the cerebellum and smaller hemorrhages being in the thalamus and subcortical white matter. On CT imaging (Figures 6-24A–C), the hemorrhages are easily appreciated as blotches of hyperdensity spread throughout the cerebellum and subcortical structures. The hemorrhages are readily identifiable on the MRI series (6-25A–D), especially the T2 FLAIR sequence with hyperintense edema surrounding the core of the hemorrhages and on GRE, with the hemorrhages identified as dark areas of blooming because of the magnetic susceptibility of blood. Diffusion imaging indicates lacuna infarction at the core of the thalamic lesion, with isotropic diffusion suggested by the dark appearance on DWI and bright appearance on ADC (arrows).

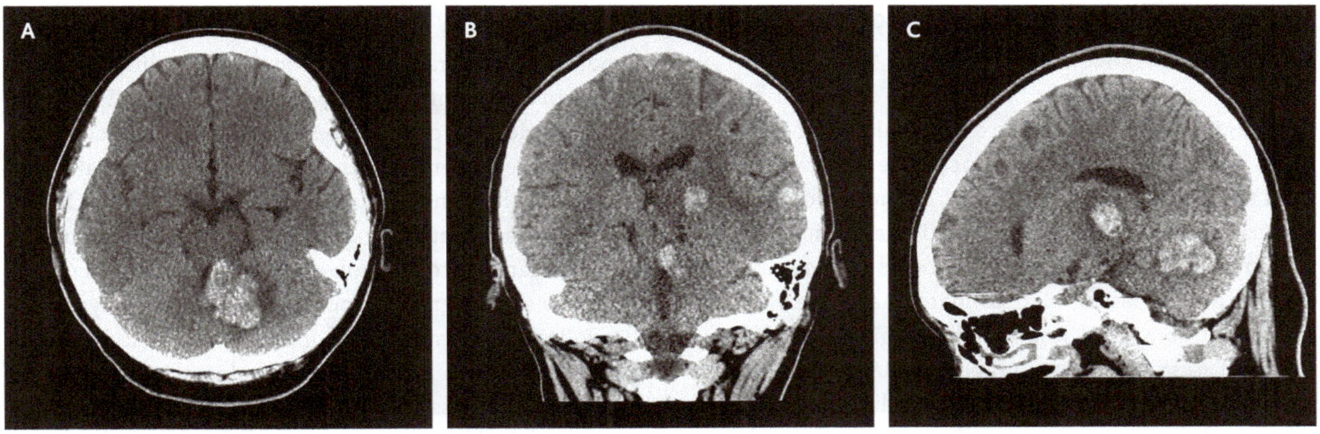

Figures 6-24A–C Clinical example Ambros: CT series of multiple Intraparenchymal hemorrhages caused by idiopathic thrombocytopenic purpura (ITP).

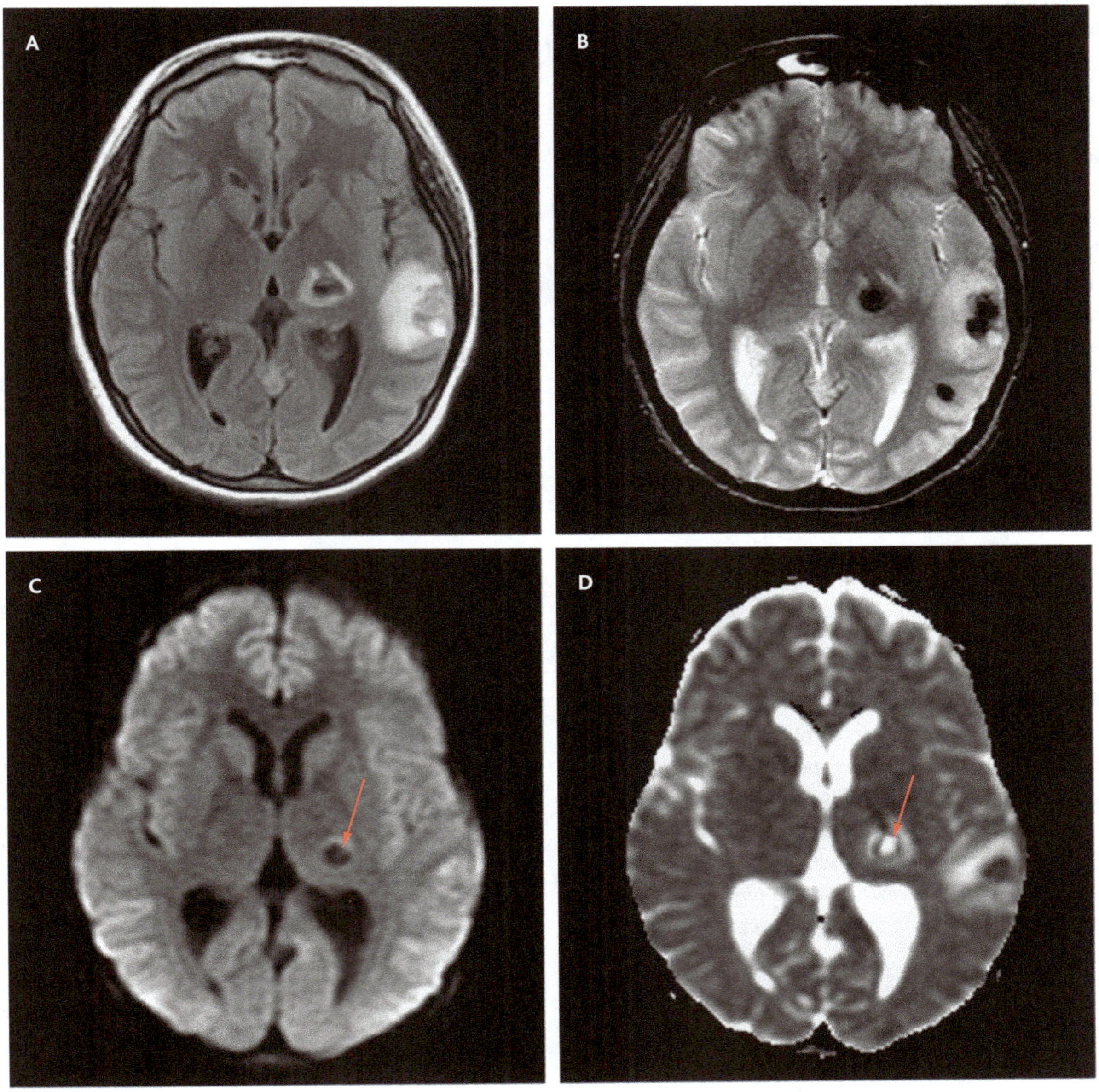

Figures 6-25A–D Clinical example Ambros: MRI series showing multiple intraparenchymal hemorrhages and lacuna infarction on diffusion imaging (arrows). **A:** T2 FLAIR. **B:** GRE. **C:** DWI. **D:** ADC.

Nonhemorrhagic and Embolic Ischemic Strokes

Nonhemorrhagic ischemic strokes resulting from reduced blood flow have a different appearance on brain imaging than that of hemorrhagic strokes. Reduced blood flow can lead to ischemic infarction of brain tissue, without the signs of hemorrhage. Sometimes an embolus or restricted flow through a vessel is visible on standard image slices, although the use of computed tomographic angiography (CTA) or magnetic resonance angiography (MRA) sequences may be required to fully appreciate the condition. Arterial flow through the larger vessels frequently results in relatively circumscribed and homogeneous damage that is isolated to the territory of the involved vessel. Hypoxic ischemic injuries to single arterial vessels have a relatively unique appearance on brain imaging. Because of the bifurcation of larger vessels to smaller vessels, the vascular territory takes on a wedge or delta shape. Ischemic injuries with a wedge appearance suggest disruption of a primary arterial vessel, such as the middle cerebral artery. With independent blood supplies flowing to the right and left internal carotid, anterior and middle cerebral arteries, single-vessel ischemic infarctions generally produce unilateral injury to the brain. The exception is the basilar artery, which supplies both sides of the brain and can result in bilateral infarction when blocked, as was evident with Brian, in the next case example.

On non-contrast CT, an embolus can appear as a hyperdense spot within the lumen of a blood vessel. Over time, with the effects of hypoxia, brain parenchyma can appear hypodense with gradual loss of gray–white differentiation at the cortical mantle. Gyri and sulci effacement is also frequently evident from the pressure effect of edema. If the hypoxia is severe enough, the transition to encephalomalacia will result in more prominent hypodensity on CT, followed by gradual atrophy over several weeks to months. If the vascular territory involves the subcortical structures, they may show signs of hypoxia with early mild hyperdensity followed by gradual loss of density, ultimately becoming hypodense over time as encephalomalacia and lacuna infarction progress. Contrast-enhanced CT imaging may be helpful in identifying occluded vessels or those with restricted flow. Perfusion CT may assist in identifying an ischemic penumbra, just as described for hemorrhagic strokes.

T1 sequences appear similar to CT sequences for ischemic infarction. Signs include edema, loss of the gray–white differentiation at the cortical mantle, effacement of the sulci–gyri pattern due to mass effect, and hypointensity within the involved area. T2-weighted imaging may show hyperintensity with the onset of edema during the acute stages; FLAIR sequences can show hyperintensity several hours earlier. The thrombus within a blood vessel may cause blooming on GRE or SWI imaging because of the increased magnetic susceptibility of the clot. A combination of DWI and ADC can be used to identify areas of ischemic infarction. MRA and CTA are useful in identifying the involved vessels or the specific vascular pathology.

CLINICAL EXAMPLE
Brian: Ischemic Infarction

Brian suffered from ischemic infarction to his midbrain, brain stem, cerebellum, and other infratentorial structures, resulting in quadraparesis and ventilator dependence. Imaging studies revealed an embolic clot within his basilar artery, visible as a white spot on CT (Figure 6-26A, arrow). For comparison, an image taken at a later time following thrombolytic therapy is included (Figure 6-26B, arrow). Note the normal black appearance of the basilar artery, indicating that it is patent with good blood flow.

Following the basilar artery thrombotic stroke, Brian suffered notable damage to his midbrain and cerebral peduncles, which was most apparent on coronal T2 and axial T2 FLAIR sequences (Figures 6-27A–C). The damage on the T2 and T2 FLAIR sequences is identified as areas of abnormal hyperintensity within the midbrain structures, especially the cerebral peduncles.

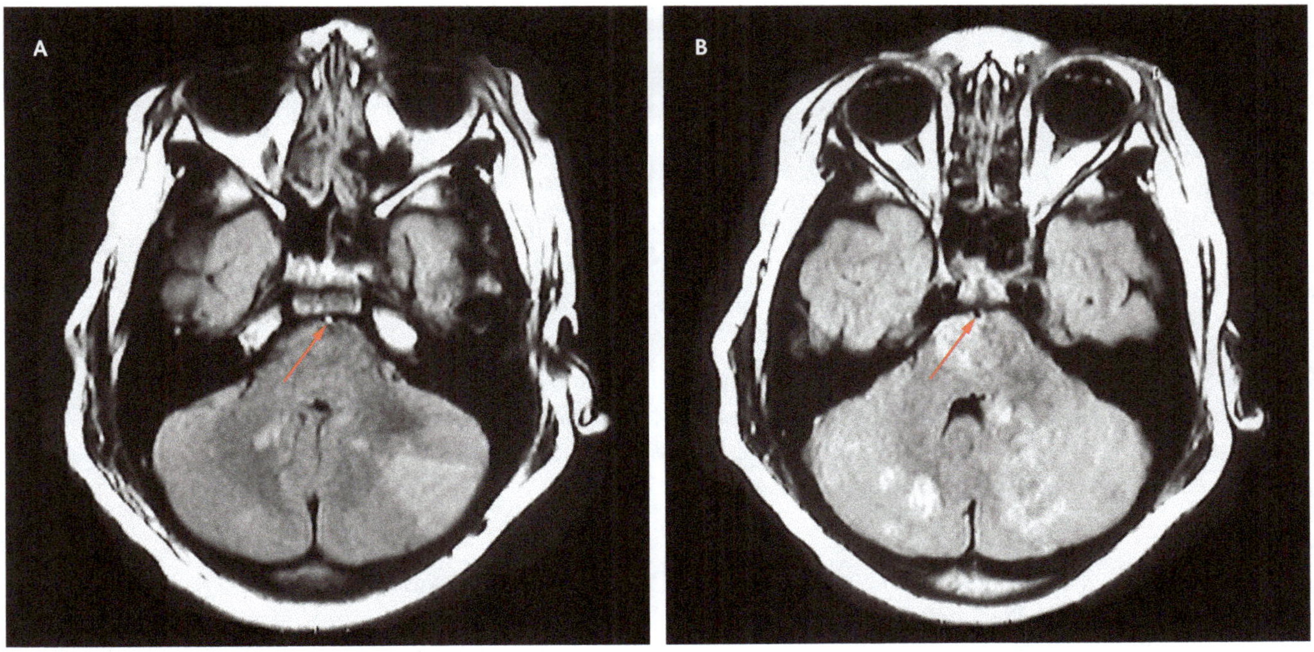

Figure 6-26A and B Clinical example Brian: axial CT imaging showing thrombotic blockage of the basilar artery that resulted in midbrain ischemic infarction. **A:** CT evidence of basilar artery blockage (arrow). **B:** CT evidence of basilar artery flow restored (arrow).

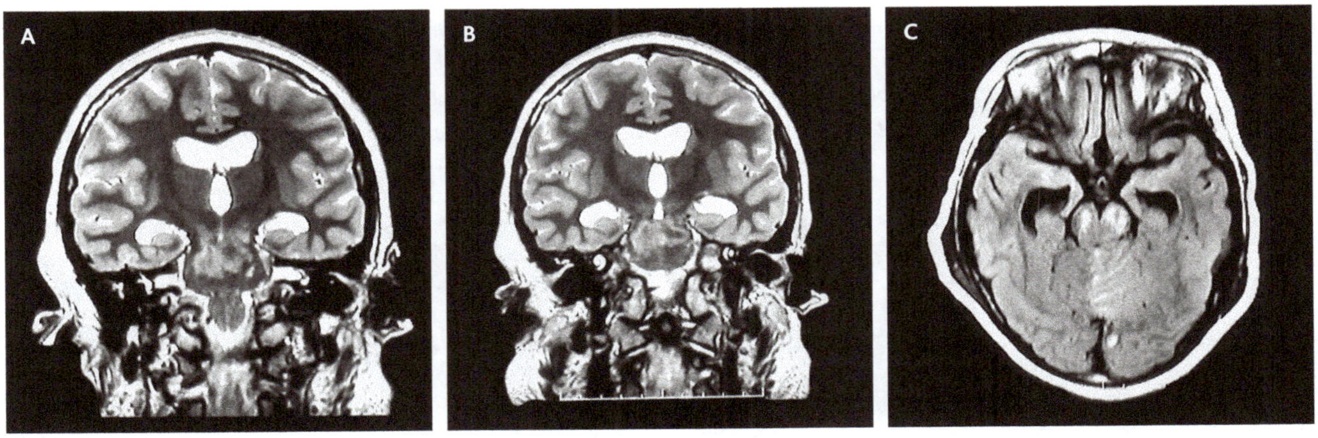

Figure 6-27A–C Clinical example Brian: damage to midbrain and cerebral peduncles resulting from a basilar artery thrombotic stroke. **A:** T2. **B:** T2. **C:** T2 FLAIR.

CLINICAL EXAMPLE

Mayleen: Left Middle Cerebral Artery Ischemic Infarction

Mayleen was hospitalized after experiencing a left middle cerebral artery (MCA) occlusion that resulted in significant ischemic infarction and functional compromise. After her stroke, Mayleen presented with a dense right hemiparesis and global aphasia involving receptive and expressive language. Over time, her global aphasia transitioned to a Broca's type or expressive aphasia, likely because the primary injury was more within the anterior MCA territory supplying Broca's area than the posterior territory supplying Wernicke's area. TOF sequences revealed an almost complete lack of flow through the left middle cerebral artery (Figures 6-28A–C). Note the occlusion of the left middle cerebral artery, suggested by the lack of left MCA hyperintensity (arrows) compared to the clear vessel hyperintensity for the right MCA (arrows). On CT imaging shortly after Mayleen's stroke, the low-density, wedge-shaped region of ischemia within the MCA territory is easily appreciated (Figure 6-29A). There is some mild midline shift due to mass effect of the edema, suggested by the asymmetrical compression of the lateral ventricles

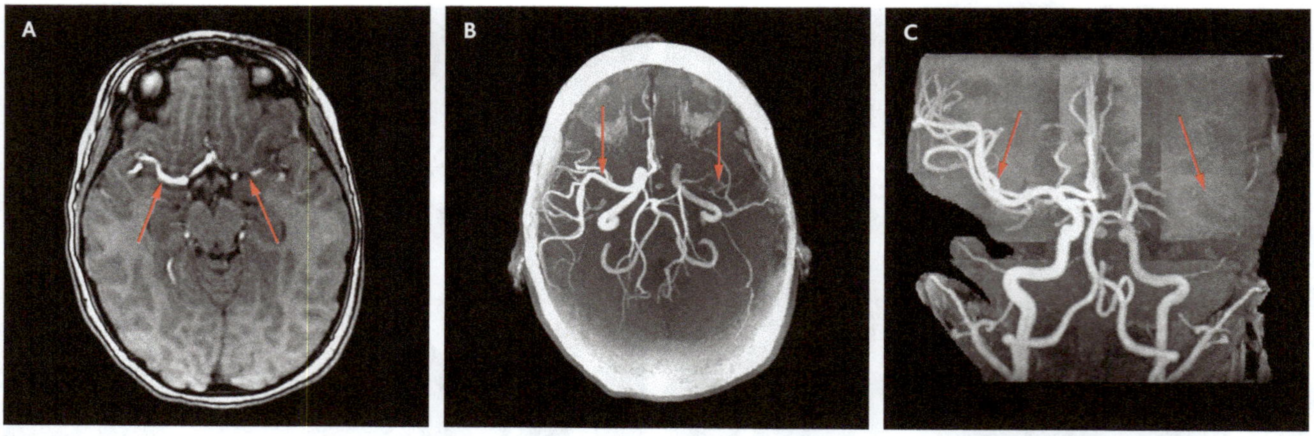

Figures 6-28A–C Clinical example Mayleen: left middle cerebral artery thrombotic occlusion resulting in ischemic infarction. Comparison between the intact right MCA and occluded left MCA is facilitated by the arrows.

and bowing of the falx cerebri. Follow-up imaging revealed notable edema with mass effect necessitating craniotomy to reduce intracranial pressure (Figure 6-29B). Diffusion MRI imaging suggested extensive disruption to diffusion, suggested by the DWI hyperintensity and ADC hypointensity, consistent with hypoxic ischemic encephalopathy within the left MCA distribution (Figures 6-29E and f).

On follow-up neuropsychological evaluation approximately 1 year post-injury Mayleen exhibited notable recovery, but with ongoing residual deficits. Mayleen presented with a moderate Broca's type aphasia, with verbal dysfluency, telegraphic speech, and limitations involving verbal formulation and word finding. Receptive language comprehension continued to improve and was within normal limits, as was verbal reasoning, once expressive limitations were accommodated. Visual–spatial and nonverbal reasoning skills ranged from average to high average without limitation or deficit. Her previous facial asymmetry had also resolved, and she was able to ambulate with an ankle-foot orthosis and right hemigait due to a mild residual hemiparesis affecting her upper extremity more than her lower extremity.

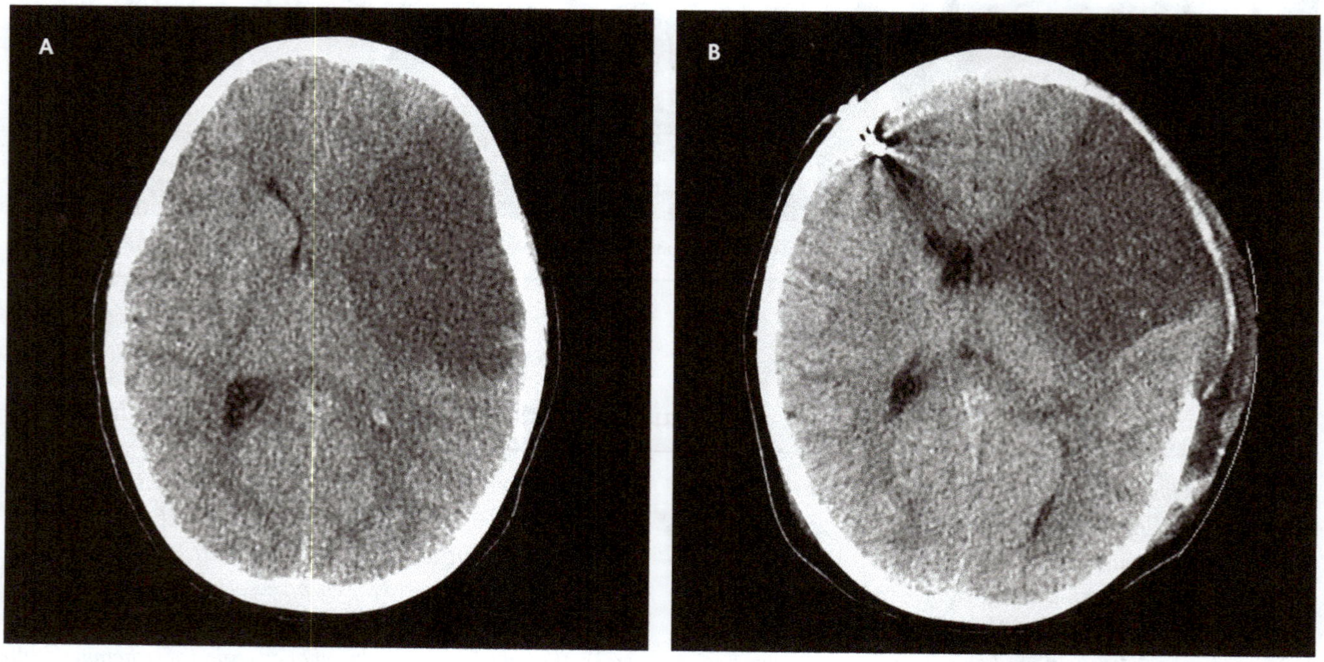

Figures 6-29A and B Clinical example Mayleen: CT series shortly after Mayleen's stroke (A) and on follow-up imaging (B) showing the classic low-density, wedge-shaped region within the left MCA territory.

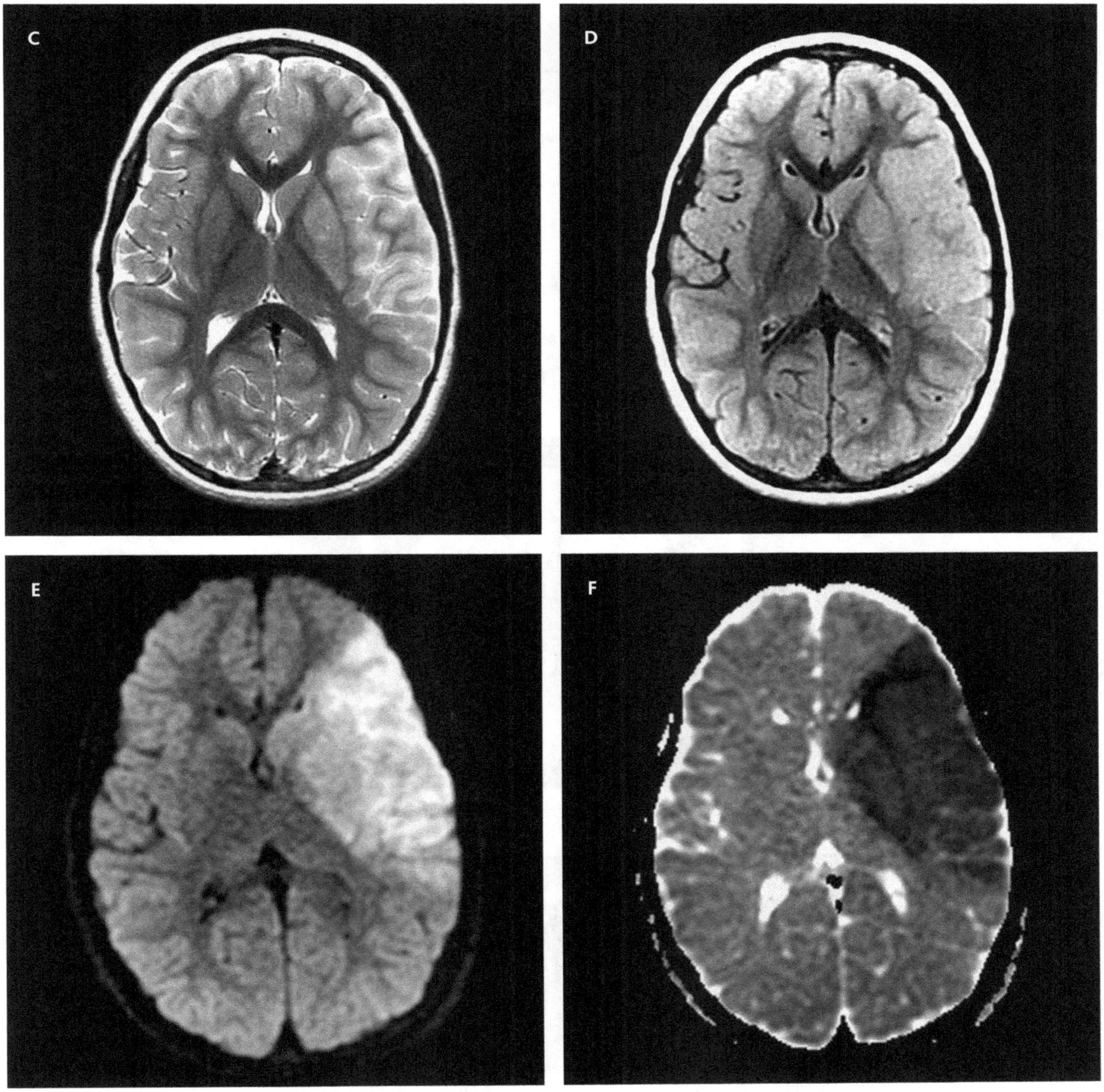

Figures 6-29C–F Clinical example Mayleen: MRI series showing the classic wedge shaped area of infarction on T2 and T2 FLAIR (hyperintense), and restricted diffusion on DWI (hyperintense) and ADC (hypointense). **C:** T2. **D:** T2 FLAIR. **E:** DWI. **F:** ADC.

Posterior cerebral artery strokes affect the occipital and inferior temporal lobes on one side of the brain (Figures 6-30A–C). While this patient recovered most functions, she continued to exhibit a right side homonymous hemianopia several years after her cerebral vascular accident. Note, In the clinical example shown in Figure 6-30A–C, the frontal epidural pneumocephalus and fluid collection are secondary to a craniotomy to control intracranial pressure, and not directly related to the stroke.

Sometimes embolic strokes are caused by surgical procedures unrelated to the region of infarction. The example shown in Figure 6-31 is from a patient who suffered a small hemorrhage and subsequent decline in blood perfusion within the left posterior cerebral artery distribution. The stroke was caused during resection of a pineal tumor. Note the bright area of T2 FLAIR hyperintensity within the left posterior cerebral artery distribution on Figure 6-31.

Clinical Example Samuel: Follow-up imaging of a PCA stroke.

Following significant loss of oxygenated blood perfusion within a specific vascular territory, follow-up imaging may show the formation of lacuna infarctions, or holes within the area supplied by the vessel. Samuel suffered from a significant

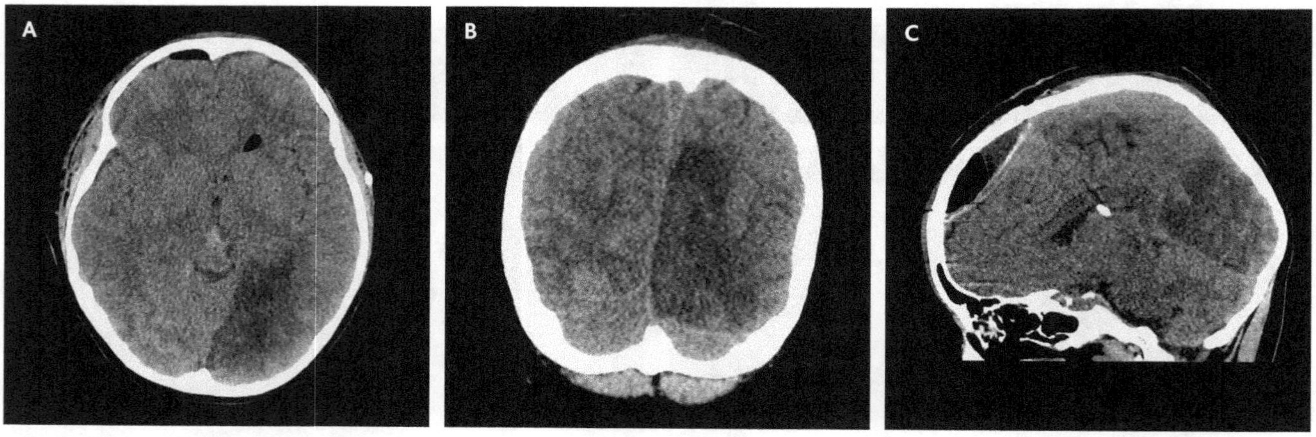

Figures 6-30A–C CT series of posterior cerebral artery stroke. Note hypodensity within the left posterior cerebral artery distribution.

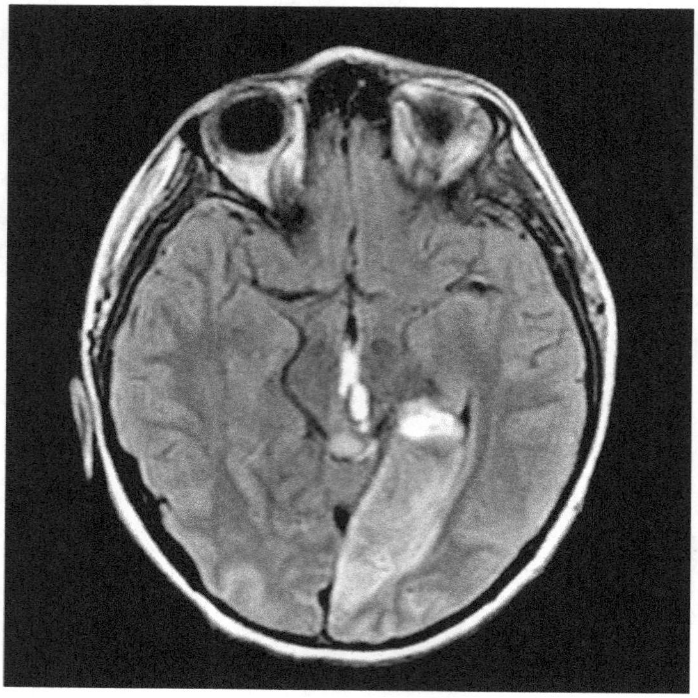

Figure 6-31 T2 FLAIR imaging from a patient who suffered a small hemorrhage and subsequent decline in blood perfusion within the left posterior cerebral artery distribution.

blockage to his right posterior cerebral artery, resulting in hypoxic ischemic injury, encephalomalacia, and, eventually, the formation of lacuna infarcts within the right posterior cerebral artery territory (Figures 6-32A–D). The lacuna infarctions are clearly evident on T2 FLAIR imaging with and without contrast (Figures 6-32A and B) as region that are isointense to CSF. The areas of lacuna infarction were also isointense to CSF on diffusion imaging, or compared to normal brain parenchyna hypointense on DWI and hyperintense on ADC (6-32C and D).

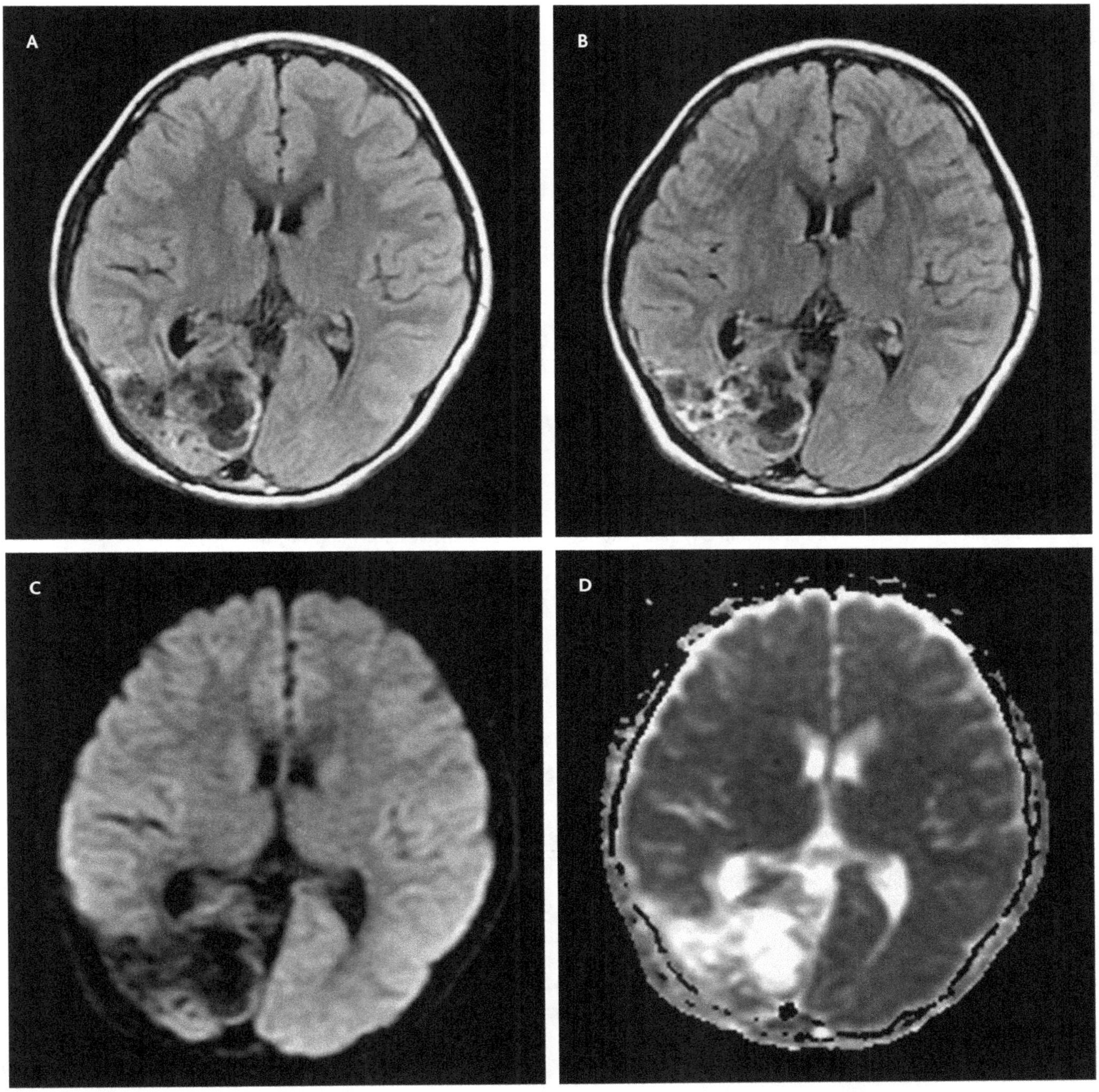

Figures 6-32A–D Clinical example Samuel: follow-up MRI imaging showing a right posterior cerebral artery stroke with formation of lacuna infarctions. **A:** T2 FLAIR. **B:** Post-contrast T2 FLAIR. **C:** DWI. **D:** ADC.

Jan: Combination of Nonhemorrhagic and Hemorrhagic Strokes

Jan had both an embolic or nonhemorrhagic stroke and a hemorrhagic stroke within the same vascular territory. Following extensive surgery to clear an arterial blockage in her abdomen, Jan had an embolic stroke within the initial segment of the left middle cerebral artery, resulting in hypoxic ischemic injury to her left peri-Sylvian region. Initial 2D TOF imaging confirmed the left middle cerebral artery embolic stroke (Figures 6-33A–C). Note flow within the right middle cerebral artery (arrows), but without comparable flow in the left hemisphere. One would think that 3D TOF imaging would give more information than 2D; however, often more detail regarding flow through specific vessels can be obtained with the higher resolution of 2D slices, and this was the case with Jan.

Following the stroke, Jan presented as globally aphasic after she awoke and began interacting with those around her. Imaging indicatted that the stroke had affected the anterior distribution of the left MCA more than the posterior distribution, resulting in a rapidly resolving Wernicke's, or fluent, aphasia, but persistence of her dense Broca's, or dysfluent, aphasia (Figures 6-34A–C). Note the location of her stroke in comparison to Broca's area, most easily visualized on the sagittal T1 FLAIR image (Figure 6-34A). T2 FLAIR and DWI imaging suggested infarction, with onset of laminar necrosis along the outer cortical rim (Figure 6-34C). No ADC images were produced for this patient, making it difficult to fully assess the restriction of diffusion on DWI without the influence of T2 shine-through. However, the excessively bright appearance of the cortical lamina suggests restricted diffusion and not just T2 shine-through. This is an area of reduced intensity on T2 FLAIR but increased intensity on DWI.

The following day, 3 days after the stroke, and with the use of thrombolytic medications, Jan recovered some minimal ability to understand simple commands and questions. Given her ongoing expressive aphasia, she responded with head shakes and nods, with eye blinks, and by squeezing and clenching her left hand. Anticoagulants were administered to prevent additional damage from the embolism within her left middle cerebral artery. Follow-up imaging 5 days later revealed evidence of hemorrhage within the left middle cerebral artery distribution, close to where the embolus was likely located most easily visualized on GRE sequences (Figures 6-35A–C arrows). Although it is difficult to confirm, it is possible that the hemorrhagic stroke was due to the use of powerful anticoagulants, combined with a damaged vessel.

Additional pathology was evident on Jan's imaging and factored into the family's decisions regarding treatment options. For example, imaging suggested the possibility of early-stage frontotemporal dementia, based on atrophy, in addition to mild diffuse white-matter injury, likely due to hypotension during Jan's extensive abdominal surgery.

Several days before Jan died, she indicated her desire to have her brain scans put into this guide to help others learn about conditions such as hers. This was one of her last communications—a wonderful gift from a wonderful woman. Jan had a long life as a schoolteacher and now gets to continue her role as a teacher long after her passing, through her brain images.

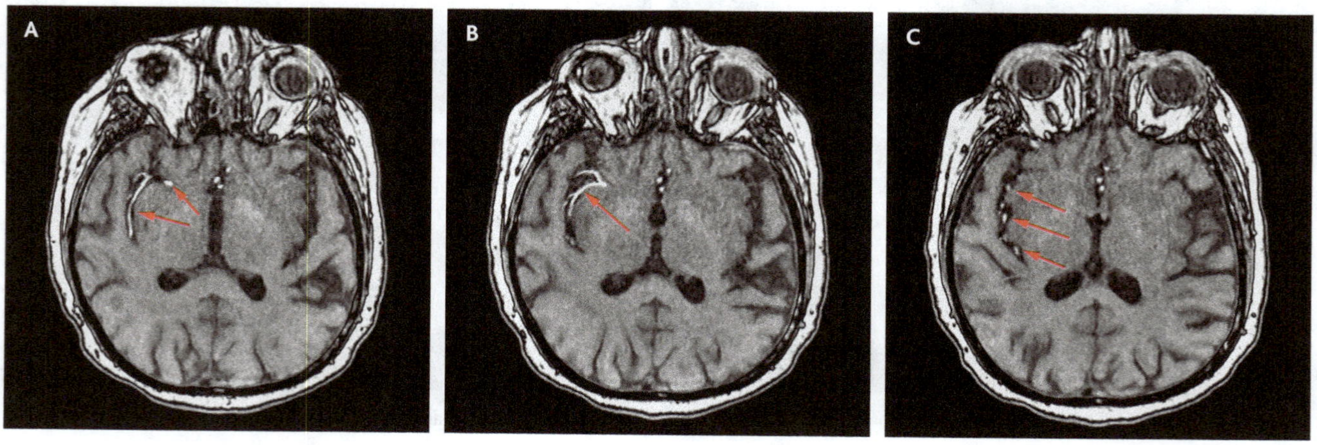

Figures 6-33A–C Clinical example Jan: MRI 2D TOF imaging showing the left middle cerebral artery embolic stroke with right MCA flow (arrows), but without comparable left MCA flow.

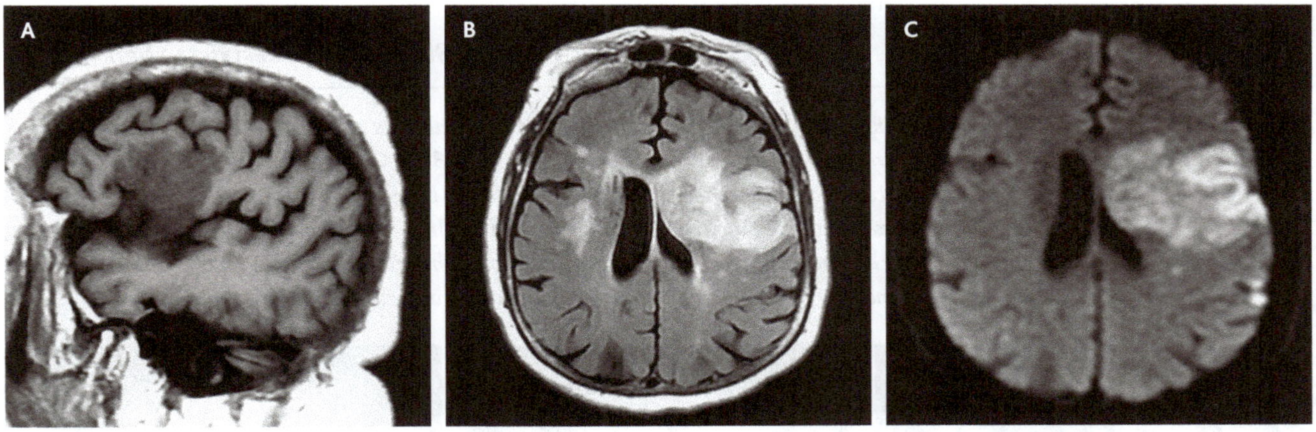

Figures 6-34A–C Clinical example Jan: MRI evidence of significant hypoxic-ischemic infarction within the left anterior MCA distribution. **A:** T1 FLAIR. **B:** T2 FLAIR. **C:** DWI.

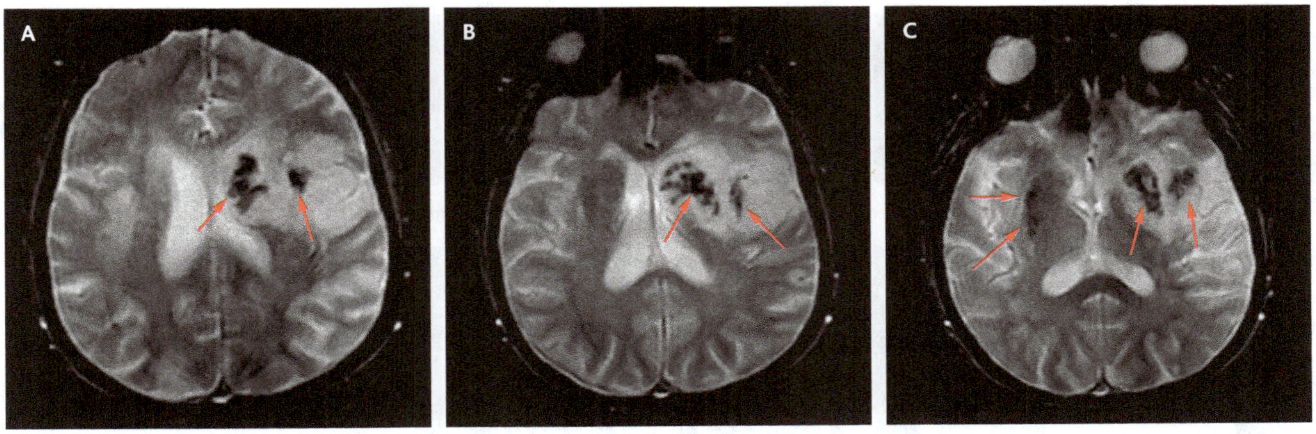

Figures 6-35A–C Clinical example Jan: follow-up GRE series 5 days post-stroke showing areas of hemorrhage as dark, blooming regions of susceptibility artifact (arrows).

Blockage of Venous Flow

With respect to blood flow, the brain can be considered a closed unit; for blood to enter the brain, an equal amount of blood must leave the brain. If there is blockage or restricted flow through the venous sinuses and veins, fresh arterial flow of blood into the brain is compromised, and hypoxic ischemic damage can result. Blockage of flow through the veins or dural sinuses can result in hemorrhagic infarctions that do not follow the usual pattern seen in arterial vascular disruption. As flow backs up into the cerebral veins, damage may become apparent in some regions but not others. Blockage of venous flow through veins or sinuses often results in a relatively heterogeneous distribution of ischemic infarction close to the location of the blockage.

Mateo experienced thrombotic disruption to blood flow through his straight sinus and internal cerebral vein of Galen. Disrupted flow was suggested by magnetic resonance venography (MRV) sequences, with the appearance of the superior sagittal, transverse and sigmoid sinuses, but not the blocked vessels (Figures 6-36A–C arrows). The primary areas of damage involved the left thalamus and bilateral basal ganglia, as indicated on Figures 6-37A–C. Note low-density within the region of the thalamus and basal ganglia. The area of greatest hypodensity corresponds to the left thalamic body. Although the CT series suggests possible ischemic infarction and evolving encephalomalacia, the hypodense appearance may also represent edema.

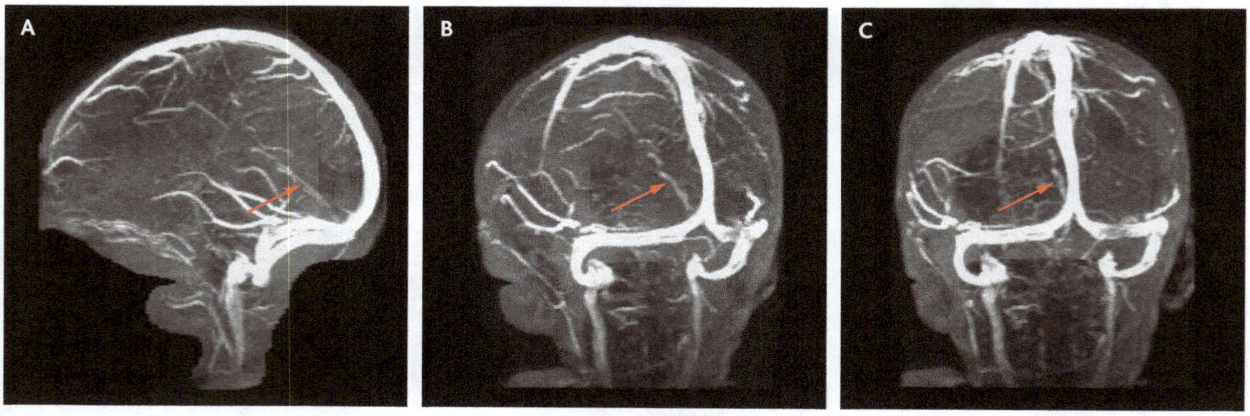

Figures 6-36A–C Clinical example Mateo: MRV series showing restricted venous flow through the straight sinus.

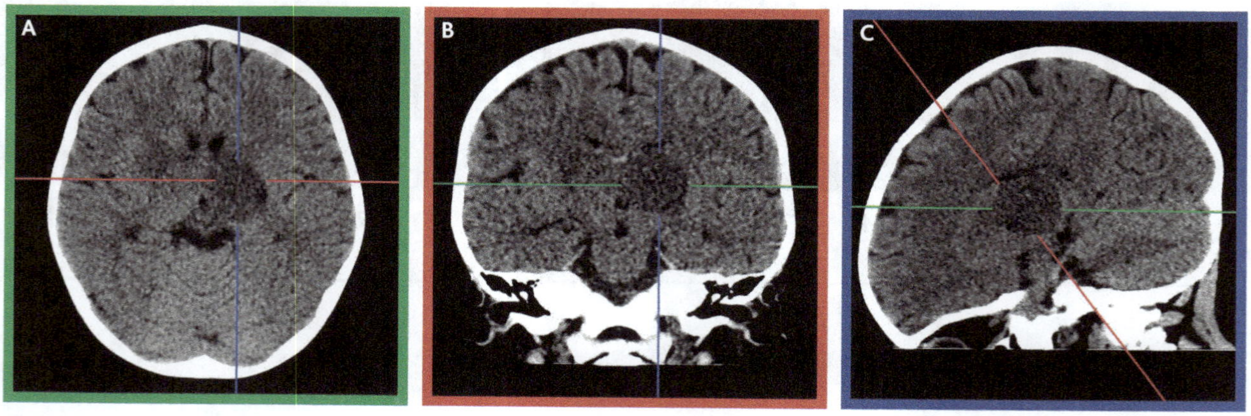

Figures 6-37A–F Clinical example Mateo: CT series showing *low-density areas of the thalamus and basal ganglia resulting from blockage of the straight sinus.*

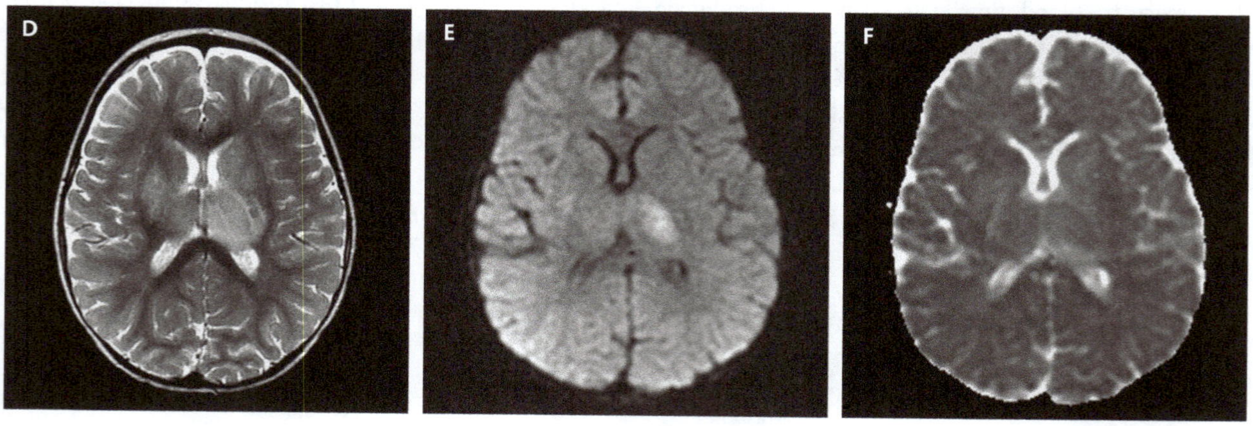

Figures 6-37D–F Clinical example Mateo: MRI series showing T2 hyperintensity within the left thalamus, with possible T2 shine-through on diffusion imaging. **D:** T2. **E:** DWI. **F:** ADC.

CLINICAL EXAMPLE
Monica: Superior Sagittal Sinus Thrombosis

Monica had reduced flow through her venous system caused by blockage of her superior sagittal sinus. Magnetic resonance venography clearly demonstrated reduced flow through the superior sagittal sinus (Figure 6-38A arrows). MRI T2 FLAIR and T1 FLAIR sequences provide evidence of significant hypoxic ischemic infarction of the superior cortical and subcortical structures, within the region of the thrombosis (Figures 6-38B and C).

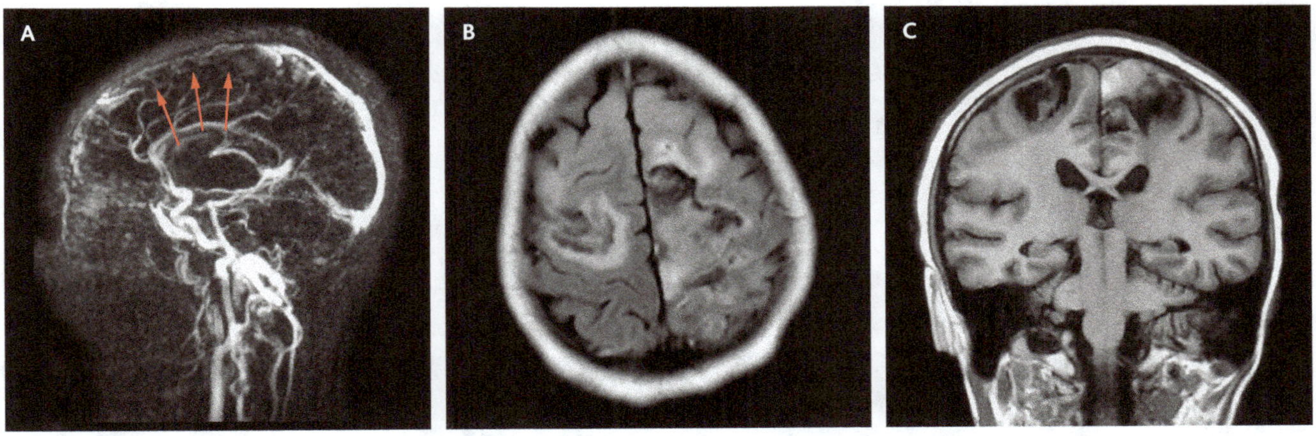

Figures 6-38A–C Clinical example Monica: MRI series showing reduced flow through the superior sagittal sinus due to thrombosis (6-38A arrows), and the resultant superior cortical and subcortical hypoxic ischemic infarctions (6-38B and C). **A:** MRV. **B:** T2 FLAIR. **C:** T1 FLAIR.

CLINICAL EXAMPLE
Jolene: Compromised Venous Drainage

Jolene presented with bilateral superior occipital-parietal nonhemorrhagic infarctions as a secondary complication of a traumatic brain injury. CT imaging suggested disrupted venous outflow from the area to the superior sagittal sinus (Figures 6-39A–D). Note that the distribution of damage is inconsistent with disruption of either the posterior or the middle cerebral arteries and is centered at the superior sagittal sinus. This distribution is highly suggestive of disrupted venous flow through the veins and superior sagittal sinus, with blood backing up into the tissue. The large craniotomy gap in the skull with mild cortical herniation is from the primary traumatic injury. The bilateral infarctions are due to a secondary complication involving venous drainage of blood. MRV imaging (Figures 6-40A–C) illustrate the lack of flow through the superior sagittal sinus (arrow 1), with compensatory flow through the falcine sinus/vein (arrow 2). The falcine sinus or vein is a structure that usually involutes after birth, although it may persist in some adults. With blockage of the superior sagittal sinus, the falcine sinus may recannulize, as was evident in Jolene. MRI imaging was used to identify the extent and severity of the injury to the posterior cortex resulting from disrupted flow through the superior sagittal sinus (Figures 6-40D–F).

Jolene's functioning was relatively preserved, with the exception of higher-level visual–spatial processing involving the localization of stimuli in visual space. For example, although Jolene was able to complete basic visual tasks, she had difficulty catching a ball or rapidly pointing to objects in front of her. While such difficulties did not prevent her normal, everyday functioning, they were of the magnitude to prevent her return to driving because of her compromised ability to visually locate structures, cars, and people around her, especially when rapidly changing, as happens when driving.

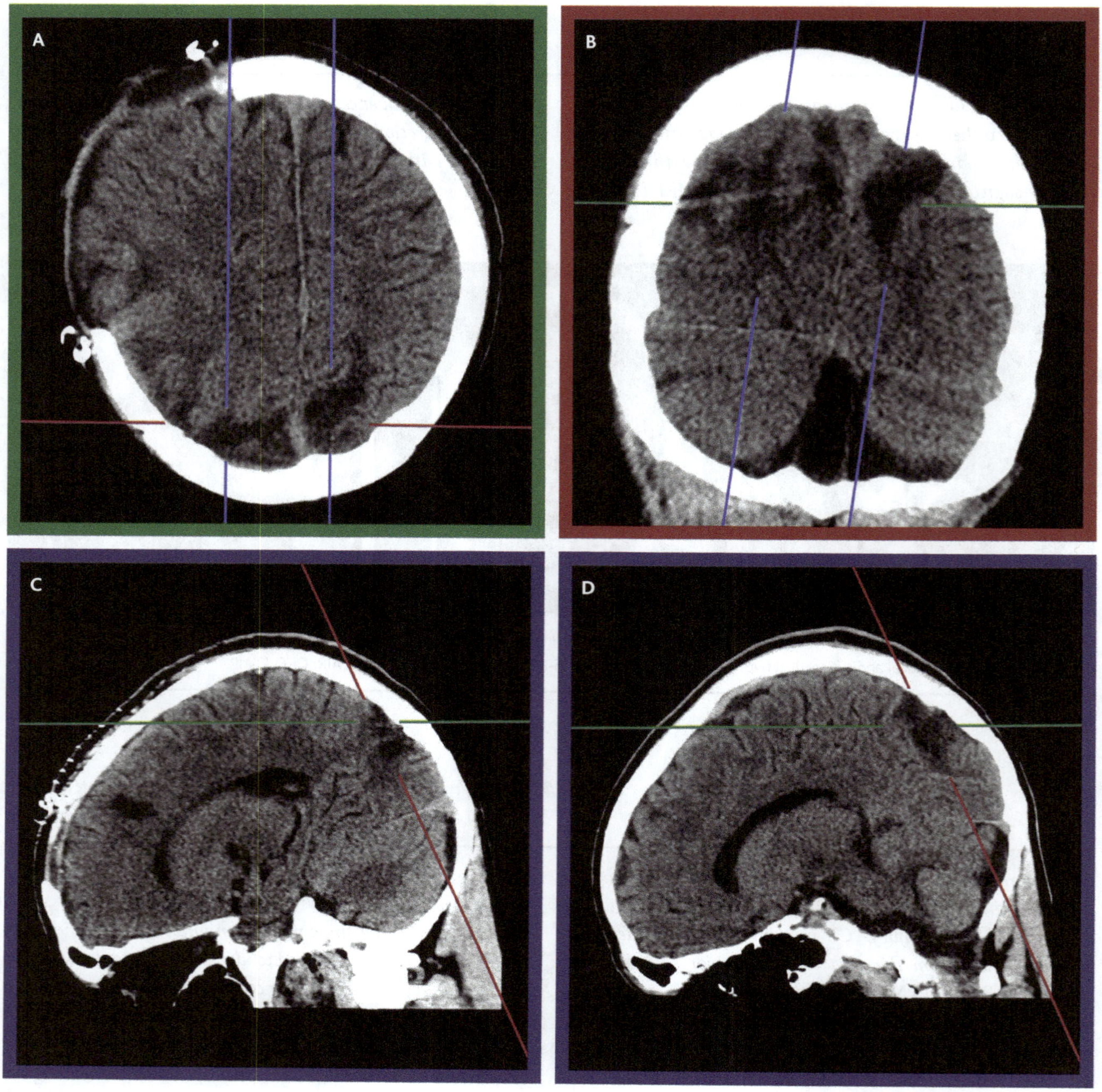

Figures 6-39A–D Clinical example Jolene: CT series of compromised venous drainage showing damage to the posterior parietal-superior occipital cortex. **A:** Axial image with right and left hemisphere sagittal reference lines. **B:** Coronal image with right and left hemisphere sagittal reference lines. **C:** Right hemisphere sagittal image. **D:** Left hemisphere sagittal image.

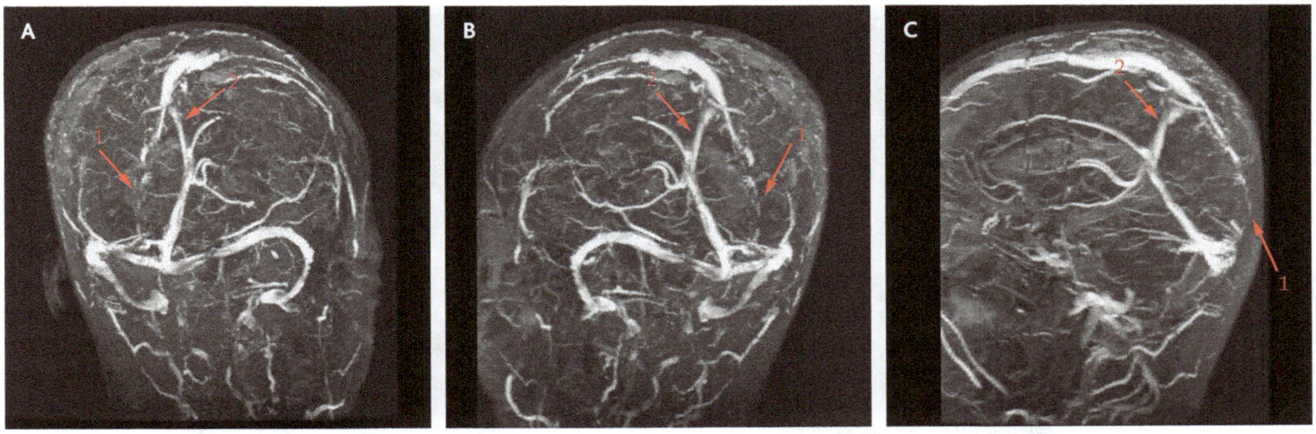

Figures 6-40A–C Clinical example Jolene: MRV series showing the reduced blood flow through the superior sagittal sinus (arrow 1), with compensatory flow through the falcine sinus/vein (arrow 2).

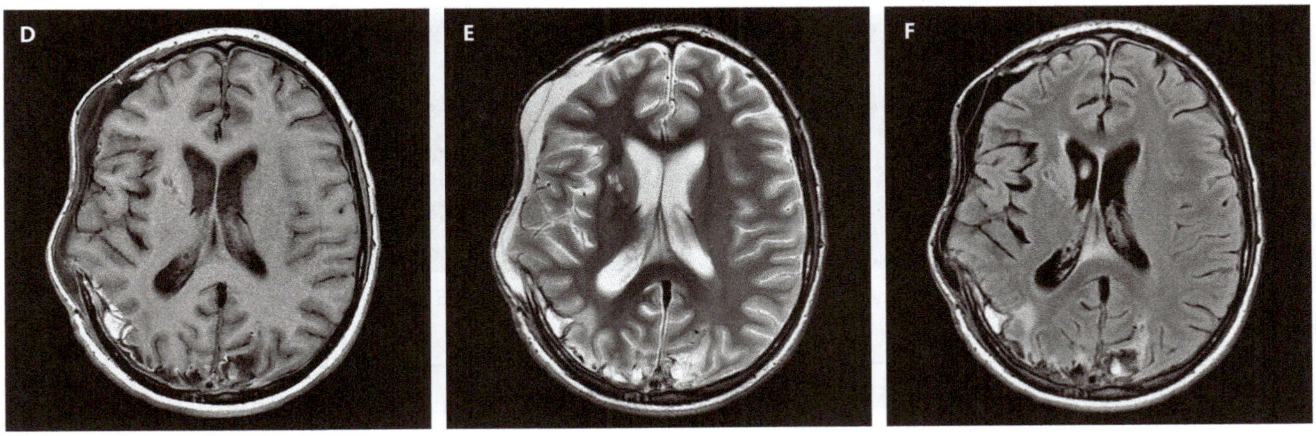

Figures 6-40D–F Clinical example Jolene: MRI series showing posterior parietal–superior occipital injury caused by restricted flow through the superior sagittal sinus. **D:** T1. **E:** T2. **F:** T2 FLAIR

Loss of Internal Carotid Flow Without Stroke-Related Symptoms

Because the vascular organization of the circle of Willis provides an anastomosis between the anterior and posterior distributions and the right and left hemisphere distributions, sometimes, damage to a major artery may not lead to a stroke. In Megan's case, presented below, compression of her right internal carotid artery did not cause any clinical symptoms; compensatory flow occurred through her posterior communicating artery.

CLINICAL EXAMPLE
Megan: Internal Carotid Artery Embolism Without Stroke Symptoms

Megan sustained a skull fracture during a fall, causing an embolism to block the blood flow through her right internal carotid artery (Figure 6-41, arrow). However, Megan experienced no functional deficits relating to the lack of flow through her right internal carotid artery, something that was unexpected. Close review of her MRA revealed that there was increased flow through her anterior and posterior communicating arteries, which form part of the circle of Willis. The right anterior cerebral artery was being supplied by the anterior communicating artery from the left internal carotid distribution. The right middle cerebral artery was receiving blood from the basilar and vertebral supply via the posterior communicating artery. Because of the natural anastomosis of the circle of Willis, Megan's right hemisphere continued to receive adequate oxygenated blood, allowing full functioning. Eventually, through vascular surgical intervention, the flow of blood was returned to the right internal carotid artery, and Megan had no further difficulties with blood flow to the brain. In Megan's case, her circle of Willis prevented a massive right-hemisphere stroke, and she left the hospital without functional deficits.

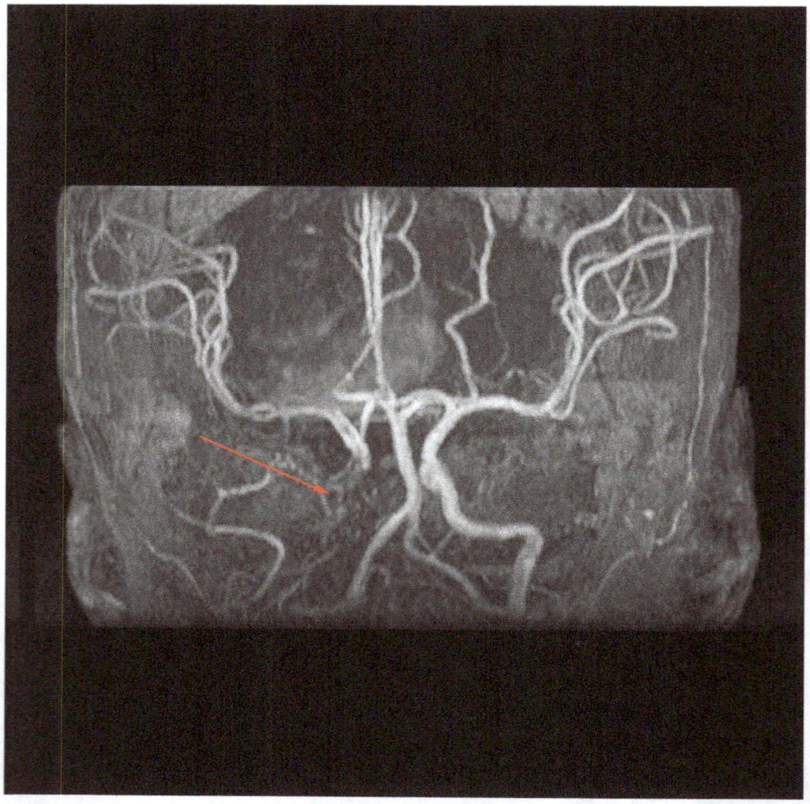

Figure 6-41 Clinical example Megan: damaged internal carotid artery without stroke symptoms due to compensatory flow through the anterior and posterior communicating arteries of the circle of Willis.

DIFFUSE HYPOXIC ENCEPHALOPATHY

Respiratory arrest, drowning accidents, or exposure to chemicals such as carbon monoxide can result in diffuse hypoxic ischemic injury to the brain. On imaging, the effects of diffuse hypoxia are similar to the focal areas of hypoxia described for traumatic brain injuries in Chapter 5, only more of the brain is involved. Both cortical and subcortical injury is evident with diffuse hypoxic encephalopathies, and in many cases, the damage is profound, permanent or even fatal.

One difficulty with the assessment of diffuse hypoxic ischemic injuries is that the appearance on imaging may differ a great deal depending on the severity and extent of damage. On CT, damage may appear as bilateral diffuse areas of low density with effacement of the sulci–gyri pattern due to edema and mass effect. Over time, loss of gray–white differentiation may become evident, followed by patches of encephalomalacia and, ultimately, atrophy. MRI is more sensitive for visualizing diffuse hypoxic injuries than CT. Hypoxic infarction often presents on MRI with bilateral T2 hyperintensity within the deep gray-matter structures of the basal ganglia and thalami, in addition to the lateral cortical convexity and insula. Over time, breakdown of the cortical mantle or laminar necrosis may occur, evident as an outline of T2 hyperintensity that follows the gyral contours. Cerebellar injury, especially in older patients, is also common, as the Purkinje cells are especially sensitive to hypoxic ischemia. Hippocampal cells are also sensitive to hypoxia and may show ischemic changes over time. T1 imaging may appear normal, although some hyperintensity may be apparent within the bilateral basal ganglia structures. DWI and ADC sequences are often the first scans to show hypoxic ischemic injury and can be positive within a few hours. However, as water diffusion changes over time, the appearance of diffusion sequences such as DWI and ADC can become confusing. The recent use of DTI fractional anisotropy (FA) maps has shown promise in assessing for diffuse white-matter breakdown.

On acute CT imaging of a patient who had nearly drowned (Figure 6-42A), there is diffuse low density in addition to loss of the gray–white differentiation. In addition, there appears to be some mild effacement of the sulci–gyri patterning, although swelling and intracranial pressure do not appear to be severe, given the visibly open perimesencephalic or quadrigeminal cistern and ventricles. Interestingly, the acute CT shown in Figure 6-42A does not have an appearance suggesting profound injury to the brain, thus predicting prognosis from this scan would be difficult. In contrast to the appearance of the scan taken acutely, the image acquired several weeks later (Figure 6-42B) indicates severe diffuse brain injury secondary to the hypoxic ischemic event. There is obvious ventricular dilation and prominence of the sulci, with thinning of the gyri suggesting diffuse atrophy. Such atrophy would be expected to continue for many weeks. If follow-up imaging were acquired, the scans would likely show an even more shriveled appearance to the brain. This patient remained severely compromised and fully dependent for all needs after the near-drowning incident.

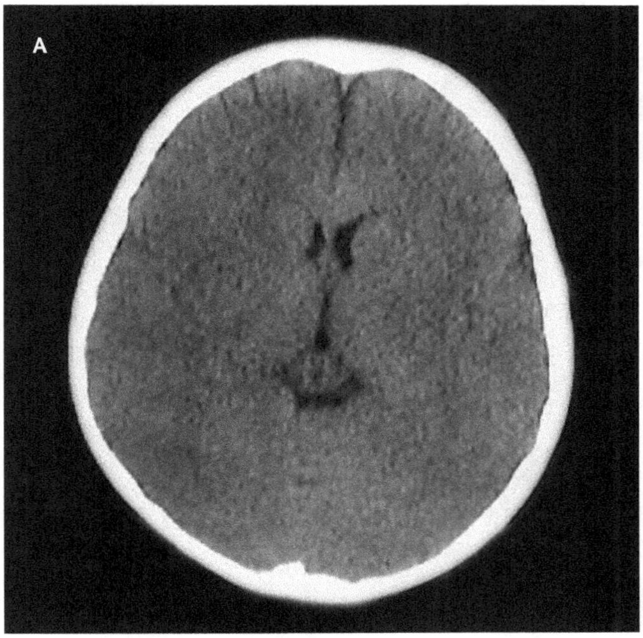

Figure 6-42A Acute CT imaging of patient after a near-drowning incident showing diffuse low-density and loss of gray-white differentiation.

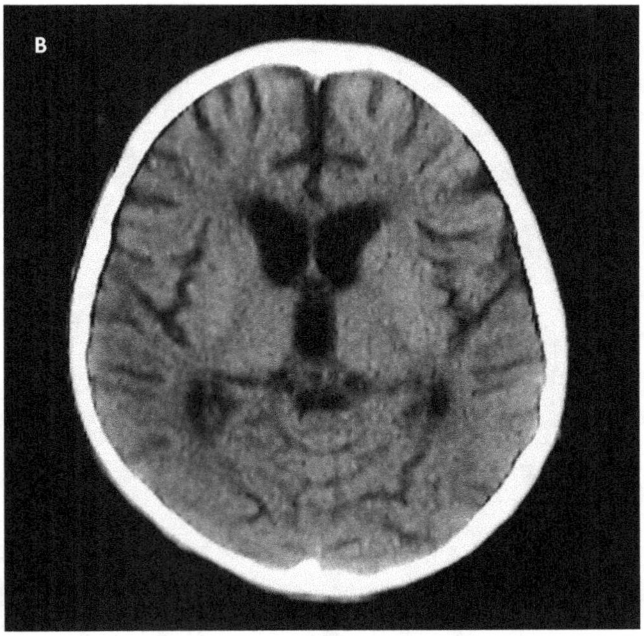

Figure 6-42B CT imaging of same patient, taken several weeks later, showing a clearly atrophic appearance due to onging diffuse hypoxic ischemic encephalopathy.

Watershed Infarctions

When viewing brain scans for diffuse hypoxic injuries, be sure to assess for watershed infarction, especially in the less severe cases. The watershed area is a region of poor blood flow at the border between the three primary vessels supplying the lateral cortex of the brain. The medial surface and the front are supplied by the anterior cerebral arteries; most of the lateral surface is supplied by the middle cerebral arteries; and the posterior and inferior temporal lobes are supplied by the posterior cerebral arteries. However, the fingers of these vessels do not meet at the border, leaving a zone of tissue with relatively poor perfusion (see Figure 3–119). Any significant loss of blood pressure, blood flow, or blood oxygenation can result in damage to the watershed region, even when other areas of the brain are unaffected. Watershed infarctions cause some very specific clinical disorders, such as transcortical aphasia due to the damage isolating the peri-Sylvian language cortices from the rest of the brain. Watershed infarctions are best appreciated on axial slices and have a dumbbell appearance. This appearance is caused by the slicing through the superior watershed area, with damage at the front and back of the slice on each side. Any injury to the subcortical gray matter will appear as a small area of infarction between the larger anterior and posterior sections, forming the handle of the dumbbell.

Pilar was trapped in a house fire and eventually passed out from reduced oxygen and a high concentration of carbon monoxide and other toxic fumes. Her T2 FLAIR imaging suggested bilateral watershed infarctions, in addition to damage to the basal ganglia, especially the head of the caudate and putamen bilaterally (Figure 6-43) resulting in the classic dumbbell appearance of hyperintensity on axial slices. Pilar experienced significant motor and cognitive compromise, with severe mixed transcortical aphasia. Pilar's transcortical aphasia was similar to a mixed or global aphasia in that she could not understand or express language to communicate. Unlike global aphasia, Pilar was able to repeat sentences, random numbers, and letters that she heard, but she could not use language functionally.

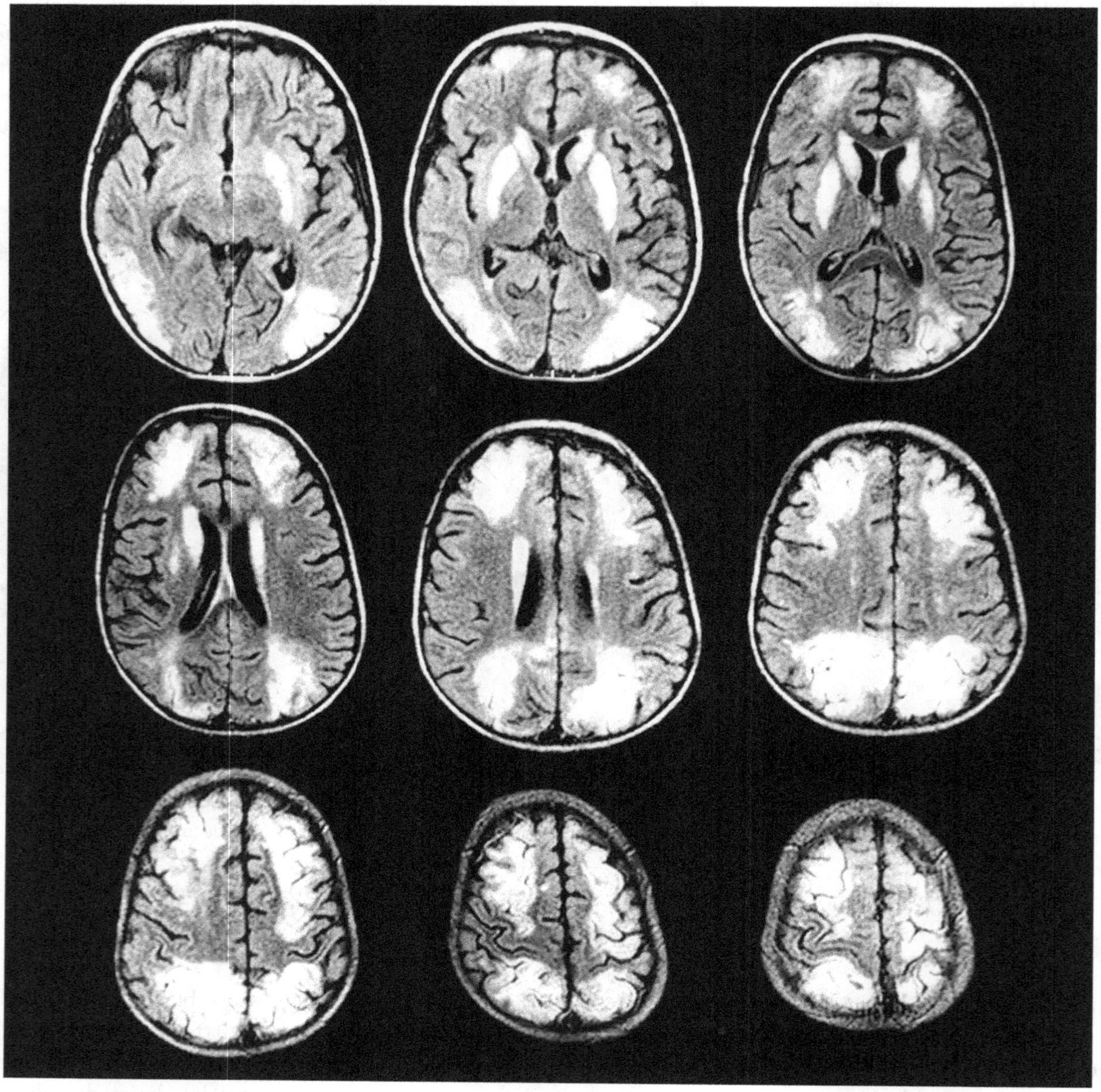

Figure 6-43 Clinical example Pilar: T2 FLAIR imaging of watershed infarction showing the classic dumbbell appearance on axial slices.

CLINICAL EXAMPLE
Cheryl: Mild Watershed Infarction

Cheryl also experienced a watershed infarction, although a much milder case than Pilar's, and she recovered to the point of being independently functional. Cheryl was injured while traveling in the back of a pick-up truck with a camper shell. The back window of the camper shell was open, and carbon monoxide from the exhaust was drawn into the camper shell, causing Cheryl to lose consciousness. Cheryl did not experience respiratory or cardiac arrest, although the high concentration of carbon monoxide did cause a mild watershed infarction, evident on T2 FLAIR (Figure 6-44A) and diffusion-weighted DWI and ADC sequences (Figure 6-44B and C). Note the subtle bilateral hyperintensities within the frontal and parietal lobes on T2 FLAIR imaging (6-44A), with commensurate hyperintensity on DWI (6-44B) and hypointensity on ADC (6-44C), in the classic dubbell pattern, suggesting hypoxic ischemia within the watershed area.

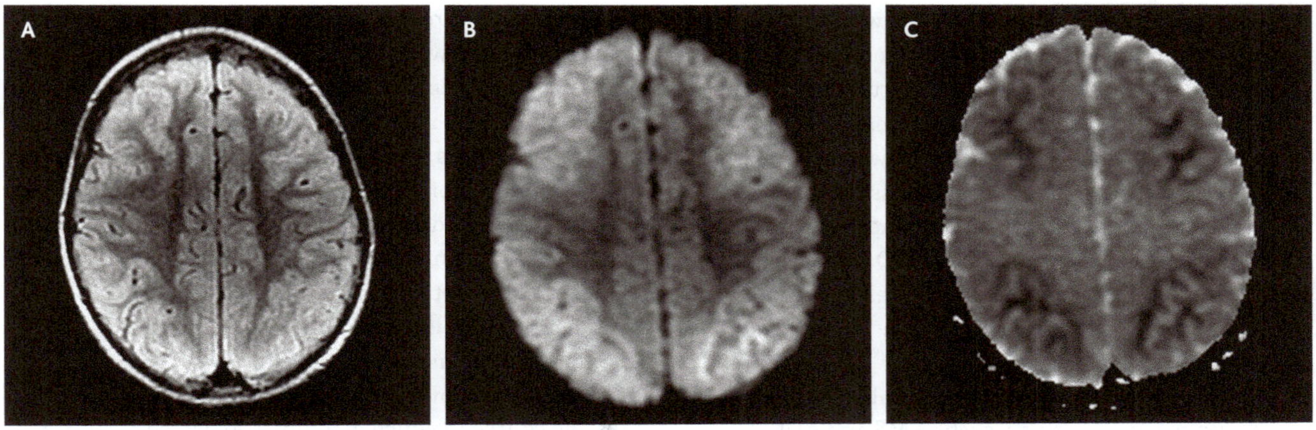

Figures 6-44A–C Clinical example Cheryl: MRI series showing the classic dumbbell appearance on axial slice, even after a relatively mild watershed infarction. **A:** T2 FLAIR. **B:** DWI. **C:** ADC.

CLINICAL EXAMPLE
Marc: Severe Unilateral Watershed Infarction

Most watershed infarctions are bilateral, resulting from disrupted oxygenation or reduced blood flow to the brain. However, reduced flow through either internal carotid artery can result in a unilateral watershed infarction. Marc suffered a basilar skull fracture following a crushing injury to his head. His left internal carotid artery was compressed by the skull fracture, reducing blood flow to his left hemisphere and resulting in a unilateral watershed infarction (Figures 6-45A–C). On CT imaging, the

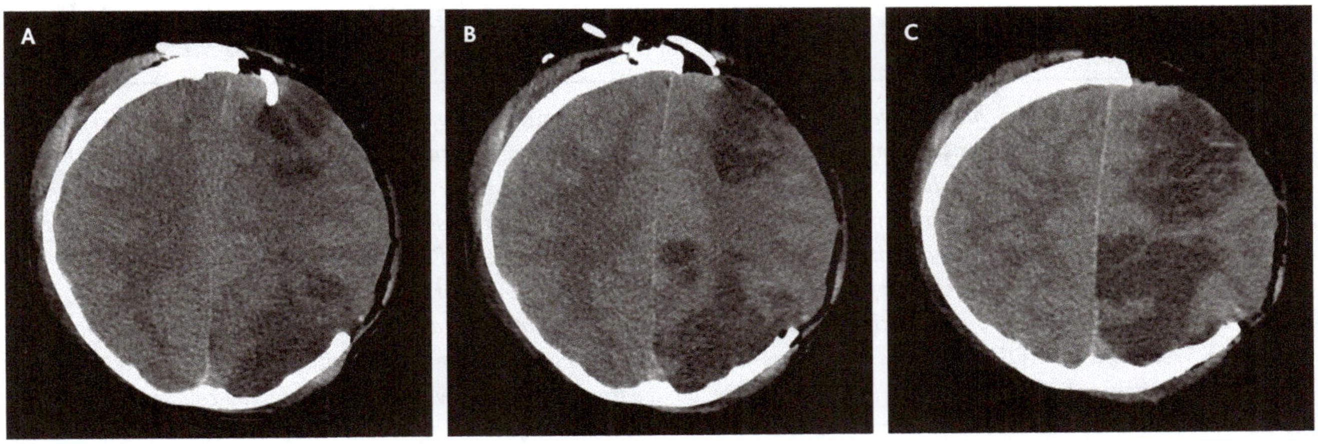

Figures 6-45A–C Clinical example Marc: CT series of severe left hemisphere unilateral watershed infarction due to compromised left internal carotid blood flow.

darker areas represent regions of significant hypoxic ischemic infarction, with reduced density due to encephalomalacia and the onset of atrophy. Note the relatively unique bumbbell appearance, suggesting damage to the watershed area, especially clear on Figure 6-45B.

The CT series was acquired shortly after a left lateral craniotomy allowing the brain parenchyma to swell outside the normal bounds of the skull, thus preventing excessive increase in intracranial pressure. Because of the craniotomy and the herniation outside the lateral cranium, there is very little pressure effect, as indicated by only slight bowing of the falx cerebri. Marc was severely compromised cognitively and functionally after this injury, with motor and sensory deficits in addition to persistent mixed or global transcortical aphasia.

WHITE-MATTER DISORDERS

Disorders of white matter can vary widely, with some patients exhibiting only subtle symptoms and others being completely incapacitated or even succumbing to the illness. The most well-known nontraumatic white matter condition is multiple sclerosis (MS), which has either a relapsing-remitting or chronic progressive course. Other white-matter disorders with similar features include acute disseminated encephalomyelitis (ADEM) and Guillain-Barré syndrome (GBS). Leukoencephalopathies and leukodystropies also come under the umbrella of nontraumatic white-matter disorders.

This section will provide some clinical examples of common white-matter disorders, such as MS and ADEM.

Multiple Sclerosis (MS)

On imaging, the only evidence of MS may be multiple tiny bilateral, asymmetrical T2 or T2 FLAIR hyperintense spots or patches. If active demyelination is taking place, these areas may be enhanced with contrast agents and show evidence of restricted diffusion. Most hyperintense areas are located within the periventricular white matter and centrum semiovale, although they can also be located within the white-matter tracts of the internal capsule, cerebral peduncles, midbrain, and brain stem. Lesions may appear isodense or hypodense on CT and T1 and during active periods of demyelination may show enhancement with contrast agents. On diffusion imaging, there may be evidence of an isotropic core (unrestricted diffusion) surrounded by an anisotropic ring (restricted diffusion). T1 imaging may be useful in assessing for changes in gross brain structures over time, especially with a chronic progressive course in which atrophy is expected.

Because the appearance of MS can be very similar to that of ADEM, assessment of the clinical course and laboratory values is necessary to accurately diagnose the condition. Unlike ADEM, MS is usually polyphasic, following a relapsing-remitting or chronic progressive course with periods of exacerbation.

CLINICAL EXAMPLE

Ray: Relapsing-Remitting and Chronic Progressive Multiple Sclerosis

Ray, a delightful 32-year-old, had a several-year history of relapsing-remitting multiple sclerosis. Contrast enhanced T1 axial images (6-46A–C) showed the lesions as bright petechial hyperintensities throughout the brain, including the brain stem, midbrain, internal capsule, and centrum semiovale. T2 and T2 FLAIR imaging provided a clearer picture of the white matter involvement (6-46D–F). Note that when comparing Figure 6-46D with 6-46E, it appears that there is more white-matter involvement in the medial left hemisphere on the T2 than on the T2 FLAIR image (arrow). This is because the T2 image shows both inflammation and CSF as hyperintense, but the FLAIR sequence attenuates CSF, only showing inflammation as hyperintense. The impression of greater left medial inflammation on the T2 image is an artifact of the slice cutting through the very top of the lateral ventricle; the most medial bright area shown by the arrow is CSF in the ventricle. In this case, the T2 FLAIR image provides a more accurate measure of white-matter involvement than the T2 image.

The acuity of Ray's condition increased over many years to the point that he was hospitalized several times a year for periods of several weeks. Over time, his course changed from relapsing-remitting to chronic progressive, with longer hospitalizations and shorter periods in between. Eventually, Ray was hospitalized continuously until he died. Over a period of

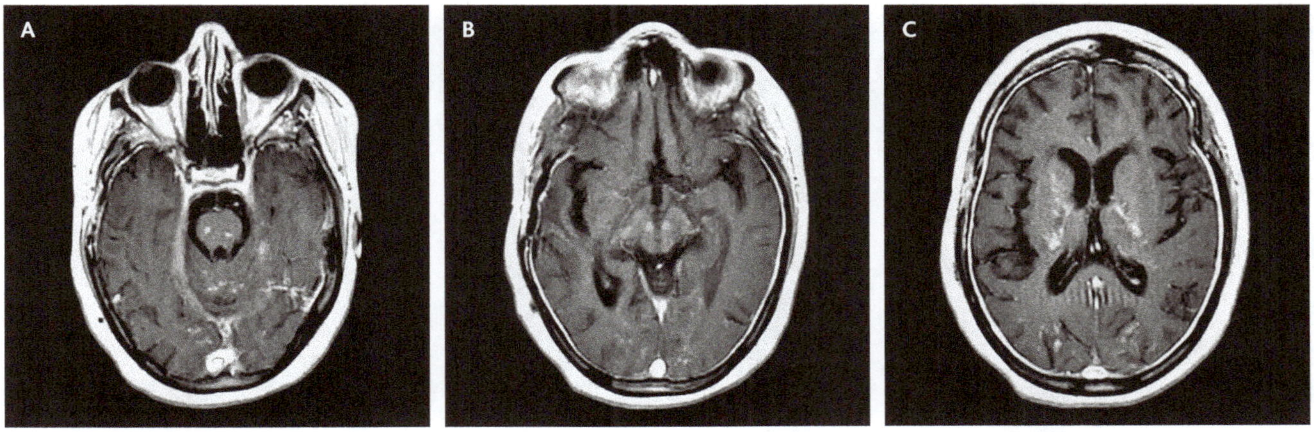

Figures 6-46A–C Clinical example Ray: Post-contrast T1 series showing white-matter lesions resulting from multiple sclerosis.

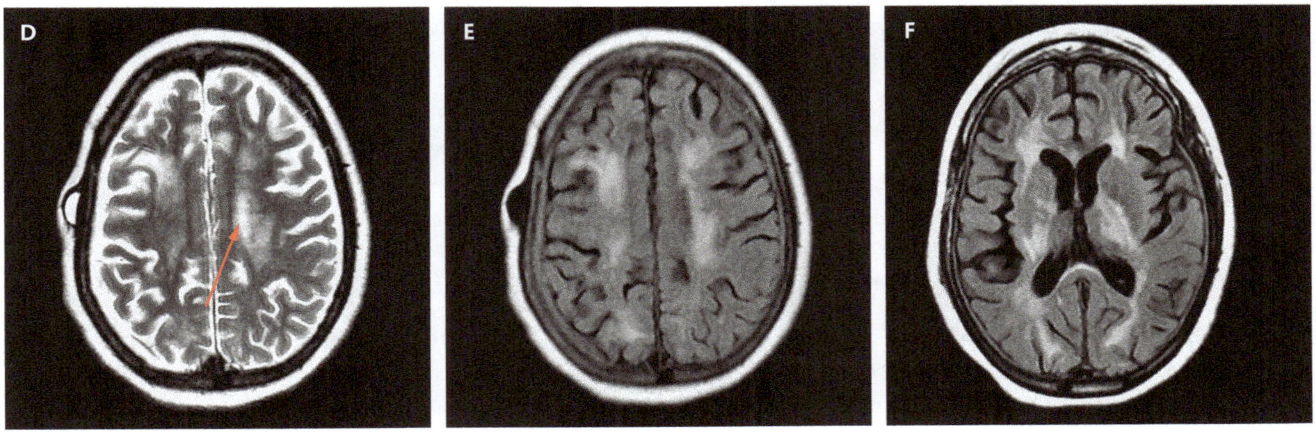

Figures 6-46A–F Clinical example Ray: *T2 and T2 FLAIR series showing white-matter involvement in multiple sclerosis.* **D:** T2. **E:** T2 FLAIR. **F:** T2 FLAIR.

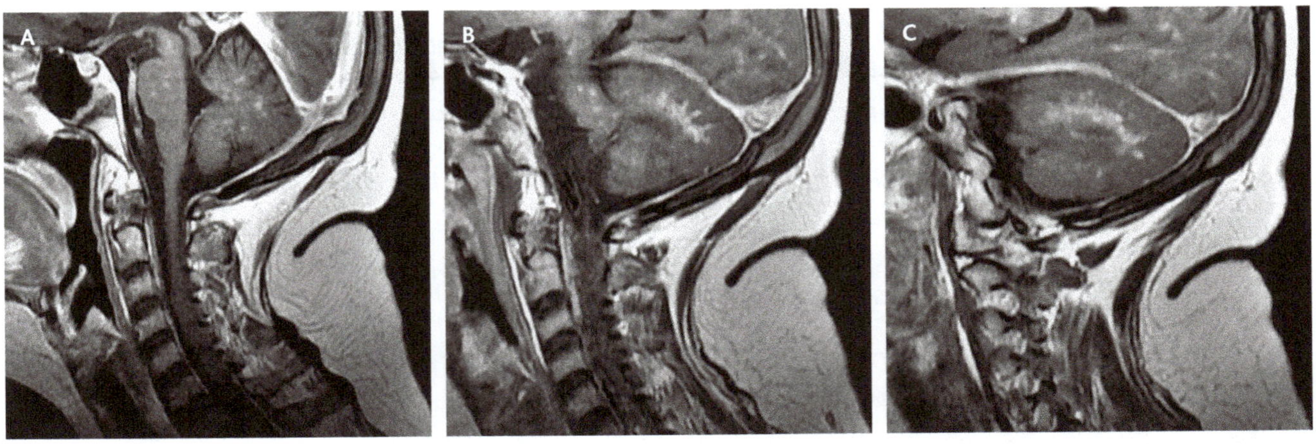

Figures 6-47A–C Clinical example Ray: T1 series showing involvement of Ray's midbrain, brain stem, and cerebellum, with lesions being due to multiple sclerosis.

several years, Ray's motor functioning declined much faster and to a greater degree than his cognitive functioning. Ray was aware that his condition was rapidly deteriorating and that he did not have long to live. As the MS progressed, involvement of the midbrain, brain stem, and cerebellum became evident on imaging (Figures 6-47A-C), with concomitant deterioration of functioning. Ultimately, Ray refused intubation during a period of respiratory compromise and bravely said goodbye to family, friends, and the hospital staff before passing away.

Review of Ray's brain imaging over the several years of his illness suggested a gradual progression of atrophic changes evident even two years prior to death (Figures 6-48A–C), with atrophy being unmistakable on imaging acquired close to his death (Figures 6-48D–F).

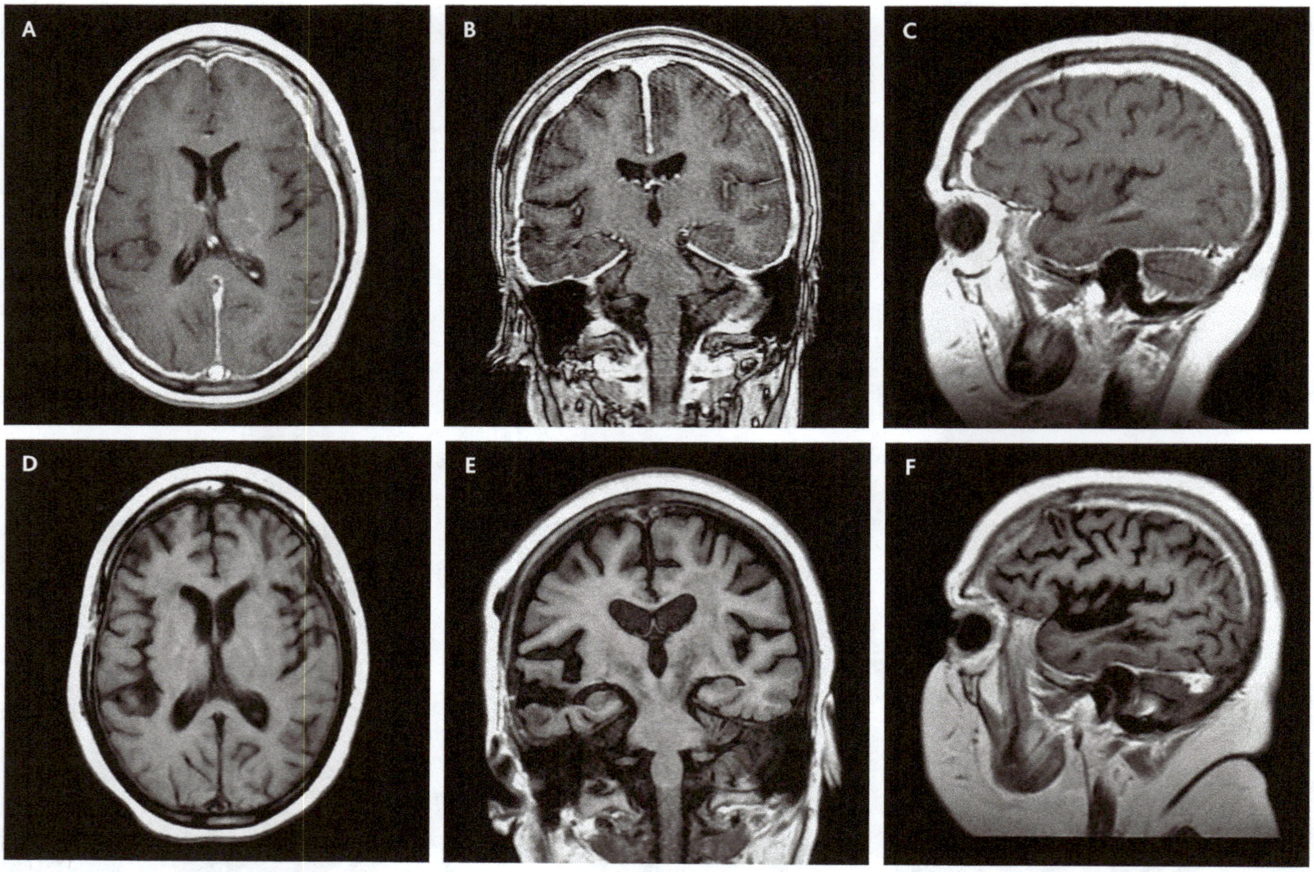

Figures 6-48A–F Clinical example Ray: T1 series 2 years before Ray died (A–C) and 2 months before Ray died (D–F), to allow for comparison of imaging over time. Note the degree of diffuse atrophy that had taken place over the two year period between the acquisition of the image series.

CLINICAL EXAMPLE

Stephanie: Focal Infarction due to Severe Multiple Sclerosis

Ray's MS resulted in many petechial and some patchy lesions throughout his brain. Sometimes demyelination from MS affects larger areas of white matter, which was the case with Stephanie. Her MS caused so much injury to the white matter of her brain that she experienced marked focal areas of infarction, clearly evident on T1 weighted imaging (Figures 6-49A–C).

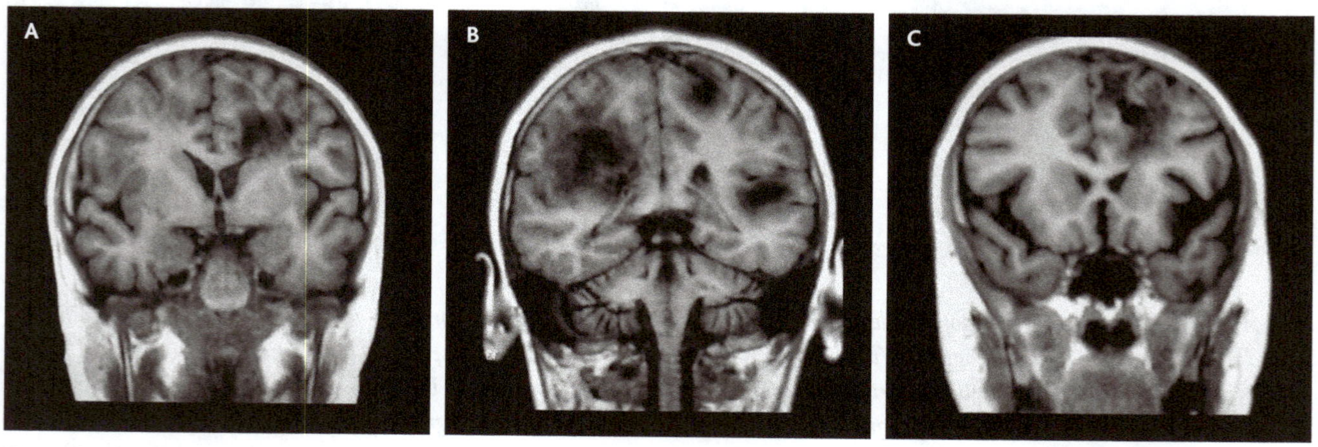

Figures 6-49A–C Clinical example Stephanie: Focal areas of severe infarction caused by MS, evident on T1 sequences as relatively large areas of hypointensity and isodensity to that of CSF in the ventricles.

Acute Disseminated Encephalomyalitis (ADEM)

Acute disseminated encephalomyelitis (ADEM) can appear very similar to MS on brain imaging, but it follows a different clinical course. ADEM presents with multiple foci of white-matter and sometimes deep gray-matter inflammation and lesions often following infectious illness. Lesions of the brain stem and posterior fossa may also be present and can result in respiratory compromise. The lesions are sometimes punctate and appear as small foci, although it is more common for the involved white matter to encompass larger areas than is seen in MS and take on a puffy cumulous cloud-like appearance. The lesions are usually bilateral and nonsymmetrical. Close to the lateral convexity, the hyperintense areas remain within the white matter and follow the sulci–gyri contours of the cortical mantle. ADEM is thought to be due to a postinfections autoimmune response resulting in demyelination. Unlike MS, ADEM is usually monophasic and does not follow a relapsing-remitting or chronic progressive course.

On non-contrast CT, it may be difficult to appreciate the condition, and the scans may be read as normal. Contrast-enhanced CT may show multifocal areas of enhancement. T1 sequences may not show the white-matter lesions, but contrast-enhanced T1 may show the affected white matter. On T2 and T2 FLAIR imaging, lesions appear hyperintense; these are often the best scans for visualizing the extent and severity of the condition. Restricted diffusion predicts a worse outcome; milder forms of the condition have normal diffusion. Lesions on DWI may appear hyperintense, a function of shine-through from the T2 weighting of the sequence, even without restricted diffusion. Use of the ADC sequence will assist in differentiating shine-through from abnormal diffusion.

CLINICAL EXAMPLE

Jamie: Acute Disseminated Encephalomyelitis

Jamie became critically ill from severe ADEM involving white matter, deep gray-matter nuclei, and brain stem structures. Recovery was protracted, and for several weeks it was unclear whether Jamie would survive her illness. Eventually, Jamie regained spontaneous respiratory functioning and began to interact with those around her. She progressed well during her hospitalization, eventually being discharged home with her parents. Imaging of Jamie's brain revealed significant white-matter involvement with additional inflammation of her brain stem and deep subcortical basal ganglia (Figures 6-50A–C). Progression of the demyelination and white-matter inflammation was evident over a 2-week period with follow-up MRI sequences showing extensive white matter involvement, clearly evident on T2 FLAIR sequences (Figures 6-51A–C). Note the progression of the white matter inflammation compared to the earlier scans, in addition to hyperintensity of the bilateral putamen and caudate nuclei. T1 non-contrast and contrast-enhanced sequences show white-matter involvement as areas of hypointensity (6-51D–F). Follow-up imaging also suggested a mild degree of diffuse atrophy with the atrophic appearance likely exacerbated by the use of high-dose steroids (Figures 6-51A–F).

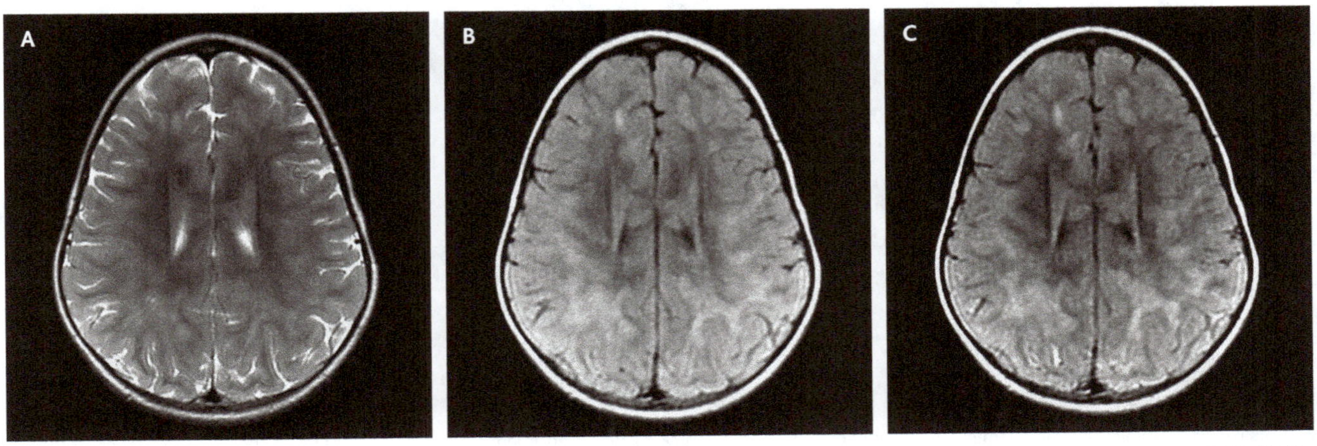

Figures 6-50A–C Clinical example Jamie: Initial MRI series showing acute disseminated encephalomyelitis, after acute hospitalization. **A:** T2. **B:** T2 FLAIR. **C:** Contrast-enhanced T2 FLAIR.

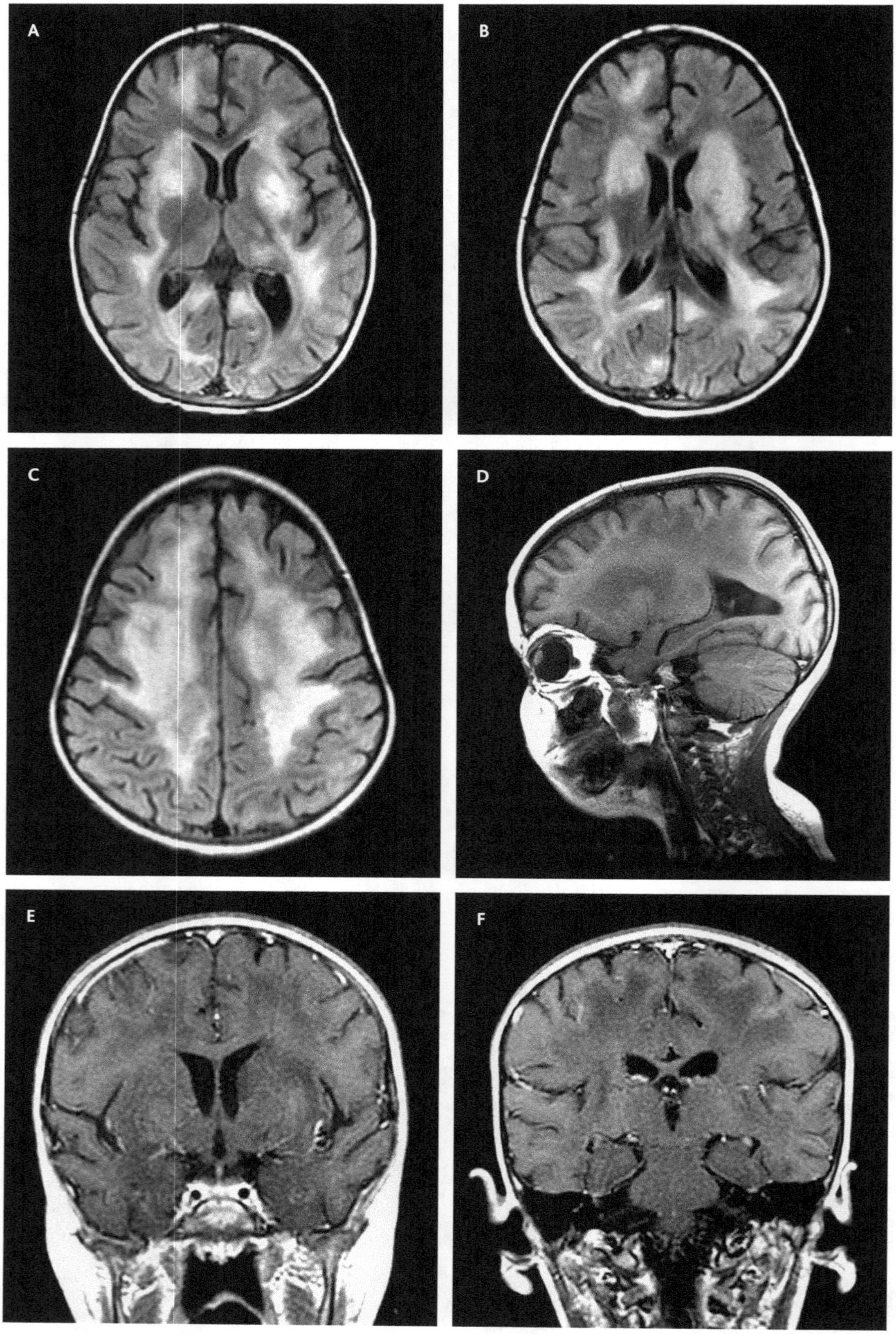

Figures 6-51A–F Clinical example Jamie: MRI series with and without contrast 2 weeks after Jamie's initial symptom onset showing progression of the illness. **A:** T2 FLAIR. **B:** T2 FLAIR. **C:** T2 FLAIR. **D:** T1. **E:** Contrast-enhanced T1 image. **F:** Contrast-enhanced T1 image.

CLINICAL CASE

Kevin: Mild Acute Disseminated Encephalomyelitis

While Jamie's case is an example of severe ADEM involving both white matter and subcortical gray matter, some cases of ADEM are so mild that it is difficult to visualize the white-matter inflammation on brain imaging, even T2 FLAIR sequences that are highly sensitive to the lesions. Kevin experienced mild ADEM with minimal cognitive, motor, and functional compromise. Only a few weeks after his illness, he was discharged home, functioning close to premorbid baseline levels. On 3-month follow-up neuropsychological examination, performance was fully intact in all domains involving cognitive, motor, and sensory functioning.

Post-contrast T2 FLAIR sequences may give one the best chance of appreciating the affected tissue in mild cases of ADEM such as Kevin's. Note the relatively normal appearance of the images, with the exception of some slight patchy hyperintensity within the white matter, mostly parietal and occipital, but also some frontal (Figure 6-52A–C, arrows).

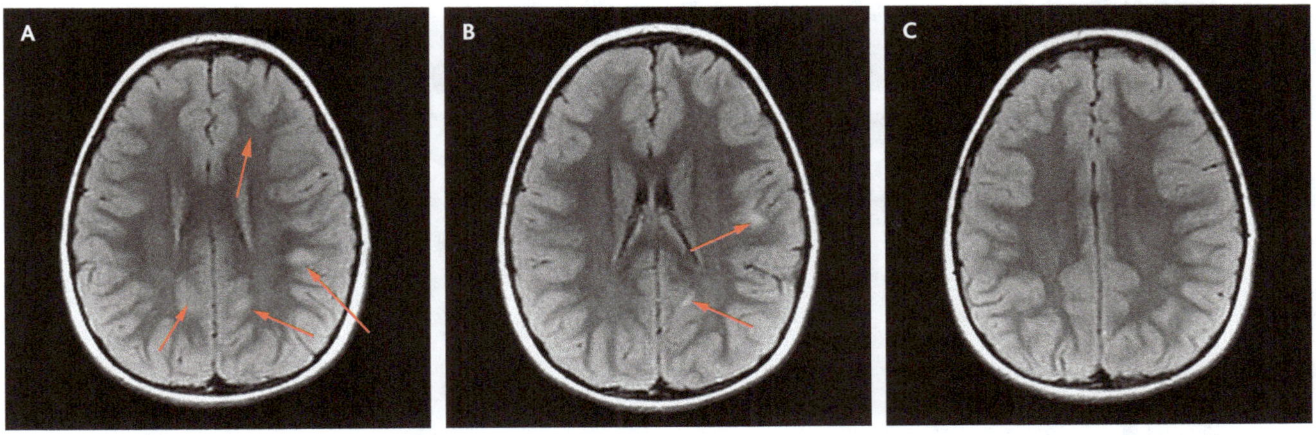

Figures 6-52A–C Clinical case Kevin: post-contrast T2 FLAIR series showing mild acute disseminated encephalomyelitis. Note slight enhancement of white matter in a relatively patchy distribution (arrows).

Toxic Damage to White Matter

White matter can also be damaged by prolonged exposure to toxic chemicals, a condition that is becoming more evident in toxic exposures from illegal methamphetamine labs.

CLINICAL EXAMPLE

Cortes: White-Matter Injury from Toxic Exposure

Cortes, a 2-year-old boy, was left in an illegal methamphetamine lab housed in an abandoned building that caught fire. The boy was discovered by fire fighters in a room filled with fumes from the volatile chemicals used in the production of methamphetamines.

Remarkably, Cortes had received CT and MRI imaging 3 months before the fire for a suspected closed-head injury, and the scans were read as normal (Figures 6-53A–C). In addition, Cortes had presented with grossly normal development and no obvious functional deficits. The availability of previous scans and clinical assessment allowed for a comparison between his premorbid findings and those obtained after the highly concentrated toxic exposure secondary to the fire (Figures 6-53D–F). It is also likely that there was some gradual injury to Cortes's brain from constant lower-level exposure; the effects of long-term exposure versus those from concentrated exposure during the fire could not be easily parsed.

On CT, the biggest difference between the premorbid scans and post-exposure scans was an obvious decrease in white-matter density encompassing almost the entire brain (Figure 6-53D). The white matter in Figure 6-53D is much darker than that in the pre-exposure scans (Figure 6-53A). Review of MRI imaging before and after toxic exposure further suggested damage to much of the white matter resulting from the exposure to toxic fumes. On T2 and T2 FLAIR sequences, the white matter appeared almost uniformly hyperintense, an appearance not common in other pathologies (Figures 6-53E and F). After exposure to the toxic chemicals, Cortes presented with marked deficits involving all cognitive and functional domains, although he retained some ability to volitionally move his upper and lower extremities.

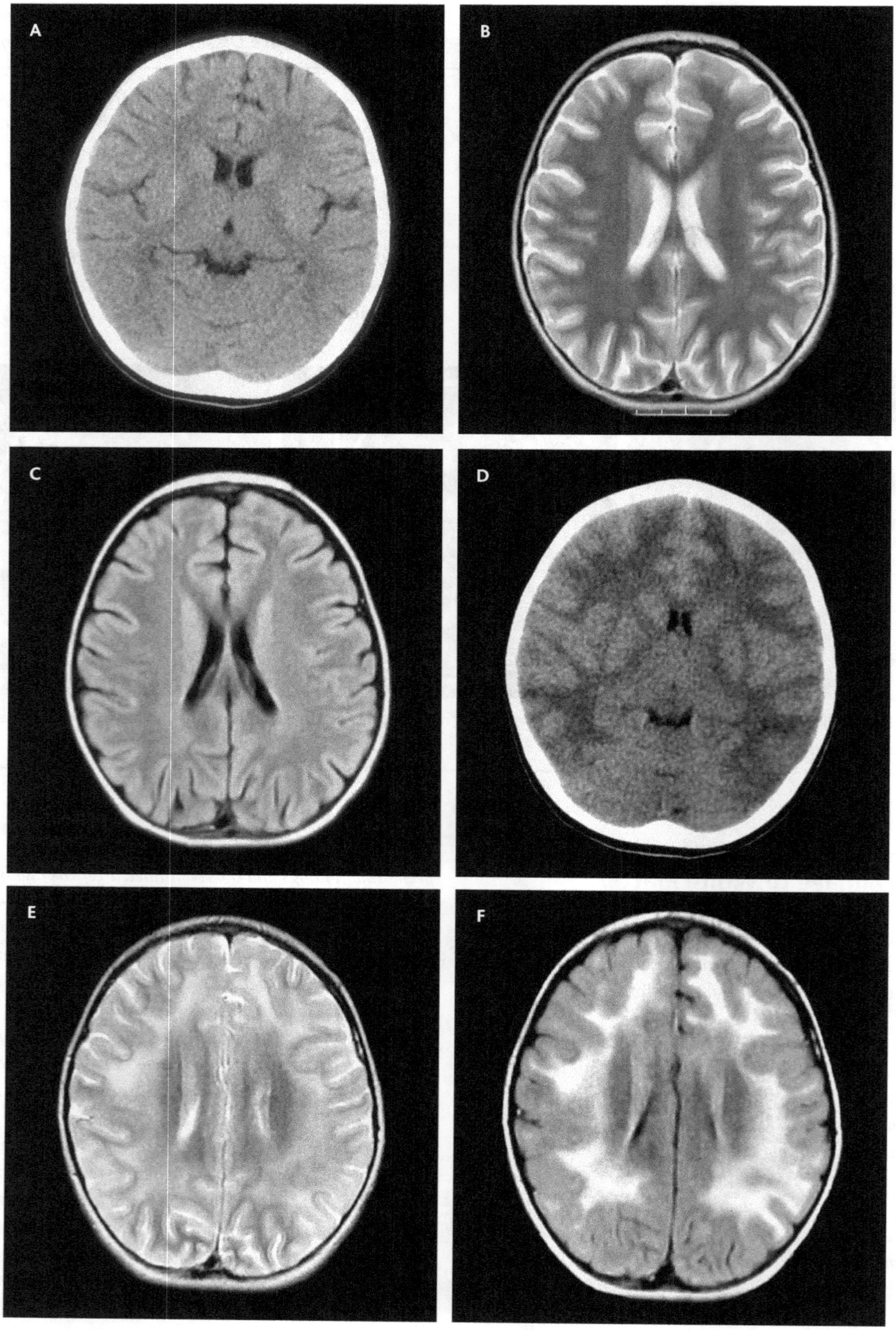

Figures 6-53A–F Clinical example Cortes: imaging prior to, and following toxic exposure showing post exposure injury to almost the entire white-matter of the brain. A–C = Pre-exposure scans. **A:** CT. **B:** T2. **C:** T2 FLAIR; D–F = Post-exposure scans. **D:** CT. **E:** T2. **F:** T2 FLAIR.

Tom exhibited mental-status changes followed by a rapid decline in his motor and cognitive abilities. MRI evidence suggested disrupted diffusion within the white matter (bright appearance on DWI and dark appearance on ADC), with sparing of the cortical lamina (Figures 6-54A–D). Interestingly, this condition has only recently been identified as a result of advances in radiology techniques. The syndrome took on a diagnostic label incorporating the radiographic presentation on DWI: "acute encephalopathy with biphasic seizures and late reduced diffusion," or AESD.

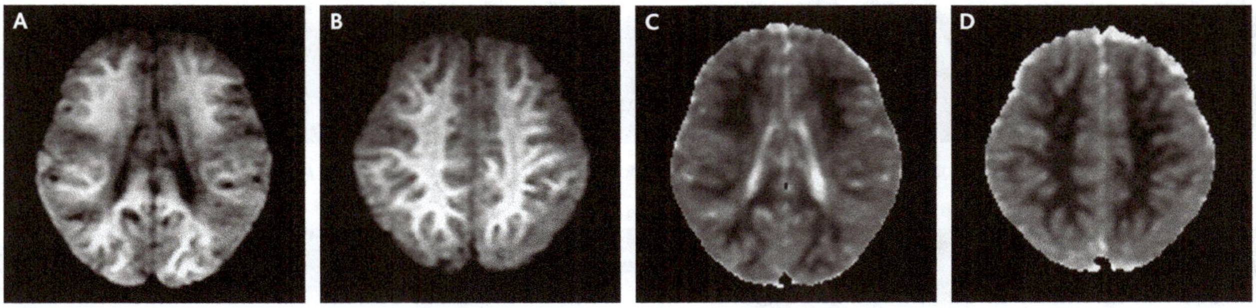

Figures 6-54A–D Diffusion series for Tom, who was identified as having acute encephalopathy with biphasic seizures and late reduced diffusion (AESD). Note appearance of restricted diffusion encompassing almost the entire white matter of the brain. **A:** DWI. **B:** DWI. **C:** ADC. **D:** ADC.

NEOPLASMS

Brain tumors are classified and graded on the basis of histological, radiological, and clinical findings. Brain imaging has become critically important in both the assessment of brain tumors and treatment decisions made by oncologists and neurosurgeons. The number and complexity of tumor types and radiological features are enormous and thus beyond the scope of this book. Instead, this section provides some examples of how tumors can appear on neuroimaging sequences. For the sake of simplicity, and by no means based on a formal classification of brain tumors, the examples are divided according to their primary anatomical and radiological features. Tumors are presented on the basis of whether they are mostly encapsulated or diffuse/infiltrating, as well as whether they show enhancement with use of contrast agents or remain unenhanced. In addition, examples of tumors resulting in secondary neurological complications due to hydrocephalus are included. The examples are provided to illustrate the variation in appearance on brain imaging for different brain tumors.

Diffuse, Infiltrating, and Nonenhancing Tumor

CLINICAL EXAMPLE

Elliott: Diffuse, Infiltrating, and Nonenhancing Tumor

Elliott was seen in the clinic for new-onset weakness of her left upper extremity. Brain imaging revealed a large right-hemisphere nonenhancing mass encompassing her lateral cortex and temporal lobe. There was uncal herniation, although this did not appear related to mass effect or pressure and was possibly due to slow growth of the tumor. Ultimately, the tumor was classified as a grade II, or low-grade, astrocytoma.

On brain imaging, low-grade astrocytomas present as a nonenhancing, relatively well-defined, but infiltrating mass found mostly within the white matter (Figures 6-55A–C). On CT and T1 sequences the mass can appear isodense to hypodense (Figures 6-55C–F), although may appear hypointense, without enhancement on post-contrast images. On T2 weighted sequences, the tumor appears hyperintense (Figures 6-55A and B). DWI images often suggest no disruption to diffusion and can appear normal.

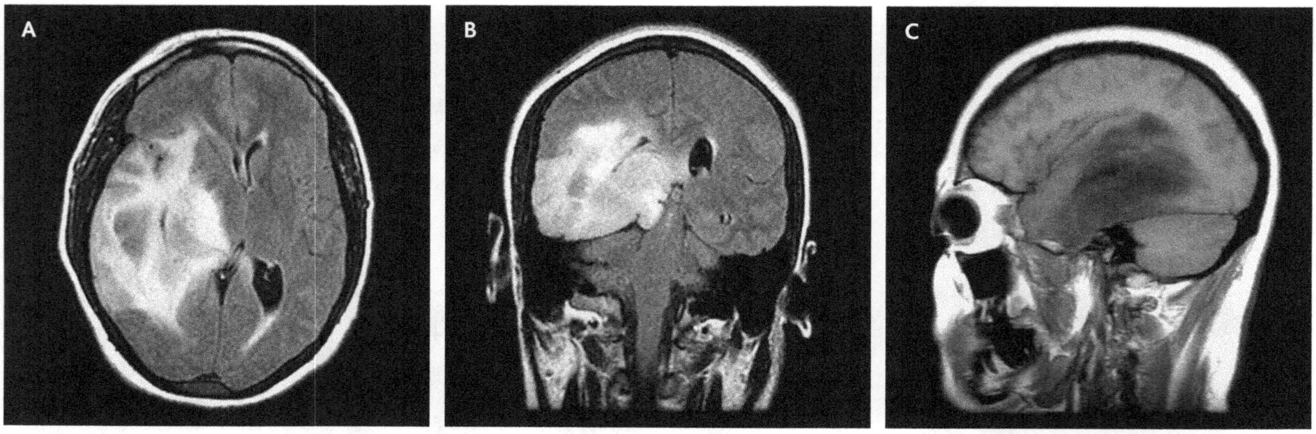

Figures 6-55A–C Clinical example Elliott: diffuse, infiltrating, and nonenhancing tumor, non-contrast MRI series. **A:** T2 FLAIR. **B:** T2 FLAIR. **C:** T1.

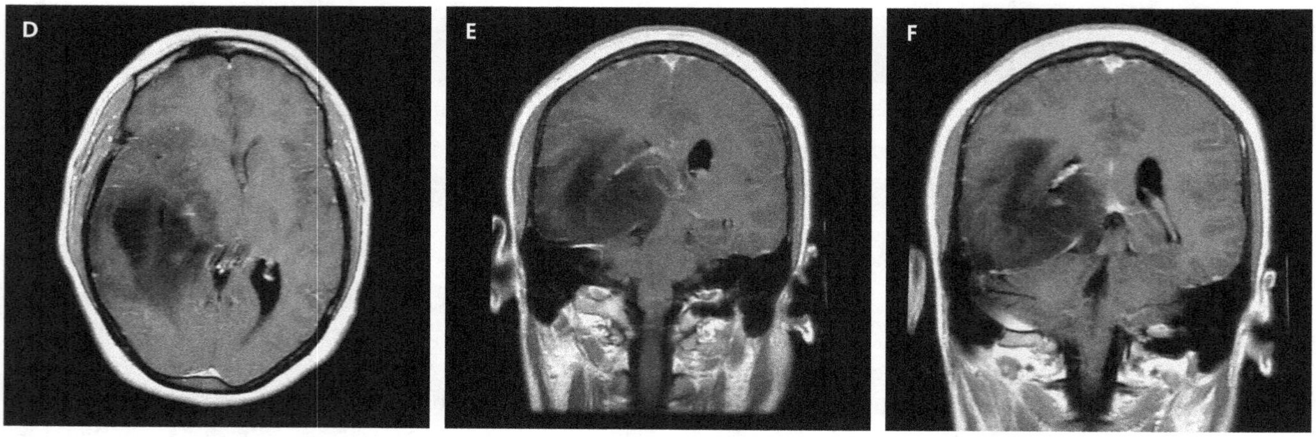

Figures 6-55A–F Clinical example Elliott: contrast-enhanced T1 FLAIR series.

Diffuse, Infiltrating, and Contrast-Enhancing Tumor

CLINICAL EXAMPLE

Jacob: Diffuse, Infiltrating, and Contrast-Enhancing Tumor

Jabob was diagnosed with a glioblastoma multiforme (GBM) in the left parietal lobe. High-grade astrocytomas such as a GBM are enhanced by the use of contrast agents. GBMs often have an enhancing border surrounding a core of necrotic brain tissue. Even though there is a border to the tumor, active malignant cells extend beyond the border and infiltrate surrounding tissue. The infiltrating cells can "seed" new areas of growth, resulting in a multifocal appearance. GBMs are highly vascular, a requirement of the rapid cellular growth of these tumors. Given the rapid growth of GBMs, mass effect and extensive edema are often features of the tumor.

On brain imaging, the mass can appear heterogeneous from the mix of tumor, necrotizing tissue, hemorrhage, and edema. On non-contrast CT and T1 imaging, the tumor can appear as a heterogeneous isodense-to-hypodense mass mostly within the white matter. On contrast-enhanced CT and T1 sequences, the most remarkable feature is the enhancing ring around a necrotic hypodense or hypointense core. T2 and T2 FLAIR sequences can be more helpful in fully appreciating the extent and severity of a GBM. On T2-weighted images, the GBM appears as a heterogeneous hyperintense mass surrounded by significant edema. DWI and ADC sequences usually suggest restricted diffusion and can be helpful in assessing for vasogenic edema. Hemorrhages may be evident on imaging studies; their appearance will vary according to the age of the bleed and the sequence used.

Because high-grade astrocytomas grow rapidly, serial imaging can be helpful in treatment planning. This was the case with Jacob, who received multiple MRI scans over a period of just a few months. Figures 6-56A–D show the GBM prior to surgical intervention on a variety of MRI sequences. Note the differing appearance of the mass on the various imaging sequences.

Two months after initial resection and debulking of Jacob's GBM, T2 and T2 FLAIR sequences show extensive involvement surrounding the cavity (Figures 6-57A and B). T1 sequences without contrast show the involvement around the resection cavity as an area of hypointensity. However, T1 imaging with contrast provides the classic appearance of the contrast enhancing ring around the resection cavity. Also note that there appears to be a metastatic lesion most evident on contrast-enhanced T1 FLAIR imaging, just medial and anterior to the resection cavity (arrow). Only a few months earlier, this lesion was not visible on imaging (Figures 6-56A–D).

Three months after initial resection and debulking of Jacob's GBM, and one month following the scans shown in Figures 5–57A–D, it was clear that there was increased edema around the surgical cavity where the tumor was debulked, and growth of the metastatic lesion (Figures 6-58A–D). GBMs are rapidly growing neoplasms and highly malignant even with ongoing chemotherapy, radiosurgery and multiple surgical resections to debulk the tumor core. Directed CyberKnife radiosurgery was successful in decreasing the size of the metastatic foci and in returning language abilities to the patient, but it is still a temporary solution to a devastating condition.

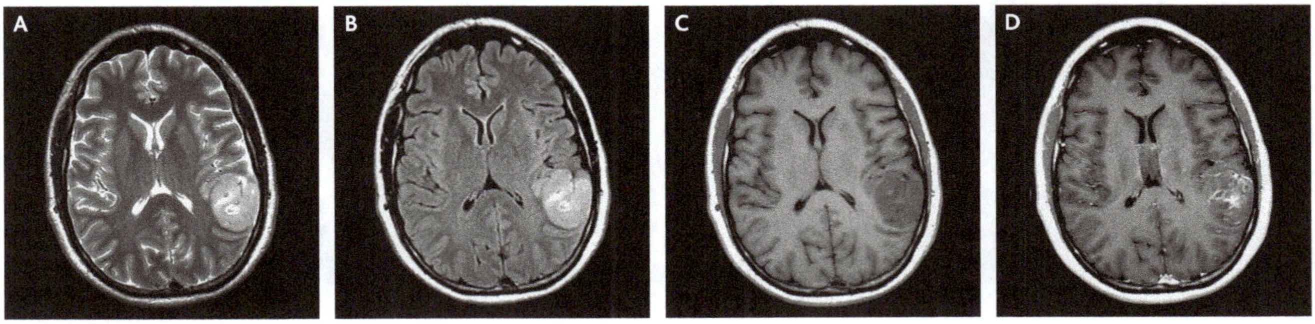

Figures 6-56A–D Clinical example Jacob: MRI series with, and without contrast showing a diffuse, infiltrating, and contrast-enhancing neoplasm prior to surgical intervention. **A:** T2. **B:** T2 FLAIR. **C:** T1 FLAIR. **D:** Contrast-enhanced T1 FLAIR.

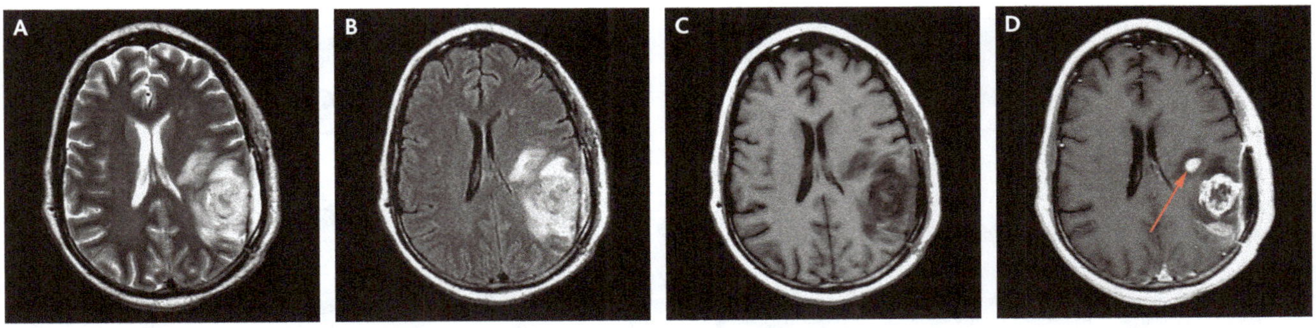

Figures 6-57A–D Clinical example Jacob: MRI series with, and without contrast 2 months after initial resection and debulking of Jacob's GBM. Note increased T2 hyperintensity, T1 hypointensity and new metastatic lesion most evident on contrast-enhanced T1 FLAIR (arrow). **A:** T2. **B:** T2 FLAIR. **C:** T1 FLAIR. **D:** Contrast-enhanced T1 FLAIR.

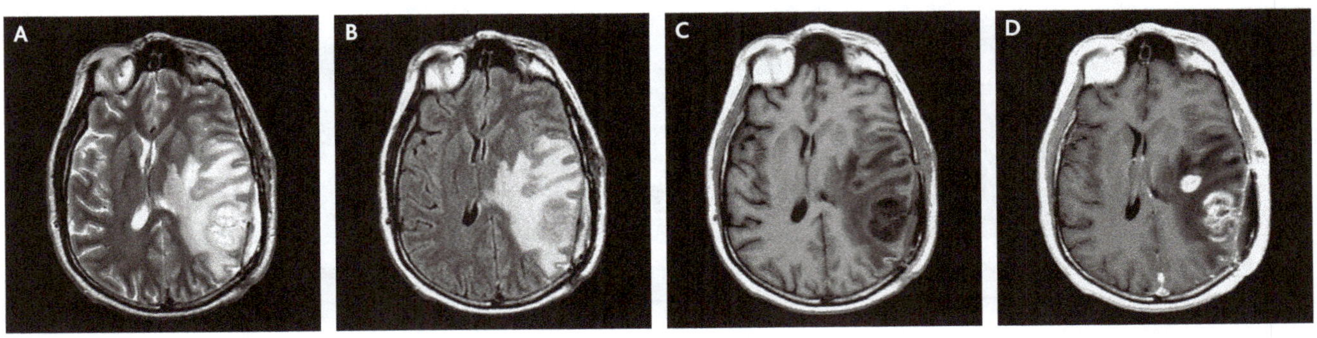

Figures 6-58A–D Clinical example Jacob: MRI series with, and without contrast 3 months after initial resection and debulking of Jacob's GBM. Note increase edema and size of the metastasis. **A:** T2. **B:** T2 FLAIR. **C:** T1 FLAIR. **D:** Contrast-enhanced T1 FLAIR.

Encapsulated Nonenhancing Cystic Tumor

CLINICAL EXAMPLE

Victoria: Encapsulated Nonenhancing Cystic Tumor

Victoria was hospitalized with new-onset seizures. Brain imaging revealed a nonenhancing, encapsulated cystic neoplasm within the right hippocampal region (Figures 6-59A–C).

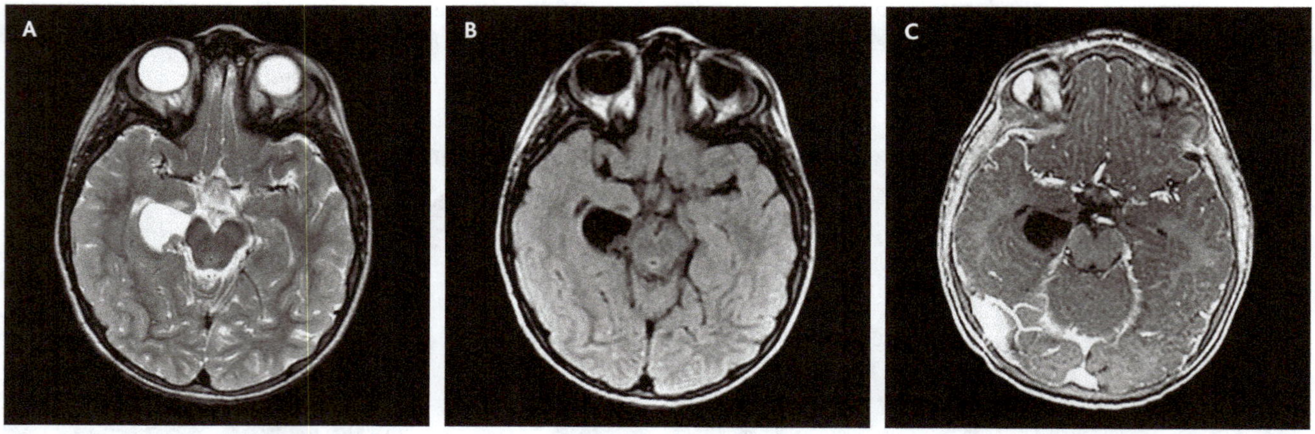

Figure 6-59A–C Clinical example Victoria: encapsulated nonenhancing cystic tumor. **A:** T2. **B:** T2 FLAIR. **C:** Contrast-enhanced T1 image.

Encapsulated Contrast-Enhancing Tumor

CLINICAL EXAMPLE

Jack: Encapsulated Contrast-Enhancing Tumor

Jack was seen in the clinic for new-onset seizures. Imaging revealed an encapsulated, contrast-enhancing mass in his left temporal lobe at the medial pole (Figures 6-60A–C). Note the bright appearance on CE T1 imaging (Figure 6-60C), in comparison to the darker appearance on non-contrast T1 (Figure 6-60B).

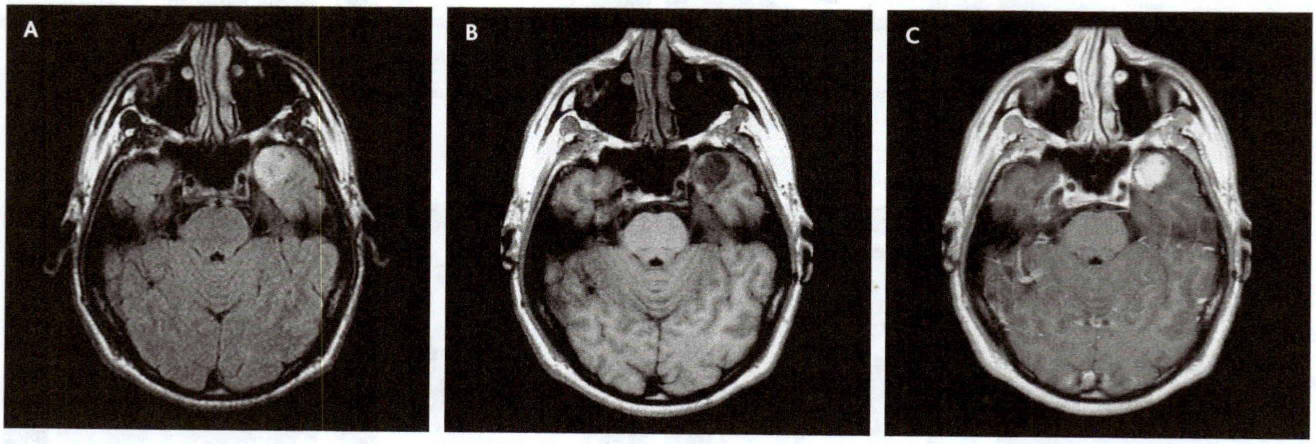

Figure 6-60A–C Clinical example Jack: encapsulated contrast-enhancing tumor. **A:** T2 FLAIR. **B:** T1 FLAIR. **C:** Contrast-enhanced T1 FLAIR.

Hydrocephalus due to Tumor Growth

Growth of tumors can result in significant mass effect within the brain. If the tumor is located away from critical structures, it can grow relatively large without notable symptoms. However, if the tumor is located close to the ventricular system, especially the thin pathways of the foramen of Monro, cerebral aqueduct of Sylvius, or foramena of Luschka or Magendie, significant hydrocephalus and ventricular dilation can occur, even with a relatively small neoplasm. Headaches, nausea, and vomiting from hydrocephalus are often the first indicators of a brain tumor located close to the ventricular system. Following are some examples of tumors that caused hydrocephalus.

CLINICAL EXAMPLE

Pinealblastoma Restricting CSF Flow

Pinealblastomas are malignant neoplasms that can rapidly grow to become a large, heterogeneous, lobulated mass originating from the pineal gland. The location of the tumor above and posterior to the third ventricle and cerebral aqueduct of Sylvius results in hydrocephalus in most if not all cases. On brain imaging, pinealblastomas can appear heterogeneous with mixed hyperdensities on CT (Figures 6-61A–C) and MRI (Figures 6-61D–F), with a somewhat heterogeneous pattern of enhancement on contrast imaging; some regions show more enhancement than others. Note the hyperdense appearance of the tumor on CT, even without the use of contrast agents. Also note the dilation of the ventricles caused by obstruction of flow through the third ventricle to the cerebral aqueduct of Sylvius.

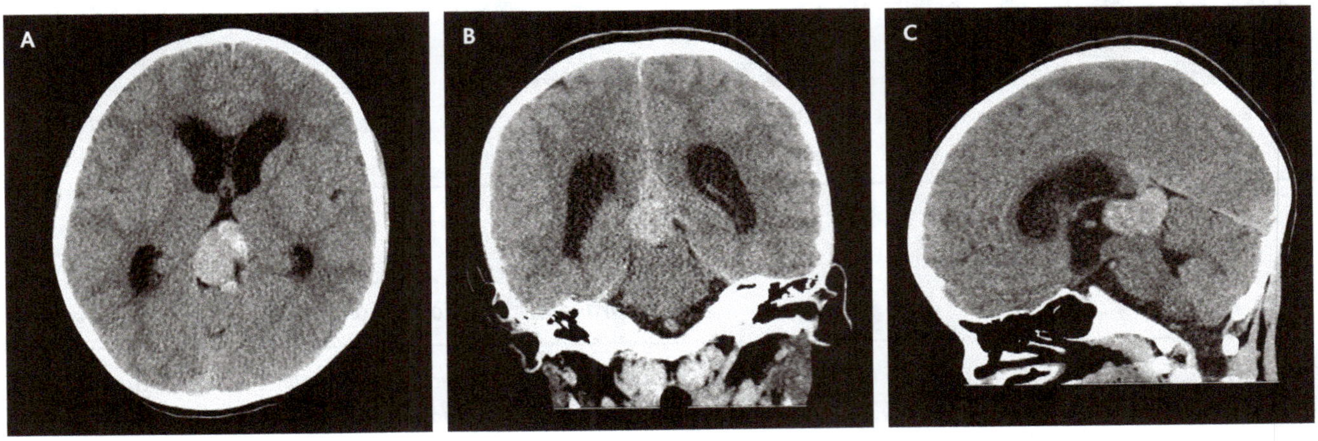

Figures 6-61A–C CT series of pinealblastoma restricting CSF flow.

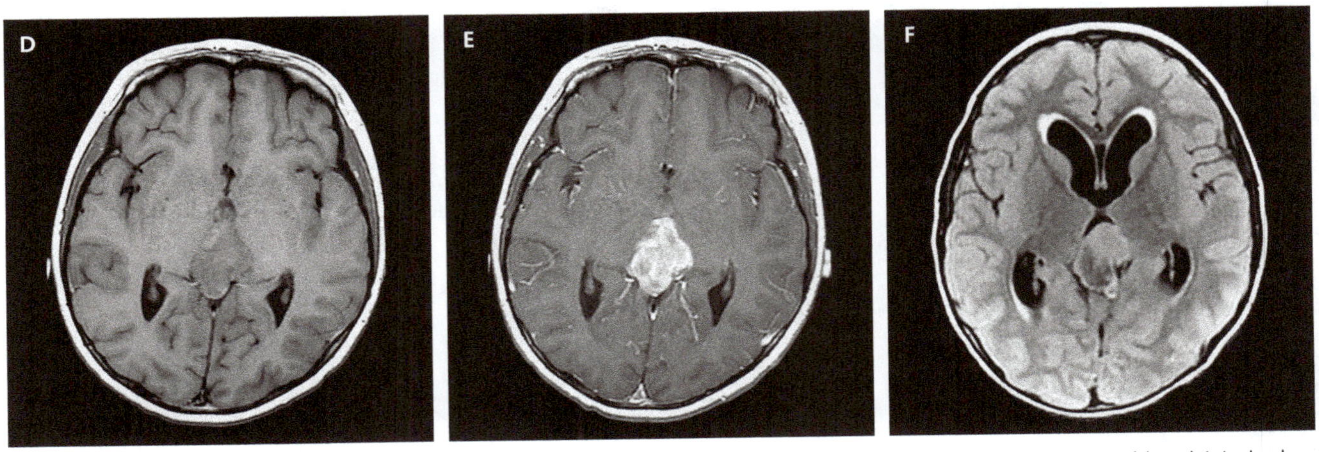

Figures 6-61D–F MRI series of pinealblastoma with, and without contrast. The tumor is difficult to appreciate on non-contrast T1, although it is clearly evident on the contrast-enhanced T1 image. **D:** T1. **E:** Contrast-enhanced T1. **F:** T2 FLAIR.

CLINICAL EXAMPLE
Mike: Suprasellar Craniopharyngioma Restricting CSF Flow

Suprasellar craniopharyngiomas, a type of adenoma, are generally benign slow-growing tumors that can reach a large size prior to discovery. They are often lobulated and cystic, giving them a heterogeneous appearance on imaging (Figures 6-62A–C). Some are so lobular that they appear like a bunch of grapes, which is the case in this example. Although the third ventricle appears completely blocked by the mass, the degree of hydrocephalus is relatively mild. This is due to the slow growth of the tumor and the use of a shunt to release intraventricular pressure. Remarkably, even with the tumor growing so large prior to discovery, Mike was still able to function normally. Primary medical issues related to his endocrine system resulting from damage to his hypothalamic and pituitary structures. He also had some visual impairment, but not of the extent to preclude normal everyday functioning.

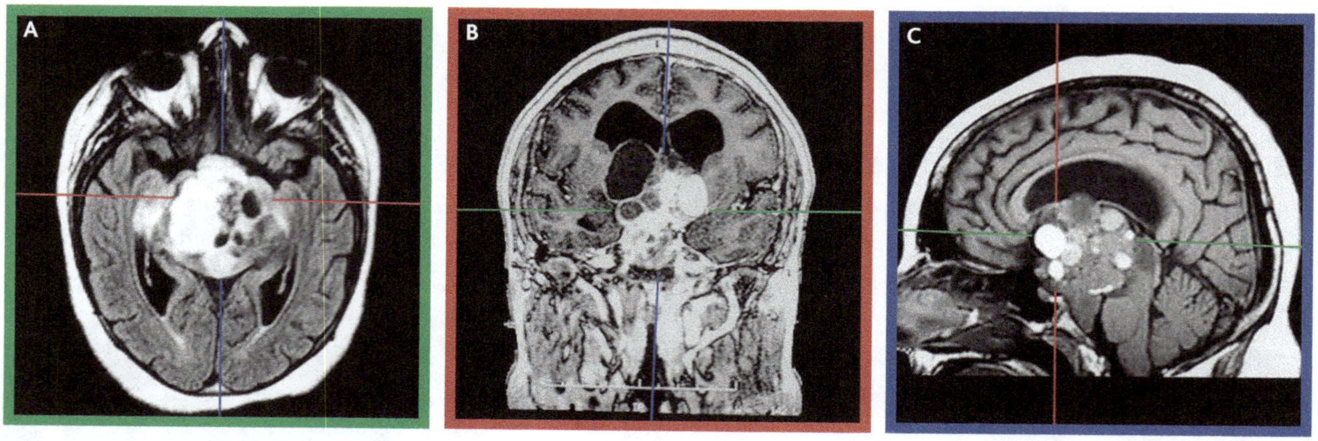

Figure 6-62A–C Clinical example Mike: Imaging of suprasellar craniopharyngioma restricting CSF flow, resulting in mild hydrocephalus due to the slow growth of the neoplasm. **A:** T2 FLAIR. **B:** T1. **C:** T1.

CLINICAL EXAMPLE
Abi: Suprasellar Craniopharyngioma Restricting CSF Flow

Not only did Abi's adenoma or tumor of the pituitary result in blockage of CSF flow, it also had a very large cystic component (Figures 6-63A–C). Remarkably, Abi experienced few symptoms, likely because of the slow growth of the neoplasm, giving her brain a chance to compensate and adapt. Not surprisingly, the primary deficits experienced by Abi were similar to

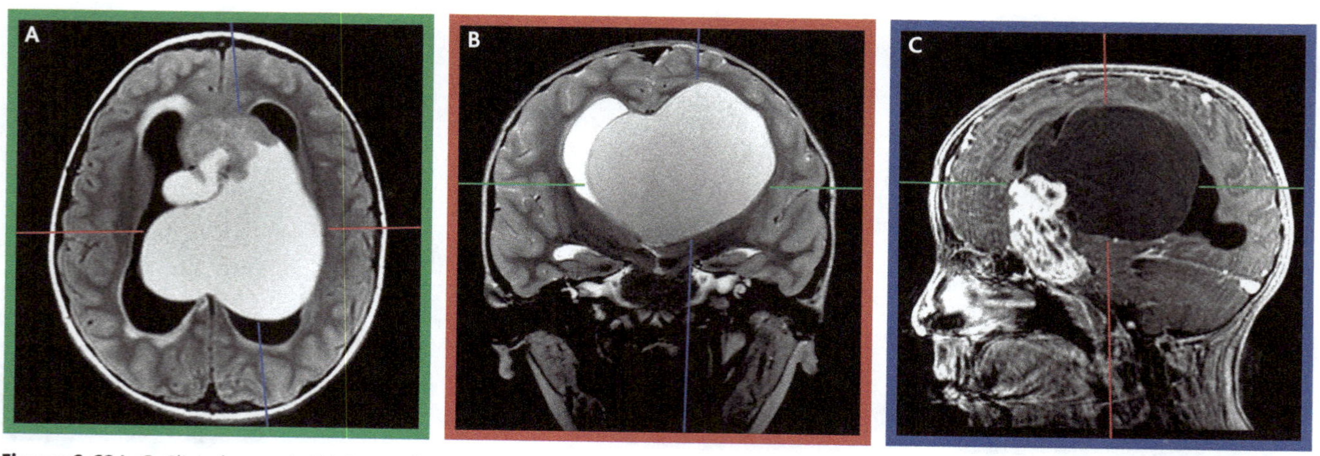

Figures 6-63A–C Clinical example Abi: Suprasellar craniopharyngioma restricting CSF flow. Note very large ventricles visible around edges of the cyst. There is also some transependymal edema most noticeable on T2 FLAIR imaging and primarily within the frontal and occipital lobes. **A:** T2 FLAIR. **B:** T2. **C:** Contrast-enhanced T1 image.

those experienced by Mike in the previous clinical example, she had disrupted endocrine functioning and visual loss. Because the patient was an infant and not yet speaking, she was unable to describe any symptoms, even those involving her vision. Her mother was concerned about her losing her vision, which precipitated the examination and brain imaging. By the time she was examined, she had limited functional vision and was unable to see small objects.

CLINICAL EXAMPLE
Amelia: Medulloblastoma Restricting CSF flow

Medulloblastomas are tumors originating from the fourth ventricle. Given the location, they frequently put pressure on the cerebral aqueduct of Sylvius and fourth ventricle, preventing CSF from flowing to the lateral foramena of Luschka and midline foramen of Magendie. The restricted flow can result in marked dilation of the lateral, third, and fouth ventricles and in increased intraventricular pressure, as was clearly evident on Amelia's brain imaging (Figures 6-64A–F). On CT, the mass can appear solid and is often hyperdense, becoming enhanced with contrast agents. On T1 and T2 sequences, the mass can appear hypointense, or slightly hyperintense on T2. Hyperintensity is greater on T2 FLAIR sequences. Just as with CT, the mass shows enhancement with the use of contrast agents. After removal of the tumor, Amelia's hydrocephalus subsided and her functioning improved. However, following her posterior fossa surgery, she experienced cerebellar mutism with severe verbal apraxia and dysphagia for several weeks. Cerebellar mutism is often temporary, lasting only a few weeks to months, and only sometimes results from posterior fossa surgeries.

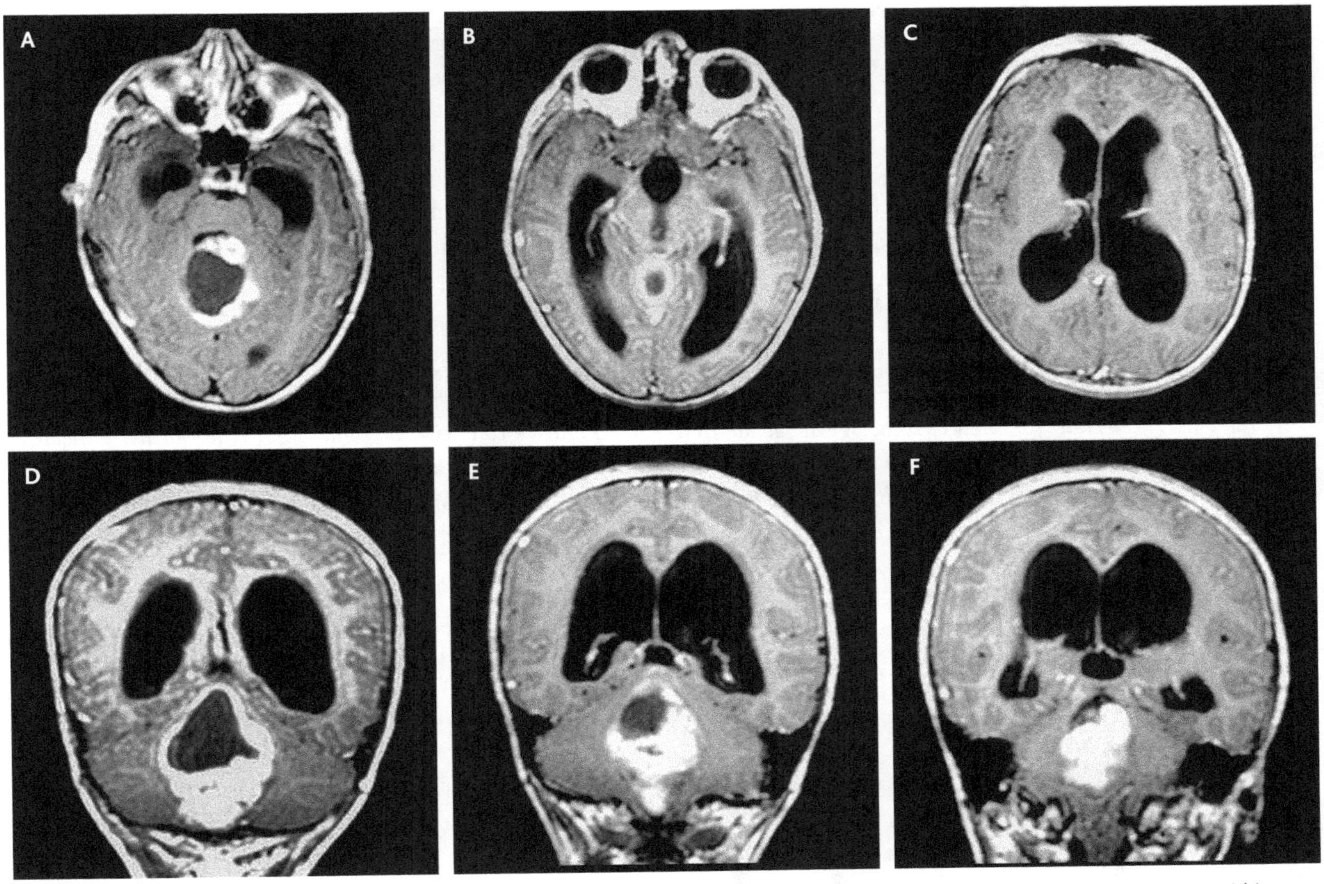

Figures 6-64A–F Clinical example Amelia: T1 contrast-enhanced MRI series of medulloblastoma restricting CSF flow. Note enhancing tumor within cerebellum at the level of the fourth ventricle and dilation of the third and lateral ventricles.

NEURODEVELOPMENTAL DISORDERS

Neurodevelopmental disorders encompass a range of conditions spanning from tiny microscopic dysplasias not visible on brain imaging to an almost complete lack of brain development. The following examples cover a range of neurodevelopmental disorders and are intended to provide you with an idea of how varied the appearance of these conditions can be on brain imaging.

Cortical Dysplasia

Many times, minor cortical dysplasia will go undiscovered, especially if the patient does not experience any symptoms. Often the discovery of an area of cortical dysplasia is incidental to another condition, such as seizures. The brain scan shown in Figure 6-65 was acquired as part of a seizure workup for a patient who had been refractory to medications. A small area of cortical dysplasia was discovered on the medial surface of the left hemisphere (arrow).

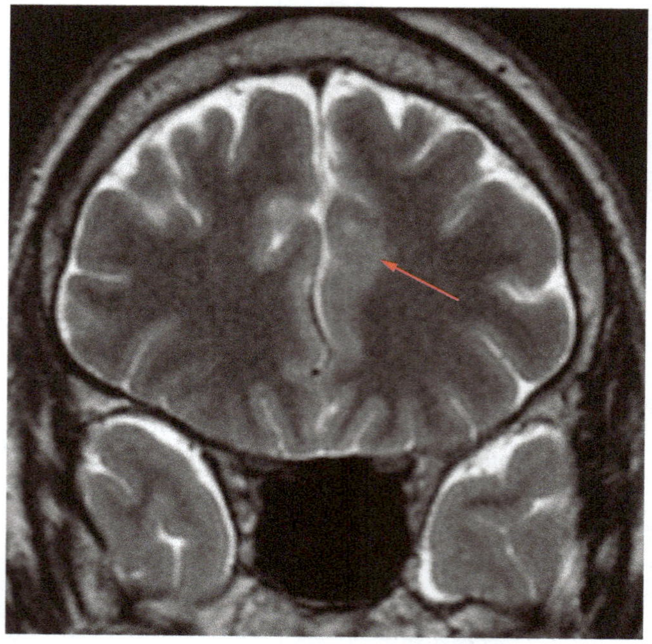

Figure 6-65 MRI T2 sequence showing and area of subtle cortical dysplasia (arrow).

Agenesis of the Corpus Callosum (ACC)

Agenesis of the corpus callosum (ACC) is a congenital disorder resulting from either partial or complete absence of corpus callosum development in utero. There is a wide range of functional presentations for this condition, with some individuals exhibiting normal intelligence and functional abilities, while others exhibit notable deficits in functioning. The general presentation is one of disrupted higher-order integrative and executive abilities, even if intelligence falls within normal limits.

CLINICAL EXAMPLE

Randy: Agenesis of the Corpus Callosum

Randy was referred for neuropsychological evaluation because he had fallen behind in school and was having increasing difficulty as he matured. As his difficulties became progressively worse over several years, he was scanned to rule out a degenerative condition or some other cause of his difficulties in school. CT imaging revealed agenesis of the corpus callosum (Figures 6-66A–C arrows), and there was no evidence that the structured had developed during fetal maturation.

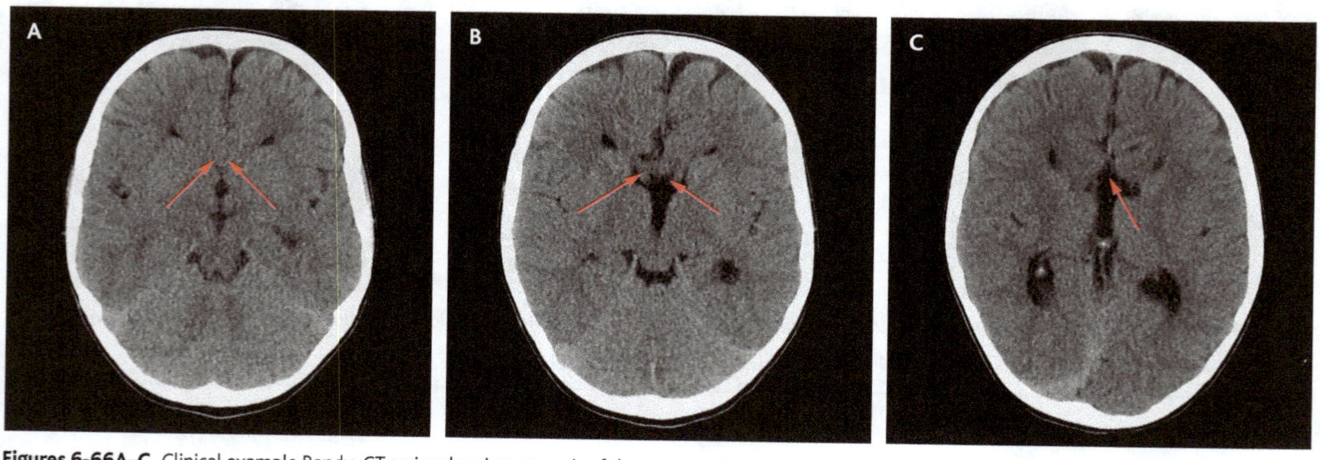

Figures 6-66A–C Clinical example Randy: CT series showing agenesis of the corpus callosum. Note absence of corpus callosum in areas identified by arrows.

Neuropsychological assessment indicated borderline to low average intelligence but with a clear deficit involving executive functioning, integrative abilities, and ability to conceptualize information abstractly. Responses were concrete and stimulus bound, and Randy had a high degree of cognitive and conceptual rigidity. Visual–motor integration and higher-order problem solving were disrupted and below that expected for his age.

It was not that Randy's abilities were deteriorating with age; it was that he was failing to develop cognitive abilities expected of his age. As he progressed through school, he was having increasing difficulty as expectations for integrative, conceptual, and abstract processing increased. Previously, he had been able to maintain good grades, as concrete processing was adequate and more appropriate to his developmental level. As his peers progressed with normal development, his brain was unable to develop integrative abilities at the same rate because of his agenesis of the corpus callosum. With the increased availability of brain imaging, anatomical correlates of cognitive and functional disabilities in children are becoming more common.

Polymicrogyria

CLINICAL EXAMPLE

Shelly: Polymicrogyria

Shelly experienced significant developmental deficits involving cognition and self-help or adaptive skills. She had required special education services since the beginning of school and was progressing slowly with basic preacademic and functional skills. Following a seizure, Shelly underwent brain imaging as part of her neurological workup. Neuroimaging revealed a highly disorganized cortical structure with many more gyri than expected and with areas of her brain where the gyri were excessively thin and compacted (Figures 6-67A–C). Polymicrogyria is a form of cortical dysplasia, in that the cortical surface and the sulci and gyri do not form appropriately. T1 sequences, especially high-contrast 3D T1 FSPGR sequences, may provide the best visualization of the cortical surface. The images in Figures 6-67A–C were produced using 3D T1 FSPGR sequences to maximize tissue resolution and facilitate viewing of the cortical structures. The crosshairs on the images highlight one of the primary areas of polymicrogyria, although areas of polymicrogyria were evident within every cortical lobe.

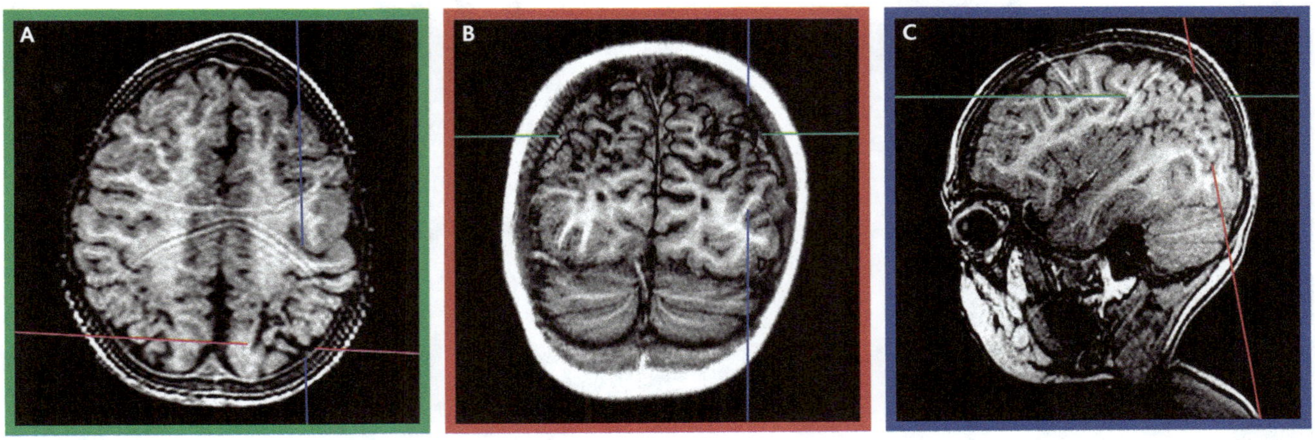

Figures 6-67A–C Clinical example Shelly: T1 3D FSPGR series showing polymicrogyria throughout most of the lateral cortex.

Anencephaly

Anencephaly is caused by a neural-tube defect involving disrupted growth of cerebral cortex and the superior part of the skull, but with development of subcortical structures such as the midbrain and brain stem. Anencephaly can result in enough subcortical tissue to sustain life, but not enough to allow cognitive or adaptive functioning.

The almost 30-year-old patient whose scan are presented here has been in a prolonged vegetative state since birth, requiring a feeding tube and full-time care. Respiratory functioning has been stable without supplemental oxygen or ventilator support. Given the lack of cortical development (Figures 6-68A–C), autonomic storming is a common occurrence requiring frequent inpatient stays for stabilization.

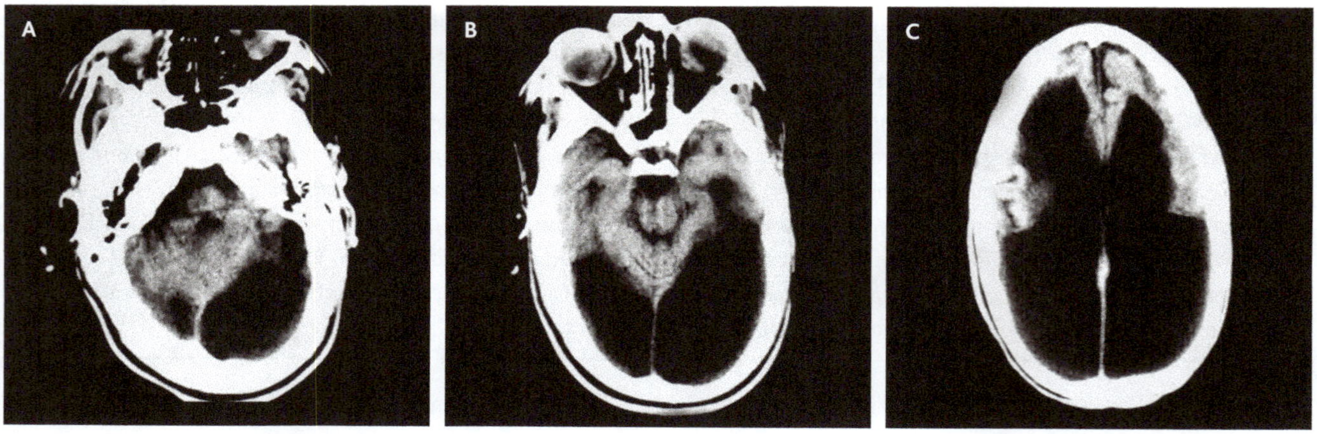

Figures 6-68A–C CT series of an adult patient with anencephaly. Note almost complete lack of lateral cortex, other than some minimal anterior temporal and frontal tissue.

Holoprosencephaly

Holoprosencephaly is a condition in which the prosencephalon of the fetus fails to develop, or atrophies. The prosencephalon or forebrain normally develops to form the telencephalon and diencephalon, and includes but is not restricted to the cerebral cortex, limbic structures, thalamus and hypothalamus, and basal ganglia. Midbrain and brain stem structures often develop, allowing for spontaneous respiratory functioning and central nervous system arousal. Holoprosencephaly is similar to anencephaly, but with development of the cranium.

The example of holoprosencephaly presented in Figures 6-69A–F may be secondary to atrophy of the forebrain,

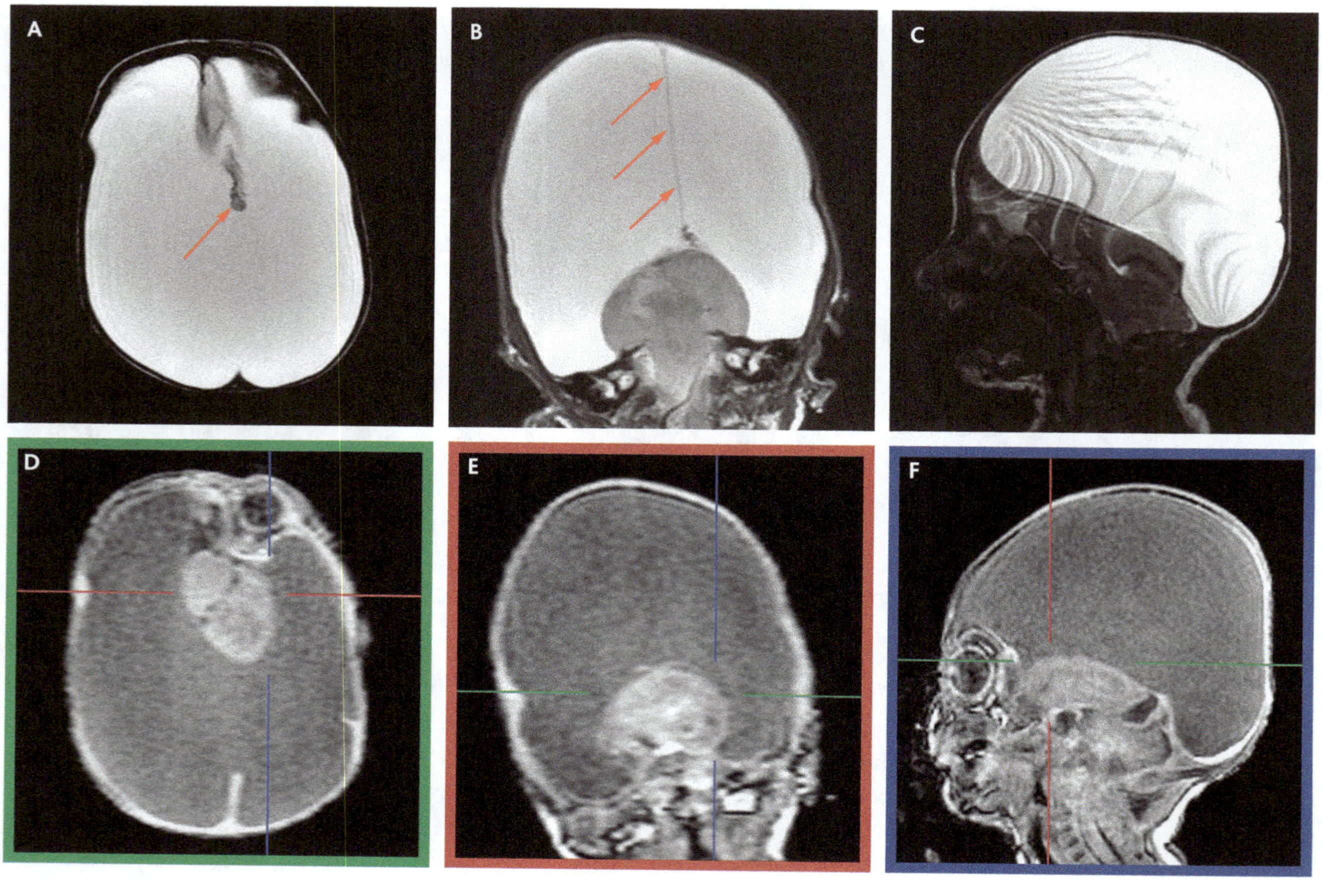

Figures 6-69A–F MRI series showing holoprosencephaly. **A:** T2. **B:** T2. **C:** FIESTA. **D:** 3D BRAVO T1. **E:** 3D BRAVO T1. **F:** 3D BRAVO T1.

not lack of development. This is suggested by the intact falx cerebri (arrows) and remnants of the choroid plexus (arrow); at one time the hemispheres may have formed, but due to some unknown pathology, they became infarcted and atrophied prior to birth.

Schizencephaly

Schizencephaly is a condition in which there are clefts between the outside of the brain and the ventricular system (Figures 6-70A–C). Schizencephaly is often the result of disrupted neuronal migration.

Multiple Neurodevelopmental Conditions

Migration defects can cause a number of neurodevelopmental conditions ranging from mild dysplasia to profound disorganization of the brain. The example shown in Figures 6-71A–F is from a baby with highly deformed

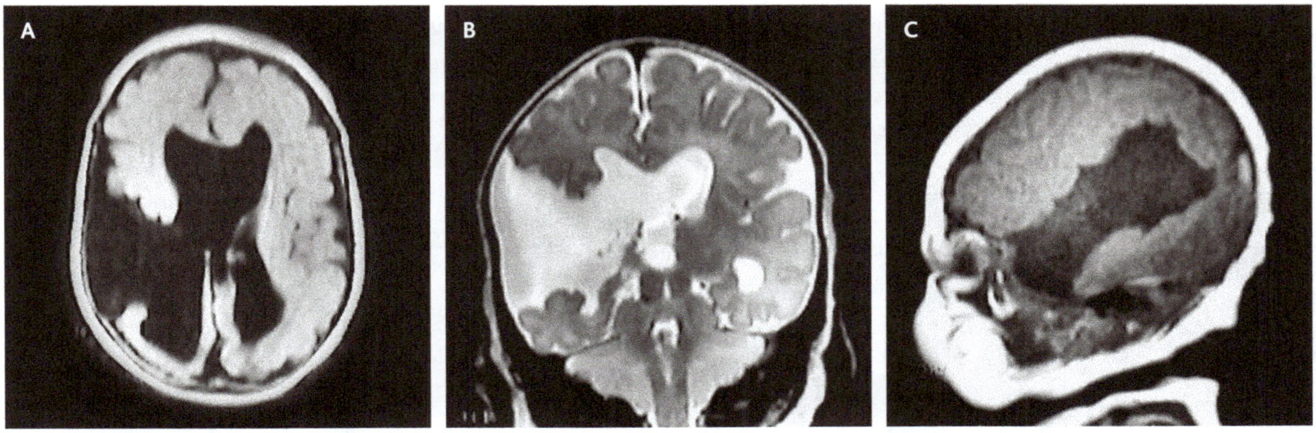

Figure 6-70A–C MRI series showing schizencephaly. **A:** T2 FLAIR. **B:** T2. **C:** T1.

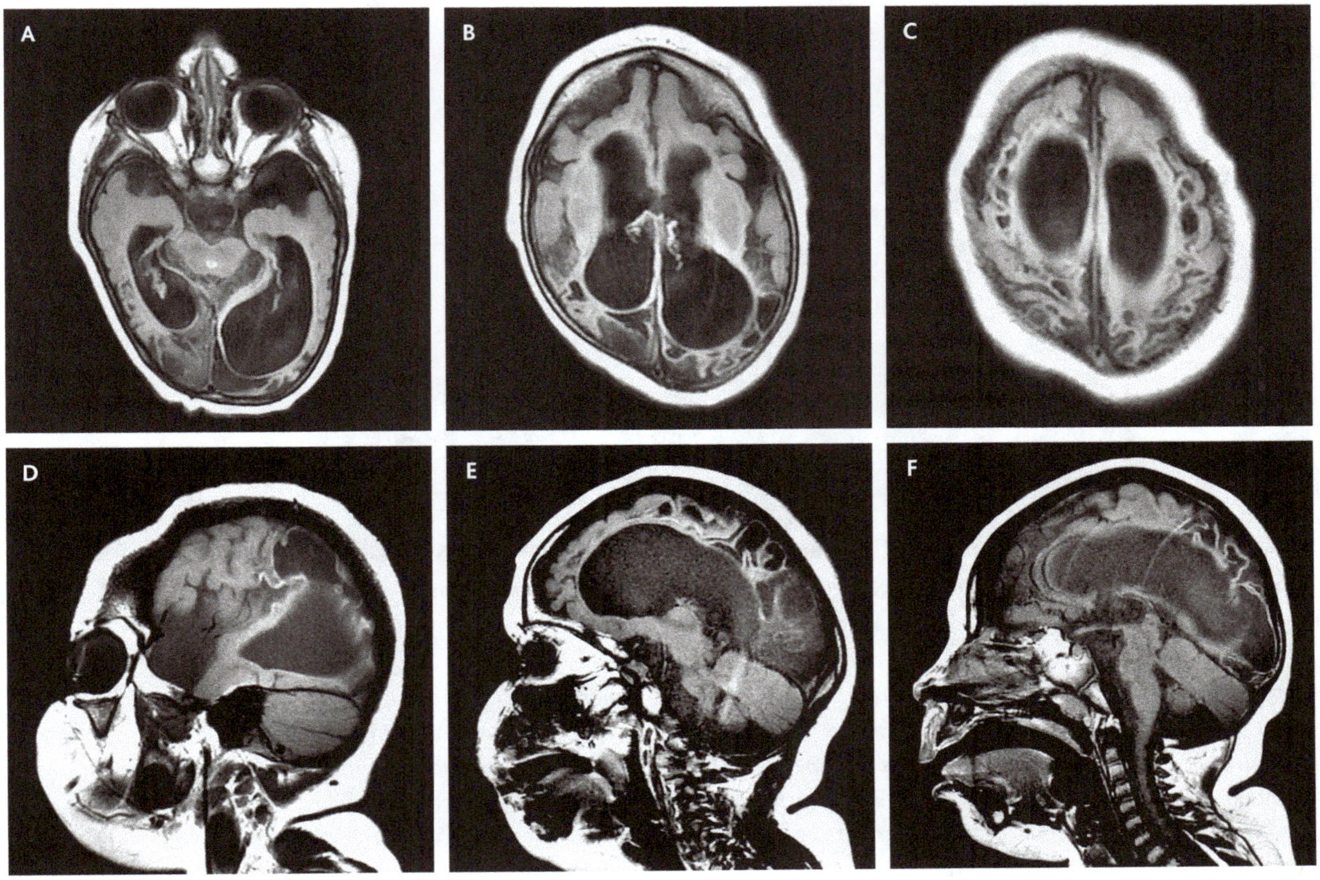

Figures 6-71A–F T2 FLAIR series (A–C) and T1 series (D–F) showing globally deformed cortical and subcortical brain structures.

cortical and subcortical structures. When babies are born with highly deformed brains, as evident in this example, it is expected that they will experience profound deficits involving all aspects of cognitive and adaptive functioning, or even death shortly following birth.

PARASITIC DISORDERS

To conclude the examples on nontraumatic pathologies, a case of a parasitic infection of the brain will be presented. This example is used to demonstrate the variability of

CLINICAL EXAMPLE

Marina: Neurocysticercosis

Marina was seen in the emergency department for new-onset seizures. A CT scan revealed a 1-cm lesion in her left parietal-occipital region with surrounding edema (Figure 6-72A). Initial impressions were that she had a rapidly growing tumor that was causing the edema and seizures. She was initially admitted to the oncology unit for a tumor workup and received medication management for her seizures. Through a clinical interview with Marina, it was learned that she had recently returned from South America, where she had lived for the past 2 years. Marina was re-evaluated with MR imaging (Figures 6-72B–F), including magnetic resonance spectroscopy (MRS), which revealed the lesion to be a small, worm-based parasite called neurocysticercosis and not neoplastic. Although the standard MRI sequences suggested the parasite, it was not until the MRS information was reviewed that the diagnosis was confirmed. Tumors have a specific profile on MRS, and Marina's MRS profile obtained from the lesion site in comparison to healthy tissue, suggested a normal spectroscopy profile, inconsistent with that expected of tumor growth.

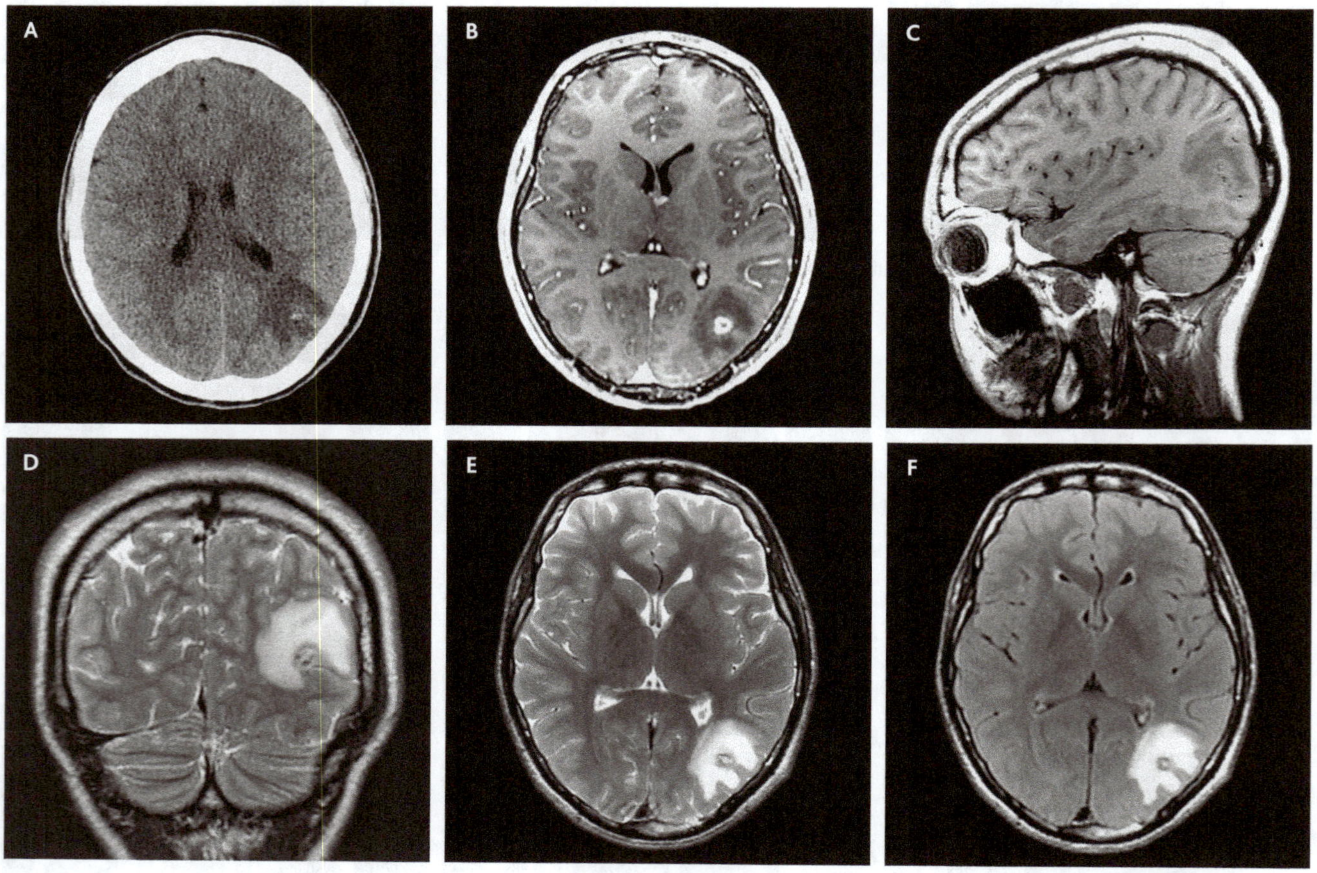

Figures 6-72A–F Clinical example Marina: neurocysticercosis. CT and MRI images showing the left parietal-occipital lesion. **A:** CT. **B:** Contrast-enhanced T1 image. **C:** T1. **D:** T2. **E:** T2. **F:** T2 FLAIR.

pathologies that you may see in a large hospital or clinic. Although parasitic infections of the brain are relatively rare in many countries, they are not uncommon in some parts of the world. Neurocysticercosis is caused by growth of the pork tapeworm, *Taenia solium*. On brain imaging, the lesions often appear similar to a cyst, but with a "dot" inside. Edema around the lesion is common in the later stages of lava breakdown. Seizures are often the first symptom of the condition and are generally the reason for imaging in these patients.

CONCLUDING REMARKS

Chapters 5 and 6 presented a number of different traumatic and nontraumatic conditions commonly seen in the clinic. It is important to understand that this guide is not intended to provide a comprehensive encyclopedia of clinical brain imaging cases. Many conditions that you encounter in your work may not be included within this text. However, even if a particular type of pathology is not included, it is helpful to recognize that the similarities between most pathological conditions outweigh the differences, and common themes are evident across cases. For example, no matter what the pathology, CT scans record density or, more precisely, the x-ray absorption properties of tissue, with greater absorption, resulting in a brighter appearance; less absorption appears darker. Blood caused by any number of conditions such as stroke, physical trauma, vascular compromise, or clotting disorders will appear similar across disorders, with relatively predictable changes in appearance over time as the blood breaks down. Edema is frequently evident after damage to brain tissue and produces changes to the brain that are often simple to interpret on a variety of brain images. For example, edema often results in tissue displacement, compression or effacement of CSF cavities, and sulci–gyri patterning, in addition to increased fluid concentration within the soft tissues of the brain. Ischemia, infarction, and encephalomalacia can appear similar across etiologies, with initial signs of inflammation or edema, then restricted diffusion, followed by gradual atrophy of tissue. Eventually, with loss of brain parenchyma, diffusion may transition from restricted to normal and, ultimately, unrestricted or isotropic. As a general rule, any structure that appears notably brighter or darker than like tissue suggests a problem in the brain, but only once artifacts have been ruled out and a determination has been made as to how the tissue should normally appear. Asymmetry is often a clue to pathology but can be misleading, especially if the head is not orthogonal in the scanner.

This guide is not a substitute for the experience and expertise of a radiologist, especially a neuroradiologist who views images from thousands of brain-related cases per year. The goal of this guide is to provide you with the basic knowledge necessary to feel confident in taking the information provided by a radiologist and supplementing it with your own review of the images and imaging reports. Interpreting imaging data from a clinical or functional perspective is often outside the role of a busy radiologist and frequently falls to the individual clinician. For example, a radiology report may not include information relevant to treatment planning, formulation of prognosis for functional recovery, or, in some cases, differential diagnosis. A lack of basic understanding of when and how to use brain images, the limitations of the technology, the different types of scanning techniques and sequences available, and knowledge of the various appearances of pathology versus normal tissue or artifact can result in faulty clinical conclusions, misinformation provided to the patient or family, and, in some cases, patient harm.

It is hoped that you have gained valuable knowledge from reading this guide and from reviewing the many clinical examples contained within this text. In addition, if your neuroanatomy skills were becoming rusty, it is hoped that a review of neuroanatomy from the perspective of brain imaging has provided you with a revision of old learning and a new way to view brain structures and anatomical regions. You may find it helpful to refer to Chapters 3 (neuroanatomy) and 7 (brain atlas) while interpreting brain scans in the clinic. Comparison of anatomical structures on brain scans with those depicted in this guide will assist you in formulating more accurate opinions regarding both pathology and anatomy. Review of Chapter 1 from time to time will remind you of the many considerations that should be taken into account before using brain scans in the clinic. Brain images should be treated like any other medical findings, and it is important that you determine the best way to communicate the information. For example, you should consider whether or not the actual images should be shown and, if so, which of the scans would best communicate the findings without the scans being misleading or causing undue emotional distress or additional confusion. It is also important to consider the many positive and negative outcomes that may result from showing brain scans to patients and family members. There is a fine balance between providing too little information and too much information, especially to those already experiencing significant trauma from the injury to themselves or a loved one.

For reference purposes, Chapter 7 provides a brain atlas to assist you in identifying many primary neuroanatomical structures on MRI and CT. Images are presented using the three primary acquisition planes with reference lines provided to help you determine the specific slice locations. Three-dimensional volume rendered images are included to assist you in visualizing the areas in three dimensions as they relate to the outside structures of the head.

7

BRAIN ATLAS

This chapter provides a basic brain atlas for many clinically relevant structures and regions. The specific slices used for the atlas images were chosen based on their locations relative to primary or critical anatomical structures of most interest to clinicians. Because of this, the spacing between slices within a particular series (axial, coronal or sagittal) is not equal, as is true for most brain imaging that you will review in the clinic. The unequal spacing was used to provide the reader with images that show the most salient anatomical structures in the most efficient manner. To assist in interpretation, additional images are provided from alternate image planes with reference lines showing the location of the slice used for the atlas. Three-dimensional volume-rendered reference images are also included as they are helpful when determining the location of the atlas slice in reference to the head. Many times, a patient or family member will point to their head and ask, "Where is the damage?" or "Where is the tumor?" Even after years of viewing brain scans, using two-dimensional (2D) images to determine a location in the head can be surprisingly difficult. Spend some time reviewing the three-dimensional volume-rendered (3D) reference images in order to form a relatively coherent spatial representation of brain structures as they relate to the outside of the head.

For the axial-image section, three-dimensional volume-rendered reference images are presented with a top-down orientation. As mentioned in Chapter 2, axial slices are acquired and viewed from a bottom-up perspective, as if the patient were lying on a bed with the clinician at the feet. As such, you will notice that the top-down 3D images are mirror-reversed when compared to the atlas images acquired using a bottom-up perspective. The top-down 3D volume-rendered images are provided to assist you in assessing the general location of the atlas image slice and how it relates to the landmarks of the head and face. Three-dimensional volume-rendered images with a bottom-up approach can be produced but are much more difficult to interpret. Many of the slices cut through the top part of the head, leaving few face and head landmarks for the viewer. Thus bottom-up 3D volume-rendered images were not used in this chapter; instead, a more easily interpreted top-down series is presented.

For the CT section, MRI images are included for reference and to offer a more detailed illustration of the anatomical areas. The MRI images were reformatted and sliced using approximately the same angle as that used in many CT scans. The reformatting to the CT angle allows for comparison between structures on a CT and an MRI, something that is not often possible because of the different slice angles used for each modality. As the brains used for the CT and MRI examples were from different patients, exact matching of some areas and structures was not possible, although most primary regions do correlate between the two images.

The MRI images used in this chapter were derived from 3D BRAVO T1 images produced using a 3T GE scanner reformatted to 0.9-mm slices. These images have excellent gray–white differentiation, are produced with a thin slice thickness, and allow for reformatting and slicing in any plane and at any angle.

AXIAL SERIES

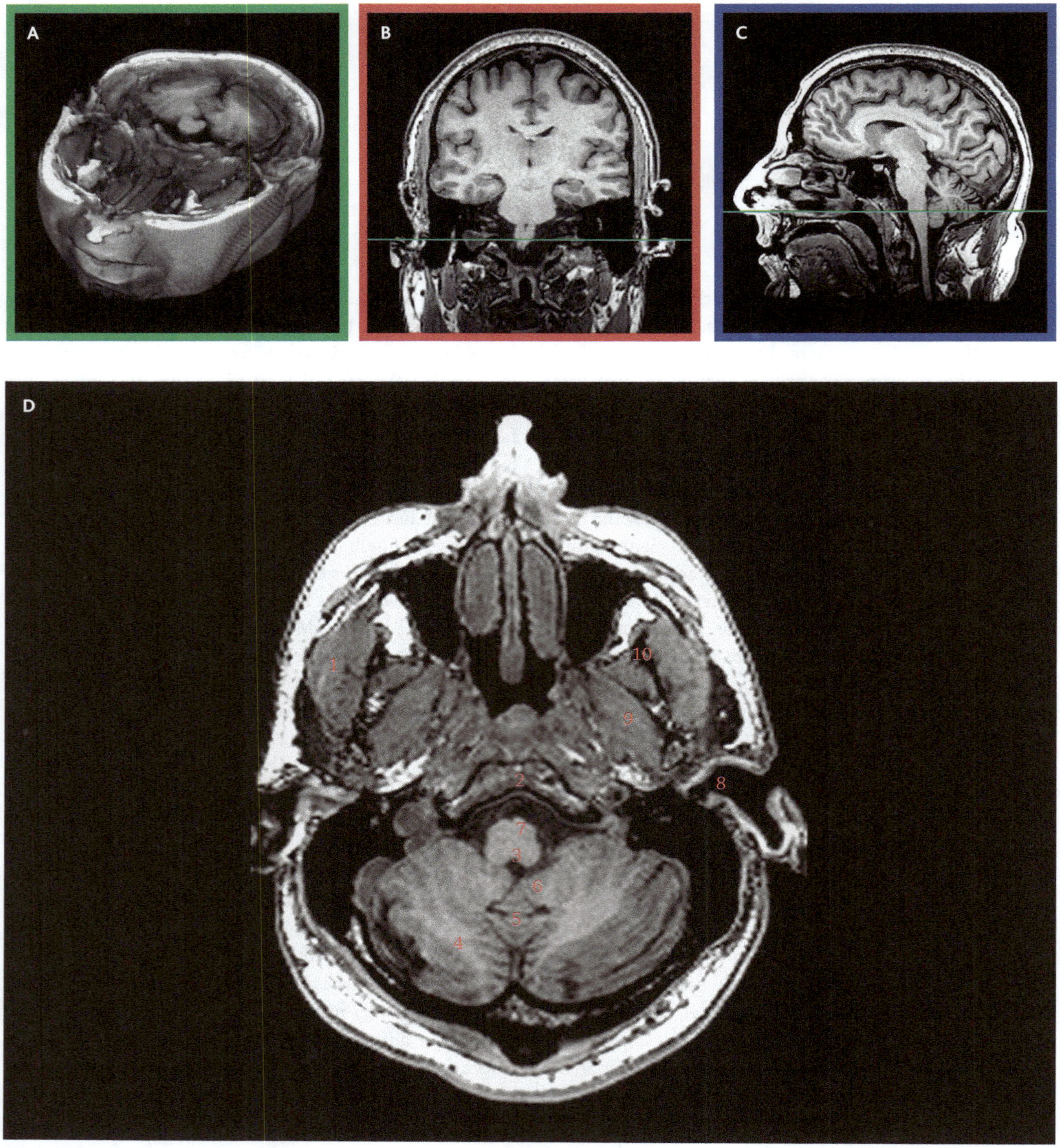

Figure 7-1 **A:** 3D view. **B:** Coronal view. **C:** Sagittal view. **D:** Axial Atlas Slice

1 Masseter Muscle
2 Clivus
3 Medulla
4 Cerebellum
5 Cerebellar Vermis
6 Cerebellar Tonsils
7 Corticospinal Tracts
8 External Auditory Canal
9 Lateral Pterygoid Muscle
10 Mandible

AXIAL SERIES

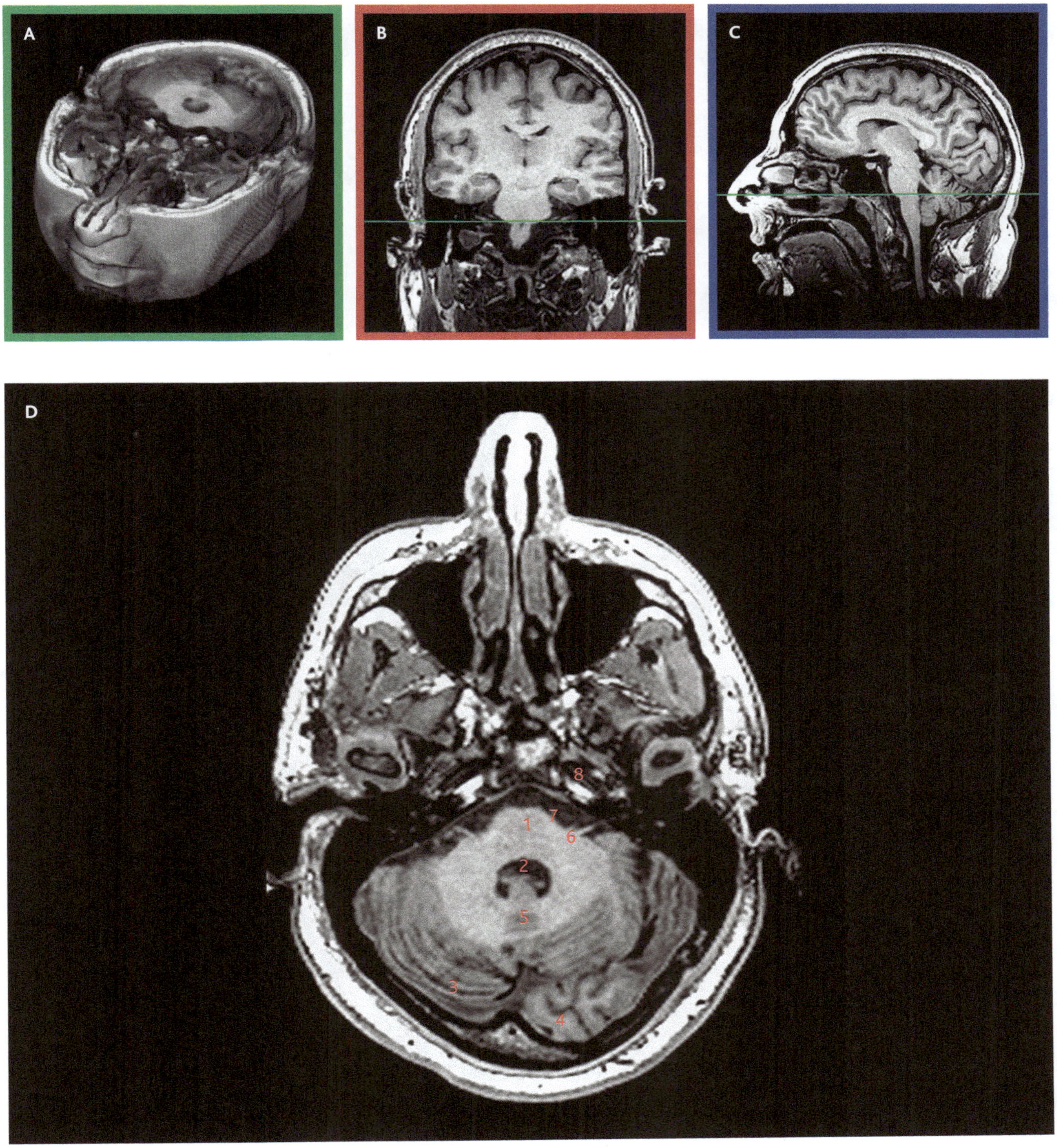

Figure 7-2 A: 3D view. **B:** Coronal view. **C:** Sagittal view. **D:** Axial Atlas Slice

1 Ponto-Medullary Junction
2 Fourth Ventricle
3 Cerebellar Folia
4 Occipital Lobe
5 Cerebellar Vermis
6 7th and 8th Cranial Nerves
7 Cerebello-Pontine Angle
8 Horizontal Internal Carotid Artery

AXIAL SERIES

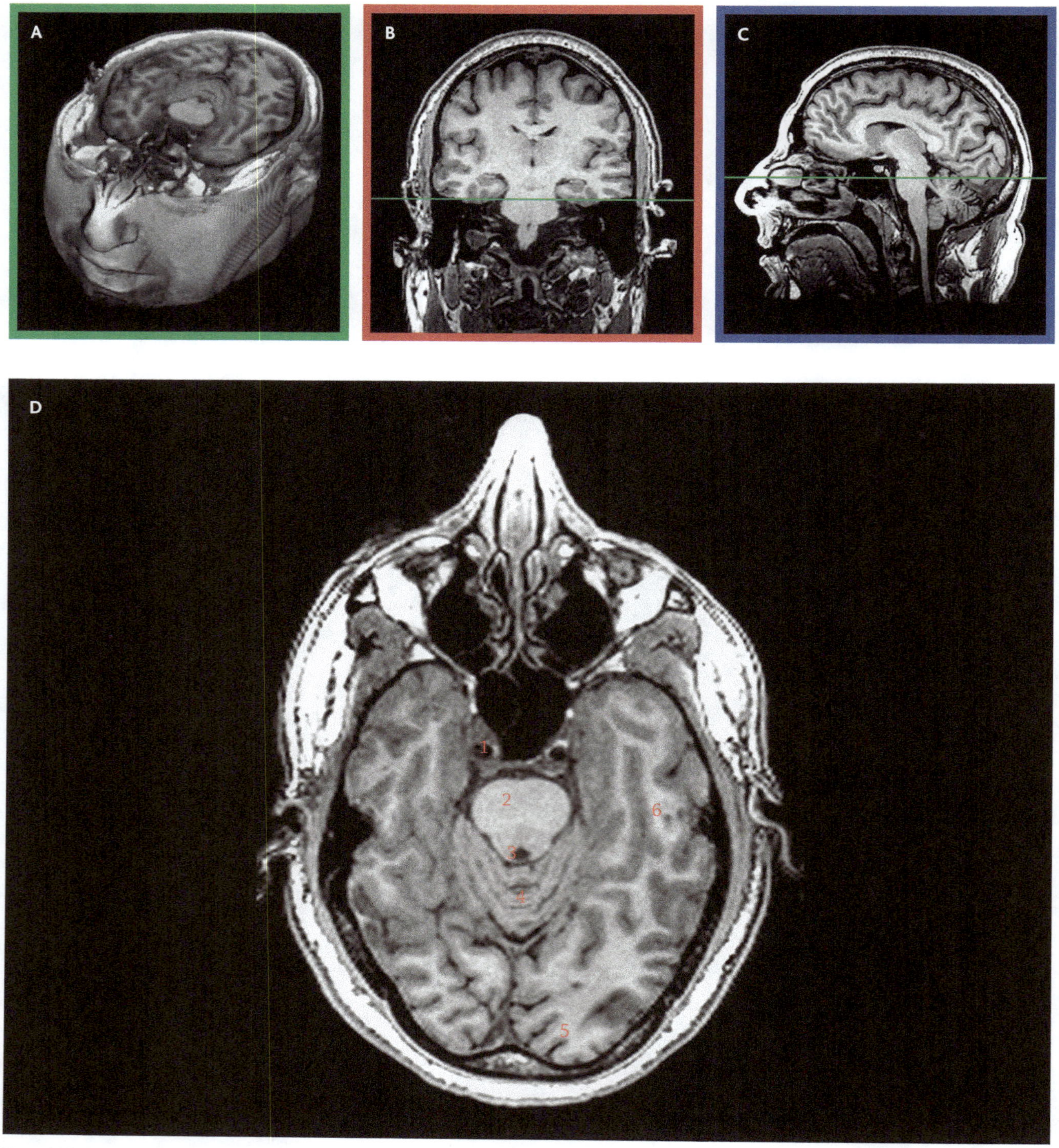

Figure 7-3 **A:** 3D view. **B:** Coronal view. **C:** Sagittal view. **D:** Axial Atlas Slice

1 Cavernous Internal Carotid Artery
2 Corticospinal Tracts in the Pons
3 Cerebral Aqueduct
4 Cerebellar Vermis
5 Occipital Lobe
6 Temporal Lobe

AXIAL SERIES

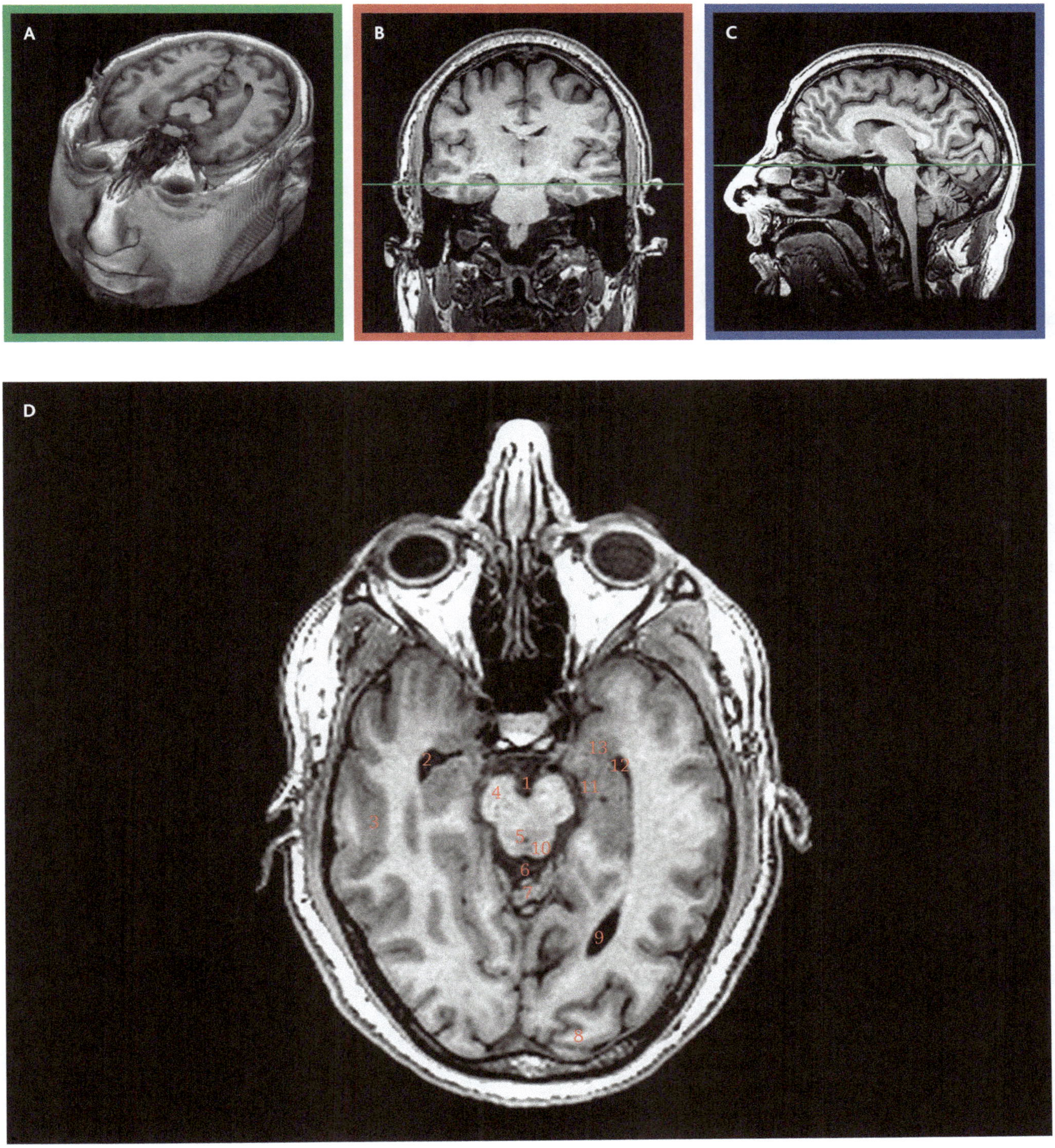

Figure 7-4 **A:** 3D view. **B:** Coronal view. **C:** Sagittal view. **D:** Axial Atlas Slice

1 Interpeduncular/Basal Cistern
2 Lateral Ventricle – Inferior/Temporal Horn
3 Temporal Lobe
4 Midbrain – Cerebral Peduncle
5 Cerebral Aqueduct – Periaqueductal Gray
6 Superior/Perimesencephalic/Quadrigeminal Cistern
7 Cerebellum
8 Occipital Lobe
9 Lateral Ventricle – Posterior/Occipital Horn
10 Tectum – Inferior Colliculus
11 Hippocampus
12 Lateral Ventricle – Inferior/Temporal Horn
13 Amygdala

AXIAL SERIES

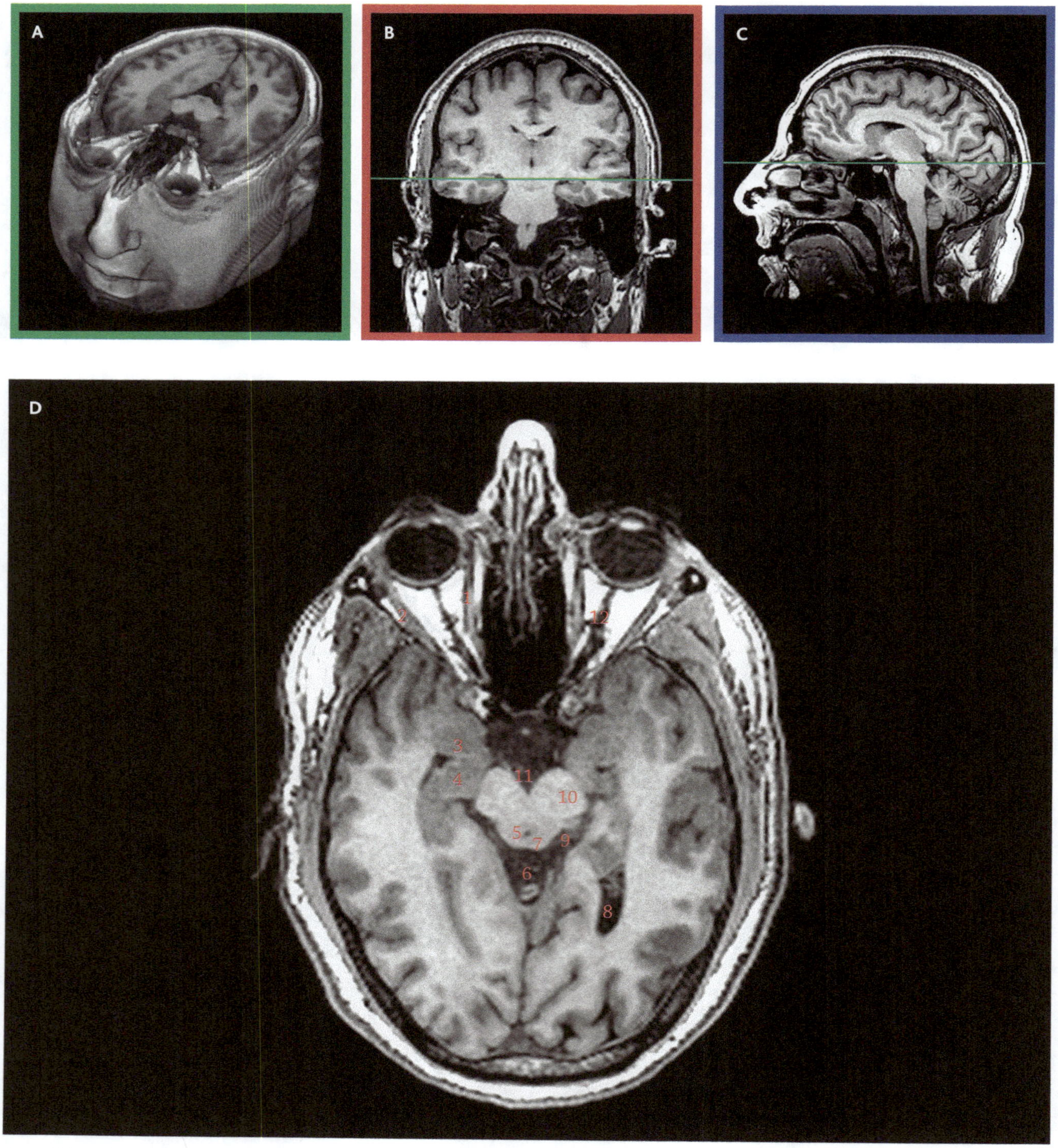

Figure 7-5 **A:** 3D view. **B:** Coronal view. **C:** Sagittal view. **D:** Axial Atlas Slice

1 Medial Rectus Muscle
2 Lateral Rectus Muscle
3 Amygdala
4 Hippocampus
5 Cerebral Aqueduct – Periaqueductal Gray
6 Superior/Perimesencephalic/Quadrigeminal Cistern
7 Tectum
8 Lateral Ventricle – Posterior/Occipital Horn
9 Ambient Cistern
10 Midbrain – Cerebral Peduncle
11 Interpeduncular/Basal Cistern
12 Optic Nerve and Sheath

AXIAL SERIES

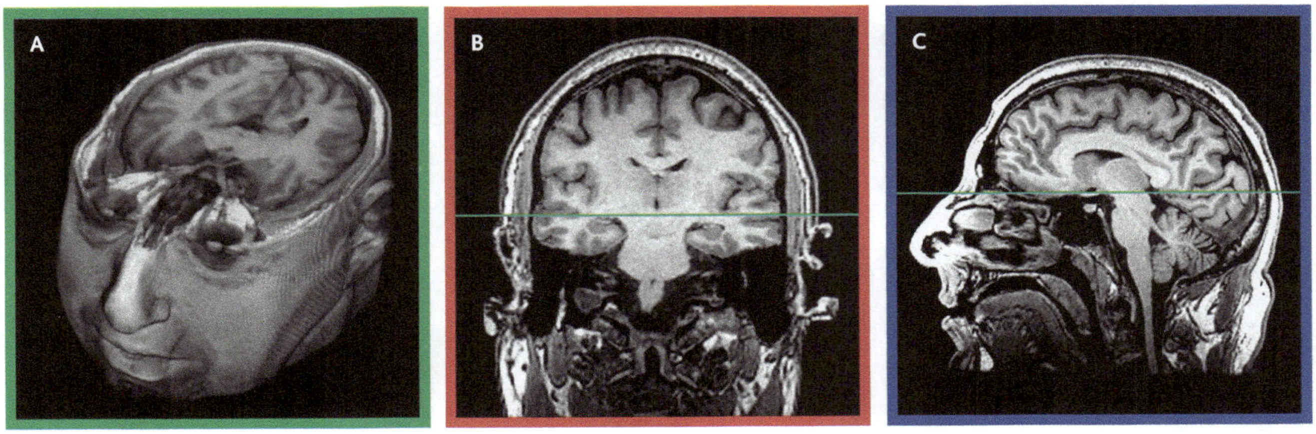

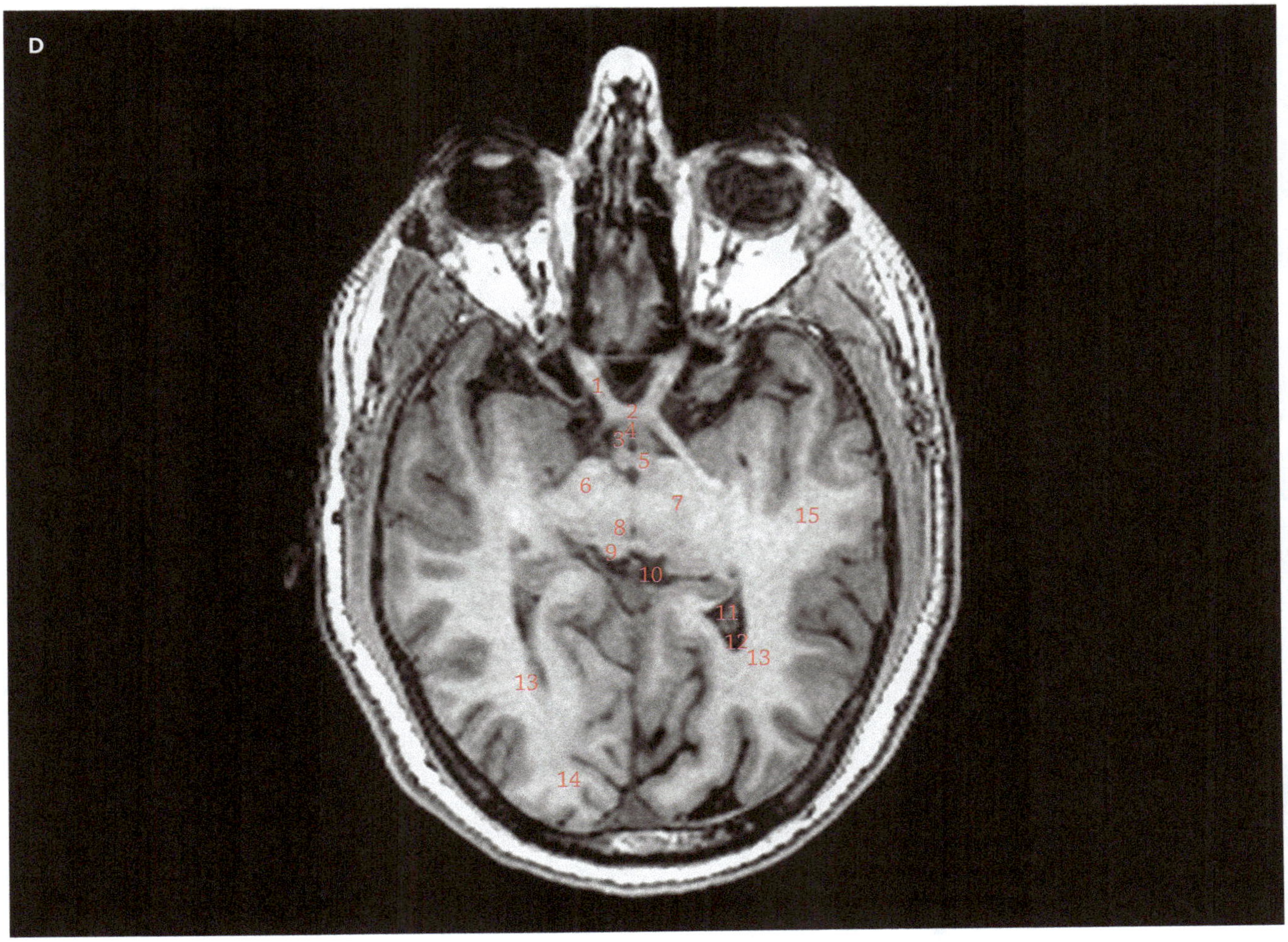

Figure 7-6 **A:** 3D view. **B:** Coronal view. **C:** Sagittal view. **D:** Axial Atlas Slice

1 Optic Nerve
2 Optic Chiasm
3 Hypothalamus
4 Third Ventricle
5 Mammillary Body
6 Midbrain – Cerebral Peduncle
7 Substantia Nigra
8 Cerebral Aqueduct – Periaqueductal Gray
9 Tectum – Superior Colliculus
10 Superior/Perimesencephalic/Quadrigeminal Cistern
11 Choroid Plexus
12 Lateral Ventricle – Atrium/Trigone to Posterior/Occipital Horn
13 Optic Radiations
14 Occipital Lobe
15 Temporal Lobe

AXIAL SERIES

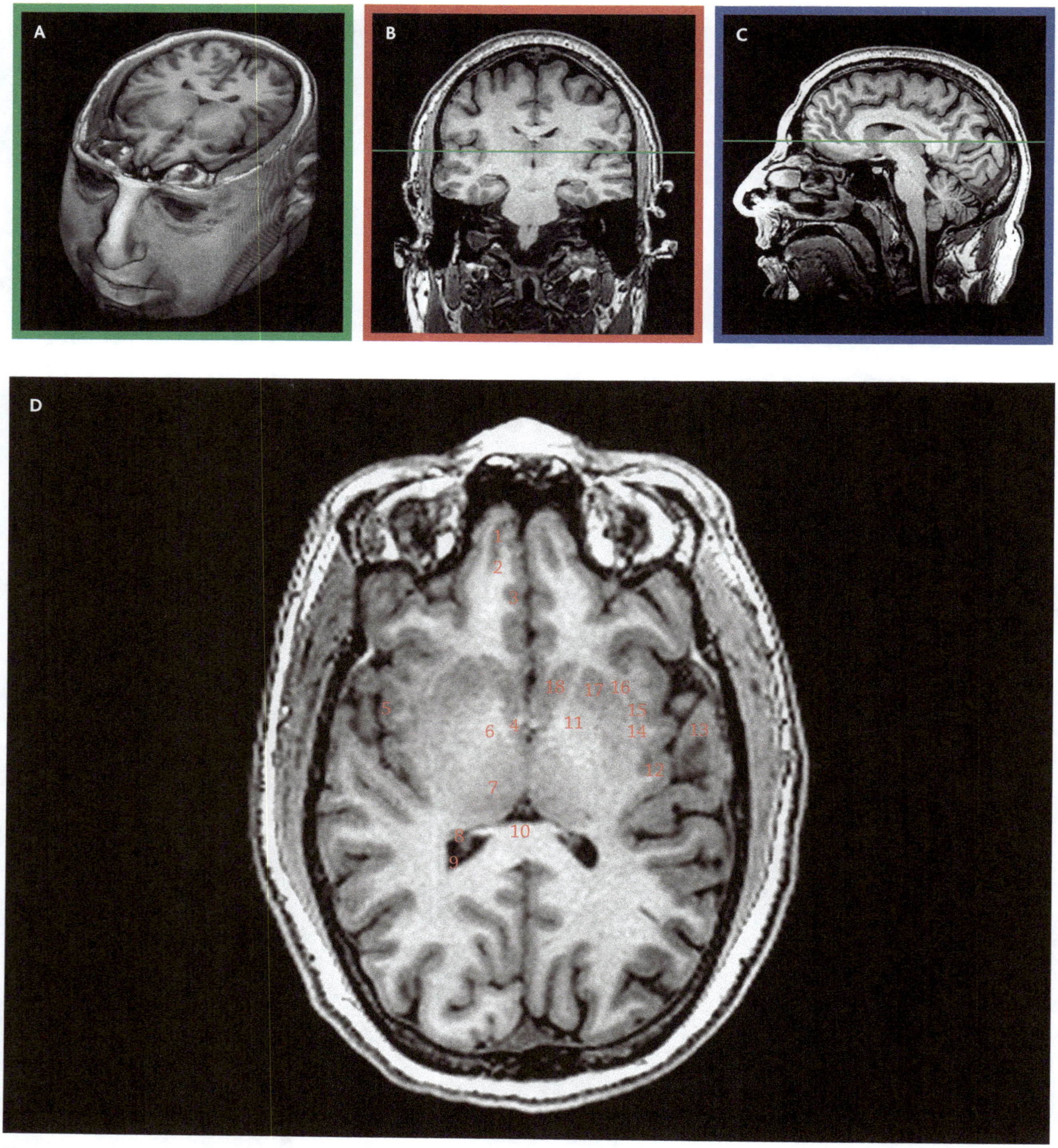

Figure 7-7 **A:** 3D view. **B:** Coronal view. **C:** Sagittal view. **D:** Axial Atlas Slice

1 Olfactory Sulcus
2 Frontal Lobe – Straight Gyrus
3 Medial Frontal Cortex
4 Fornix
5 Insula
6 Internal Capsule
7 Thalamus
8 Choroid Plexus
9 Lateral Ventricle – Atrium/Trigone
10 Corpus Callosum – Splenium
11 Globus Pallidus
12 Insula
13 Temporal Lobe
14 Claustrum
15 Extreme Capsule
16 External Capsule
17 Putamen
18 Caudate Nucleus – Head

AXIAL SERIES

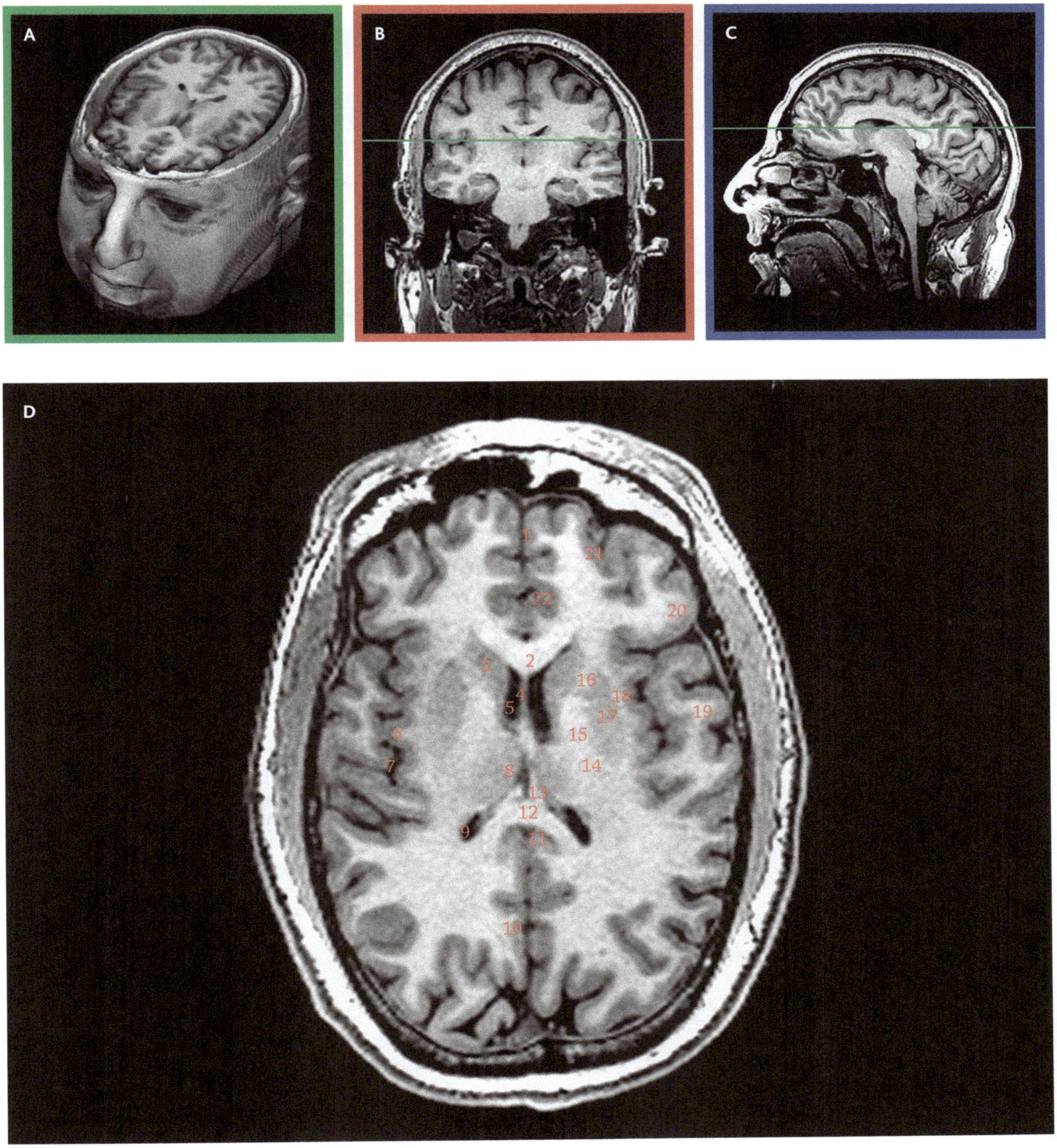

Figure 7-8 **A:** 3D view. **B:** Coronal view. **C:** Sagittal view. **D:** Axial Atlas Slice

1 Interhemispheric or Longitudinal Fissure
2 Corpus Callosum – Genu
3 Caudate Nucleus – Head
4 Septum Pellucidum
5 Lateral Ventricle – Body
6 Insula
7 Sylvian Fissure
8 Thalamus
9 Lateral Ventricle – Atrium/Trigone
10 Cuneus
11 Cingulate Gyrus – Posterior
12 Corpus Callosum – Splenium
13 Fornix
14 Internal Capsule – Posterior Limb
15 Internal Capsule – Genu
16 Internal Capsule – Anterior Limb
17 Putamen
18 External Capsule
19 Frontal Lobe – Inferior and Operculum
20 Broca's Gyrus
21 Orbital Frontal Lobe
22 Cingulate Gyrus – Anterior

AXIAL SERIES

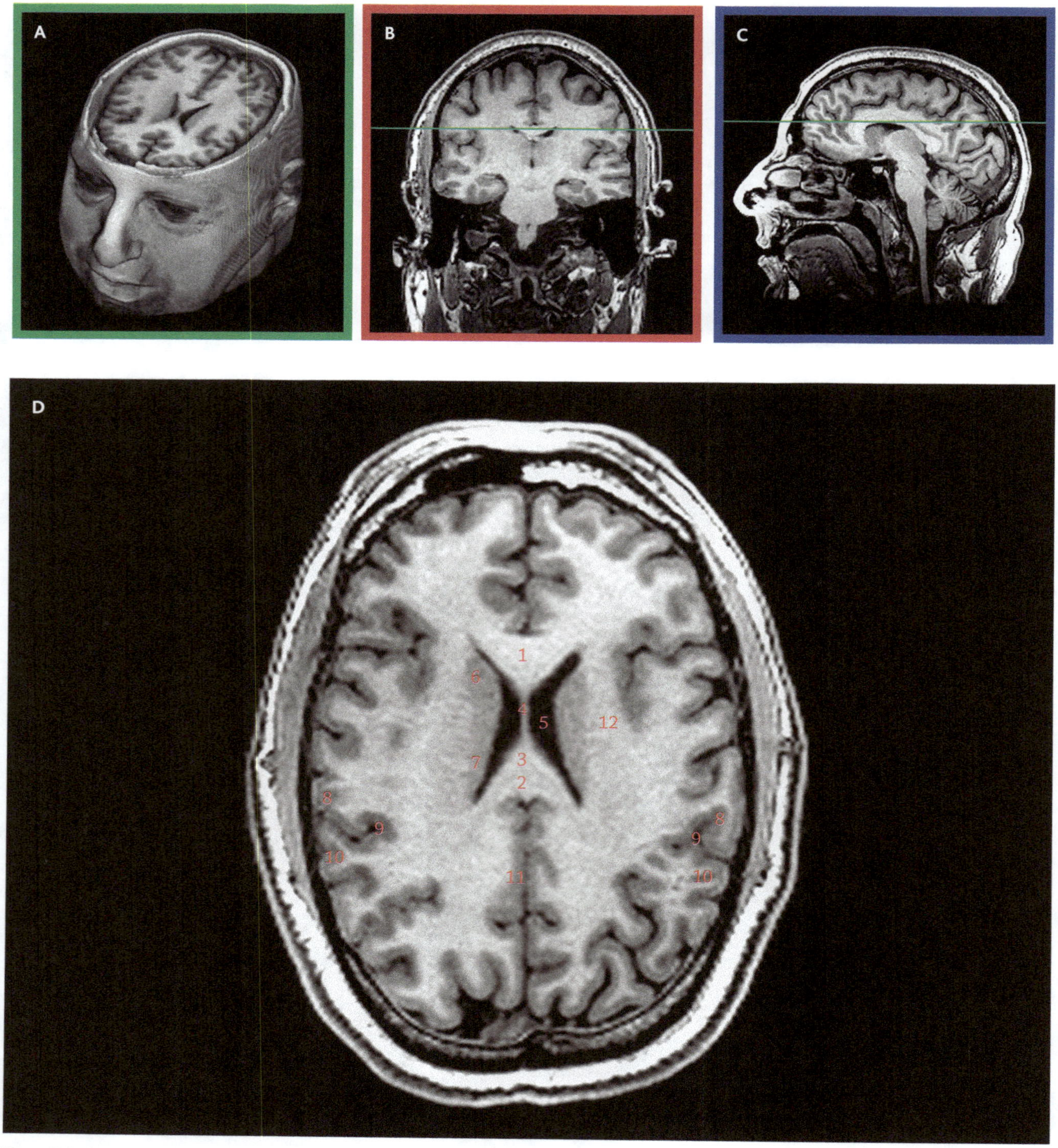

Figure 7-9 **A:** 3D view. **B:** Coronal view. **C:** Sagittal view. **D:** Axial Atlas Slice

1 Corpus Callosum – Genu
2 Corpus Callosum – Splenium
3 Fornix
4 Septum Pellucidum
5 Lateral Ventricle – Body
6 Caudate Nucleus – Head
7 Caudate Nucleus – Tail
8 Pre-Central Gyrus
9 Central Sulcus
10 Post-Central Gyrus
11 Pre-Cuneus
12 Corona Radiata

CORONAL SERIES

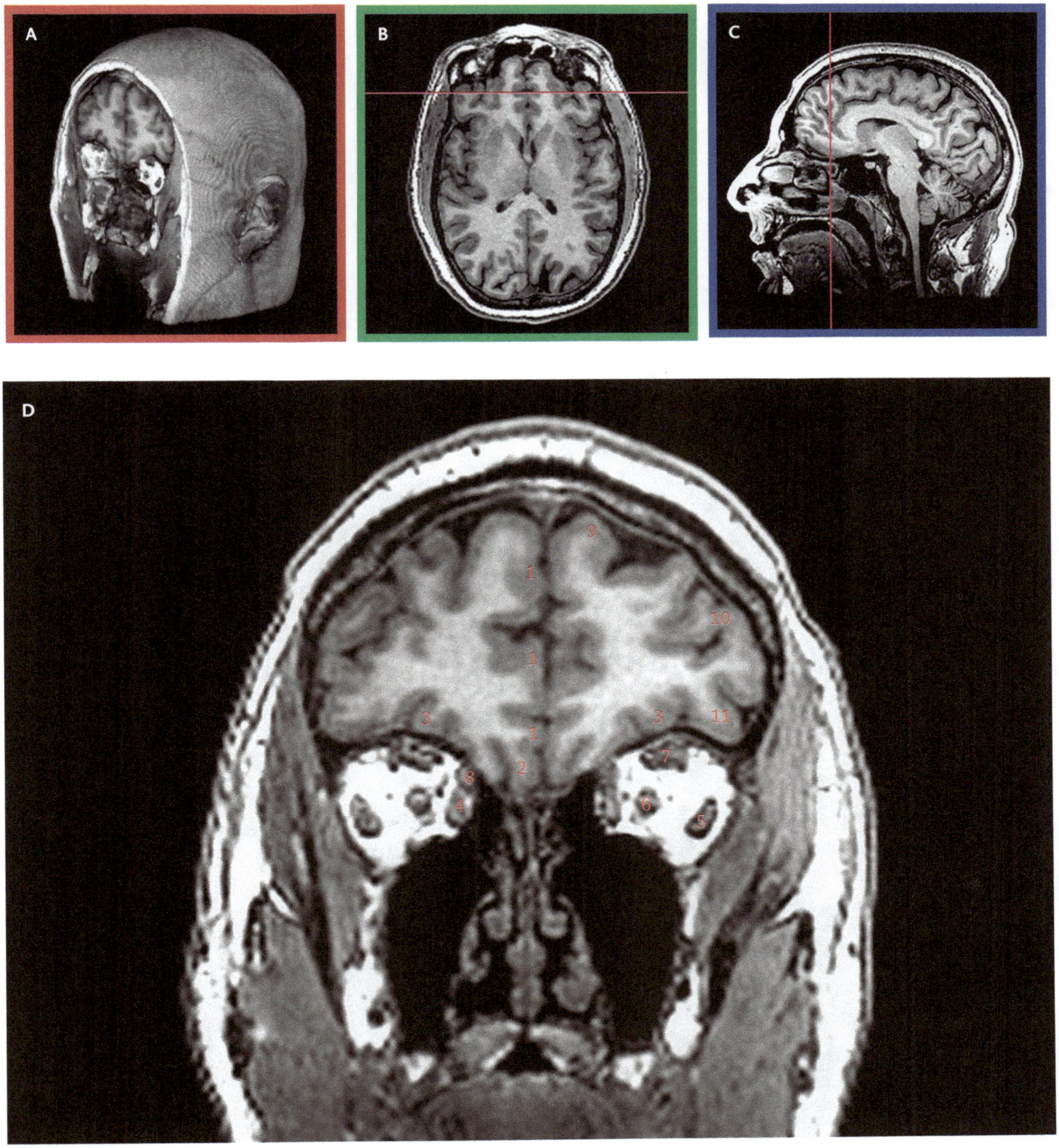

Figure 7-10 **A:** 3D view. **B:** Axial view. **C:** Sagittal view. **D:** Coronal Atlas Slice

1 Frontal Lobe – Medial
2 Frontal Lobe – Straight Gyrus
3 Frontal Lobe – Orbital
4 Medial Rectus Muscle
5 Lateral Rectus Muscle
6 Optic Nerve
7 Superior Rectus Muscle
8 Superior Oblique Muscle
9 Superior Frontal Gyrus
10 Middle Frontal Gyrus
11 Inferior Frontal Gyrus

CORONAL SERIES

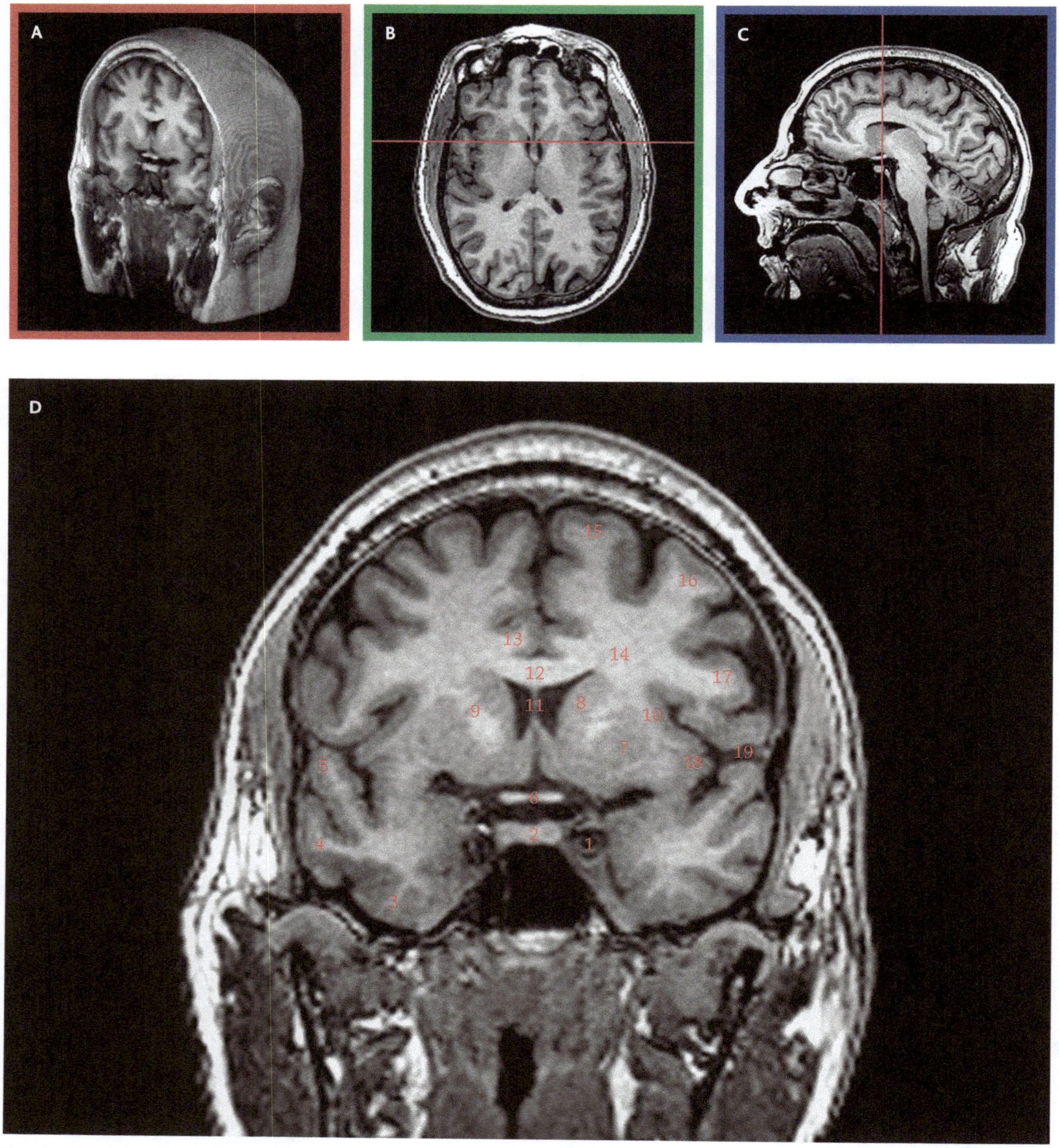

Figure 7-11 **A:** 3D view. **B:** Axial view. **C:** Sagittal view. **D:** Coronal Atlas Slice

1 Cavernous Internal Carotid Artery
2 Pituitary
3 Inferior Temporal Gyrus
4 Middle Temporal Gyrus
5 Superior Temporal Gyrus
6 Optic Chiasm
7 Putamen
8 Caudate Nucleus – Head
9 Internal Capsule – Anterior Limb
10 External Capsule
11 Septum Pellucidum
12 Corpus Callosum – Body
13 Cingulate Gyrus
14 Corona Radiata
15 Superior Frontal Gyrus
16 Middle Frontal Gyrus
17 Pre-Central Gyrus
18 Insula
19 Sylvian Fissure

CORONAL SERIES

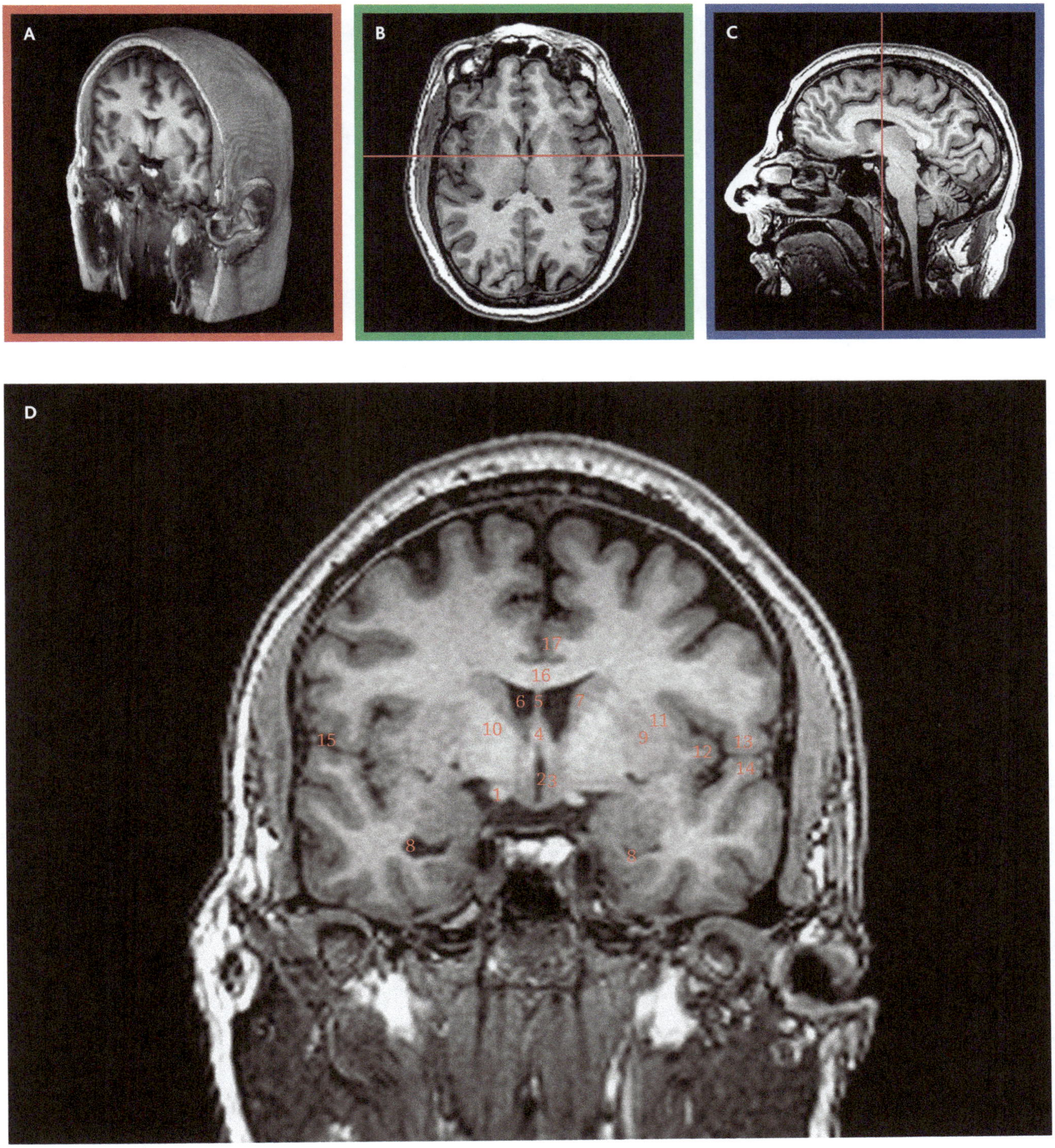

Figure 7-12 **A:** 3D view. **B:** Axial view. **C:** Sagittal view. **D:** Coronal Atlas Slice

1 Optic Nerve
2 Third Ventricle
3 Hypothalamus
4 Fornix
5 Septum Pellucidum
6 Lateral Ventricle – Body
7 Caudate Nucleus – Head
8 Lateral Ventricle – Inferior/Temporal Horn
9 Putamen
10 Internal Capsule – Genu
11 External Capsule
12 Insula
13 Frontal Operculum
14 Temporal Operculum
15 Sylvian Fissure
16 Corpus Callosum – Body
17 Cingulate Gyrus

CORONAL SERIES

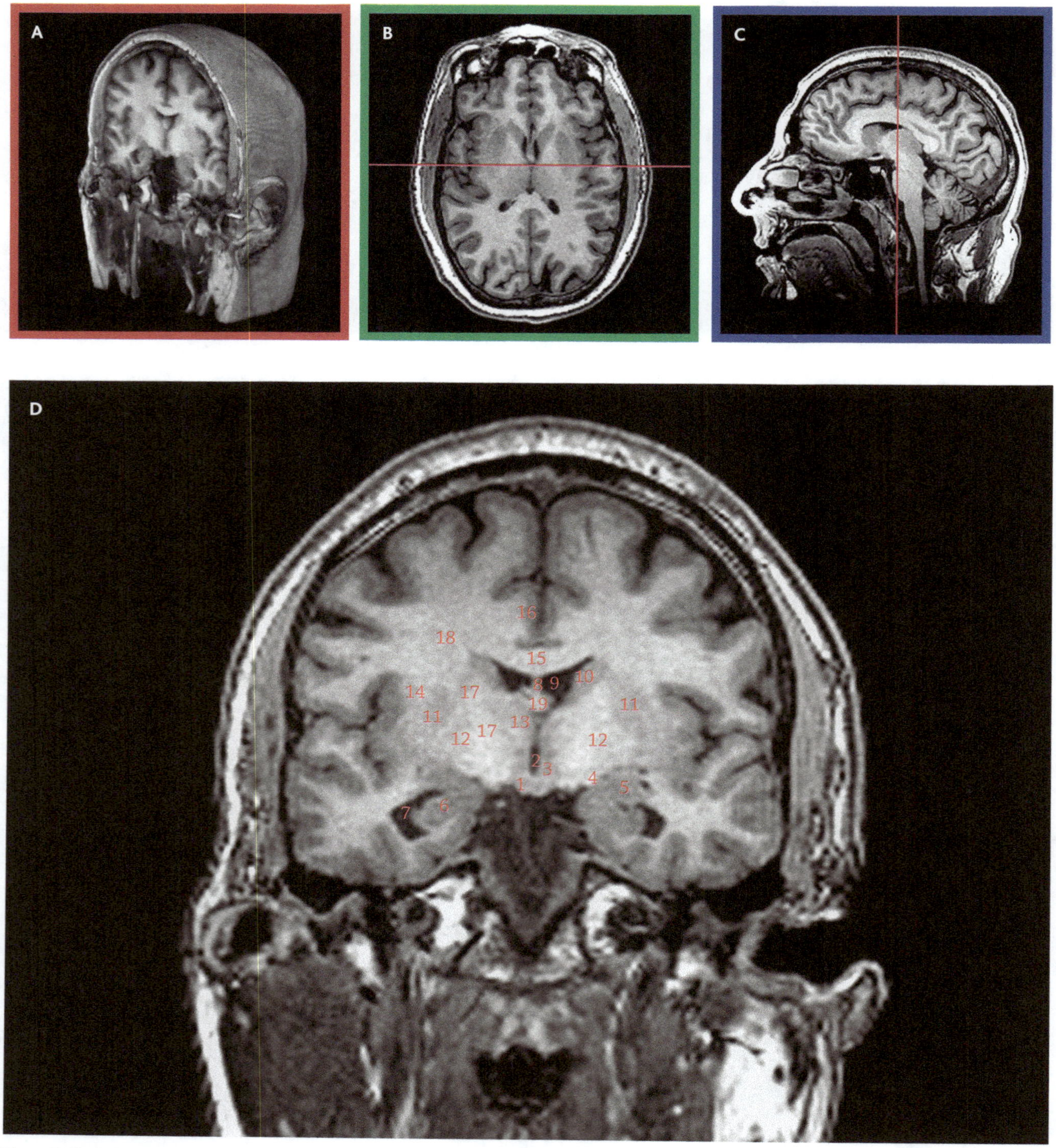

Figure 7-13 **A:** 3D view. **B:** Axial view. **C:** Sagittal view. **D:** Coronal Atlas Slice

1 Mammillary Bodies
2 Third Ventricle
3 Hypothalamus
4 Optic Tract
5 Amygdala
6 Hippocampus
7 Lateral Ventricle – Inferior/Temporal Horn
8 Septum Pellucidum
9 Lateral Ventricle – Body
10 Caudate Nucleus – Head
11 Putamen
12 Globus Pallidus
13 Thalamus
14 External Capsule
15 Corpus Callosum
16 Cingulate Gyrus
17 Internal Capsule – Genu
18 Corona Radiata
19 Fornix

CORONAL SERIES

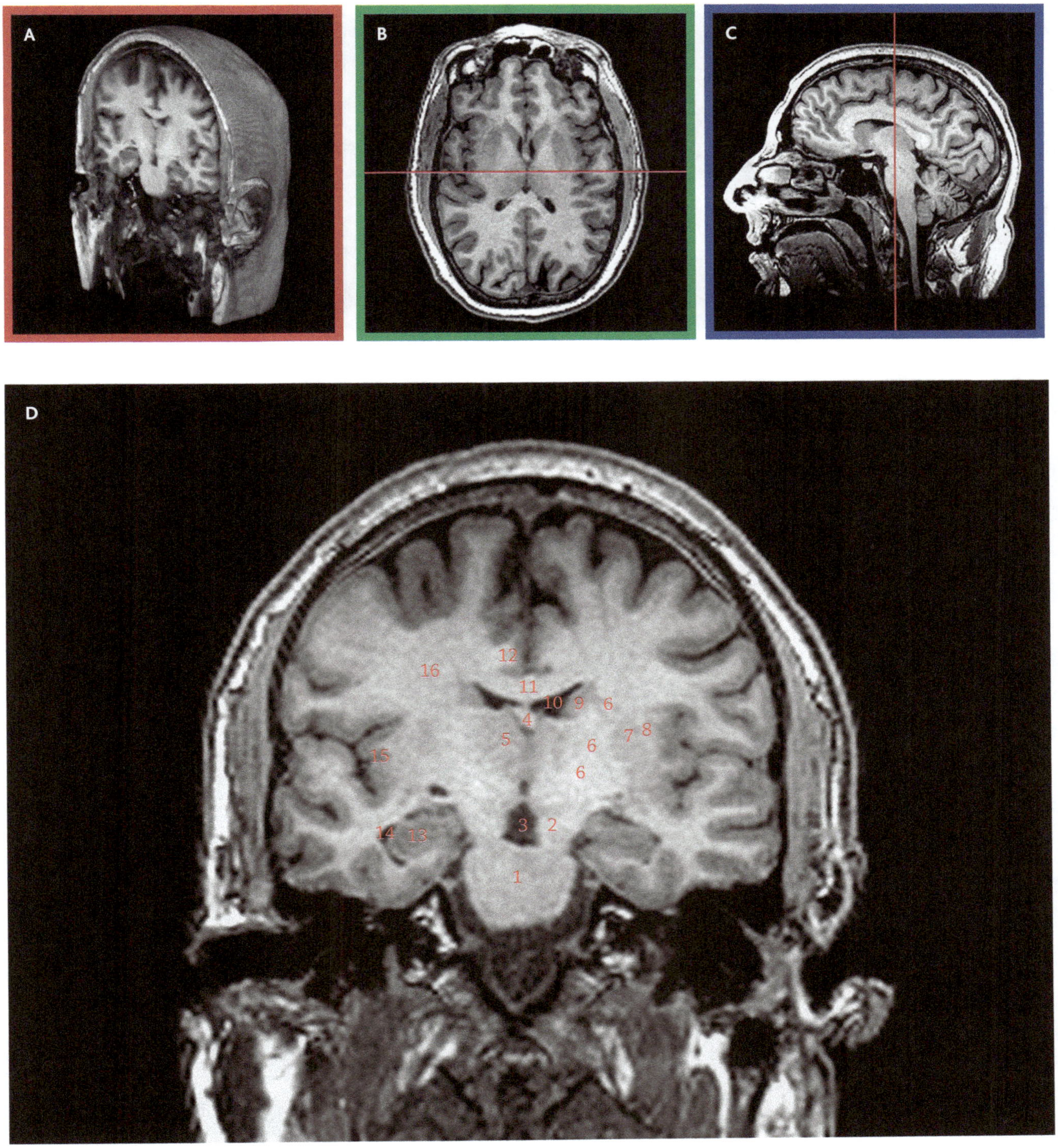

Figure 7-14 **A:** 3D view. **B:** Axial view. **C:** Sagittal view. **D:** Coronal Atlas Slice

1 Pons
2 Cerebral Peduncle
3 Interpeduncular/Basal Cistern
4 Fornix
5 Thalamus
6 Internal Capsule – Posterior Limb
7 Putamen
8 External Capsule
9 Caudate Nucleus – Body
10 Lateral Ventricle – Body
11 Corpus Callosum – Body
12 Cingulate Gyrus
13 Hippocampus
14 Lateral Ventricle – Inferior/Temporal Horn
15 Insula
16 Corona Radiata

CORONAL SERIES

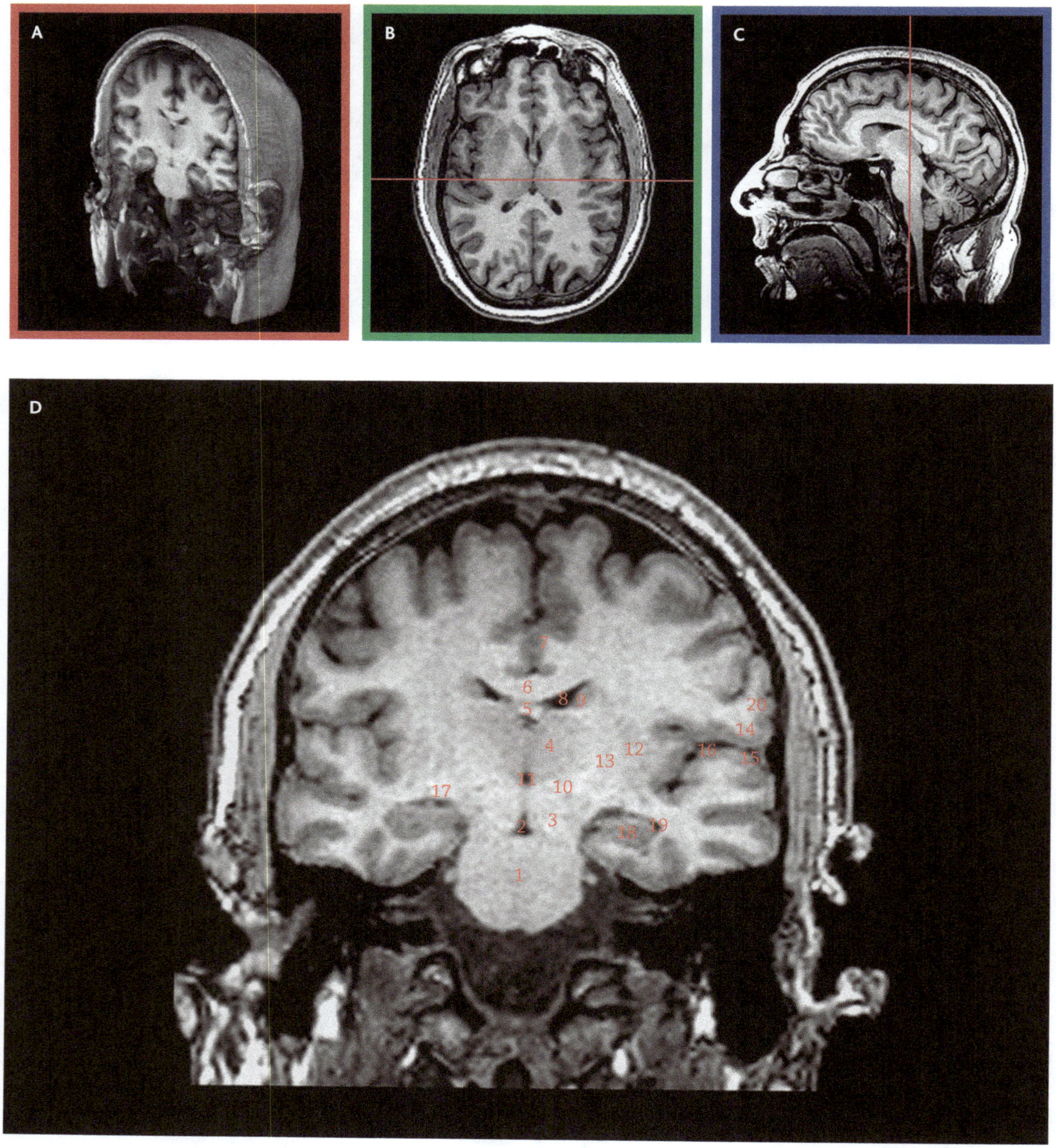

Figure 7-15 **A:** 3D view. **B:** Axial view. **C:** Sagittal view. **D:** Coronal Atlas Slice

1 Pons
2 Interpeduncular/Basal Cistern
3 Cerebral Peduncle
4 Thalamus
5 Fornix
6 Corpus Callosum – Body
7 Cingulate Gyrus
8 Lateral Ventricle – Body
9 Caudate Nucleus – Body
10 Internal Capsule – Posterior Limb
11 Third Ventricle
12 Putamen
13 Globus Pallidus
14 Parietal Operculum
15 Temporal Operculum
16 Sylvian Fissure
17 Optic Tract
18 Hippocampus
19 Lateral Ventricle – Inferior/Temporal Horn
20 Post-Central Gyrus

CORONAL SERIES

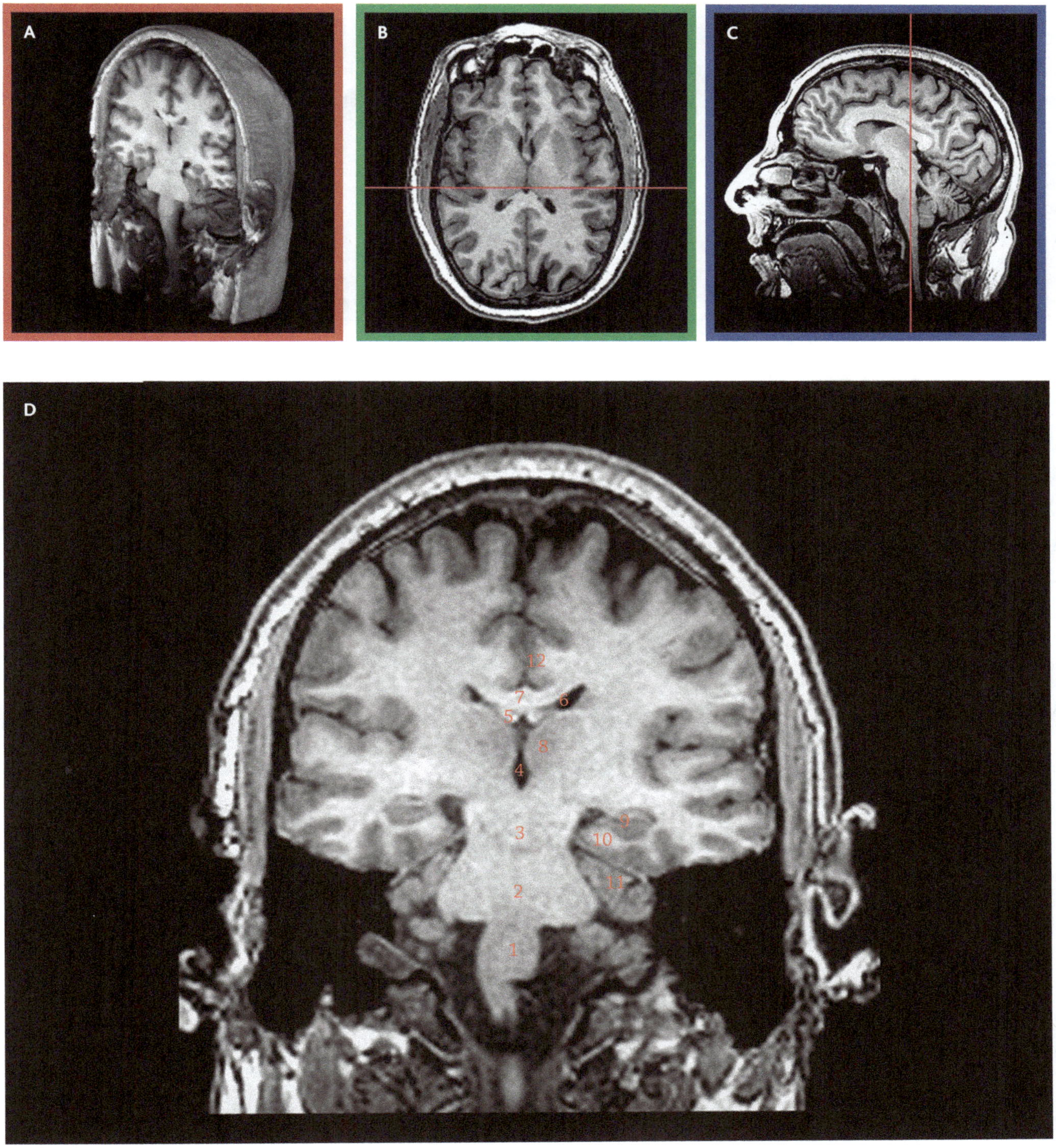

Figure 7-16 **A:** 3D view. **B:** Axial view. **C:** Sagittal view. **D:** Coronal Atlas Slice

1 Medulla Oblongata
2 Pons
3 Midbrain
4 Third Ventricle
5 Fornix
6 Lateral Ventricle – Body
7 Corpus Callosum – Isthmus
8 Thalamus
9 Hippocampus
10 Parahippocampal Gyrus
11 Cerebellum
12 Cingulate Gyrus

CORONAL SERIES

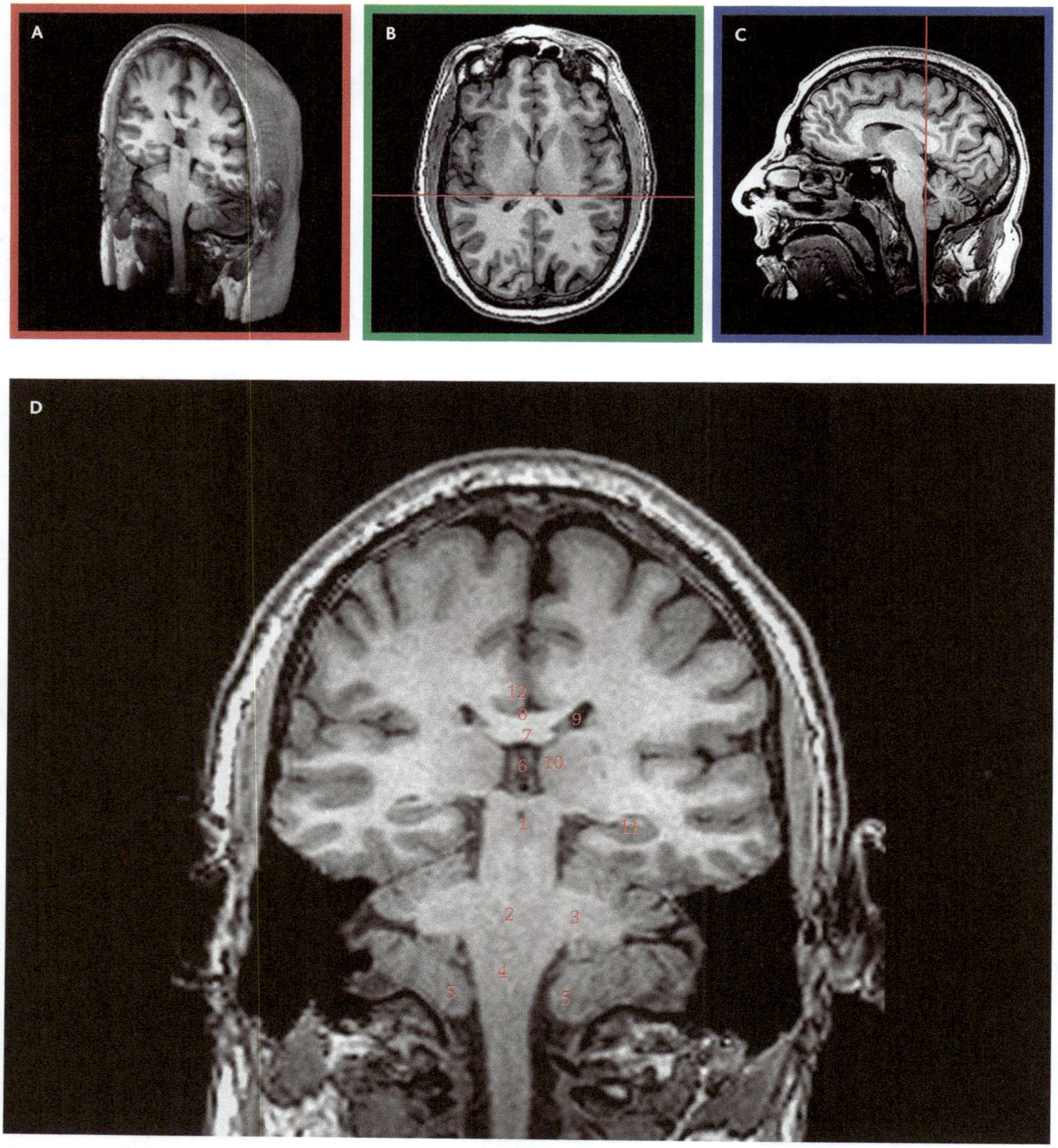

Figure 7-17 **A:** 3D view. **B:** Axial view. **C:** Sagittal view. **D:** Coronal Atlas Slice

1 Cerebral Aqueduct of Sylvius
2 Pons
3 Middle Cerebellar Peduncle
4 Medulla Oblongata
5 Cerebellar Tonsils
6 Superior/Perimesencephalic/ Quadrigeminal Cistern
7 Commissure of the Fornix
8 Corpus Callosum
9 Lateral Ventricle – Atrium/Trigone
10 Thalamus
11 Hippocampus
12 Cingulate Gyrus

CORONAL SERIES

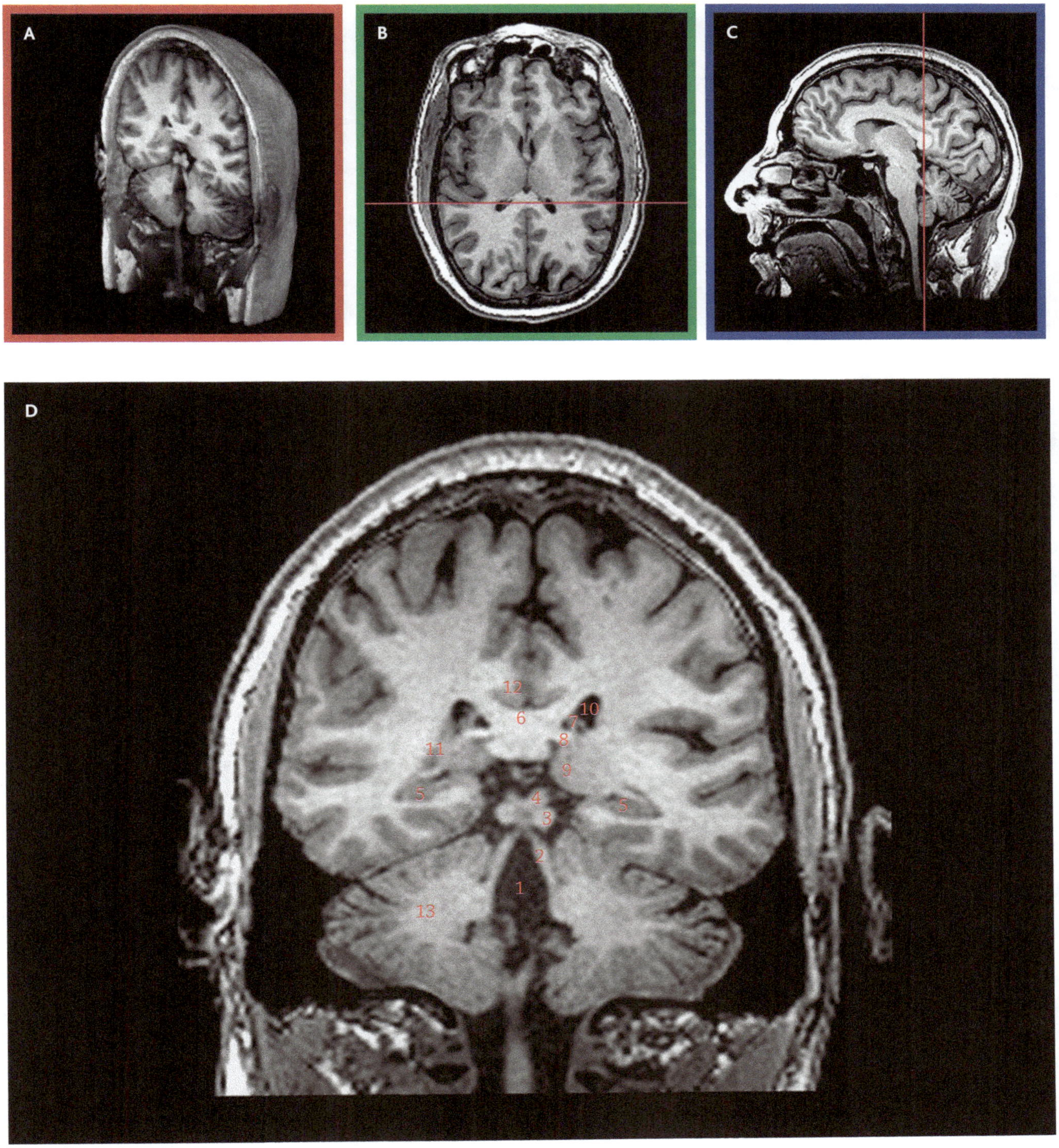

Figure 7-18 **A:** 3D view. **B:** Axial view. **C:** Sagittal view. **D:** Coronal Atlas Slice

1 Fourth Ventricle
2 Superior Cerebellar Peduncle
3 Tectum – Inferior Colliculus
4 Tectum – Superior Colliculus
5 Hippocampus
6 Corpus Callosum – Splenium
7 Choroid Plexus
8 Fornix
9 Thalamus
10 Lateral Ventricle -Atrium/Trigone
11 Caudate Nucleus – Tail
12 Cingulate Gyrus
13 Cerebellum

CORONAL SERIES

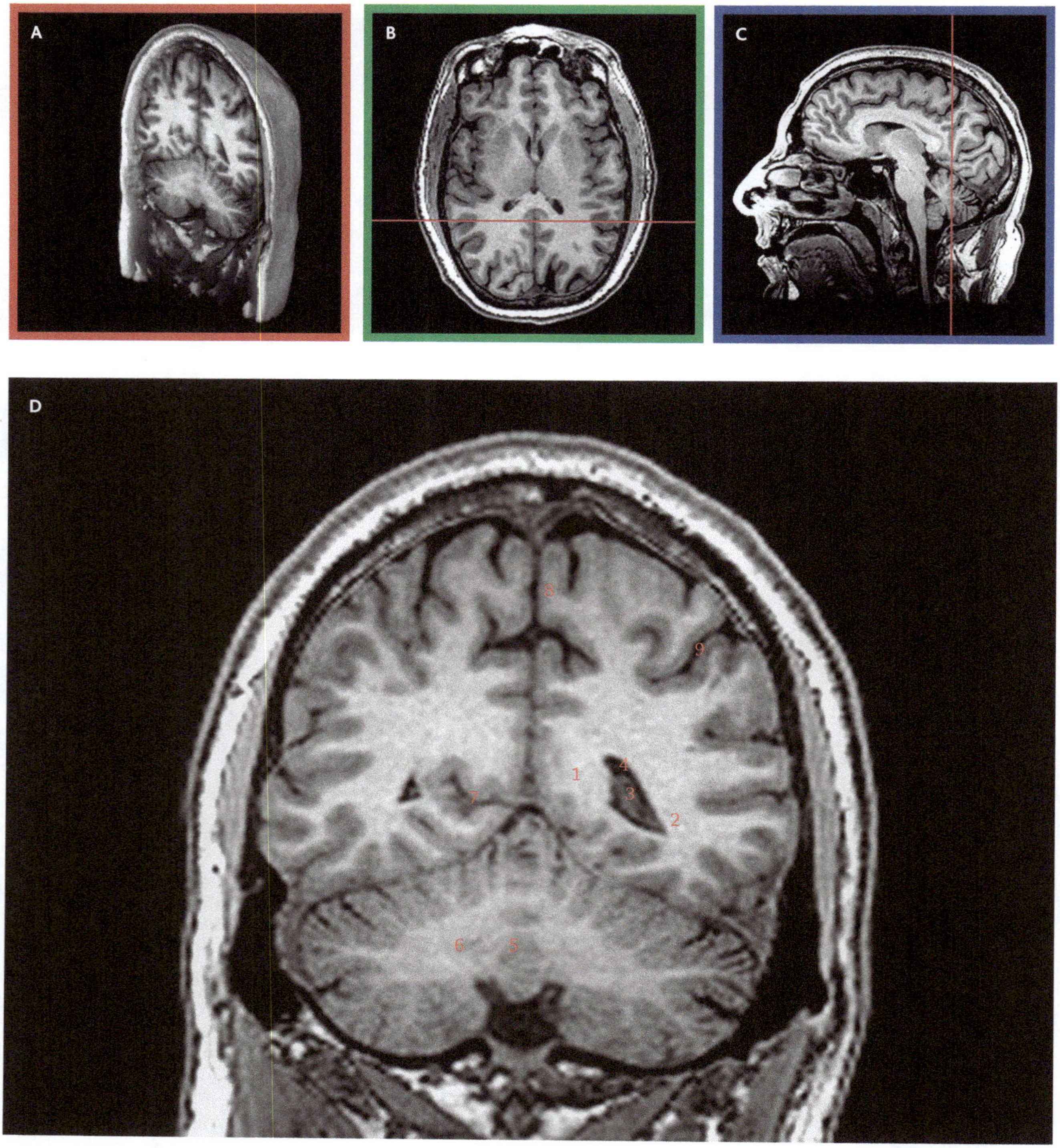

Figure 7-19 **A:** 3D view. **B:** Axial view. **C:** Sagittal view. **D:** Coronal Atlas Slice

1 Radiations of the Corpus Callosum
2 Optic Radiations
3 Choroid Plexus
4 Lateral Ventricle – Atrium/Trigone to Posterior/Occipital Horn
5 Cerebellar Vermis
6 Dentate Nucleus of Cerebellum
7 Calcarine Fissure
8 Precuneus
9 Intraparietal Sulcus

SAGITTAL SERIES

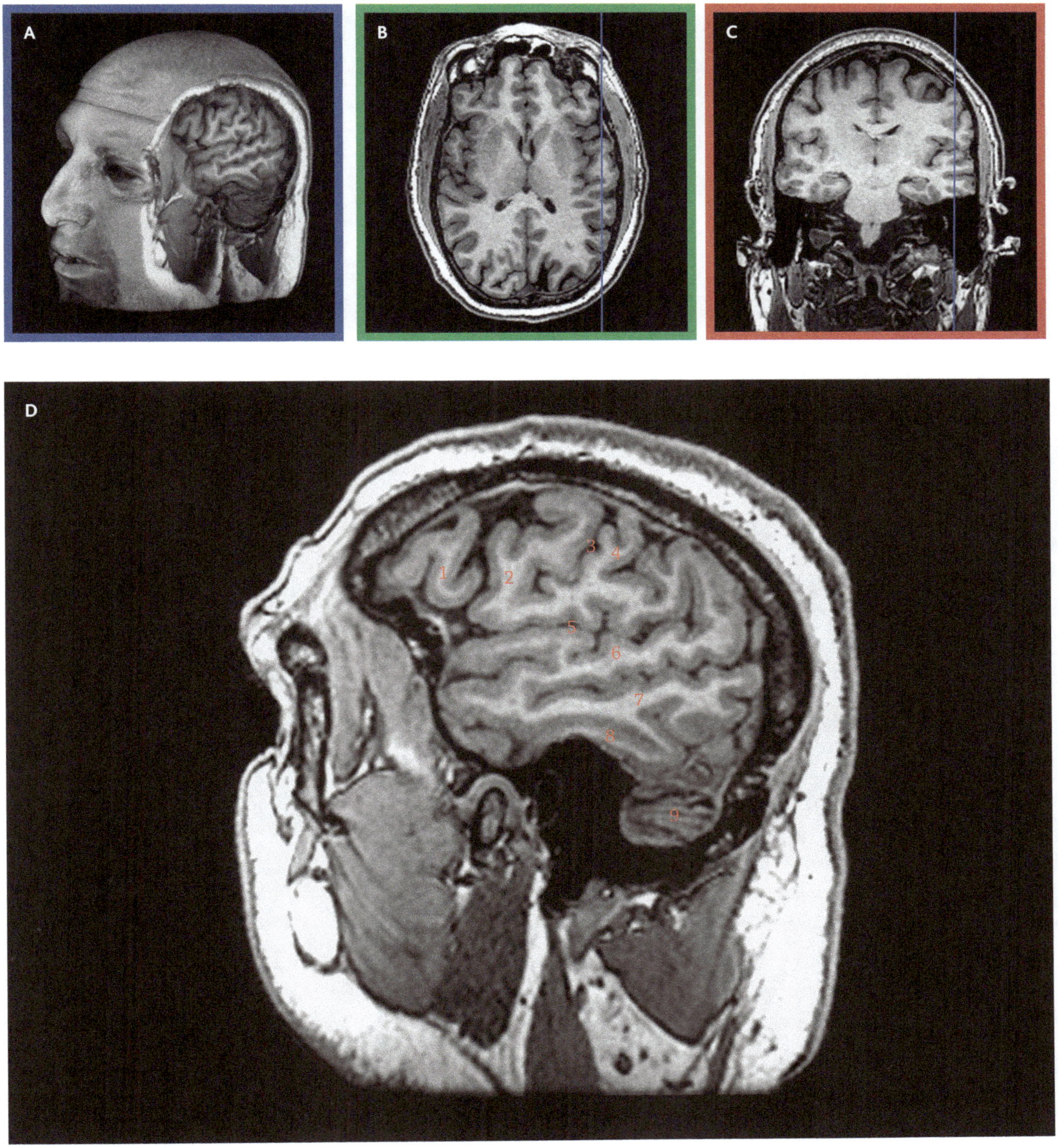

Figure 7-20 **A:** 3D view. **B:** Axial view. **C:** Coronal view. **D:** Sagittal Atlas Slice

1 Frontal Lobe
2 Pre-Central Gyrus
3 Central Sulcus
4 Post-Central Gyrus
5 Sylvian Fissure
6 Superior Temporal Gyrus
7 Middle Temporal Gyrus
8 Inferior Temporal Gyrus
9 Cerebellum

SAGITTAL SERIES

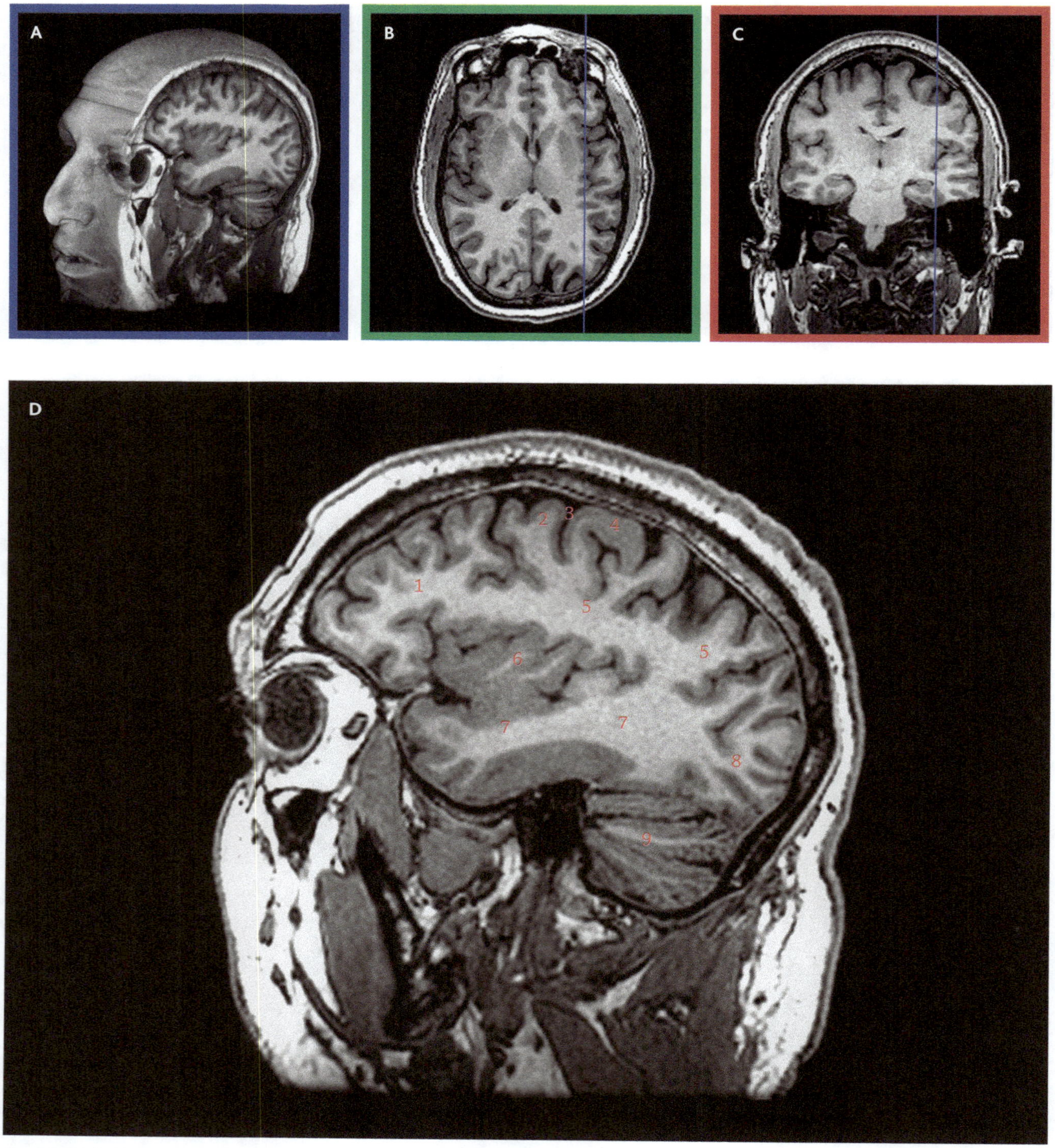

Figure 7-21 A: 3D view. **B:** Axial view. **C:** Coronal view. **D:** Sagittal Atlas Slice

1 Frontal Lobe
2 Pre-Central Gyrus
3 Central Sulcus
4 Post-Central Gyrus
5 Parietal Lobe
6 Insula
7 Temporal Lobe
8 Occipital Lobe
9 Cerebellum

SAGITTAL SERIES

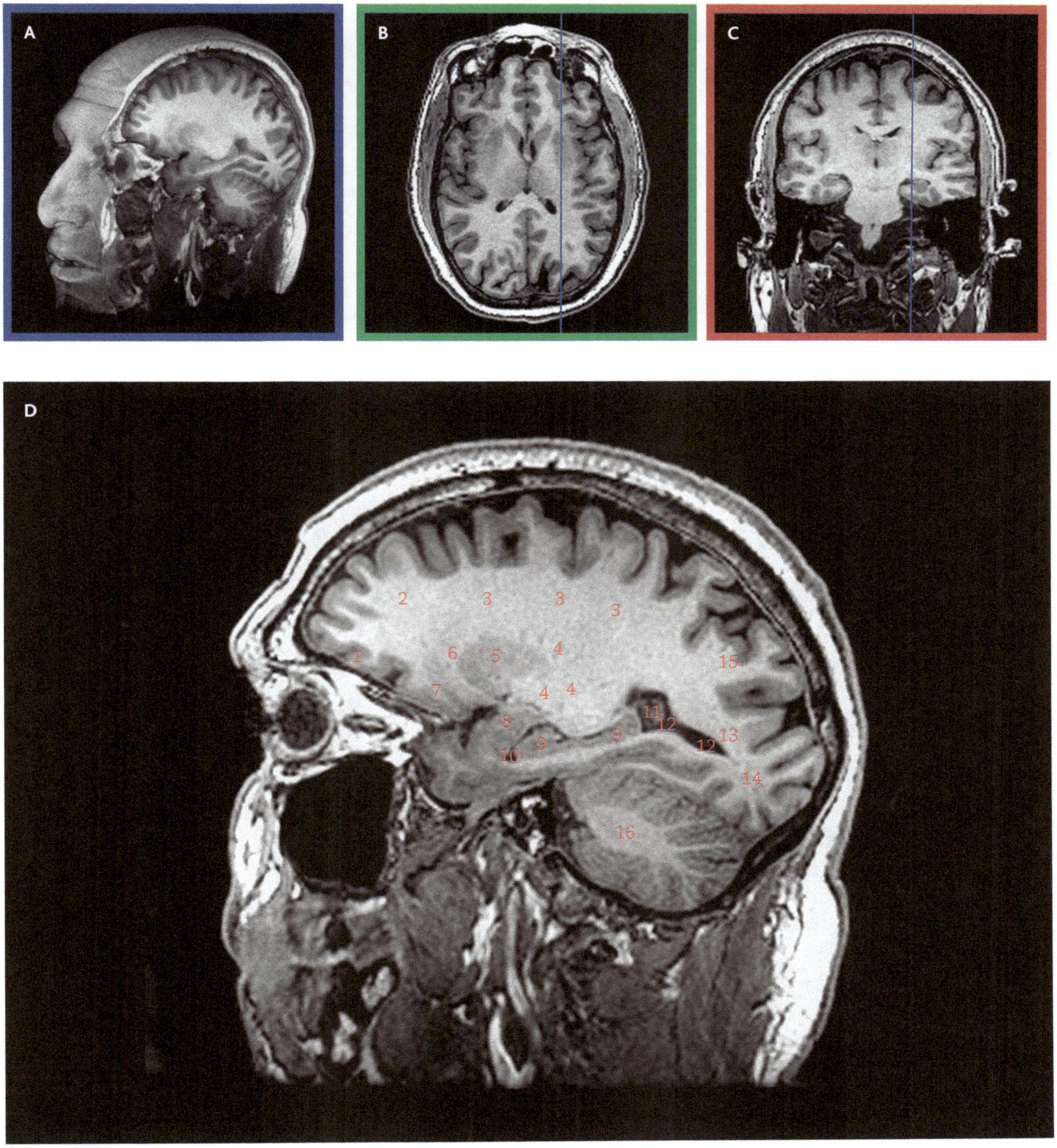

Figure 7-22 **A:** 3D view. **B:** Axial view. **C:** Coronal view. **D:** Sagittal Atlas Slice

1 Frontal Lobe – Orbital
2 Frontal Lobe
3 Corona Radiata
4 Internal Capsule
5 Putamen
6 External Capsule
7 Extreme Capsule
8 Amygdala
9 Hippocampus
10 Lateral Ventricle – Inferior/Temporal Horn
11 Choroid Plexus
12 Lateral Ventricle – Posterior/Occipital Horn
13 Optic Radiations
14 Occipital Lobe
15 Parietal Lobe

SAGITTAL SERIES

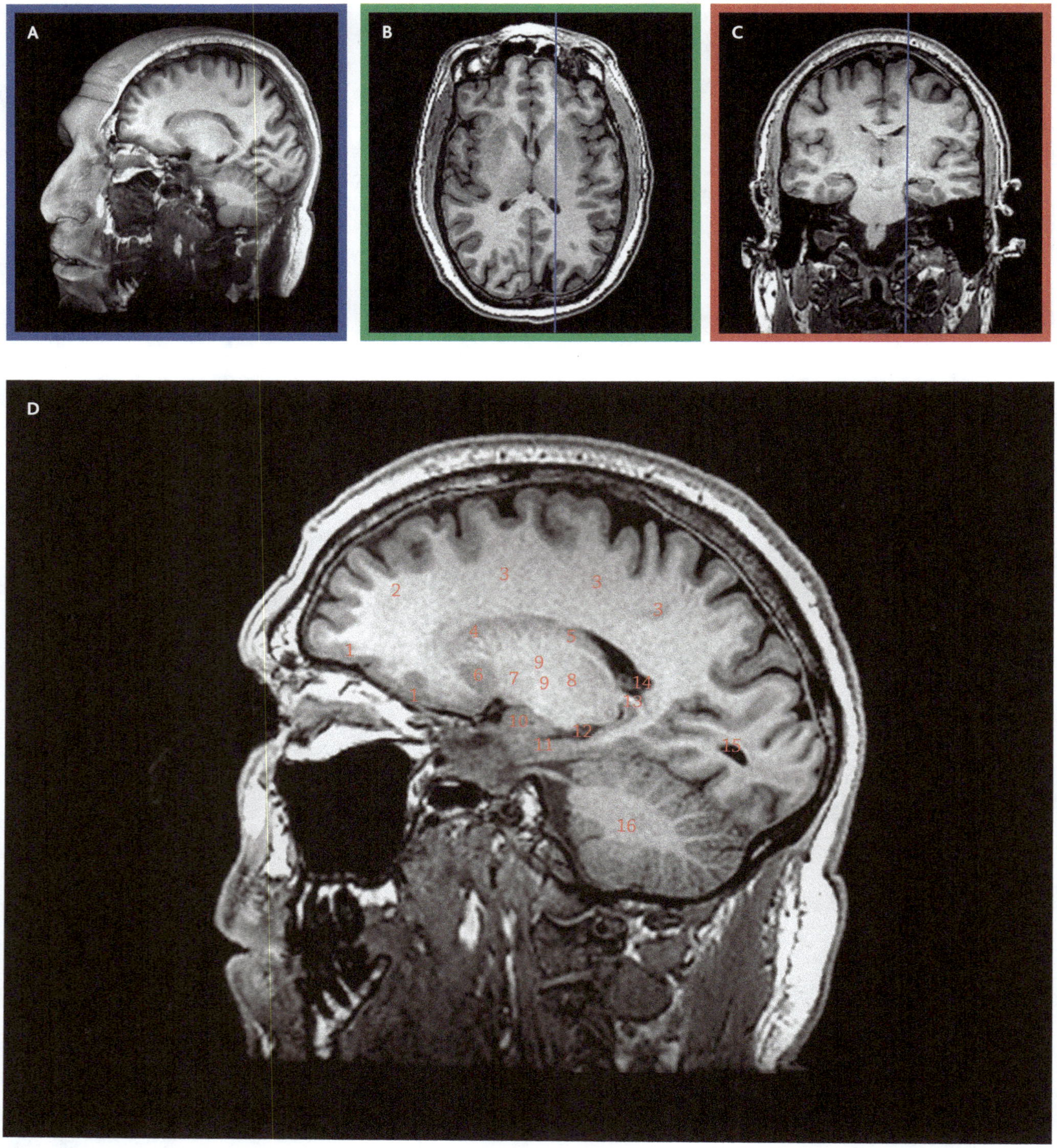

Figure 7-23 **A:** 3D view. **B:** Axial view. **C:** Coronal view. **D:** Sagittal Atlas Slice

1 Frontal Lobe – Orbital
2 Frontal Lobe
3 Corona Radiata
4 Caudate Nucleus – Head
5 Caudate Nucleus – Tail
6 Putamen
7 Globus Pallidus
8 Thalamus
9 Internal Capsule – Genu
10 Amygdala
11 Hippocampus
12 Lateral Ventricle – Inferior/Temporal Horn
13 Fornix
14 Lateral Ventricle – Atrium/Trigone
15 Lateral Ventricle – Posterior/Occipital Horn
16 Cerebellum

SAGITTAL SERIES

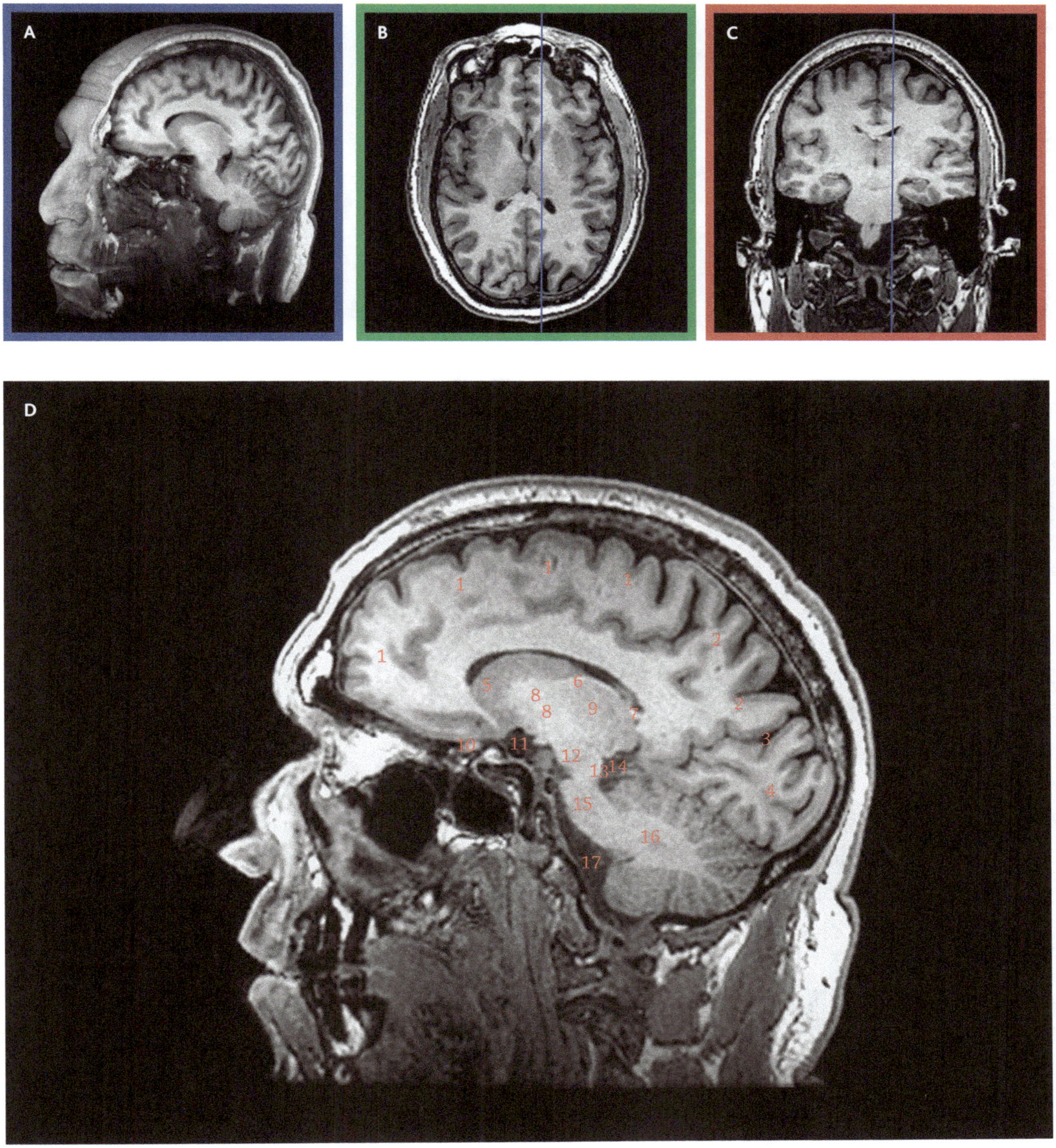

Figure 7-24 **A:** 3D view. **B:** Axial view. **C:** Coronal view. **D:** Sagittal Atlas Slice

1 Frontal Lobe
2 Parietal Lobe
3 Parieto-Occipital Sulcus
4 Occipital Lobe
5 Caudate Nucleus – Head
6 Caudothalamic Notch
7 Fornix
8 Internal Capsule – Genu
9 Thalamus
10 Optic Tract
11 Interpeduncular/Basal Cistern
12 Midbrain
13 Tectum – Superior/Inferior Colliculi
14 Superior/Perimesencephalic/Quadrigeminal Cistern
15 Middle Cerebellar Peduncle
16 Dentate Nucleus of the Cerebellum
17 Fourth Ventricle

SAGITTAL SERIES

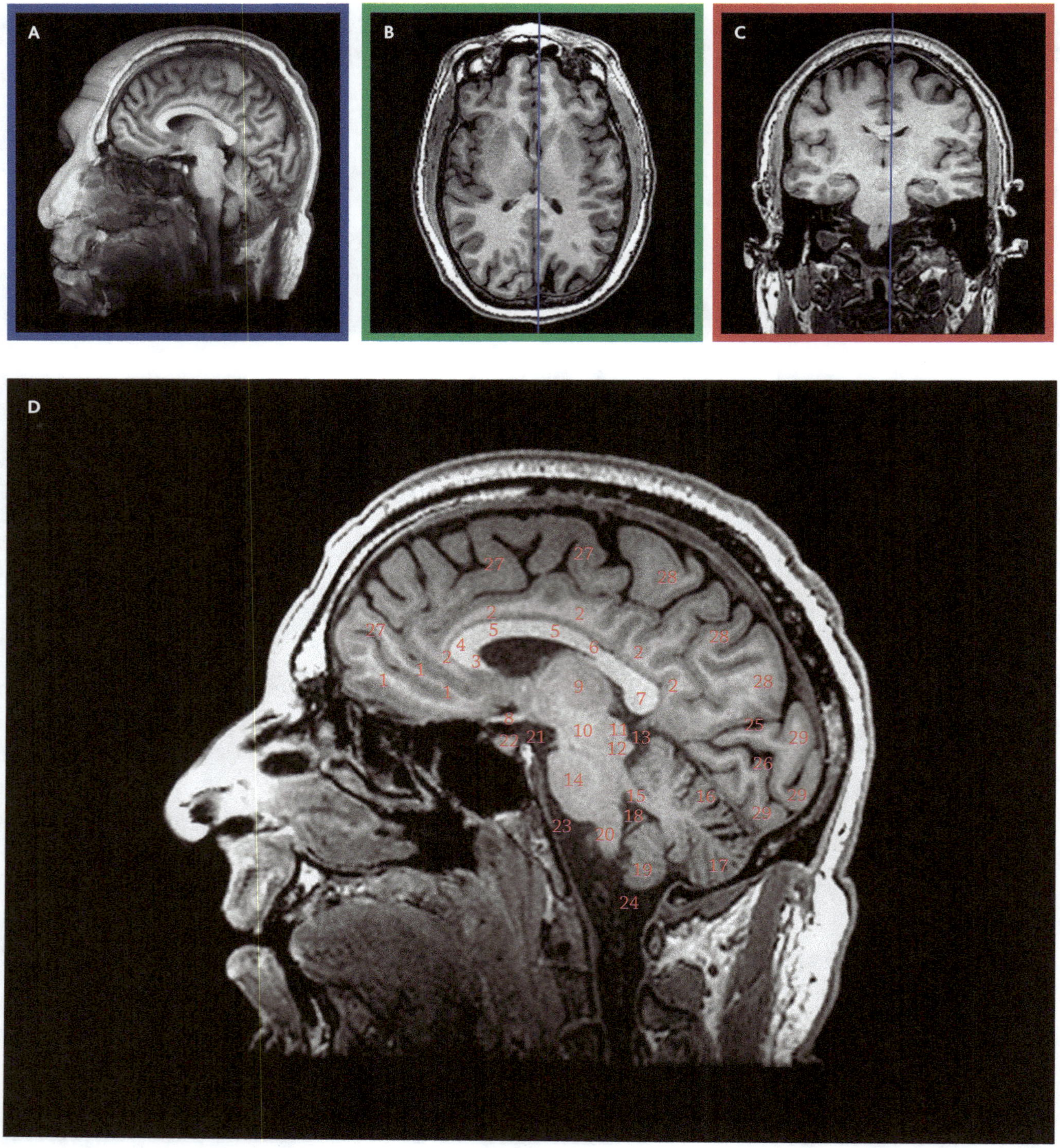

Figure 7-25 **A:** 3D view. **B:** Axial view. **C:** Coronal view. **D:** Sagittal Atlas Slice

1 Frontal Lobe – Medial
2 Cingulum within the Cingulate Gyrus
3 Corpus Callosum – Rostrum
4 Corpus Callosum – Genu
5 Corpus Callosum – Body
6 Corpus Callosum – Isthmus
7 Corpus Callosum – Splenium
8 Optic Chiasm
9 Thalamus
10 Midbrain
11 Tectum – Superior Colliculus
12 Tectum – Inferior Colliculus
13 Superior/Perimesencephalic/Quadrigeminal Cistern
14 Pons
15 Superior Cerebellar Peduncle
16 Cerebellar Vermis Folia
17 Cerebellar Folia
18 Fourth Ventricle
19 Cerebellar Tonsils
20 Medulla Oblongata
21 Interpeduncular/Basal Cistern
22 Pituitary
23 Pontine Cistern
24 Cisterna Magna
25 Parieto-Occipital Sulcus
26 Calcarine Fissure
27 Frontal Lobe
28 Parietal Lobe
29 Occipital Lobe

SAGITTAL SERIES

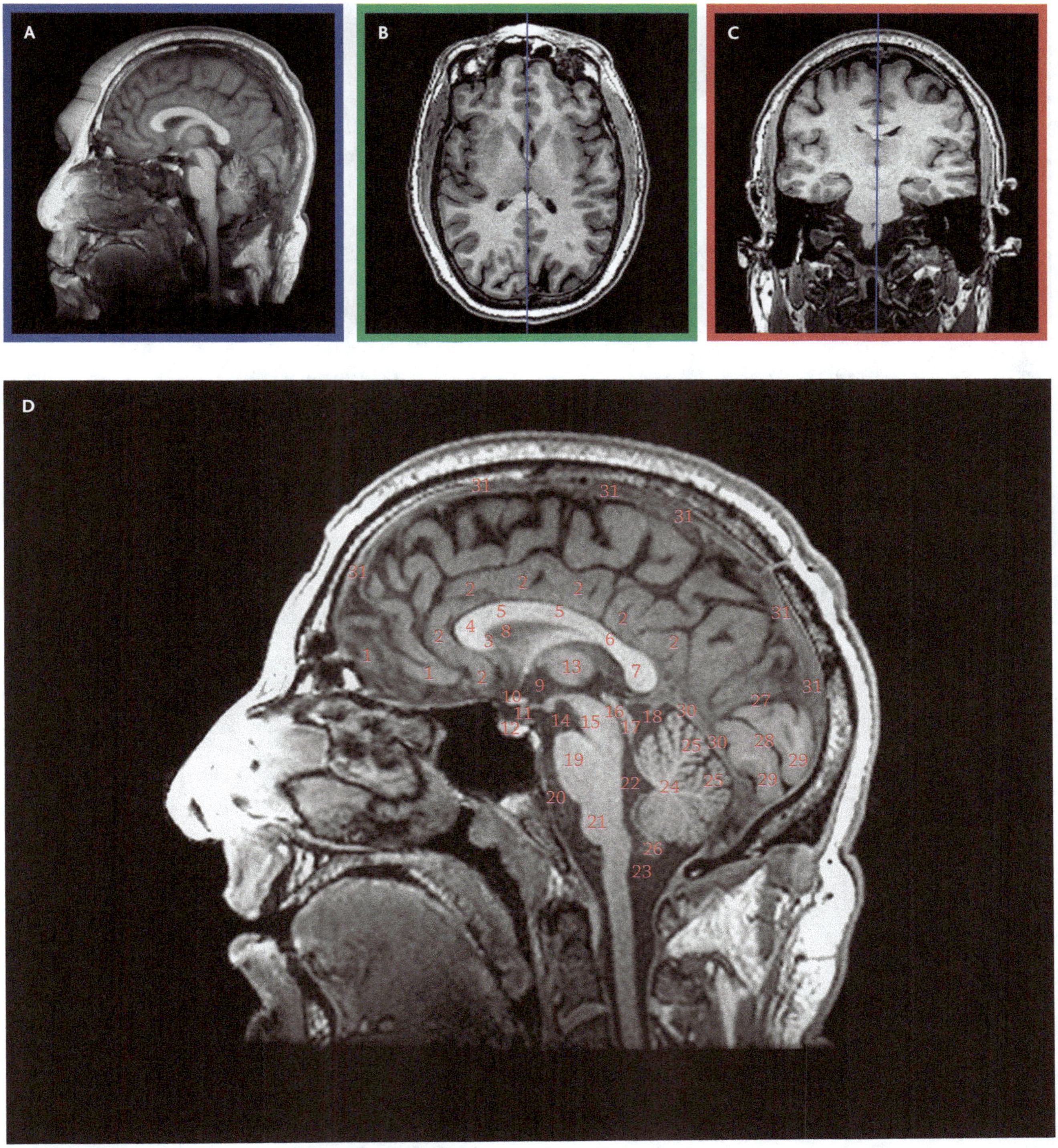

Figure 7-26 **A:** 3D view. **B:** Axial view. **C:** Coronal view. **D:** Sagittal Atlas Slice

1 Medial Frontal Lobe
2 Cingulate Gyrus
3 Corpus Callosum – Rostrum
4 Corpus Callosum – Genu
5 Corpus Callosum – Body
6 Corpus Callosum – Isthmus
7 Corpus Callosum – Splenium
8 Lateral Ventricle – Body
9 Third Ventricle
10 Optic Chiasm
11 Infundibulum
12 Pituitary
13 Thalamus
14 Interpeduncular/Basal Cistern
15 Midbrain
16 Cerebral Aqueduct of Sylvius
17 Tectum
18 Superior/Perimesencephalic/Quadrigeminal Cistern
19 Pons
20 Pontine Cistern
21 Medulla Oblongata
22 Fourth Ventricle
23 Cisterna Magna
24 Cerebellum – Arbor Vitae
25 Cerebellar Vermis – Folia
26 Cerebellar Tonsils
27 Parieto-Occipital Sulcus
28 Calcarine Fissure
29 Occipital Lobe
30 Tentorium Cerebelli
31 Superior Sagittal Sinus

CT AXIAL SERIES WITH MRI REFERENCE

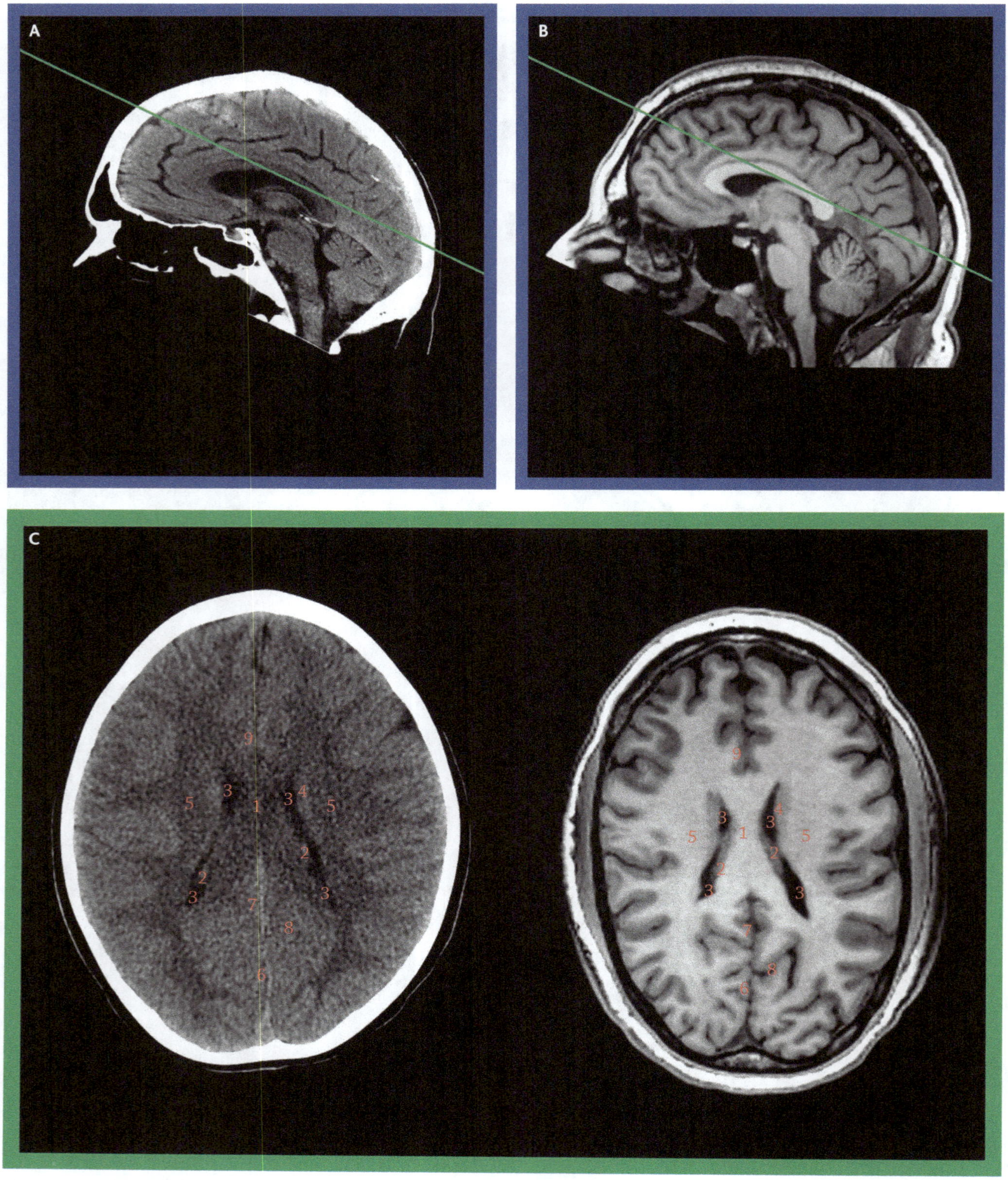

Figure 7-27 **A:** CT sagittal reference. **B:** MRI sagittal reference. **C:** Axial CT and MRI Atlas Slices

1 Corpus Callosum – Body
2 Choroid Plexus
3 Lateral Ventricles – Body
4 Caudate Nucleus – Head
5 Corona Radiata
6 Cuneus
7 Precuneus
8 Parieto-Occipital Sulcus
9 Cingulate Gyrus

CT AXIAL SERIES WITH MRI REFERENCE

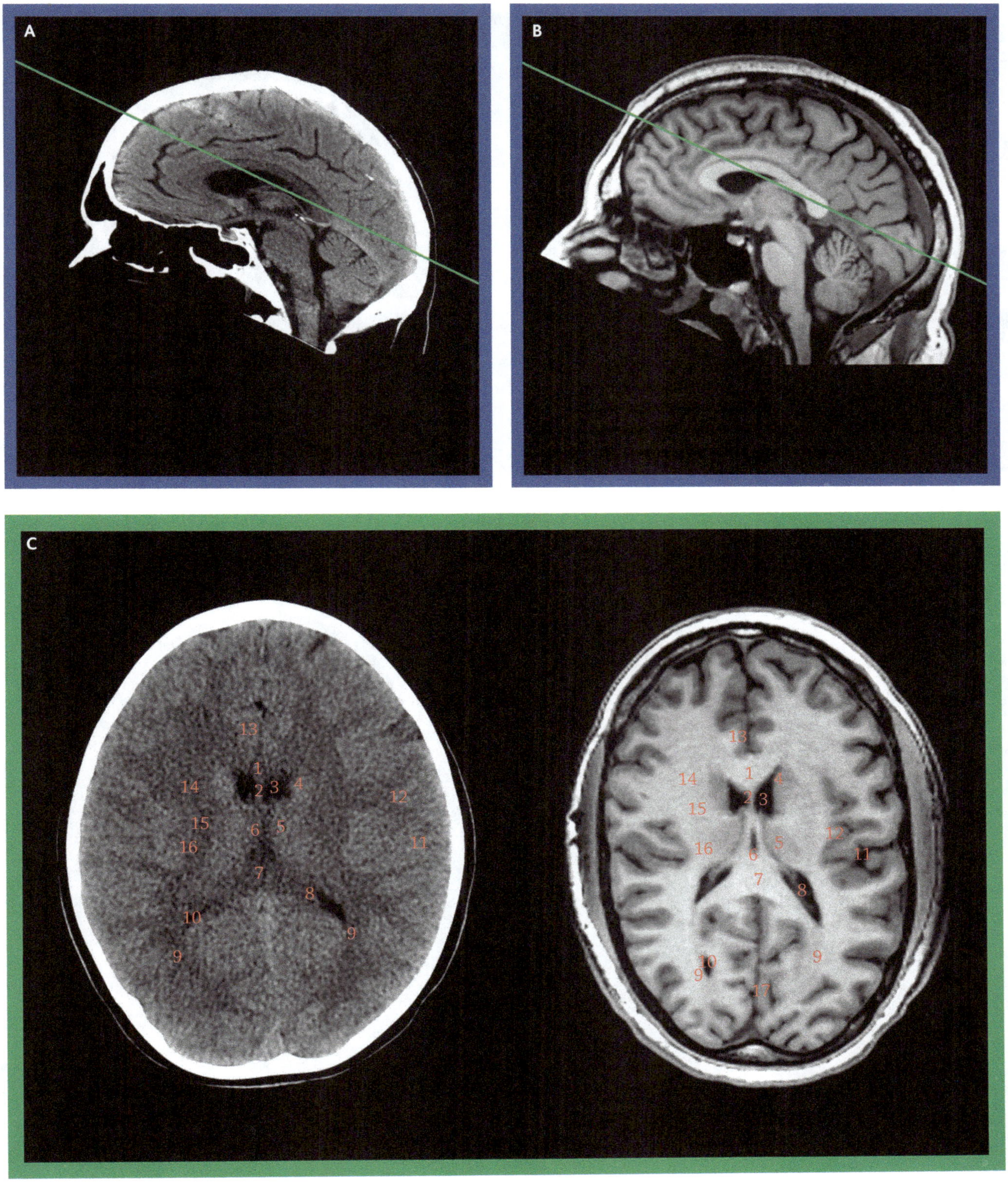

Figure 7-28 A: CT sagittal reference. **B:** MRI sagittal reference. **C:** Axial CT and MRI Atlas Slices

1 Corpus Callosum – Genu
2 Septum Pellucidum
3 Lateral Ventricle – Frontal Horn
4 Caudate Nucleus – Head
5 Thalamus
6 Fornix
7 Corpus Callosum – Splenium
8 Choroid Plexus
9 Optic Radiations
10 Lateral Ventricle – Posterior/ Occipital Horn
11 Sylvian Fissure
12 Insula
13 Cingulate Gyrus
14 Internal Capsule – Anterior Limb
15 Internal Capsule – Genu
16 Internal Capsule – Posterior Limb

CT AXIAL SERIES WITH MRI REFERENCE

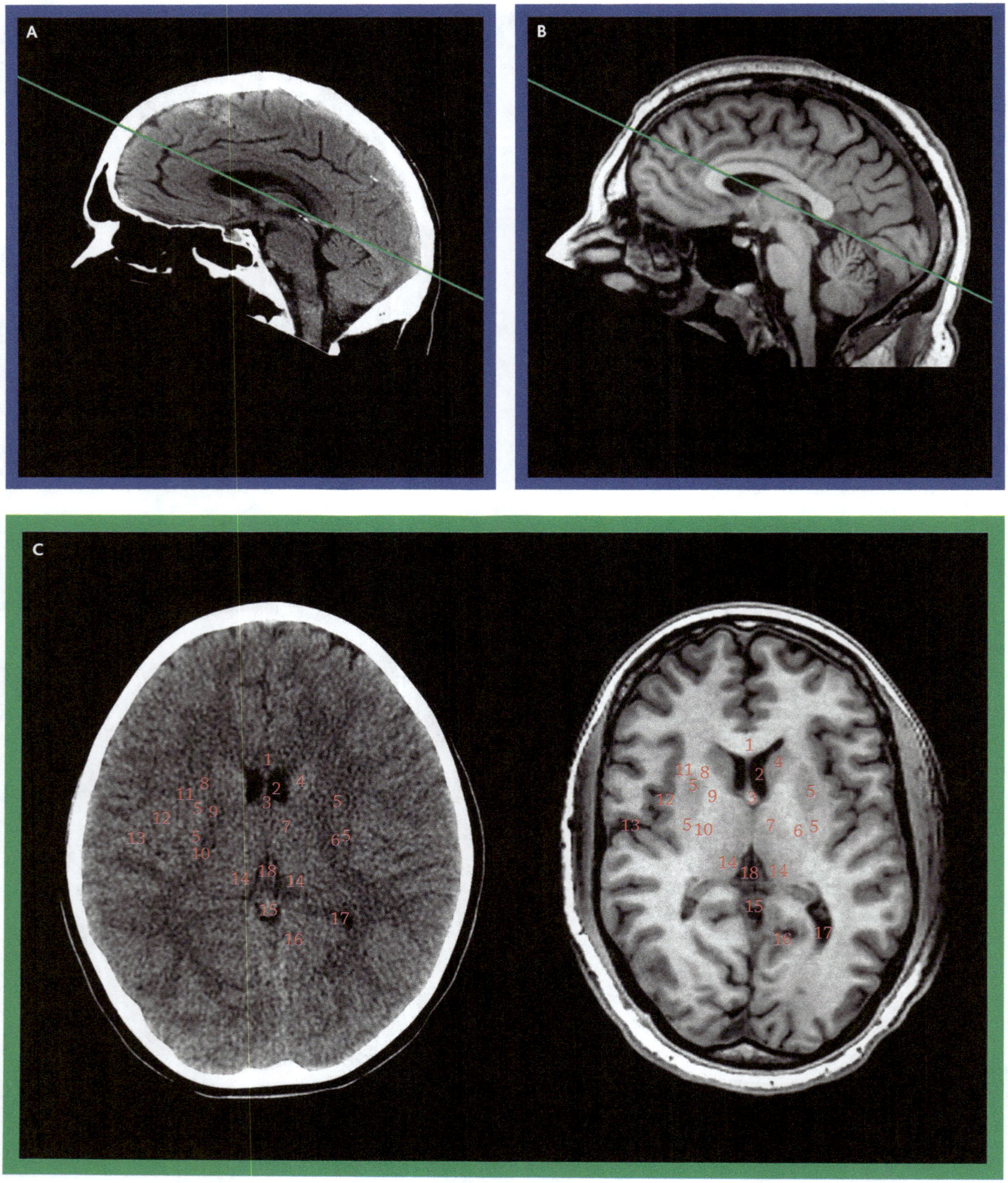

Figure 7-29 **A:** CT sagittal reference. **B:** MRI sagittal reference. **C:** Axial CT and MRI Atlas Slices

1 Corpus Callosum – Genu
2 Lateral Ventricle – Frontal Horn
3 Fornix
4 Caudate Nucleus – Head
5 Putamen
6 Globus Pallidus
7 Thalamus
8 Internal Capsule – Anterior Limb
9 Internal Capsule – Genu
10 Internal Capsule – Posterior Limb
11 External Capsule
12 Insula
13 Sylvian Fissure
14 Thalamus – Pulvinar
15 Pineal
16 Parieto-Occipital Sulcus
17 Lateral Ventricle - Posterior/ Occipital Horn
18 Superior/Perimesencephalic/ Quadrigeminal Cistern

CT AXIAL SERIES WITH MRI REFERENCE

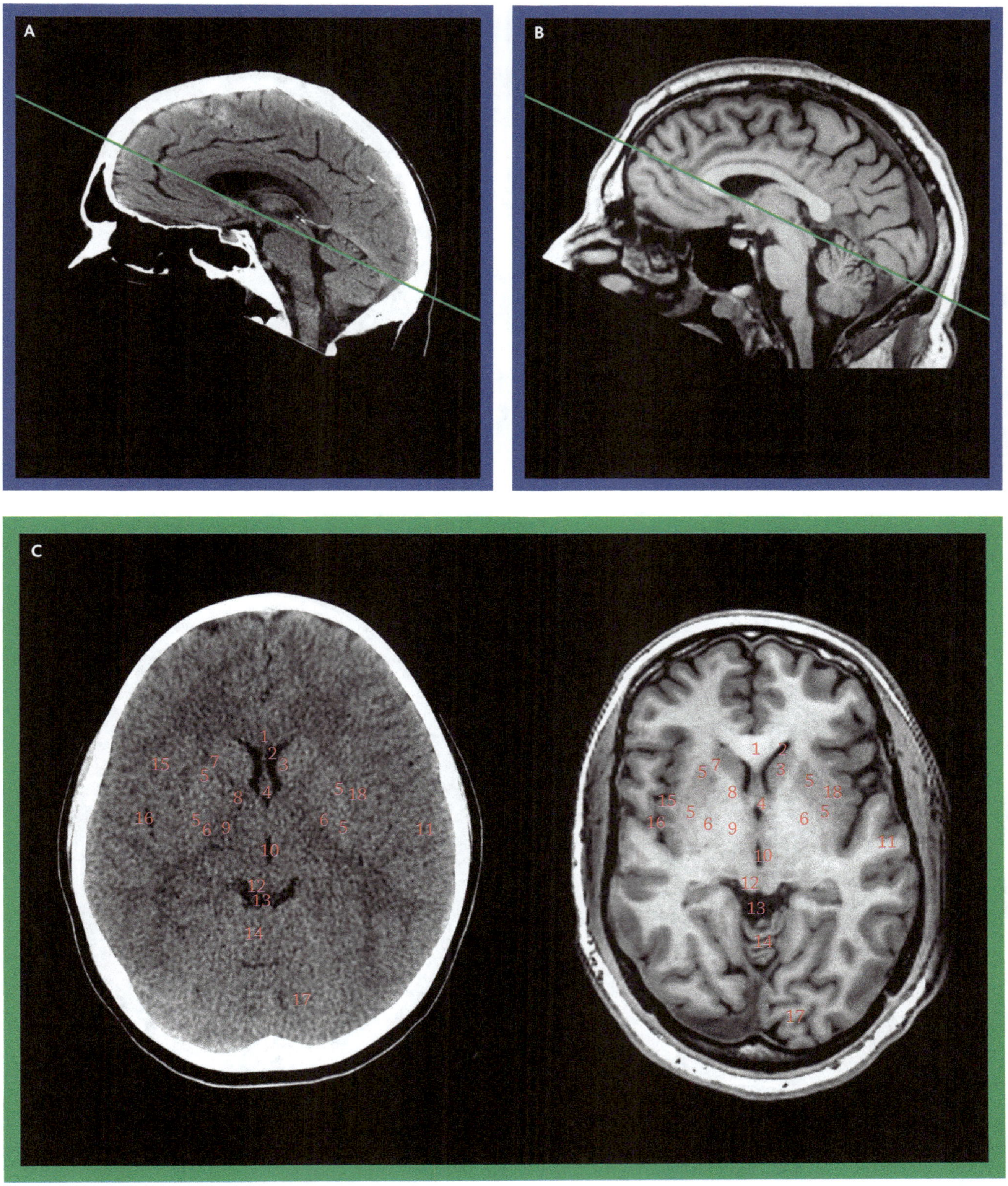

Figure 7-30 **A:** CT sagittal reference. **B:** MRI sagittal reference. **C:** Axial CT and MRI Atlas Slices

1 Corpus Callosum – Genu
2 Lateral Ventricle – Frontal Horn
3 Caudate Nucleus – Head
4 Fornix
5 Putamen
6 Globus Pallidus
7 Internal Capsule – Anterior Limb
8 Internal Capsule – Genu
9 Internal Capsule – Posterior Limb
10 Third Ventricle
11 Temporal Lobe
12 Tectum – Superior Colliculus
13 Superior/Perimesencephalic/ Quadrigeminal Cistern
14 Cerebellar Vermis
15 Insula
16 Sylvian Fissure
17 Occipital Lobe
18 Claustrum

CT AXIAL SERIES WITH MRI REFERENCE

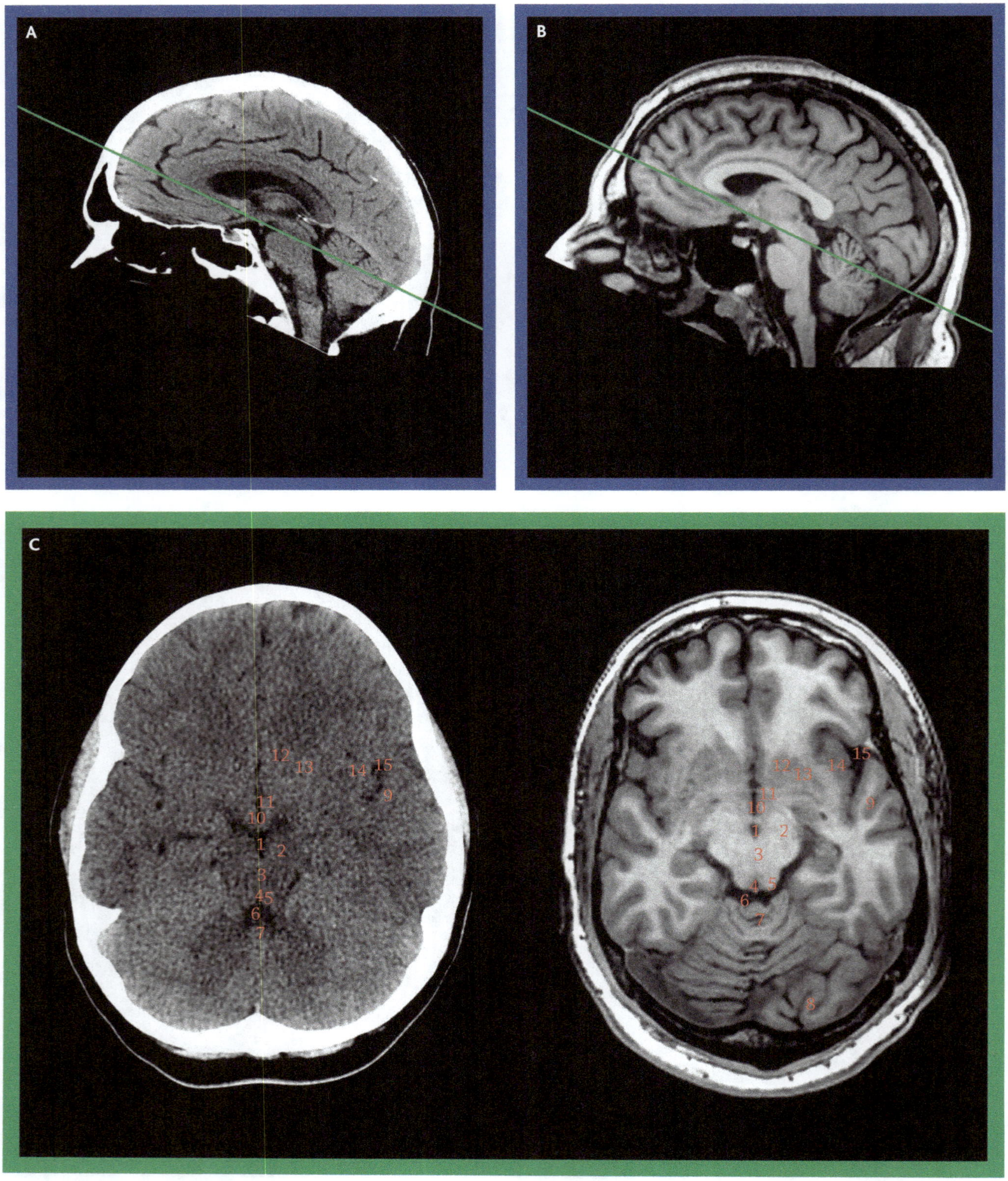

Figure 7-31 A: CT sagittal reference. **B:** MRI sagittal reference. **C:** Axial CT and MRI Atlas Slices

1 Interpeduncular/Basal Cistern
2 Cerebral Peduncle
3 Midbrain
4 Cerebral Aqueduct of Sylvius
5 Tectum – Inferior Colliculus
6 Superior/Perimesencephalic/Quadrigeminal Cistern
7 Cerebellar Vermis
8 Occipital Lobe
9 Temporal Lobe
10 Third Ventricle
11 Hypothalamus
12 Caudate Nucleus – Head
13 Putamen
14 Insula
15 Sylvian Fissure

CT AXIAL SERIES WITH MRI REFERENCE

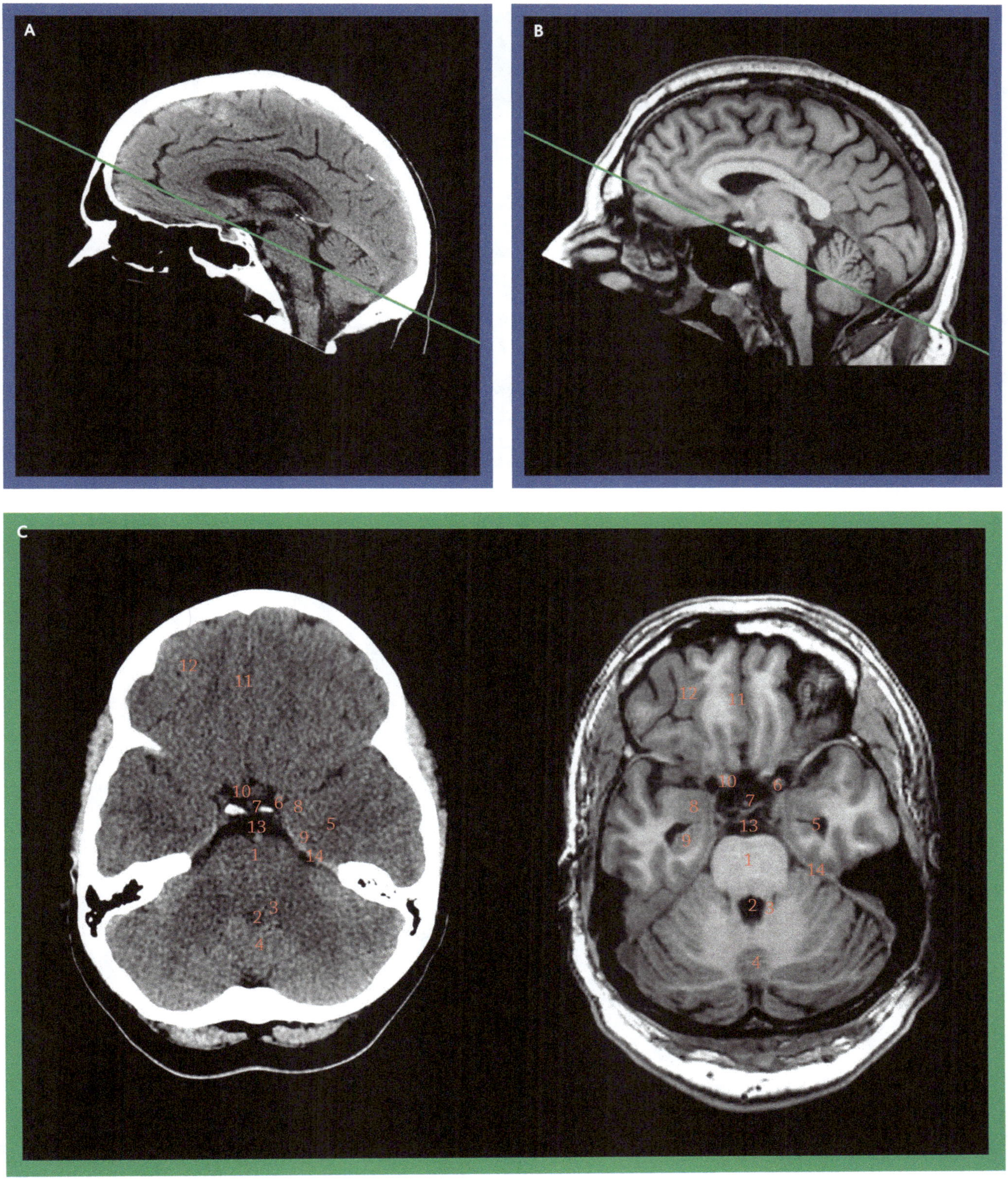

Figure 7-32 **A:** CT sagittal reference. **B:** MRI sagittal reference. **C:** Axial CT and MRI Atlas Slices

1 Pons
2 Fourth Ventricle
3 Superior Cerebellar Peduncle
4 Cerebellar Vermis
5 Lateral Ventricle – Inferior/ Temporal Horn
6 Internal Carotid Artery
7 Infundibulum
8 Amygdala
9 Hippocampus
10 Optic Nerve
11 Frontal Lobe – Medial
12 Frontal Lobe – Orbital
13 Basilar Artery
14 Tentorium Cerebelli

INDEX

INDEX OF CLINICAL EXAMPLES

Printed in the USA
CPSIA information can be obtained
at www.ICGtesting.com
CBHW071432290124
3750CB00034B/388

9 780190 239060